Targeting Notch in Cancer

Lucio Miele • Spyros Artavanis-Tsakonas
Editors

Targeting Notch in Cancer

From the Fruit Fly to the Clinic

Springer

Editors
Lucio Miele
Department of Genetics
Louisiana State University Health
Sciences Center
New Orleans, LA, USA

Spyros Artavanis-Tsakonas
Department of Cell Biology
Harvard Medical School
Boston, MA, USA

ISBN 978-1-4939-8857-0 ISBN 978-1-4939-8859-4 (eBook)
https://doi.org/10.1007/978-1-4939-8859-4

Library of Congress Control Number: 2018957844

This Springer imprint is published by the registered company Springer Science+Business Media, LLC part of Springer Nature.
The registered company address is: 233 Spring Street, New York, NY 10013, U.S.A.

Preface

In 1991, a rare chromosomal translocation affecting chromosomes 9 and 7 was described in T-cell lymphoblastic leukemia. The translocation involved TAN-1, a previously unknown human locus highly homologous to *Drosophila* Notch, a gene well known to developmental biologists as a determinant of cell fate during development. This serendipitously discovered link between developmental biology and cancer biology touched off a veritable explosion of discoveries on the role of Notch in human malignancy. Today, major pharmaceutical and biotechnology companies have Notch programs and have developed investigational drugs and biologics targeting Notch signaling. Notch ligands have been used successfully to expand human cord blood progenitor cells for transplantation purposes. Studies of Notch signaling and its crosstalk with other developmental pathways have revealed a remarkably complex network of molecular interactions at the core of the cell fate-controlling machinery. Interest in this field has steadily increased, and today Notch signaling is known to play roles in virtually every aspect of cancer biology, from control of differentiation, proliferation, and apoptosis in transformed cells to angiogenesis, tumor-stroma interaction, and anticancer immune responses. A number of observations have revealed a role of Notch in the self-renewal of "cancer stem-like cells" or "tumor-initiating cells" that are thought to be a major cause of treatment failure in cancer. It is not unreasonable to speculate that pharmacological manipulation of Notch signaling could alter the practice of medicine in the treatment of many human malignancies. This does not mean that targeting Notch in the clinic will be easy or straightforward. The notorious context dependence of Notch effects, well known to developmental biologists but frustrating to pharmacologists and cancer biologists, means that the question "what does Notch *do* in cancer and what is the best strategy to target it" does not have a simple answer.

Advances in genomics have revealed that human cancers are remarkably plastic, particularly during and after treatment with chemo- or radiotherapy or even targeted therapy: many cancers undergo a process of quasi-Darwinian clonal evolution, selecting cellular clones with more stem-like characteristics. Phenotypic plasticity due to tumor microenvironmental effects can also alter the biology of cancer cells through metabolic and/or epigenetic effects. These aberrant cell fate decisions prominently involve developmental pathways including Notch.

Efforts to translate our growing but still incomplete understanding of Notch biology in cancer will have to take these complexities into account. A detailed understanding of the intricate crosstalk between Notch and other pathways of therapeutic interest will be necessary to design rational drug combinations for specific diseases and disease subsets. The multiple classes of agents currently in various stages of development have different advantages and disadvantages. It is still unclear what the best agents are or what drug combinations are most promising in individual indications. Determining the status of Notch signaling in tumor samples is a challenge in its own right, with four Notch paralogs, five ligands, a host of co-ligands, as well as canonical and noncanonical Notch target genes that are differentially affected in different cell types. These hurdles are not insurmountable, but they need to be considered by those approaching the clinical development of Notch-targeting agents if we are to avoid unpleasant surprises.

Genetic experiments in model organisms have revealed much about genes and pathways that modify the effects of Notch signaling in tumorigenesis. These invaluable insights are now being translated to human tumor biology and experimental oncology.

This volume is an attempt at describing the current state of the art in the field of Notch signaling in cancer, with a specific focus on targeting Notch signaling for therapeutic purposes. Internationally known experts in the Notch field have contributed chapters to what we hope will be a comprehensive discussion.

No single book can encompass all aspects of a vast and growing field of biomedical research, and this volume is no exception. We hope that the reader will be left with a clear view of the field's complexity, a clear understanding of what is known, and a sense of what remains unknown. We thank the readers for their interest in our work and hope that our effort will stimulate further interest in this fascinating field of biomedical research.

New Orleans, LA, USA — Lucio Miele
Boston, MA, USA — Spyros Artavanis-Tsakonas

Contents

Chapter 1
Structural Biology of Notch Signaling

Kelly L. Arnett, Tom C. M. Seegar, and Stephen C. Blacklow

Abstract The conserved Notch signaling pathway plays a central role in development and adult tissue homeostasis. Notch signaling is initiated by binding to a transmembrane ligand. E3 ubiquitin ligase-mediated ligand endocytosis enables release of the negative regulatory region (NRR) of Notch from autoinhibition, which then allows metalloprotease cleavage within the NRR, followed by intramembrane cleavage by the γ-secretase complex. After release from the membrane, the Notch intracellular domain translocates to the nucleus to form a transcriptionally active complex and initiate transcription of Notch-responsive genes. Structural studies of Notch and Notch-associated molecules, which have advanced our understanding of each of these steps in the Notch signaling pathway, are reviewed here.

Keywords Notch · DSL · Receptor signaling · Protein biochemistry · Structural biology · Regulated intramembrane proteolysis · Transcription

1.1 Introduction

Notch receptors bind transmembrane ligands on neighboring cells and transduce signals, playing an essential role in cell-fate decisions during development and tissue homeostasis. In mouse, fly, and worm models, severe deficiencies in Notch signaling lead to embryonic lethality. Abnormal decreases and increases in Notch

K. L. Arnett · T. C. M. Seegar · S. C. Blacklow (✉)
Department of Biological Chemistry and Molecular Pharmacology, Harvard Medical School, Boston, MA, USA

Department of Cancer Biology, Dana Farber Cancer Institute, Boston, MA, USA
e-mail: Kelly_Arnett@hms.harvard.edu; Tom_Seegar@hms.harvard.edu; Stephen_Blacklow@hms.harvard.edu

L. Miele, S. Artavanis-Tsakonas (eds.), *Targeting Notch in Cancer*,
https://doi.org/10.1007/978-1-4939-8859-4_1

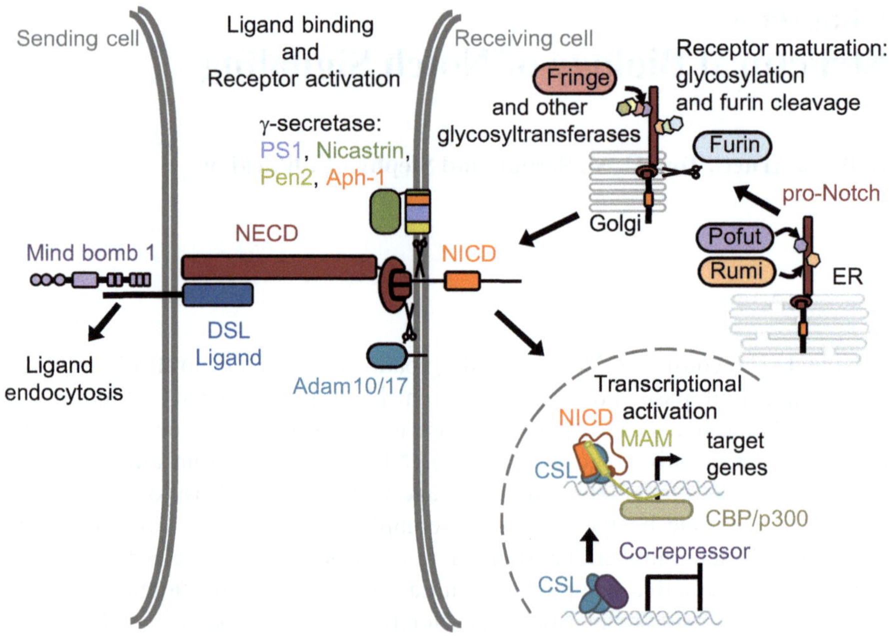

Fig. 1.1 Overview of major events in Notch signaling. Notch is expressed as a pro-protein precursor and undergoes a series of posttranslational modifications during maturation, including O-linked glycosylation and processing at site S1 by a furin-like protease. Signals are initiated by the engagement of ligand on the signal-sending cell with the extracellular part of Notch (NECD) on the signal-receiving cell. Ligand endocytosis promotes relief of Notch autoinhibition allowing metalloprotease cleavage by an ADAM family metalloprotease at site S2. This proteolytic step allows the cleavage of Notch by the γ-secretase complex at site S3 within the transmembrane domain and release of the Notch intracellular domain (NICD) from the membrane. Upon translocation to the nucleus, NICD enters into a transcriptional activation complex with the DNA-binding transcription factor CSL and coactivator Mastermind (MAM)

signaling are associated with human developmental abnormalities and disease, and cancer-associated mutations have been found which produce both constitutively active and inactive forms of Notch. Notch receptors, their ligands, and many accessory proteins are essential for transducing a Notch signal, which proceeds through a series of connected events: (1) ligand binding, (2) ligand endocytosis, (3) release from autoinhibition, (4) metalloprotease cleavage, (5) intramembrane cleavage, and (6) transcriptional activation (Fig. 1.1).

Notch receptors are large modular transmembrane proteins with distinct regions playing specific roles in each of these steps (Fig. 1.2a). The N-terminal region of Notch receptors consists of a series of epidermal growth factor (EGF)-like repeats that bind ligands of the Delta and Serrate families and initiate the Notch signal [28, 94]. C-terminal to the EGF repeats, a region known as the negative regulatory region (NRR) of Notch holds Notch receptors in an autoinhibited conformation prior to ligand engagement [35, 95]. Ligand binding and endocytosis of the ligand, stimulated by Mind bomb or Neuralized E3 ubiquitin ligases, are required for release

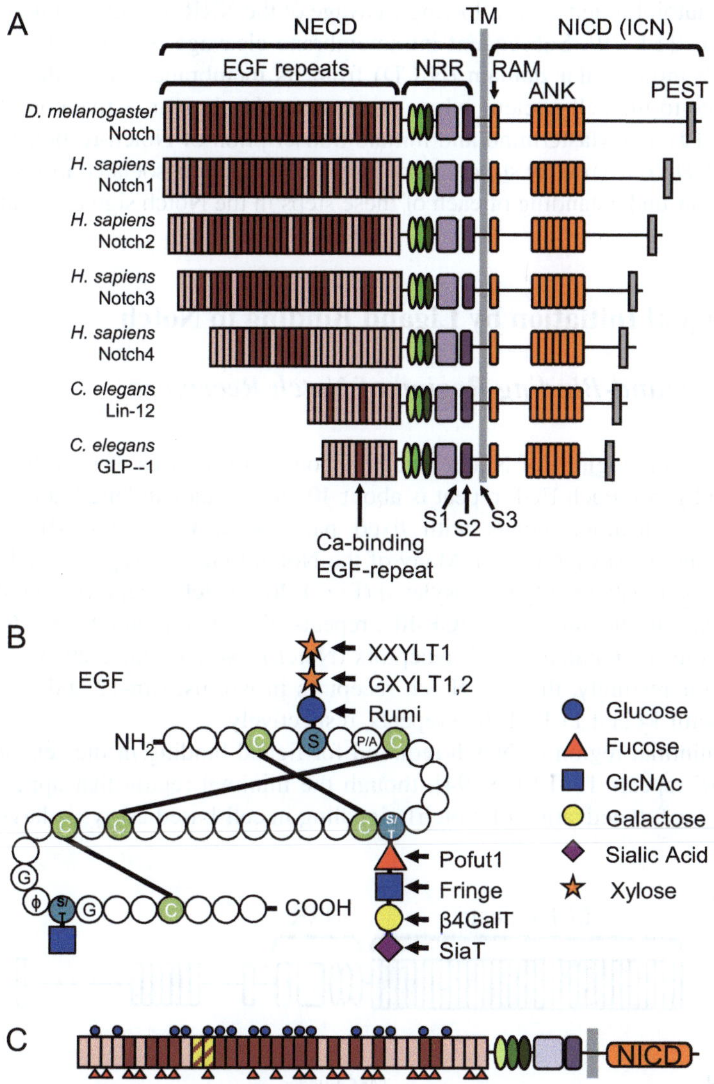

Fig. 1.2 Domain organization of Notch receptors. (**a**) Domain organization of Notch receptors and DSL family ligands from fly, human, and worm. Notch extracellular domain (NECD), Notch intracellular domain (NICD), epidermal growth factor-like repeats (EGF), transmembrane region (TM), negative regulatory region (NRR), RBPJ-associated module (RAM), ankyrin repeats (ANK), and C-terminal PEST domain are indicated. Calcium-binding EGF repeats are in a dark shade, and non-calcium-binding EGF repeats are in a light shade. (**b**) Schematic of a Notch EGF domain showing sugar modifications. N-acetylglucosamine (GlcNac), xyloside xylosyltransferase 1 (XXYLT1), glucoside xylosyltransferases 1,2 (GXYLT1,2), β-1,4-galactosyltransferase (β4GalT), sialyltransferase (SaiT). (**c**) Domain organization of Notch1 showing positions of glucose addition by Rumi (blue circles) and fucose addition by Pofut1 (red triangles). Ligand-binding EGF repeats 11–12 are indicated in yellow

from the autoinhibited state, allowing cleavage of the NRR by ADAM family metalloproteases [14, 79]. Subsequent intramembrane cleavage by γ-secretase releases the Notch intracellular domain (NICD) from its membrane tether, allowing it to translocate to the cell nucleus where it can assemble into an active complex with CSL (RBPJ) and Mastermind and initiate transcription of Notch-responsive genes [90, 122]. Here we review structures of Notch and Notch-associated molecules that advance our understanding of each of these steps in the Notch signaling pathway.

1.2 Signal Initiation by Ligand Binding to Notch

1.2.1 Ligand-Binding Region of Notch Receptors

The N-terminal regions of Notch receptors consist of a series of EGF-like repeats that bind ligand. Each EGF repeat is about 40 amino acids in length and has three intradomain disulfide bonds with fixed pairings of Cys(I)–Cys(III), Cys(II)–Cys(IV), and Cys(V)–Cys(VI). Many of the Notch EGF-like repeats bind calcium and are posttranslationally glycosylated (Fig. 1.2b). Notch receptors from different species vary in the number of EGF-like repeats. *Drosophila* Notch has 36 repeats, and the four mammalian Notch receptors (Notch1–Notch4) have 29–36 EGF-like repeats. Interestingly, the two Notch receptors in worms, Lin-12 and GLP-1, are smaller with 14 and 11 EGF-like repeats, respectively.

The minimal region of Notch required for ligand binding in flies encompasses only EGF repeats 11–12 [28, 94], though the minimal region that appears to be required for full activation of Notch1 signaling in cell-based assays is larger and is

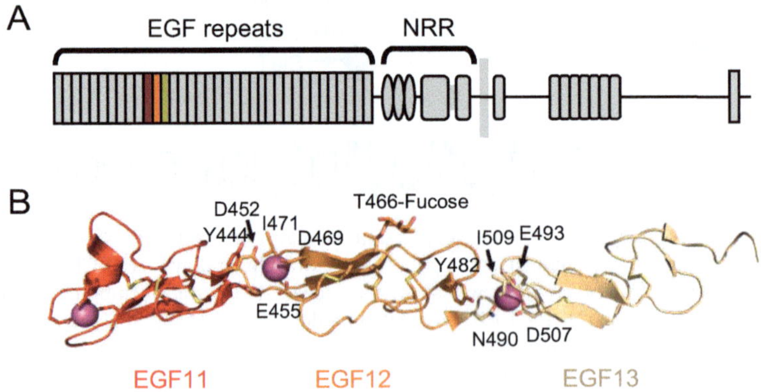

Fig. 1.3 Structure of the ligand-binding region of Notch1. (**a**) Domain organization of Notch1, highlighting EGF repeats 11–13. (**b**) Ribbon diagram of human Notch1 EGF repeats 11–13. EGF repeat 11 (red), EGF12 (orange), and EGF13 (straw) are shown. Acidic resides that coordinate calcium ions (magenta) and resides involved in packing between EGF repeats are labeled. T466 of EGF12, which has a fucose adduct, is labeled (PDB code 4CUD)

encompassed by EGF repeats 6–15 [1, 126]. Structures inclusive of the minimal ligand-binding region from human Notch1, spanning repeats 11–13, have been determined by NMR and X-ray crystallography [21, 40]. The X-ray structure of Notch1 EGF repeats 11–13 (Fig. 1.3) shows that the modules are in an extended rodlike conformation. The interdomain arrangements in this three-repeat structure are defined by the coordination of Ca^{2+} ions at the interface between adjacent repeats as well as by hydrophobic packing of residues at the interdomain interface.

1.2.2 Notch Ligands

There are two families of canonical Notch ligands, homologous to the parent molecules Delta and Serrate in flies. In mammals, there are three homologs of Delta, Delta-like (DLL)1, DLL3, and DLL4, and two of Serrate, Jagged1 (Jag1) and Jagged2 (Jag2). Whereas DLL1, DLL4, Jag1, and Jag2 activate Notch signaling, it is believed that DLL3 is a decoy ligand that does not stimulate signaling [42, 60].

All of these proteins in mammals are single-pass, type 1 transmembrane proteins with a modular extracellular domain organization and intracellular tail (Fig. 1.4). Both Serrate and Delta family members contain a module at the N-terminus of

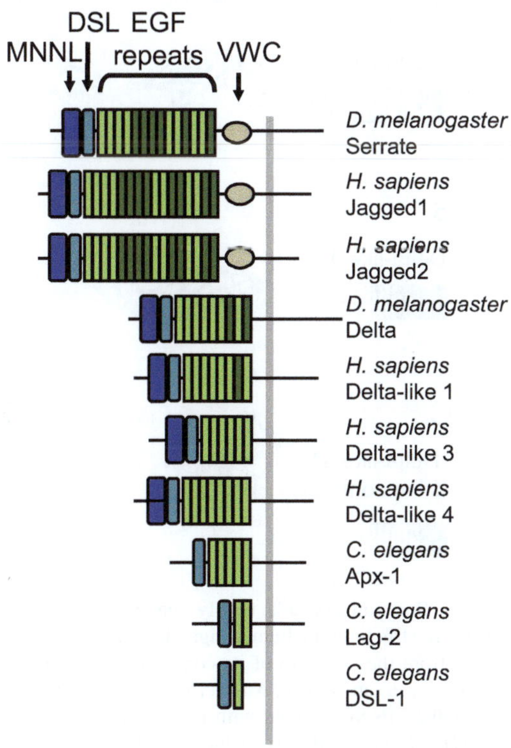

Fig. 1.4 Domain organization of Notch ligands. Domain organization of DSL family ligands from fly, human, and worm. Module at the N-terminus of Notch ligands (MNNL), Delta/Serrate/Lag-2 domain (DSL), von Willebrand factor type C domain (VWC). Calcium-binding EGF repeats are in a dark shade, and non-calcium-binding EGF repeats are in a light shade

Notch ligand (MNNL) domain, followed by a Delta-Serrate-Lag-2 (DSL) domain and a variable number of additional EGF-like repeats. The Serrate class of ligands diverges from the Delta-like proteins in the inclusion of a cysteine-rich domain homologous to the von Willebrand factor C domain immediately proximal to the transmembrane region. All of the activating ligands contain C-terminal intracellular tails that contain recognition motifs for Mind bomb and Neuralized E3 ligases and that are predicted to be predominantly unstructured in isolation.

Structures have been reported for fragments of the DLL1 and Jagged1 extracellular domains and for a modified fragment of DLL4 in complex with ligand-binding repeats EGF11–13 of Notch1 [17, 21, 52, 72, 109]. In the reported X-ray structures (Fig. 1.5), the three ligand molecules (unbound and Notch-bound) adopt an extended conformation, and studies of the DLL1 and Jagged1 proteins using velocity sedimentation and other methods also support the conclusion that the overall architecture of these molecules remains extended in solution [17, 52]. In the larger DLL1 fragment, which includes almost the complete extracellular region of the protein, electron density is visible for the region spanning from the N-terminal MNNL domain through EGF-like repeat six. Intriguingly, the interdomain interface between EGF repeats five and six generates a ~90-degree bend in the protein, suggesting that simple representation of the ligands as extended sticks orthogonal to

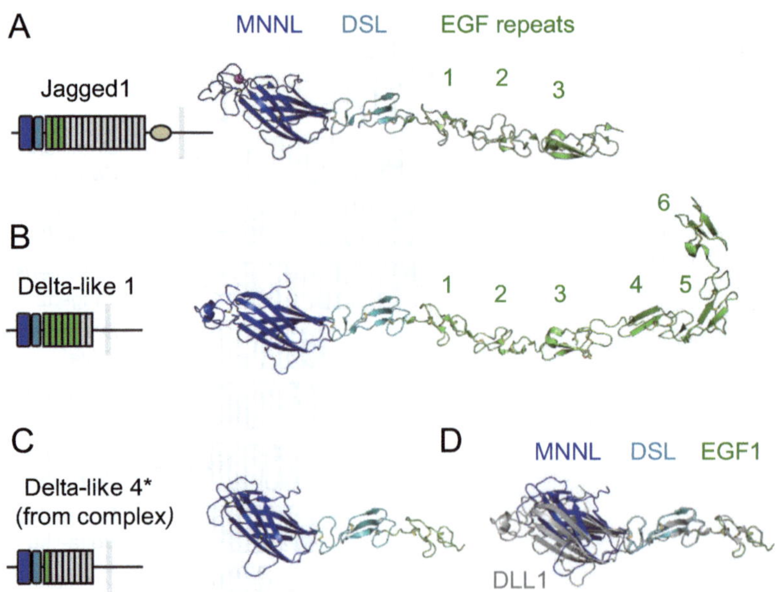

Fig. 1.5 Structures of DSL family ligands. Domain organization and ribbon diagrams representing X-ray structures of human ligands: Jagged1 (**a**), Delta-like 1, DLL1 (**b**), and Delta-like 4, DLL4, from the structure of its complex with Notch1 (**c**). MNNL (blue), DSL (teal), and EGF repeats (green) are shown. An overlay of DLL4 and DLL1 (**d**) reveals a difference in the orientation of the MNNL domain with respect to the DSL and EGF1 domains in the two structures. Jagged1 (PDB code 4CC0), Delta-like1 (PDB code 4XBM), Delta-like4 (PDB code 4XL1)

the plane of the plasma membrane does not accurately reflect the configuration of the ligand molecules on the cell surface. Structures of the smaller Jagged1 and DLL4 fragments superimpose on the larger DLL1 structure with root mean square deviations of 1.9 and 3.1 Å, respectively.

Key structural elements of the ligand ectodomains, in addition to the canonical EGF-like repeats, are their MNNL and DSL modules. The MNNL domain of the ligands folds into a β-sandwich resembling the C2 domains found in proteins such as syntaxin, Munc13, and PTEN. In these other proteins, C2 domains can bind calcium and are often involved in membrane localization by facilitating binding to membrane lipids or phosphoinositides [64, 102]. The structure of the N-terminal fragment of Jag1 revealed a bound calcium ion in the MNNL tip, and calcium is reported to stabilize binding of Jag1 to phospholipid bilayers [17]. Although a similar lipid-binding function was proposed for DLL1, Ca^{2+} is not observed in the X-ray structures of either DLL1 in isolation or DLL4 in the DLL4-Notch1 complex nor are the residues involved in calcium and lipid binding conserved in the DLL proteins [8, 52, 72]. The DSL domain, immediately C-terminal to the MNNL module, is a variant EGF-like domain unique to members of the Delta, Serrate, and Lag-2 family of Notch ligands, and numerous biochemical and mutational studies highlight the importance of this domain in receptor recognition [21, 52, 89, 101].

1.2.3 Initiation of Notch Activation by Notch/Ligand Interactions

For many years, complexes between Notch and ligand resisted crystallization, presumably due to the relatively low affinity between the small minimal binding regions that were produced for biochemical and structural studies [21, 118]. Using yeast display, Luca and colleagues [72] evolved a high-affinity variant of DLL4 that forms a stable complex with a minimal ligand-binding fragment of Notch1 and solved the X-ray structure of this DLL4-Notch1 complex, which includes the MNNL-EGF2 region of DLL4 and the EGF11–13 region of Notch1 (Fig. 1.6). In the complex, the Notch1 and DLL4 molecules are each in an extended conformation and aligned in an antiparallel orientation with about 1100 $Å^2$ of surface area buried at the interface. The Notch1 EGF11–13 fragment does not undergo a substantial conformational change upon binding [72]. In contrast, the MNNL domain in the bound DLL4 complex rotates substantially with respect to the adjacent DSL domain when compared to the unbound DLL1 structure, which results in the engagement of DLL4 with Notch1 at two discontinuous surfaces, first between the MNNL domain and EGF12 and second between the DSL domain and EGF11. In agreement with biochemical assays identifying the minimal ligand-binding region of Notch, the observed binding surface is localized to just these two sites, referred to as site 1, between EGF12 and the MNNL domain, and site 2, between EGF11 and the DSL domain.

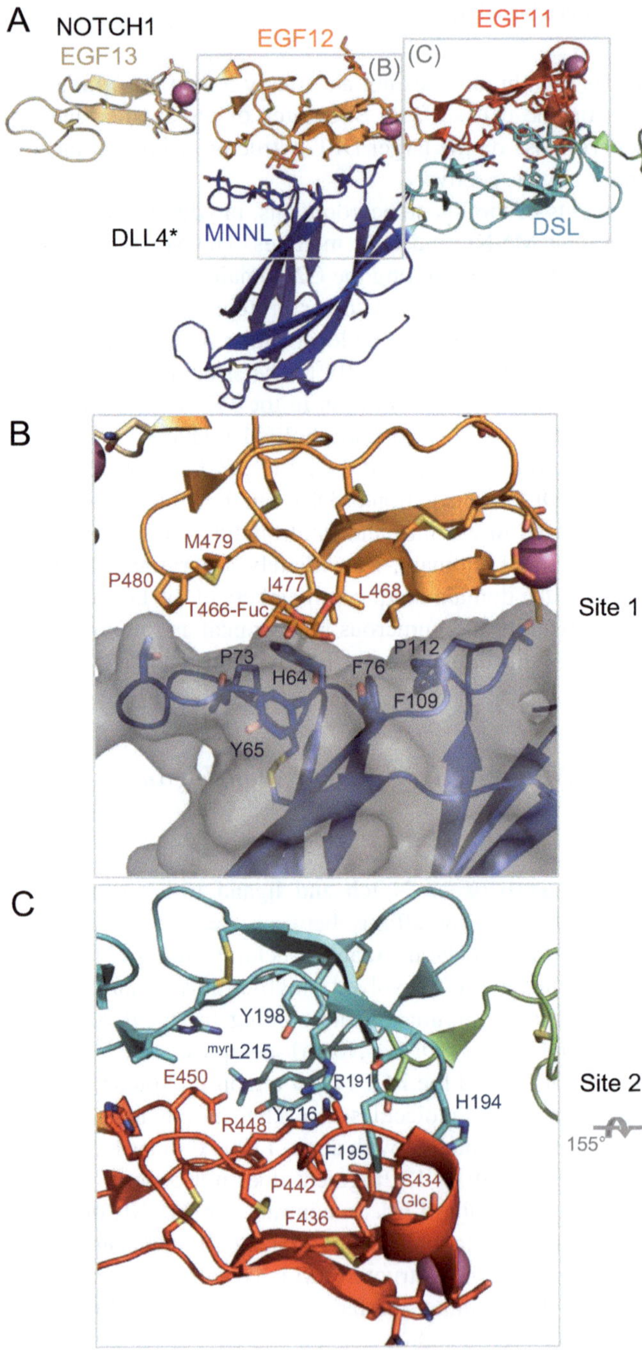

Fig. 1.6 Structure of a complex between Notch1 and an affinity-matured DLL4 ligand. (**a**) Ribbon diagram of the X-ray structure of a complex between rat Notch1 (EGF11–13) and DLL4 (MNNL-EGF1), colored as in Figs. 1.3 and 1.4, reveals a bipartite binding mode. The MNNL domain of DLL4 binds EGF12 of Notch1 at site 1 (**b**), and the DSL domain binds Notch1 EGF11 at site 2 (**c**). Contact resides are labeled (PDB code 4XL1)

Site 1 includes the glycosylated surface of EGF12 and the cysteine-tethered loop of the DLL4 MNNL domain. A hydrophobic pocket at the base of the MNNL loop is generated by the convergence of His64, Phe76, and Phe109, which contact Leu468 and Ile477 of EGF12. Leu468 and Ile477 appear to make critical contributions to ligand binding, as alanine substitutions at these residues interfere with ligand binding and receptor activation [118].

O-linked fucosylation of Notch receptors exerts an important influence on Notch signaling [85, 97, 99, 125, 126]. Genetic deletion of the enzyme that catalyzes this posttranslational modification in mice (POFUT1) is embryonically lethal and gives rise to Notch loss-of-function phenotypes [99]. Within the ligand-binding region of Notch1, even the point mutation of Thr466 in Notch EGF12, which is an O-fucosylation site within the ligand-binding region, results in embryonic lethality when paired with a null allele. This mutation also impairs Notch1 activation by Jag1 and DLL1 ligands in signaling assays [32, 93].

In the structure of the DLL4-Notch1 complex, His74 and Tyr65 in the DLL4 MNNL loop pack against the fucose on Thr466 of Notch1, sandwiching the sugar moiety at the interface [72]. Addition of an N-acetylglucosamine (GlcNac) to the fucose moiety by fringe glycosyltransferases fine-tunes the responsiveness of Notch receptors to Delta and Serrate family ligands [55]. Recent biochemical data investigating the binding of Notch1 fragments to Dll1, DLL4, and Jag1 show that GlcNac addition to the fucose at Thr466 results in higher affinity for DLL1 and Jag1 [109], and modeling of a GlcNac added onto the fucosylated T466 in the X-ray structure of the complex is consistent with the idea that the presence of the sugar will extend the protein-protein interface [72]. These results nicely complement previous functional studies pointing to enhanced responsiveness of Fringe-modified Notch to Delta in flies [125, 126].

The second major point of contact in the Notch1-DLL4 structure involves the interface between the DSL module of DLL4 and the EGF11 domain of Notch1. The binding interface between these modules is highly conserved across a wide range of Notch receptors and ligands. Functional studies probing the interaction between Serrate and Notch in flies point to the particular importance of Arg191 and Phe195 of the ligand in specific recognition [21]. Perhaps the conserved interaction at the DSL-EGF11 interface serves as a primary anchor in ligand binding, with the MNNL-EGF12 interface responsible for tuning ligand specificity for the various mammalian Notch receptors [1, 116] or modulating the strength of the various receptors more generally for all ligands.

1.3 Ligand Endocytosis Mediated by E3 Ubiquitin Ligases

Ubiquitination-mediated endocytosis of ligand into the signal-sending cell is required for Notch activation and signal transduction in the receiving cell [80]. Removal of the cytoplasmic tails from Delta and Serrate results in Notch loss-of-function phenotypes in flies [106]. Two structurally distinct families of E3 ligases,

Mind bomb (Mib) and Neuralized (Neur), can catalyze ubiquitination of ligand cytoplasmic tails [23, 45, 62, 63, 77]. Since Mind bomb1 (Mib1) is the primary E3 ligase implicated in ligand endocytosis and Notch signal transduction in mammals [53, 54], only it will be discussed herein.

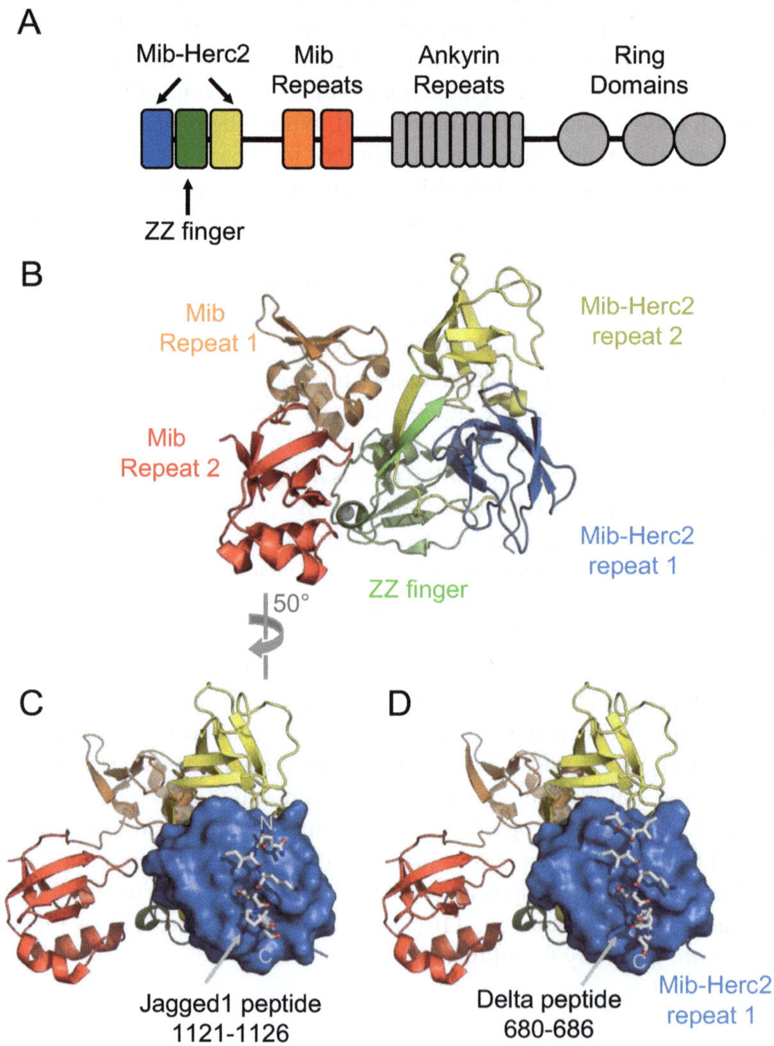

Fig. 1.7 Structure of the Mind bomb1 ligand-binding region. (**a**) Domain organization of Mib1, highlighting the MZM, REP, ANK, and RNG regions of the protein. (**b**) Ribbon diagram of the X-ray structure of the human MZM-REP region of Mib1, colored by domain. The two Zn2+ ions in the ZZ domain are represented by gray spheres. Surface representation of Mib-Herc2 repeat 1 showing the binding of the N-box peptide from human Jagged1 (**c**) and fly Delta (**d**). Mib1 MZM-REP (PDB code 4XI6), Mib1 MZM-REP/Jagged1 N-box (PDB code 4XI7), Mib1 MZM-REP/Delta N-box (PDB code 4XIB)

Mind bomb proteins have four structural regions: an N-terminal MZM region consisting of a ZZ zinc finger (ZZ) domain flanked by two Mib-Herc2 domains, a REP region with two Mib-repeat domains, an ankyrin repeat domain (ANK), and a C-terminal region with three RING domains (Fig. 1.7). The MZM and REP regions are required for ligand binding [16, 45, 77], whereas the RING domains are presumed to associate with the ubiquitin (Ub)-conjugated E2 required for Ub transfer.

The human Mib1 MZM-REP region, the structure of which was recently solved by X-ray crystallography [77], adopts a compact architecture (Fig. 1.7). The MZM region forms an integrated structural unit with extensive interdomain contacts. The Mib-Herc2 domains exhibit the overall topology of SH3 domains. As in other ZZ zinc finger domains, the Mib1 ZZ module includes two structured Zn^{++} ions that are coordinated by a Cys_2 X Cys_2 motif and Cys_2 X His_2 motif. Each of the two Mib repeats shares structural features with the Mib-Herc2 domains (and thus with SH3 domains), packing against the MZM over a small interface area, but not with each other. Small-angle X-ray scattering data suggest that in solution the MZM-REP is sampling conformations that are more open than the compact structure observed in the crystal.

Notch ligands from flies to mammals share a conserved “N-box” near the transmembrane region [22]. N-box peptides from human Jagged1 and fly Delta each bind in a shallow groove on the first Mib-Herc2 domain of the MZM (Fig. 1.7). Jagged ligands also contain a second Mib1-binding site near the ligand C-terminus, denoted as the “C-box.” The human Jagged1 C-box peptide binds to the Mib repeats and contributes substantially to the overall binding affinity, creating a bipartite binding mode [77]. It is proposed that this binding mode enables optional positioning of the lysine-containing loop between the two binding sites for ubiquitination. Although an analogous C-box peptide in the Delta family of ligands is not readily apparent from informatics analysis, the bipartite mode of recognition also seems to apply for these molecules as well (SCB, unpublished data).

1.4 Release from Autoinhibition in the Negative Regulatory Region of Notch

The negative regulatory region (NRR) of Notch lies between the ligand-binding EGF repeats and the transmembrane domain and keeps Notch in an autoinhibited state prior to ligand engagement [35, 38, 56, 95]. Transcriptionally active Notch molecules (NICD) are created by intramembrane proteolysis of membrane-bound Notch by the γ-secretase complex, which is preceded by cleavage at the S2 cleavage site [14, 79] by metalloproteases of the ADAM family, most notably ADAM10. The metalloprotease-sensitive S2 site is located in the NRR within the heterodimerization domain (HD), so named for the presence of the furin S1 cleavage site [9, 68], which

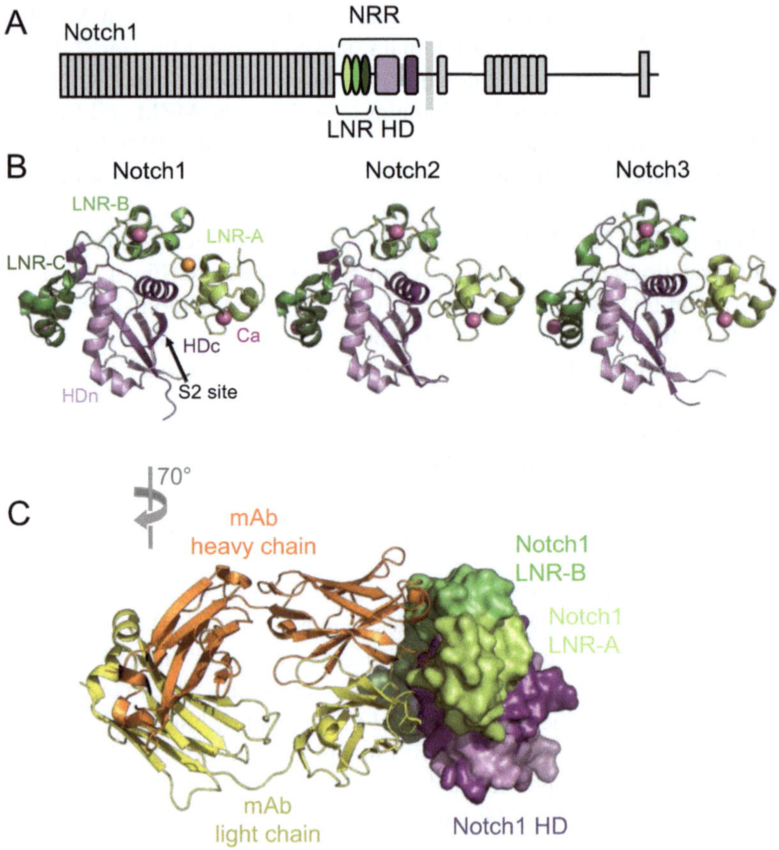

Fig. 1.8 Notch negative regulatory region (NRR) structures. (**a**) Domain organization of Notch, highlighting the NRR. (**b**) Ribbon diagrams of X-ray structures of Notch1 NRR (left), Notch 2 NRR (center), and Notch 3 NRR (right). Lin-12/Notch (LNR) repeats are colored in shades of green. Heterodimerization (HD) domain is colored in shades of violet. (**c**) Complex between an inhibitory anti-Notch1 NRR antibody (yellow, orange) showing how the antibody stabilizes the closed conformation of the NRR. Notch1 NRR (PDB code 3I08), Notch 2 NRR (PDB code 2OO4), Notch 3 NRR (PDB code 4ZLP), and Notch1/antibody (PDB code 3L95)

upon cleavage creates an obligate heterodimer from the pro-Notch precursor in many Notch family members.

Structures of the human Notch1, Notch2, and Notch3 NRRs (Fig. 1.8) adopt the same architecture, in which the HD domain folds into an α-/β-sandwich and is capped by three Lin-12/Notch repeats that each share a fold characterized by three disulfide bonds and a coordinated calcium ion [34–36, 127]. The LNRs stabilize the HD and prevent access to the buried S2 site [110, 111]. Many of the constitutively active cancer-associated mutations found in Notch1 in patients with T-cell acute lymphoblastic leukemia (T-ALL) are localized to the hydrophobic core of the HD and are shown to destabilize the NRR [34, 75]. Notch3 appears to have a higher constitutive amount of basal activity than either Notch1 or Notch2 [127], and this difference seems to correlate with a less stable autoinhibited conformation of its NRR.

Many lines of evidence suggest a mechanotransduction model for release of autoinhibition, in which ligand endocytosis provides a pulling force on the NRR [37, 84, 88, 98]. This pulling force may peel the three LNR domains away from the HD, allowing partial unfolding of the HD and exposure of the S2 site to ADAM metalloproteases.

Several antagonist antibodies that bind to the Notch1 NRR have been described [3, 123]. For one of these antibodies, the structure of the antibody in complex with the Notch1 NRR shows that it bridges from the LNR "cap" to the HD domain "stem" (Fig. 1.8c), stabilizing the NRR in a closed conformation [123].

1.5 Cleavage by ADAM Family Metalloproteases at Site S2

Exposure of the S2 site within the NRR allows cleavage by ADAM family metalloproteases. Though ADAM10 and ADAM17 both appear to be able to cleave Notch1 between Ala1710 and Val1711, the importance of ADAM10 in the proteolytic processing of Notch receptors was first recognized in *Drosophila* from the overlapping phenotypes observed due to the loss of Notch and the transcriptional silencing of the ADAM10 homolog, *kuzbanian* [87, 103]. In both cases, mosaic sensory organ neural progenitor cells deficient in *kuzbanian* or *notch* fail to become epithelial, causing a deficiency in wing margin and sensory organ formation. In mice, genetic ablation of ADAM10 in endothelial, neuronal progenitor, or epithelial cells attenuates Notch1 transcriptional targets, resulting in prenatal death [33, 50, 115]. *Adam10*$^{-/-}$ and *notch*$^{-/-}$ organisms have similar phenotypes and die during development. ADAM10 has other substrates and other proteases may also process Notch. ADAM17, which shares 29% sequence identity with ADAM10, appears to selectively process certain Notch1 receptors that have leukemia-associated activating mutations, though the origin of this selectivity remains unclear [12].

The ADAMs are type 1 membrane proteins with a modular domain organization (Fig. 1.9). Each ADAM contains an N-terminal signal sequence, followed by pro-, metalloprotease, disintegrin, cysteine-rich domains, a transmembrane segment, and cytoplasmic tail. All ADAMs except ADAM10 and ADAM17 also contain an additional EGF-like domain between the cysteine-rich and transmembrane domains. The structure of the catalytically inactive ADAM22 (Fig. 1.9b) shows the metalloprotease-like domain resting within an "open-cup" structure adopted by the disintegrin/cysteine-rich domains [67]. This overall globular structure places the metalloprotease domain in close proximity to the disintegrin domain, with the cysteine-rich domain functioning as a rigid scaffold held together by a conserved disulfide bond network.

The metalloprotease domain of ADAMs shares a characteristic reprolysin-type active site (HEXGHXXGXXHD) with coordination of a catalytic zinc ion followed

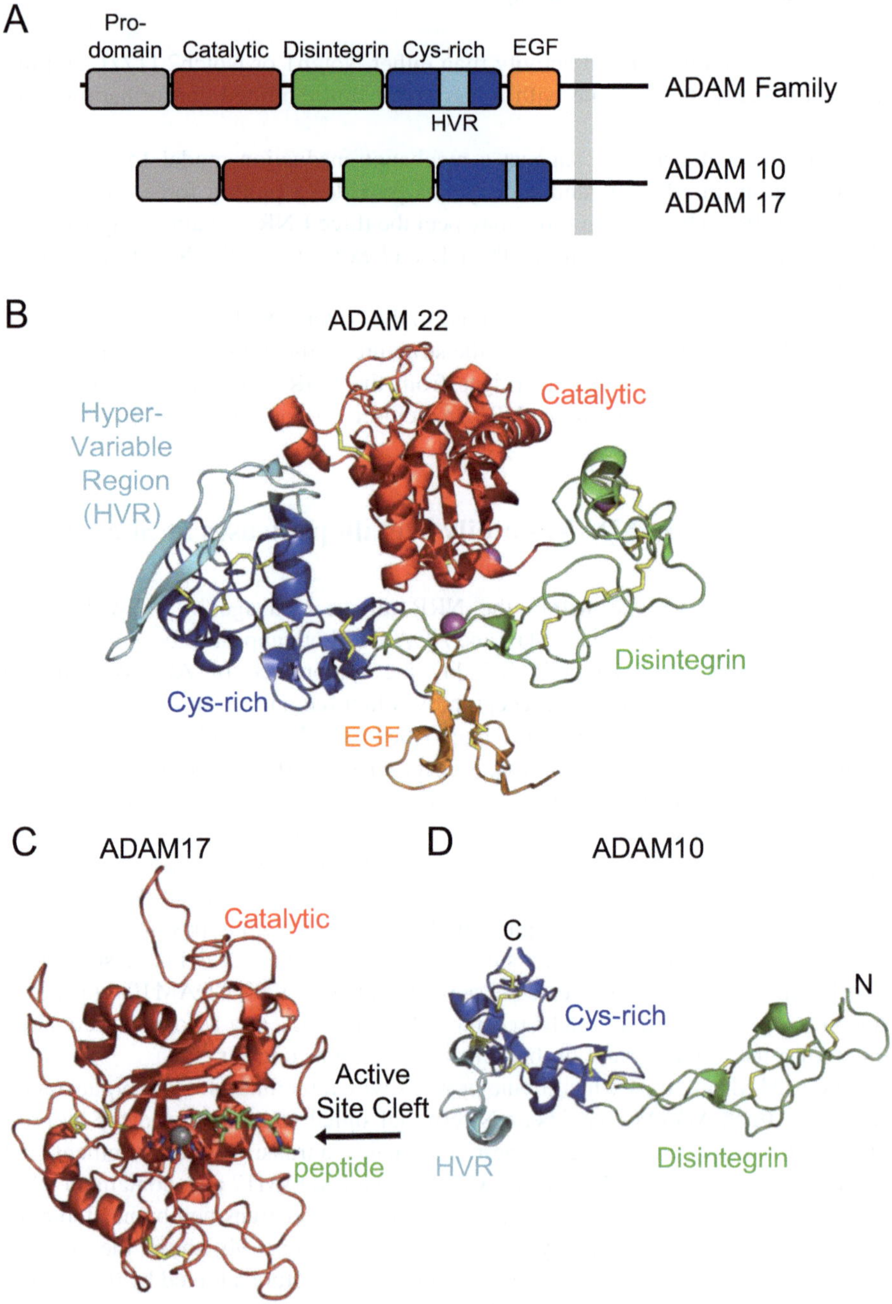

Fig. 1.9 ADAM family metalloprotease structures. (**a**) Domain organization of ADAM family metalloproteases, showing prodomain (gray), catalytic domain (red), disintegrin domain (green), cysteine-rich (Cys-rich, blue), hypervariable region (HVR, light blue), and EGF domain (orange). Adam10 and Adam17, implicated in Notch signaling, share a domain organization distinct from other family members, lacking the EGF domain. (**b**) Ribbon diagram of the catalytically inactive human ADAM22 ectodomain. (**c**) Ribbon diagram of bovine ADAM10 disintegrin and cysteine-rich domains. (**d**) Ribbon diagram of human ADAM17 catalytic domain. ADAM22 (PDB code 3G5C). ADAM10 disintegrin/Cys-rich (PDB code 2AO7), ADAM17 catalytic domain (PDB code 1BKC)

by a conserved methionine (Met-turn). Structures of bound peptide-like inhibitors to the ADAM17 (Fig. 1.9c) metalloprotease domain reveal an elongated substrate bound to a catalytic cleft, extending the core antiparallel β-sheet by an additional β-strand [76]. The disintegrin domain contains an insertion of 17–55 amino acids with low sequence conservation across the ADAM family called the hypervariable region (HVR). This domain may also direct enzymatic activity by binding directly to proteolytic substrates: binding of an acidic surface in the cysteine-rich domain of ADAM10 (Fig. 1.9c) to an ephrin-A5/EphA3 complex has been described, and this interaction has been proposed to position the metalloprotease domain optimally for ephrin-5A cleavage [46]. Furthermore, the importance of the disintegrin/cysteine-rich domains of ADAM10 in Notch signaling is observed in transgenic flies expressing a truncated form of ADAM10 that lacks the metalloprotease domain. These flies acquire a phenotype resembling Notch and ADAM10 knockouts, suggesting that disintegrin/cysteine-rich region may act as a dominant-negative modulator of Notch signaling by interfering with the activity of the endogenous metalloprotease [87].

1.6 Cleavage by γ-Secretase at Site S3

Cleavage at S2 by an ADAM family protease creates a membrane-tethered Notch molecule with about ten extracellular residues remaining exterior to the plasma membrane (12 in the case of Notch1). This Notch extracellular truncation (NEXT) is a substrate for γ-secretase, an intramembrane-cleaving aspartyl protease. The γ-secretase complex consists of four proteins. The catalytic subunit, called presenilin, has nine transmembrane segments, is cleaved between TM6 and TM7 during maturation, and contains the two essential aspartates forming the active site. In humans, two homologous forms of presenilin are made, PS1 and PS2. Aph-1, also expressed in two forms Aph-1a and Aph-1b, is proposed to play a role as a scaffold protein and has seven TM segments. Pen-2, essential for catalytic activity and in stimulating autoproteolysis of PS1, has three TM segments. Nicastrin, which has a single TM segment and a large, heavily glycosylated head group, was previously proposed to be required for substrate recognition [96], although this proposed role has been called into question by recent biochemical and structural studies [5, 6, 10, 69, 104, 105, 130].

Recent cryo-electron microscopy studies have elucidated atomic resolution structures (Fig. 1.10) of the entire human γ-secretase [5, 6, 105]. The large extracellular domain of Nicastrin sits on top of the intramembrane region of γ-secretase making contact with the two ends of the horseshoe shape created by the TM segments of the four proteins. The large glycosylated Nicastrin headpiece cantilevers over PS1 and sterically blocks the interaction of Notch substrates with large ectodomains [10]. The single TM segment of Nicastrin forms one end of the horseshoe, and PEN-2, with three TM segments, forms the other end; Aph-1 is adjacent to Nicastrin. PS1 sits between Aph-1 and PEN-2 and forms the convex side of the complex. Among γ-secretase subunits, PS1 has the greatest conformational variability. In initial high-resolution models, TM2 and TM6 of PS1 are largely disordered. The two catalytic aspartates, D257 on TM6 and D385 on TM7, are

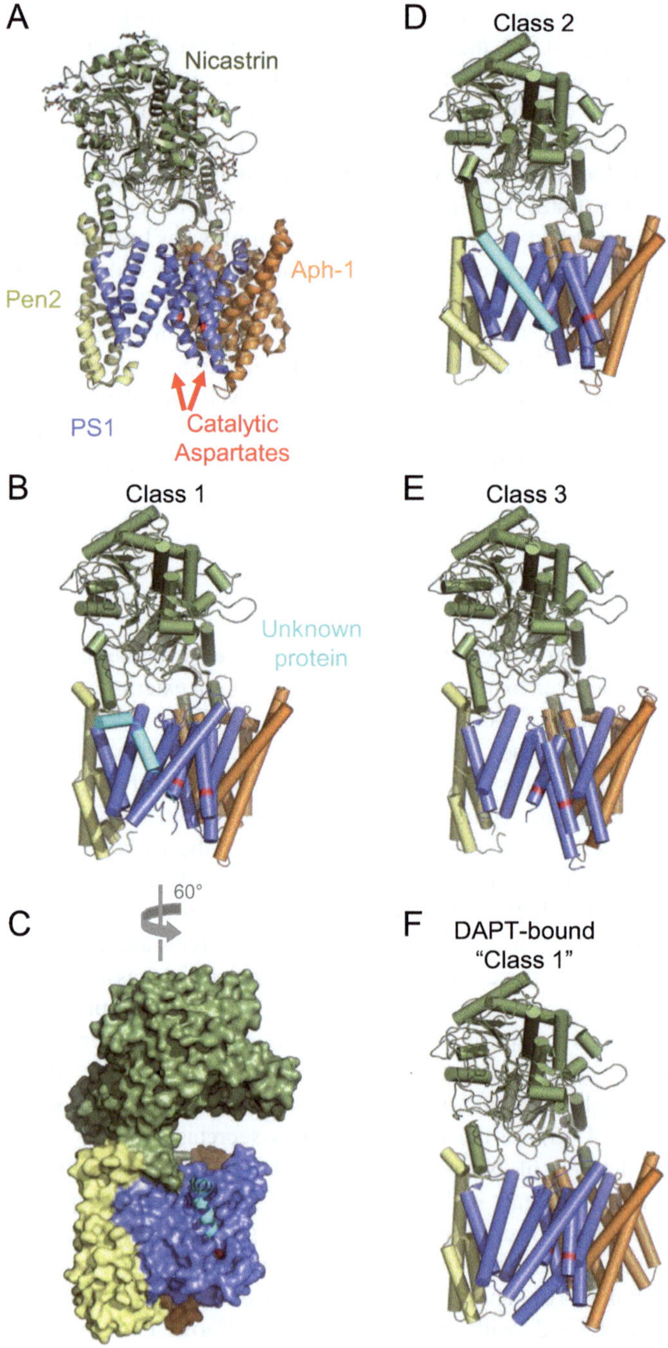

Fig. 1.10 Structures of the γ-secretase complex. (**a**) Ribbon diagram of the human γ-secretase complex, determined by cryo-EM. The complex includes Nicastrin (green), presenilin 1 (PS1, lavender), Pen-2 (yellow), and Aph-1 (orange). Cartoon representations of three classifications of

located near the highly conserved PAL motif (433–435) on TM9, shown to be required for γ-secretase catalytic activity [114], and surrounded by other conserved residues. In the high-resolution 3.4 Å structure (PDB code 5a63), however, D257 and D385 are too far apart to catalyze proteolysis, and thus this structure likely represents an inactive conformation (Table. 1.1).

Application of masked classification to the high-resolution dataset allowed three conformational snapshots to be observed [5]. Notably, TM6 is in a different location in each of these models. TM2 is only observed in class 1. In class 3, PEN-2 rotates away from PS1, and there is significant rearrangement of TM3–TM6 of PS1. In class 1, TM2, TM3, and TM5 create a cavity lined with residues mutated in an early-onset familial form of Alzheimer's disease (FAD). Within this cavity, helical density that cannot be attributed to γ-secretase is observed. Additional helical density is also observed in class 2, but is best ordered in class 1, where the density is modeled as a kinked helix that ends in an extended conformation approaching the active site of PS1. This density, presumably from a mixture of copurified peptides, may mimic substrate binding. In a structure solved with the γ-secretase inhibitor DAPT, there is less flexibility in PS1, and one well-ordered class is observed, which resembles class 1 of the apo complex. DAPT occupies the base of the cavity near the active site.

1.7 Transcriptional Activation and Assembly of Notch Nuclear Complexes

Intramembrane proteolysis by the γ-secretase complex releases Notch from the membrane, allowing the intracellular portion of Notch (NICD) to translocate to the nucleus. In the nucleus, NICD interacts with the DNA-binding protein CSL and a member of the Mastermind (MAM) family [90, 121] to form a transcriptionally active complex. NICD consists of a high-affinity RBPJ-associated module (RAM), an ankyrin repeat domain (ANK), and a C-terminal region including a PEST sequence involved in Notch turnover. The only region of intracellular Notch with known secondary structure is the ANK domain.

Progress toward visualizing Notch nuclear complexes began with reports of the X-ray structures of the ankyrin repeat (ANK) domains from fly Notch and human Notch1 [26, 82, 134]. The conserved ANK region includes 7 ankyrin repeats, the first of which is largely disordered in fly and human proteins when they are not bound to the CSL transcription factor. Each ankyrin repeat motif consists of two antiparallel α-helices followed by an extended β-hairpin. These repeats stack against each other in a conserved manner to form a curved solenoid-type structure with both a convex and a concave face.

Fig. 1.10 (continued) γ-secretase complex structures, class 1 (**b, c**), class 2 (**d**), and class 3 (**e**), and of the DAPT-bound complex (**f**), which adopts a "class 1" conformation. Panel **c** shows a surface representation of the class 1 structure with the Nicastrin headpiece extended over the TM region of the complex, blocking access to the catalytic site. γ-Secretase (PDB code 5A63), class 1 (PDB code 5FN3), class 2 (PDB code 5FN4), class 3 (PDB code 5FN5), DAPT complex (PDB code 5FN2)

Table 1.1 Atomic resolution structures of Notch pathway-related proteins and their complexes

Description	PDB	Species	Method	Reference
Notch EGF region				
Notch1 EGF11–13 (ligand binding)	1TOZ	*H. sapiens*	NMR	[40]
Notch1 EGF11–13 (ligand binding)	2VJ3	*H. sapiens*	X-ray	[21]
Notch1 EGF12	2RR0	*M. musculus*	NMR	[43]
Notch1 EGF12, O-fucosylated	2RR2	*M. musculus*	NMR	[43]
Notch1 EGF12, sugar modified	2RQZ	*M. musculus*	NMR	[43]
Notch1 EGF11–13, T466 O-fucosylated	4CUD	*H. sapiens*	X-ray	[109]
Notch1 EGF11–13, T466 sugar modified	4D0E	*H. sapiens*	X-ray	[109]
Notch1 EGF11–13, T466V	4CUE	*H. sapiens*	X-ray	[109]
Notch1 EGF11–13, T466A	4D0F	*H. sapiens*	X-ray	[109]
Notch1 EGF11–13, T466S	4CUF	*H. sapiens*	X-ray	[109]
DSL ligands				
Jagged1 DSL-EGF3	2VJ2	*H. sapiens*	X-ray	[21]
Jagged1 EGF2	2KB9	*H. sapiens*	NMR	[91]
Jagged1 MNNL-EGF3	4CC0	*H. sapiens*	X-ray	[17]
Jagged1 MNNL-EGF3	4CBZ	*H. sapiens*	X-ray	[17]
Jagged1 MNNL-EGF3	4CC1	*H. sapiens*	X-ray	[17]
Delta-like1 N-terminal MNNL-EGF6	4XBM	*H. sapiens*	X-ray	[52]
Jagged1 + anti-Jagged1 Fab	5BO1	*H. sapiens*	X-ray	[61]
Notch/ligand complex				
Notch1 EGF11–13 + affinity-matured Delta-like4 MNNL-EGF1	4XL1	*R. norvegicus*	X-ray	[72]
Notch1 EGF11–13 + affinity-matured Delta-like4 MNNL-EGF2	4XLW	*R. norvegicus*	X-ray	[72]
Notch negative regulatory region				
Notch1 LNR-A domain	1PB5	*H. sapiens*	NMR	[112]
Notch2 NRR (LNR-HD)	2OO4	*H. sapiens*	X-ray	[35]
Notch1 NRR	3ETO	*H. sapiens*	X-ray	[34]
Notch1 NRR, S1-cleaved	3I08	*H. sapiens*	X-ray	[36]
Notch1 NRR + antagonist antibody fragment	3L95	*H. sapiens*	X-ray	[123]
Notch3 NRR	4ZLP	*H. sapiens*	X-ray	[127]
Extracellular/TM Notch-associated molecules				
Adam17 (TACE) catalytic domain + inhibitor	1BKC	*H. sapiens*	X-ray	[76]
Manic Fringe	2J0A	*M. musculus*	X-ray	[48]
Manic Fringe + UDP/Mn	2J0B	*M. musculus*	X-ray	[48]
Adam10 disintegrin and Cys-rich domain	2AO7	*B. taurus*	X-ray	[46]
Adam17 + N-TIMP-3	3CKI	*H. sapiens*	X-ray	[120]
Adam17 membrane proximal domain	2M2F	*H. sapiens*	NMR	[25]
Nicastrin extracellular domain	4R12	*D. purpureum*	X-ray	[124]
γ-Secretase complex (PS1, Nicastrin, APH-1, Pen-2)	5A63	*H. sapiens*	EM	[6]
γ-Secretase complex	4UIS	*H. sapiens*	EM	[105]

(continued)

Table 1.1 (continued)

Description	PDB	Species	Method	Reference
γ-Secretase complex + DAPT	5FN2	*H. sapiens*	EM	[5]
γ-Secretase complex, structure class 1	5FN3	*H. sapiens*	EM	[5]
γ-Secretase complex, structure class 2	5FN4	*H. sapiens*	EM	[5]
γ-Secretase complex, structure class 3	5FN5	*H. sapiens*	EM	[5]
Xyloside α-1,3-xylosyltransferase(XXYLT1) + human factor IX (hFA9)	4WM0	*M. musculus/H. sapiens*	X-ray	[128]
XXYLT1 + hFA9 + UDP	4WMI	*M. musculus/H. sapiens*	X-ray	[128]
XXYLT1 +hFA9 + UDP	4WMK	*M. musculus/H. sapiens*	X-ray	[128]
XXYLT1+ hFA9 + UDP	4WN2	*M. musculus/H. sapiens*	X-ray	[128]
XXYLT1 +hFA9 + UDP-glucose	4MWA	*M. musculus/H. sapiens*	X-ray	[128]
XXYLT1 + hFA9 + UDP-xylose	4WNH	*M. musculus/H. sapiens*	X-ray	[128]
Intracellular ligand-associated molecules				
Neuralized NHR domain	2E63	*H. sapiens*	NMR	[41]
Neuralized NHR domain	2YUE	*D. melanogaster*	NMR	[41]
Neuralized NHR1 domain	4KG0	*D. melanogaster*	X-ray	[39]
Mind bomb1 REP (Mib repeat domain)	4TSE	*H. sapiens*	X-ray	[77]
Mind bomb1 MZM-REP	4XI6	*H. sapiens*	X-ray	[77]
Mind bomb1 MZM-REP + Jagged1 N-box peptide	4XI7	*H. sapiens*	X-ray	[77]
Mind bomb1 MZM-REP + Delta N-box peptide	4XIB	*H. sapiens/D. melanogaster*	X-ray	[77]
Intracellular Notch nuclear complex				
Notch ANK	1OT8	*D. melanogaster*	X-ray	[134]
Lag-1 (CSL) + DNA	1TTU	*C. elegans*	X-ray	[57]
Notch1 ANK repeats 3–7	1YMP	*M. musculus*	X-ray	[71]
Notch1 ANK	1YYH	*H. sapiens*	X-ray	[26]
Notch1 ANK	2F8Y	*H. sapiens*	X-ray	[82]
Notch1 ANK+ MAML+ RBPJ (CSL) + DNA	2F8X	*H. sapiens*	X-ray	[82]
Lin12 RAMANK (Notch)+ Sel8 (MAM) + Lag-1(CSL) + DNA	2FO1	*C. elegans*	X-ray	[119]
Notch1 ANK, Hydroxylated	2QC9	*H. sapiens*	X-ray	[19]
RBPJ (CSL) + DNA	3BRG	*M. musculus*	X-ray	[30]
Lin12 RAM (Notch) + Lag-1 (CSL) + DNA	3BRD	*C. elegans*	X-ray	[30]
Lin12 RAM (Notch) + Lag-1 (CSL) + DNA	3BRF	*C. elegans*	X-ray	[30]
RBPJ (CSL) + DNA (HES1 non-consensus)	3IAG	*M. musculus*	X-ray	[29]
Notch1 ANK + MAML RBPJ (CSL) + DNA (HES1 paired site)	3NBN	*H. sapiens*	X-ray	[2]
Notch1 ANK + Notch1 RAM + MAML + RBPJ (CSL) + DNA	3 V79	*H. sapiens*	X-ray	[18]

(continued)

Table 1.1 (continued)

Description	PDB	Species	Method	Reference
Intracellular Notch-associated molecules				
Su(dx) WW domains 3–4	1TK7	*D. melanogaster*	NMR	[27]
Deltex WWE domain	2A90	*D. melanogaster*	X-ray	[133]
Su(dx) WW domain 4 + phosphorylated Notch peptide	2JMF	*D. melanogaster*	NMR	[47]
Factor Inhibiting HIF-1 (FIH) + Notch1 peptide	3P3N	*H. sapiens/M. musculus*	X-ray	[19]
FIH + Notch1 peptide	3P3P	*H. sapiens/M. musculus*	X-ray	[19]
KyoT2 + RBPJ (CSL) + DNA	4J2X	*M. musculus/H. sapiens*	X-ray	[20]
Suppressor of Hairless (Su(H)) + hairless (H)	5E24	*D. melanogaster*	X-ray	[129]

1.7.1 The DNA-Binding Protein CSL

CSL, named for CBF1 in humans (gene name RBPJ) and Suppressor of Hairless in flies (Su(H)) and Lag-1 in worms, is the DNA-binding protein associated with Notch. CSL consists of a conserved core with three structured domains, an N-terminal immunoglobulin-like Rel homology region (NTD), a β-trefoil domain (BTD), and a C-terminal Rel homology region (CTD), which are linked by a long β-strand that spans all three domains [57]. The NTD and BTD together form an electropositive surface that binds DNA. The NTD inserts a β-hairpin into the major groove of DNA to recognize the GGGA base pairs that form the core of the consensus binding motif (C/t)(G/a/c)TG(G/t/a)GA(A/g). The BTD provides additional DNA contacts in the major and minor grooves. Unlike other Rel family proteins, which use both their N- and C-terminal domains to contact cognate DNA sequences, the CTD does not contact DNA but rather sits above the BTD and NTD providing essential contacts with Notch.

1.7.2 Assembly of the Notch Transcription Complex (NTC)

The architecture of the NTC is illustrated by complexes of human and worm Notch, CSL, and MAM on DNA [18, 82, 119]. The 7-repeat ankyrin domain of Notch is the minimal region of Notch required for assembly with CSL and MAM (Fig. 1.11).

Fig. 1.11 Structures of nuclear Notch transcription complexes (NTC). (**a**) Domain organization of human Notch1, MAML1, and RBPJ (CSL) proteins. Ribbon diagrams of X-ray structures of the human NTC (**b**) and worm NTC (**c**) showing Notch (human Notch1 and worm Lin12) ankyrin domain (ANK, orange), CSL (human RBPJ and worm Lag-1), N-terminal domain (NTD), β-trefoil domain (BTD), and C-terminal domain (CTD) (shades of teal) and Mastermind (human MAML1 and worm Lag-3) (yellow) bound to a segment of the HES1 promoter (gray). (**d**) Structure of a dimer of NTC trimers on a Suppressor of Hairless Paired Site (SPS, or sequence-paired site), shown with one NTC as a ribbon diagram and one as a surface representation. Human NTC (PDB code 3 V79), worm NTC (PDB code 2FO1); dimeric NTC/SPS (PDB code 3NBN)

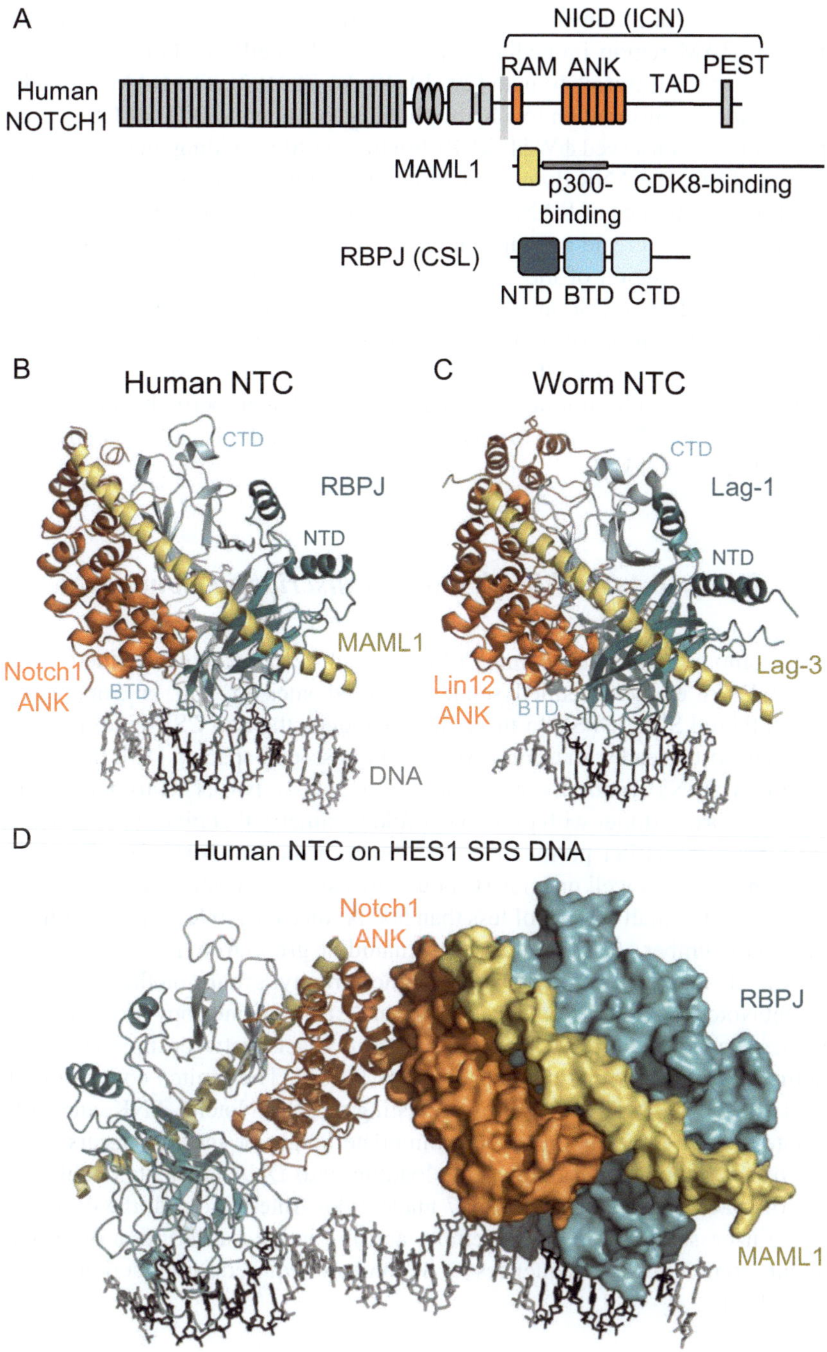

Fig. 1.11 (continued)

However, the high-affinity interaction between Notch and CSL is driven by the conserved RAM region immediately internal to the cell membrane, which binds exclusively to the β-trefoil domain [29, 30, 49, 59, 70, 107]. The RAM region binds in an extended conformation to a hydrophobic groove in the BTD of CSL, with the tryptophan of a conserved ϕWϕP RBPJ-binding motif providing most of the energy of binding [49]. The ANK domain of Notch, which has only weak intrinsic affinity for CSL in the absence of RAM [4, 24], contacts the NTD and CTD Rel homology domains of CSL to create a composite binding surface for MAM [82, 119]. Only a short N-terminal region of the 1016 amino acid MAML1 (13–74) is required for cooperative binding to CSL and Notch, and this natively unstructured region adopts a kinked helical conformation upon binding to CSL and Notch. When fused to a carrier protein domain like GFP, this N-terminal region of MAML1 acts as a strong dominant-negative inhibitor of Notch signaling [117], a property that has been used to probe the role of Notch in a variety of different physiologic and pathophysiologic contexts [e.g., [78, 131]].

1.7.3 Dimeric Assembly of Notch Transcription Complexes

In the promoter region of a number of key Notch-responsive genes, there are specialized DNA elements called sequence-paired sites [7, 83] or Suppressor of Hairless Paired Sites (SPS). In these SPS elements, the two CSL-binding sites are oriented head-to-head with a conserved 15–17 base-pair spacing [15]. In the crystal structure of an NTC/paired-site complex (Fig. 1.11d), two NTC trimers assemble together to form a dimer with pseudo twofold symmetry that binds cooperatively to an SPS from the HES1 promoter region. Each of the two NTC complexes in the dimer superimposes well on an NTC bound to a single site [2]. The dimer interface is restricted to a small surface of less than 500 $Å^2$ on each ANK domain, with a relatively small number of key contacts. The guanidine group from R1984 of one Notch molecule fits into a pocket lined by backbone carbonyl groups on the surface of the adjacent Notch molecule. Residues K1945 and E1949 of one copy form salt bridges with the second copy, as seen in the crystal contacts between monomers in the structure of a single trimeric Notch complex [2, 81]. The limited contact interface allows the two rigid NTC structures consisting of CSL, Notch1-ANK, and MAML to rotate relative to each other to accommodate longer or shorter spacers between the two CSL-binding sites, supporting loading onto DNA elements readily over a range of spacer lengths from 15 to 17 nucleotides. Interactions at the dimer interface are necessary for dimeric assembly and for active transcription on promoter elements containing SPS sequences [2, 81] and are required for induction of T-ALL in mice [66].

1.7.4 *Intracellular Notch Repressor Complexes*

CSL also interacts with a number of corepressors in the absence of Notch [11]. CSL corepressors are typically part of larger multiprotein complexes, many of which include histone-modifying components responsible for placing repressive marks on local chromatin. Known repressors include KyoT2, MINT/SHARP, SMRT, SKIP, and CIR in mammals and Hairless in flies [44, 51, 58, 65, 86, 92, 100, 108, 132].

The structure of the KyoT2 in complex with CSL reveals that this corepressor competes directly with Notch for binding to CSL [20]. KyoT2, which shares the conserved ϕWϕP motif found in the RAM region of Notch, fills the hydrophobic groove in the CSL BTD domain with high affinity and in a manner similar to the mammalian Notch1 and worm Lin12 RAM regions (Fig. 1.12). The transition from a KyoT2 repressed to a Notch active complex thus requires either exchange of molecules or loading of new Notch-bound complexes onto DNA, as Notch and KyoT2 binding are mutually exclusive through direct competition.

In flies, the protein Hairless (H) binds Suppressor of Hairless, Su(H), the fly ortholog of CSL, to form a corepressor complex [13, 73]. Hairless and NICD binding to CSL are also mutually exclusive [74], but the mechanism of binding of Hairless to Su(H) is fundamentally different from that of KyoT2 and other corepressors that bind to the BTD (Fig. 1.13). Hairless binds exclusively to the CTD of Su(H) in a unique way [129]. Upon binding the Su(H) CTD, the natively unstructured region of Hairless that binds adopts a β-hairpin that is wedged between the first and last β-strand of the CTD β-sandwich. This rearrangement induces a significant conformational change in CSL, producing steric clashes that would prevent binding to the ankyrin domain of Notch and to MAM.

1.8 Summary

Since the first Notch structures in 2003 of the ankyrin domain of fly Notch [134] and LNR-A of human Notch1 [112], there has been an explosion of structural and biochemical data that have helped to elucidate molecular mechanistic detail for many major steps in Notch signaling, including ligand binding, ligand endocytosis, release from autoinhibition, metalloprotease cleavage, intramembrane cleavage, and transcriptional activation. A clear picture is emerging of the mechanism of Notch autoinhibition, the minimal requirements for ligand binding by Notch, and the assembly of intracellular Notch into transcriptionally active complexes. Structures of a growing list of Notch-related proteins and complexes have been solved and are shedding new light on modulators of signaling, such as ligand-associated E3 ligases, Notch-modifying glycosyltransferases, Notch-activating proteases (including the γ-secretase intramembrane protease), and CSL corepressors. While all of these structures have contributed greatly to our current understanding of Notch signaling, there are still some important, and as yet unsolved, structural

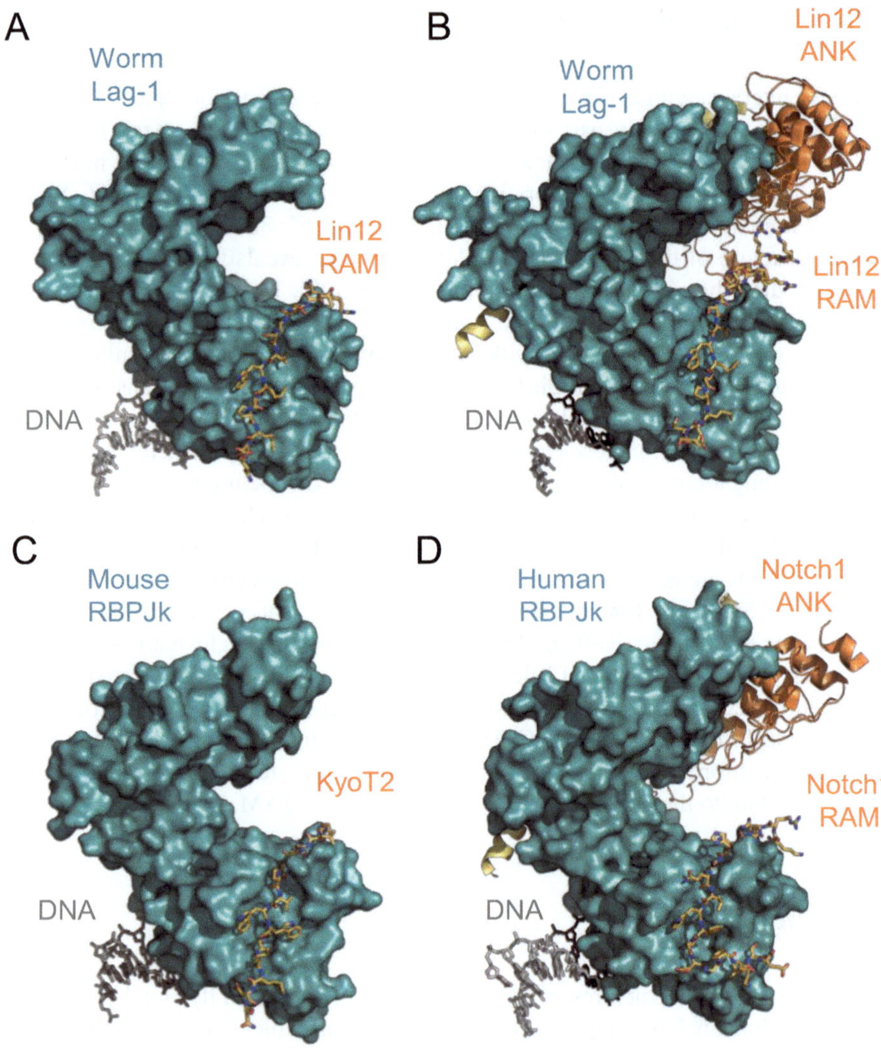

Fig. 1.12 Structures of RAM and corepressor KyoT2 peptides bound to CSL. Surface representations of worm Lag-1 bound to Lin12 RAM in the absence (**a**) and presence (**b**) of Lin12 and Lag-3 colored as in Fig. 1.10. (**c**) Surface representations of corepressor KyoT2 bound to mouse RBPJ and (**d**) human Notch1 RAM peptide bound to human RBPJ. The conserved binding groove for RAM and for the KyoT2 peptide is in the CSL β-trefoil domain. Worm Lag-1/Lin12 RAM (PDB code 3BRD), worm Lag-1/Lin12 RAMANK/Lag-3 (PDB code 2FO1), mouse RBPJ/KyoT2 (PDB code 4J2X), and human RBPJ/Notch RAM/Notch ANK/MAML1 (PDB code 3V79)

questions to be answered. How Notch is recognized for modification by glycosyltransferases remains relatively poorly understood at a detailed structural level. Similarly, the current view of Notch-ligand complexes is limited to a the "minimal-interacting" region between Notch1 and DLL4, leaving unanswered how these interacting regions on the two proteins are presented to each other in the context of

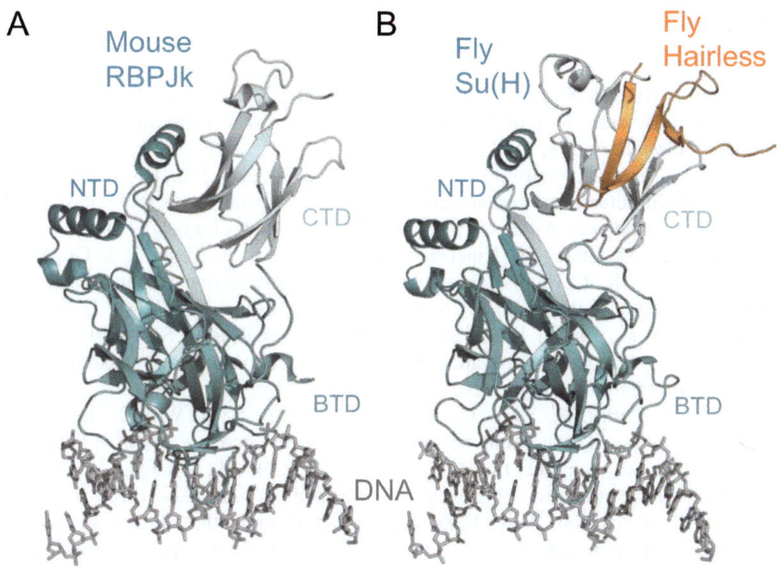

Fig. 1.13 Structure of Hairless bound to Suppressor of Hairless, Su(H). (**a**) Ribbon diagram of mouse RBPJ bound to DNA, colored as in Fig. 1.10. (**b**) Ribbon diagram of fly Hairless (orange) bound to Su(H). Insertion of Hairless remodels the CTD of Su(H). Mouse RBPJ (PDB code 3BRG), fly Su(H)/Hairless (PDB code 5E24)

full-length molecules or ectodomains. The unusual interdomain orientation in DLL1 also suggests the tantalizing possibility that Notch-ligand complexes might exhibit catch-bond behavior, as the kink in the structure could serve as a hook that strengthens the ligand-receptor interaction when force is applied. Binding of ligand tails by the E3 ligase Mind bomb1 is understood, at least in part, but how it transfers ubiquitin to the ligand tail and promotes ubiquitin-mediated endocytosis remain elusive. Partial structures for metalloproteases ADAM17 and ADAM10 have been solved, but an intact enzyme and the mechanism of Notch recognition and cleavage are still unknown. Notch modulators, such as NRARP and the Hes family proteins, play important roles in Notch signaling, but their structures and mechanism of action are largely unknown. Transcriptional activation of Notch-responsive genes is also dependent on the recruitment of additional coactivators linked to the general transcription machinery, such as p300 (E1A-binding protein p300) or CREB-binding protein (CBP) [31, 113], but little is known about the structure or mechanism of these interactions. Thus, there is much to occupy the attention of mechanistic biochemists in the Notch field for a number of years to come.

Note added in proof Since this chapter was written, a structure of a JAG1-Notch1 complex was reported (V.C. Luca et al., Science 10.1126/science.aaf9739;2017), the structure of an ADAM10 ectodomain was reported (T.C.M. Seegar et al., Cell 171, 1638–1648.e7;2017), and new structures of DLL4 and JAG2 isolated ligand fragments were reported (Suckling, R.J., et al. EMBO J 36(15): 2204–2215;2017).

References

1. Andrawes, M. B., Xu, X., Liu, H., Ficarro, S. B., Marto, J. A., Aster, J. C., & Blacklow, S. C. (2013). Intrinsic selectivity of Notch 1 for Delta-like 4 over Delta-like 1. *The Journal of Biological Chemistry, 288*, 25477–25489.
2. Arnett, K. L., Hass, M., Mcarthur, D. G., Ilagan, M. X. G., Aster, J. C., Kopan, R., & Blacklow, S. C. (2010). Structural and mechanistic insights into cooperative assembly of dimeric Notch transcription complexes. *Nature Structural and Molecular Biology, 17*, 1312–1317.
3. Aste-Amézaga, M., Zhang, N., Lineberger, J. E., Arnold, B. A., Toner, T. J., Gu, M., Huang, L., Vitelli, S., Vo, K. T., Haytko, P., et al. (2010). Characterization of Notch1 antibodies that inhibit signaling of both normal and mutated Notch1 receptors. *PLoS One, 5*, e9094.
4. Aster, J. C., Xu, L., Karnell, F. G., Patriub, V., Pui, J. C., & Pear, W. S. (2000). Essential roles for ankyrin repeat and transactivation domains in induction of T-cell leukemia by notch1. *Molecular and Cellular Biology, 20*, 7505–7515.
5. Bai, X.-C., Rajendra, E., Yang, G., Shi, Y., & Scheres, S. H. W. (2015). Sampling the conformational space of the catalytic subunit of human γ-secretase. *eLife, 4*, e11182.
6. Bai, X.-C., Yan, C., Yang, G., Lu, P., Ma, D., Sun, L., Zhou, R., Scheres, S. H. W., & Shi, Y. (2015). An atomic structure of human γ-secretase. *Nature, 525*, 212–217.
7. Bailey, A. M., & Posakony, J. W. (1995). Suppressor of hairless directly activates transcription of enhancer of split complex genes in response to Notch receptor activity. *Genes and Development, 9*, 2609–2622.
8. Blacklow, S. C. (2013). Refining a Jagged edge. *Structure, 21*, 2100–2101.
9. Blaumueller, C. M., Qi, H., Zagouras, P., & Artavanis-Tsakonas, S. (1997). Intracellular cleavage of Notch leads to a heterodimeric receptor on the plasma membrane. *Cell, 90*, 281–291.
10. Bolduc, D. M., Montagna, D. R., Gu, Y., Selkoe, D. J., & Wolfe, M. S. (2016). Nicastrin functions to sterically hinder γ-secretase-substrate interactions driven by substrate transmembrane domain. *Proceedings of the National Academy of Sciences, 113*, E509–E518.
11. Borggrefe, T., & Oswald, F. (2009). The Notch signaling pathway: Transcriptional regulation at Notch target genes. *Cellular and Molecular Life Sciences: CMLS, 66*, 1631–1646.
12. Bozkulak, E. C., & Weinmaster, G. (2009). Selective use of ADAM10 and ADAM17 in activation of Notch1 signaling. *Molecular and Cellular Biology, 29*, 5679–5695.
13. Bray, S., & Furriols, M. (2001). Notch pathway: Making sense of suppressor of hairless. *Current Biology, 11*, R217–R221.
14. Brou, C., Logeat, F., Gupta, N., Bessia, C., LeBail, O., Doedens, J. R., Cumano, A., Roux, P., Black, R. A., & Israël, A. (2000). A novel proteolytic cleavage involved in Notch signaling: The role of the disintegrin-metalloprotease TACE. *Molecular Cell, 5*, 207–216.
15. Cave, J. W., Loh, F., Surpris, J. W., Xia, L., & Caudy, M. A. (2005). A DNA transcription code for cell-specific gene activation by notch signaling. *Current Biology, 15*, 94–104.
16. Chen, W., & Casey Corliss, D. (2004). Three modules of zebrafish Mind bomb work cooperatively to promote Delta ubiquitination and endocytosis. *Developmental Biology, 267*, 361–373.
17. Chillakuri, C. R., Sheppard, D., Ilagan, M. X. G., Holt, L. R., Abbott, F., Liang, S., Kopan, R., Handford, P. A., & Lea, S. M. (2013). Structural analysis uncovers lipid-binding properties of Notch ligands. *Cell Reports, 5*, 861–867.
18. Choi, S. H., Wales, T. E., Nam, Y., O'Donovan, D. J., Sliz, P., Engen, J. R., & Blacklow, S. C. (2012). Conformational locking upon cooperative assembly of notch transcription complexes. *Structure, 20*, 340–349.
19. Coleman, M. L., McDonough, M. A., Hewitson, K. S., Coles, C., Mecinovic, J., Edelmann, M., Cook, K. M., Cockman, M. E., Lancaster, D. E., Kessler, B. M., et al. (2007). Asparaginyl hydroxylation of the Notch ankyrin repeat domain by factor inhibiting hypoxia-inducible factor. *The Journal of Biological Chemistry, 282*, 24027–24038.

20. Collins, K. J., Yuan, Z., & Kovall, R. A. (2014). Structure and function of the CSL-KyoT2 corepressor complex: A negative regulator of Notch signaling. *Structure, 22*, 70–81.
21. Cordle, J., Johnson, S., Tay, J. Z. Y., Roversi, P., Wilkin, M. B., de Madrid, B. H., Shimizu, H., Jensen, S., Whiteman, P., Jin, B., et al. (2008). A conserved face of the Jagged/Serrate DSL domain is involved in Notch trans-activation and cis-inhibition. *Nature Structural and Molecular Biology, 15*, 849–857.
22. Daskalaki, A., Shalaby, N. A., Kux, K., Tsoumpekos, G., Tsibidis, G. D., Muskavitch, M. A. T., & Delidakis, C. (2011). Distinct intracellular motifs of Delta mediate its ubiquitylation and activation by Mindbomb1 and Neuralized. *The Journal of Cell Biology, 195*, 1017–1031.
23. Deblandre, G. A., Lai, E. C., & Kintner, C. (2001). Xenopus neuralized is a ubiquitin ligase that interacts with XDelta1 and regulates Notch signaling. *Developmental Cell, 1*, 795–806.
24. Del Bianco, C., Aster, J. C., & Blacklow, S. C. (2008). Mutational and energetic studies of Notch 1 transcription complexes. *Journal of Molecular Biology, 376*, 131–140.
25. Düsterhöft, S., Jung, S., Hung, C.-W., Tholey, A., Sönnichsen, F. D., Grötzinger, J., & Lorenzen, I. (2013). Membrane-proximal domain of a disintegrin and metalloprotease-17 represents the putative molecular switch of its shedding activity operated by protein-disulfide isomerase. *Journal of the American Chemical Society, 135*, 5776–5781.
26. Ehebauer, M. T., Chirgadze, D. Y., Hayward, P., Martinez-Arias, A., & Blundell, T. L. (2005). High-resolution crystal structure of the human Notch 1 ankyrin domain. *The Biochemical Journal, 392*, 13–20.
27. Fedoroff, O. Y., Townson, S. A., Golovanov, A. P., Baron, M., & Avis, J. M. (2004). The structure and dynamics of tandem WW domains in a negative regulator of notch signaling, suppressor of deltex. *The Journal of Biological Chemistry, 279*, 34991–35000.
28. Fehon, R. G., Kooh, P. J., Rebay, I., Regan, C. L., Xu, T., Muskavitch, M. A., & Artavanis-Tsakonas, S. (1990). Molecular interactions between the protein products of the neurogenic loci Notch and Delta, two EGF-homologous genes in Drosophila. *Cell, 61*, 523–534.
29. Friedmann, D. R., & Kovall, R. A. (2010). Thermodynamic and structural insights into CSL-DNA complexes. *Protein Science, 19*, 34–46.
30. Friedmann, D. R., Wilson, J. J., & Kovall, R. A. (2008). RAM-induced allostery facilitates assembly of a notch pathway active transcription complex. *The Journal of Biological Chemistry, 283*, 14781–14791.
31. Fryer, C. J., Lamar, E., Turbachova, I., Kintner, C., & Jones, K. A. (2002). Mastermind mediates chromatin-specific transcription and turnover of the Notch enhancer complex. *Genes and Development, 16*, 1397–1411.
32. Ge, C., & Stanley, P. (2008). The O-fucose glycan in the ligand-binding domain of Notch1 regulates embryogenesis and T cell development. *Proceedings of the National Academy of Sciences of the United States of America, 105*, 1539–1544.
33. Glomski, K., Monette, S., Manova, K., De Strooper, B., Saftig, P., & Blobel, C. P. (2011). Deletion of Adam10 in endothelial cells leads to defects in organ-specific vascular structures. *Blood, 118*, 1163–1174.
34. Gordon, W. R., Roy, M., Vardar-Ulu, D., Garfinkel, M., Mansour, M. R., Aster, J. C., & Blacklow, S. C. (2009). Structure of the Notch1-negative regulatory region: Implications for normal activation and pathogenic signaling in T-ALL. *Blood, 113*, 4381–4390.
35. Gordon, W. R., Vardar-Ulu, D., Histen, G., Sanchez-Irizarry, C., Aster, J. C., & Blacklow, S. C. (2007). Structural basis for autoinhibition of Notch. *Nature Structural and Molecular Biology, 14*, 295–300.
36. Gordon, W. R., Vardar-Ulu, D., L'heureux, S., Ashworth, T., Malecki, M. J., Sanchez-Irizarry, C., Mcarthur, D. G., Histen, G., Mitchell, J. L., Aster, J. C., et al. (2009). Effects of S1 cleavage on the structure, surface export, and signaling activity of human Notch1 and Notch2. *PLoS One, 4*, e6613.
37. Gordon, W. R., Zimmerman, B., He, L., Miles, L. J., Huang, J., Tiyanont, K., Mcarthur, D. G., Aster, J. C., Perrimon, N., Loparo, J. J., et al. (2015). Mechanical allostery: Evidence for a force requirement in the proteolytic activation of Notch. *Developmental Cell, 33*, 729–736.

38. Greenwald, I., & Seydoux, G. (1990). Analysis of gain-of-function mutations of the lin-12 gene of Caenorhabditis elegans. *Nature, 346*, 197–199.
39. Gupta, D., Beaufils, S., Vie, V., Paboeuf, G., Broadhurst, B., Schweisguth, F., L Blundell, T., & M Bolanos-Garcia, V. (2013). Crystal structure, biochemical and biophysical characterisation of NHR1 domain of E3 Ubiquitin ligase neutralized. *Advances in Enzyme Research, 01*, 61–75.
40. Hambleton, S., Valeyev, N. V., Muranyi, A., Knott, V., Werner, J. M., McMichael, A. J., Handford, P. A., & Downing, A. K. (2004). Structural and functional properties of the human notch-1 ligand binding region. *Structure, 12*, 2173–2183.
41. He, F., Saito, K., Kobayashi, N., Harada, T., Watanabe, S., Kigawa, T., Güntert, P., Ohara, O., Tanaka, A., Unzai, S., et al. (2009). Structural and functional characterization of the NHR1 domain of the Drosophila neuralized E3 ligase in the notch signaling pathway. *Journal of Molecular Biology, 393*, 478–495.
42. Heuss, S. F., Ndiaye-Lobry, D., Six, E. M., Israël, A., & Logeat, F. (2008). The intracellular region of Notch ligands Dll1 and Dll3 regulates their trafficking and signaling activity. *Proceedings of the National Academy of Sciences of the United States of America, 105*, 11212–11217.
43. Hiruma-Shimizu, K., Hosoguchi, K., Liu, Y., Fujitani, N., Ohta, T., Hinou, H., Matsushita, T., Shimizu, H., Feizi, T., & Nishimura, S.-i. (2010). Chemical synthesis, folding, and structural insights into O-fucosylated epidermal growth factor-like repeat 12 of mouse Notch-1 receptor. *Journal of the American Chemical Society, 132*, 14857–14865.
44. Hsieh, J. J., Zhou, S., Chen, L., Young, D. B., & Hayward, S. D. (1999). CIR, a corepressor linking the DNA binding factor CBF1 to the histone deacetylase complex. *Proceedings of the National Academy of Sciences of the United States of America, 96*, 23–28.
45. Itoh, M., Kim, C.-H., Palardy, G., Oda, T., Jiang, Y.-J., Maust, D., Yeo, S.-Y., Lorick, K., Wright, G. J., Ariza-McNaughton, L., et al. (2003). Mind bomb is a ubiquitin ligase that is essential for efficient activation of Notch signaling by Delta. *Developmental Cell, 4*, 67–82.
46. Janes, P. W., Saha, N., Barton, W. A., Kolev, M. V., Wimmer-Kleikamp, S. H., Nievergall, E., Blobel, C. P., Himanen, J.-P., Lackmann, M., & Nikolov, D. B. (2005). Adam meets Eph: An ADAM substrate recognition module acts as a molecular switch for ephrin cleavage in trans. *Cell, 123*, 291–304.
47. Jennings, M. D., Blankley, R. T., Baron, M., Golovanov, A. P., & Avis, J. M. (2007). Specificity and autoregulation of Notch binding by tandem WW domains in suppressor of Deltex. *The Journal of Biological Chemistry, 282*, 29032–29042.
48. Jinek, M., Chen, Y.-W., Clausen, H., Cohen, S. M., & Conti, E. (2006). Structural insights into the Notch-modifying glycosyltransferase Fringe. *Nature Structural and Molecular Biology, 13*, 945–946.
49. Johnson, S. E., Ilagan, M. X. G., Kopan, R., & Barrick, D. (2010). Thermodynamic analysis of the CSL x Notch interaction: Distribution of binding energy of the Notch RAM region to the CSL beta-trefoil domain and the mode of competition with the viral transactivator EBNA2. *Journal of Biological Chemistry, 285*, 6681–6692.
50. Jorissen, E., Prox, J., Bernreuther, C., Weber, S., Schwanbeck, R., Serneels, L., Snellinx, A., Craessaerts, K., Thathiah, A., Tesseur, I., et al. (2010). The disintegrin/metalloproteinase ADAM10 is essential for the establishment of the brain cortex. *The Journal of Neuroscience, 30*, 4833–4844.
51. Kao, H. Y., Ordentlich, P., Koyano-Nakagawa, N., Tang, Z., Downes, M., Kintner, C. R., Evans, R. M., & Kadesch, T. (1998). A histone deacetylase corepressor complex regulates the Notch signal transduction pathway. *Genes and Development, 12*, 2269–2277.
52. Kershaw, N., Church, N., Griffin, M., Luo, C., Adams, T., & Burgess, A. (2015). Notch ligand Delta-like1: X-ray crystal structure and binding affinity. *The Biochemical Journal, 468*, 159–166.

53. Koo, B.-K., Lim, H.-S., Song, R., Yoon, M.-J., Yoon, K.-J., Moon, J.-S., Kim, Y.-W., Kwon, M.-C., Yoo, K.-W., Kong, M.-P., et al. (2005). Mind bomb 1 is essential for generating functional Notch ligands to activate Notch. *Development, 132*, 3459–3470.
54. Koo, B.-K., Yoon, M.-J., Yoon, K.-J., Im, S.-K., Kim, Y.-Y., Kim, C.-H., Suh, P.-G., Jan, Y. N., & Kong, Y.-Y. (2007). An obligatory role of mind bomb-1 in notch signaling of mammalian development. *PLoS One, 2*, e1221.
55. Kopan, R., & Ilagan, M. X. G. (2009). The canonical Notch signaling pathway: Unfolding the activation mechanism. *Cell, 137*, 216–233.
56. Kopan, R., Schroeter, E. H., Weintraub, H., & Nye, J. S. (1996). Signal transduction by activated mNotch: Importance of proteolytic processing and its regulation by the extracellular domain. *Proceedings of the National Academy of Sciences of the United States of America, 93*, 1683–1688.
57. Kovall, R. A., & Hendrickson, W. A. (2004). Crystal structure of the nuclear effector of Notch signaling, CSL, bound to DNA. *The EMBO Journal, 23*, 3441–3451.
58. Kuroda, K., Han, H., Tani, S., Tanigaki, K., Tun, T., Furukawa, T., Taniguchi, Y., Kurooka, H., Hamada, Y., Toyokuni, S., et al. (2003). Regulation of marginal zone B cell development by MINT, a suppressor of Notch/RBP-J signaling pathway. *Immunity, 18*, 301–312.
59. Kurooka, H., Kuroda, K., & Honjo, T. (1998). Roles of the ankyrin repeats and C-terminal region of the mouse notch1 intracellular region. *Nucleic Acids Research, 26*, 5448–5455.
60. Ladi, E., Nichols, J. T., Ge, W., Miyamoto, A., Yao, C., Yang, L.-T., Boulter, J., Sun, Y. E., Kintner, C., & Weinmaster, G. (2005). The divergent DSL ligand Dll3 does not activate Notch signaling but cell autonomously attenuates signaling induced by other DSL ligands. *The Journal of Cell Biology, 170*, 983–992.
61. Lafkas, D., Shelton, A., Chiu, C., de Leon Boenig, G., Chen, Y., Stawicki, S. S., Siltanen, C., Reichelt, M., Zhou, M., Wu, X., et al. (2015). Therapeutic antibodies reveal Notch control of transdifferentiation in the adult lung. *Nature, 528*, 127–131.
62. Lai, E. C., Deblandre, G. A., Kintner, C., & Rubin, G. M. (2001). Drosophila neuralized is a ubiquitin ligase that promotes the internalization and degradation of delta. *Developmental Cell, 1*, 783–794.
63. Lai, E. C., Roegiers, F., Qin, X., Jan, Y. N., & Rubin, G. M. (2005). The ubiquitin ligase Drosophila Mind bomb promotes notch signaling by regulating the localization and activity of Serrate and Delta. *Development, 132*, 2319–2332.
64. Lee, J. O., Yang, H., Georgescu, M. M., Di Cristofano, A., Maehama, T., Shi, Y., Dixon, J. E., Pandolfi, P., & Pavletich, N. P. (1999). Crystal structure of the PTEN tumor suppressor: Implications for its phosphoinositide phosphatase activity and membrane association. *Cell, 99*, 323–334.
65. Liefke, R., Oswald, F., Alvarado, C., Ferres-Marco, D., Mittler, G., Rodriguez, P., Dominguez, M., & Borggrefe, T. (2010). Histone demethylase KDM5A is an integral part of the core Notch-RBP-J repressor complex. *Genes and Development, 24*, 590–601.
66. Liu, H., Chi, A. W. S., Arnett, K. L., Chiang, M. Y., Xu, L., Shestova, O., Wang, H., Li, Y.-M., Bhandoola, A., Aster, J. C., et al. (2010). Notch dimerization is required for leukemogenesis and T-cell development. *Genes and Development, 24*, 2395–2407.
67. Liu, H., Shim, A., & He, X. (2009). Structural characterization of the ectodomain of a disintegrin and metalloproteinase-22 (ADAM22), a neural adhesion receptor instead of metalloproteinase: Insights on ADAM function. *The Journal of Biological Chemistry, 284*, 29077–29086.
68. Logeat, F., Bessia, C., Brou, C., LeBail, O., Jarriault, S., Seidah, N. G., & Israël, A. (1998). The Notch1 receptor is cleaved constitutively by a furin-like convertase. *Proceedings of the National Academy of Sciences of the United States of America, 95*, 8108–8112.
69. Lu, P., Bai, X.-C., Ma, D., Xie, T., Yan, C., Sun, L., Yang, G., Zhao, Y., Zhou, R., Scheres, S. H. W., et al. (2014). Three-dimensional structure of human γ-secretase. *Nature, 512*, 166–170.

70. Lubman, O. Y., Ilagan, M. X. G., Kopan, R., & Barrick, D. (2007). Quantitative dissection of the Notch:CSL interaction: Insights into the Notch-mediated transcriptional switch. *Journal of Molecular Biology, 365*, 577–589.
71. Lubman, O. Y., Kopan, R., Waksman, G., & Korolev, S. (2005). The crystal structure of a partial mouse Notch-1 ankyrin domain: Repeats 4 through 7 preserve an ankyrin fold. *Protein Science, 14*, 1274–1281.
72. Luca, V. C., Jude, K. M., Pierce, N. W., Nachury, M. V., Fischer, S., & Garcia, K. C. (2015). Structural biology. Structural basis for Notch1 engagement of Delta-like 4. *Science (New York NY), 347*, 847–853.
73. Maier, D. (2006). Hairless: The ignored antagonist of the Notch signalling pathway. *Hereditas, 143*, 212–221.
74. Maier, D., Kurth, P., Schulz, A., Russell, A., Yuan, Z., Gruber, K., Kovall, R. A., & Preiss, A. (2011). Structural and functional analysis of the repressor complex in the Notch signaling pathway of Drosophila melanogaster. *Molecular Biology of the Cell, 22*, 3242–3252.
75. Malecki, M. J., Sanchez-Irizarry, C., Mitchell, J. L., Histen, G., Xu, M. L., Aster, J. C., & Blacklow, S. C. (2006). Leukemia-associated mutations within the NOTCH1 heterodimerization domain fall into at least two distinct mechanistic classes. *Molecular and Cellular Biology, 26*, 4642–4651.
76. Maskos, K., Fernandez-Catalan, C., Huber, R., Bourenkov, G. P., Bartunik, H., Ellestad, G. A., Reddy, P., Wolfson, M. F., Rauch, C. T., Castner, B. J., et al. (1998). Crystal structure of the catalytic domain of human tumor necrosis factor-alpha-converting enzyme. *Proceedings of the National Academy of Sciences of the United States of America, 95*, 3408–3412.
77. McMillan, B. J., Schnute, B., Ohlenhard, N., Zimmerman, B., Miles, L., Beglova, N., Klein, T., & Blacklow, S. C. (2015). A tail of two sites: A bipartite mechanism for recognition of Notch ligands by mind bomb E3 ligases. *Molecular Cell, 57*, 912–924.
78. Mercher, T., Cornejo, M. G., Sears, C., Kindler, T., Moore, S. A., Maillard, I., Pear, W. S., Aster, J. C., & Gilliland, D. G. (2008). Notch signaling specifies megakaryocyte development from hematopoietic stem cells. *Cell Stem Cell, 3*, 314–326.
79. Mumm, J. S., Schroeter, E. H., Saxena, M. T., Griesemer, A., Tian, X., Pan, D. J., Ray, W. J., & Kopan, R. (2000). A ligand-induced extracellular cleavage regulates gamma-secretase-like proteolytic activation of Notch1. *Molecular Cell, 5*, 197–206.
80. Musse, A. A., Meloty-Kapella, L., & Weinmaster, G. (2012). Notch ligand endocytosis: Mechanistic basis of signaling activity. *Seminars in Cell and Developmental Biology., 23*, 429.
81. Nam, Y., Sliz, P., Pear, W. S., Aster, J. C., & Blacklow, S. C. (2007). Cooperative assembly of higher-order Notch complexes functions as a switch to induce transcription. *Proceedings of the National Academy of Sciences of the United States of America, 104*, 2103–2108.
82. Nam, Y., Sliz, P., Song, L., Aster, J. C., & Blacklow, S. C. (2006). Structural basis for cooperativity in recruitment of MAML coactivators to Notch transcription complexes. *Cell, 124*, 973–983.
83. Nellesen, D. T., Lai, E. C., & Posakony, J. W. (1999). Discrete enhancer elements mediate selective responsiveness of enhancer of split complex genes to common transcriptional activators. *Developmental Biology, 213*, 33–53.
84. Nichols, J. T., Miyamoto, A., Olsen, S. L., D'Souza, B., Yao, C., & Weinmaster, G. (2007). DSL ligand endocytosis physically dissociates Notch1 heterodimers before activating proteolysis can occur. *The Journal of Cell Biology, 176*, 445–458.
85. Okajima, T., & Irvine, K. D. (2002). Regulation of notch signaling by o-linked fucose. *Cell, 111*, 893–904.
86. Oswald, F., Kostezka, U., Astrahantseff, K., Bourteele, S., Dillinger, K., Zechner, U., Ludwig, L., Wilda, M., Hameister, H., Knöchel, W., et al. (2002). SHARP is a novel component of the Notch/RBP-Jkappa signalling pathway. *The EMBO Journal, 21*, 5417–5426.
87. Pan, D., & Rubin, G. M. (1997). Kuzbanian controls proteolytic processing of Notch and mediates lateral inhibition during Drosophila and vertebrate neurogenesis. *Cell, 90*, 271–280.

88. Parks, A. L., Klueg, K. M., Stout, J. R., & Muskavitch, M. A. (2000). Ligand endocytosis drives receptor dissociation and activation in the Notch pathway. *Development, 127*, 1373–1385.
89. Parks, A. L., Stout, J. R., Shepard, S. B., Klueg, K. M., Dos Santos, A. A., Parody, T. R., Vaskova, M., & Muskavitch, M. A. T. (2006). Structure-function analysis of delta trafficking, receptor binding and signaling in Drosophila. *Genetics, 174*, 1947–1961.
90. Petcherski, A. G., & Kimble, J. (2000). LAG-3 is a putative transcriptional activator in the C. Elegans Notch pathway. *Nature, 405*, 364–368.
91. Pintar, A., Guarnaccia, C., Dhir, S., & Pongor, S. (2009). Exon 6 of human JAG1 encodes a conserved structural unit. *BMC Structural Biology, 9*, 43.
92. Qin, H., Wang, J., Liang, Y., Taniguchi, Y., Tanigaki, K., & Han, H. (2004). RING1 inhibits transactivation of RBP-J by Notch through interaction with LIM protein KyoT2. *Nucleic Acids Research, 32*, 1492–1501.
93. Rampal, R., Arboleda-Velasquez, J. F., Nita-Lazar, A., Kosik, K. S., & Haltiwanger, R. S. (2005). Highly conserved O-fucose sites have distinct effects on Notch1 function. *The Journal of Biological Chemistry, 280*, 32133–32140.
94. Rebay, I., Fleming, R. J., Fehon, R. G., Cherbas, L., Cherbas, P., & Artavanis-Tsakonas, S. (1991). Specific EGF repeats of Notch mediate interactions with Delta and Serrate: Implications for Notch as a multifunctional receptor. *Cell, 67*, 687–699.
95. Sanchez-Irizarry, C., Carpenter, A. C., Weng, A. P., Pear, W. S., Aster, J. C., & Blacklow, S. C. (2004). Notch subunit heterodimerization and prevention of ligand-independent proteolytic activation depend, respectively, on a novel domain and the LNR repeats. *Molecular and Cellular Biology, 24*, 9265–9273.
96. Shah, S., Lee, S.-F., Tabuchi, K., Hao, Y.-H., Yu, C., LaPlant, Q., Ball, H., Dann, C. E., Südhof, T., & Yu, G. (2005). Nicastrin functions as a gamma-secretase-substrate receptor. *Cell, 122*, 435–447.
97. Shao, L., Moloney, D. J., & Haltiwanger, R. (2003). Fringe modifies O-fucose on mouse Notch1 at epidermal growth factor-like repeats within the ligand-binding site and the Abruptex region. *The Journal of Biological Chemistry, 278*, 7775–7782.
98. Shergill, B., Meloty-Kapella, L., Musse, A. A., Weinmaster, G., & Botvinick, E. (2012). Optical tweezers studies on Notch: Single-molecule interaction strength is independent of ligand endocytosis. *Developmental Cell, 22*, 1313–1320.
99. Shi, S., & Stanley, P. (2003). Protein O-fucosyltransferase 1 is an essential component of Notch signaling pathways. *Proceedings of the National Academy of Sciences of the United States of America, 100*, 5234–5239.
100. Shi, Y., Downes, M., Xie, W., Kao, H. Y., Ordentlich, P., Tsai, C. C., Hon, M., & Evans, R. M. (2001). Sharp, an inducible cofactor that integrates nuclear receptor repression and activation. *Genes and Development, 15*, 1140–1151.
101. Shimizu, K., Chiba, S., Kumano, K., Hosoya, N., Takahashi, T., Kanda, Y., Hamada, Y., Yazaki, Y., & Hirai, H. (1999). Mouse Jagged1 physically interacts with notch2 and other notch receptors. Assessment by quantitative methods. *The Journal of Biological Chemistry, 274*, 32961–32969.
102. Shin, O.-H., Lu, J., Rhee, J.-S., Tomchick, D. R., Pang, Z. P., Wojcik, S. M., Camacho-Perez, M., Brose, N., Machius, M., Rizo, J., et al. (2010). Munc13 C2B domain is an activity-dependent Ca2+ regulator of synaptic exocytosis. *Nature Structural and Molecular Biology, 17*, 280–288.
103. Sotillos, S., Roch, F., & Campuzano, S. (1997). The metalloprotease-disintegrin Kuzbanian participates in Notch activation during growth and patterning of Drosophila imaginal discs. *Development, 124*, 4769–4779.
104. Sun, L., Li, X., & Shi, Y. (2016). Structural biology of intramembrane proteases: Mechanistic insights from rhomboid and S2P to γ-secretase. *Current Opinion in Structural Biology, 37*, 97–107.

105. Sun, L., Zhao, L., Yang, G., Yan, C., Zhou, R., Zhou, X., Xie, T., Zhao, Y., Wu, S., Li, X., et al. (2015). Structural basis of human γ-secretase assembly. *Proceedings of the National Academy of Sciences, 112*, 6003–6008.
106. Sun, X., & Artavanis-Tsakonas, S. (1996). The intracellular deletions of Delta and Serrate define dominant negative forms of the Drosophila Notch ligands. *Development, 122*, 2465–2474.
107. Tamura, K., Taniguchi, Y., Minoguchi, S., Sakai, T., Tun, T., Furukawa, T., & Honjo, T. (1995). Physical interaction between a novel domain of the receptor Notch and the transcription factor RBP-J kappa/Su(H). *Current Biology, 5*, 1416–1423.
108. Taniguchi, Y., Furukawa, T., Tun, T., Han, H., & Honjo, T. (1998). LIM protein KyoT2 negatively regulates transcription by association with the RBP-J DNA-binding protein. *Molecular and Cellular Biology, 18*, 644–654.
109. Taylor, P., Takeuchi, H., Sheppard, D., Chillakuri, C., Lea, S. M., Haltiwanger, R. S., & Handford, P. A. (2014). Fringe-mediated extension of O-linked fucose in the ligand-binding region of Notch1 increases binding to mammalian notch ligands. *Proceedings of the National Academy of Sciences, 111*, 7290–7295.
110. Tiyanont, K., Wales, T. E., Aste-Amézaga, M., Aster, J. C., Engen, J. R., & Blacklow, S. C. (2011). Evidence for increased exposure of the Notch1 metalloprotease cleavage site upon conversion to an activated conformation. *Structure, 19*, 546–554.
111. Tiyanont, K., Wales, T. E., Siebel, C. W., Engen, J. R., & Blacklow, S. C. (2013). Insights into Notch3 activation and inhibition mediated by antibodies directed against its negative regulatory region. *Journal of Molecular Biology, 425*, 3192–3204.
112. Vardar, D., North, C. L., Sanchez-Irizarry, C., Aster, J. C., & Blacklow, S. C. (2003). Nuclear magnetic resonance structure of a prototype Lin12-Notch repeat module from human Notch1. *Biochemistry, 42*, 7061–7067.
113. Wallberg, A. E., Pedersen, K., Lendahl, U., & Roeder, R. G. (2002). p300 and PCAF act cooperatively to mediate transcriptional activation from chromatin templates by notch intracellular domains in vitro. *Molecular and Cellular Biology, 22*, 7812–7819.
114. Wang, J., Brunkan, A. L., Hecimovic, S., Walker, E., & Goate, A. (2004). Conserved "PAL" sequence in presenilins is essential for gamma-secretase activity, but not required for formation or stabilization of gamma-secretase complexes. *Neurobiology of Disease, 15*, 654–666.
115. Weber, S., Niessen, M. T., Prox, J., Lüllmann-Rauch, R., Schmitz, A., Schwanbeck, R., Blobel, C. P., Jorissen, E., De Strooper, B., Niessen, C. M., et al. (2011). The disintegrin/metalloproteinase Adam10 is essential for epidermal integrity and Notch-mediated signaling. *Development, 138*, 495–505.
116. Weisshuhn, P. C., Sheppard, D., Taylor, P., Whiteman, P., Lea, S. M., Handford, P. A., & Redfield, C. (2016). Non-linear and flexible regions of the human Notch1 extracellular domain revealed by high-resolution structural studies. *Structure, 24*, 555–566.
117. Weng, A. P., Nam, Y., Wolfe, M. S., Pear, W. S., Griffin, J. D., Blacklow, S. C., & Aster, J. C. (2003). Growth suppression of pre-T acute lymphoblastic leukemia cells by inhibition of notch signaling. *Molecular and Cellular Biology, 23*, 655–664.
118. Whiteman, P., de Madrid, B. H., Taylor, P., Li, D., Heslop, R., Viticheep, N., Tan, J. Z., Shimizu, H., Callaghan, J., Masiero, M., et al. (2013). Molecular basis for Jagged-1/Serrate ligand recognition by the Notch receptor. *Journal of Biological Chemistry, 288*, 7305–7312.
119. Wilson, J. J., & Kovall, R. A. (2006). Crystal structure of the CSL-Notch-Mastermind ternary complex bound to DNA. *Cell, 124*, 985–996.
120. Wisniewska, M., Goettig, P., Maskos, K., Belouski, E., Winters, D., Hecht, R., Black, R., & Bode, W. (2008). Structural determinants of the ADAM inhibition by TIMP-3: Crystal structure of the TACE-N-TIMP-3 complex. *Journal of Molecular Biology, 381*, 1307–1319.
121. Wu, L., Aster, J. C., Blacklow, S. C., Lake, R., Artavanis-Tsakonas, S., & Griffin, J. D. (2000). MAML1, a human homologue of Drosophila mastermind, is a transcriptional co-activator for NOTCH receptors. *Nature Genetics, 26*, 484–489.

122. Wu, L., Sun, T., Kobayashi, K., Gao, P., & Griffin, J. D. (2002). Identification of a family of mastermind-like transcriptional coactivators for mammalian notch receptors. *Molecular and Cellular Biology, 22*, 7688–7700.
123. Wu, Y., Cain-Hom, C., Choy, L., Hagenbeek, T. J., de Leon, G. P., Chen, Y., Finkle, D., Venook, R., Wu, X., Ridgway, J., et al. (2010). Therapeutic antibody targeting of individual Notch receptors. *Nature, 464*, 1052–1057.
124. Xie, T., Yan, C., Zhou, R., Zhao, Y., Sun, L., Yang, G., Lu, P., Ma, D., & Shi, Y. (2014). Crystal structure of the γ-secretase component nicastrin. *Proceedings of the National Academy of Sciences, 111*, 13349–13354.
125. Xu, A., Haines, N., Dlugosz, M., Rana, N. A., Takeuchi, H., Haltiwanger, R. S., & Irvine, K. D. (2007). In vitro reconstitution of the modulation of Drosophila Notch-ligand binding by Fringe. *The Journal of Biological Chemistry, 282*, 35153–35162.
126. Xu, A., Lei, L., & Irvine, K. D. (2005). Regions of Drosophila Notch that contribute to ligand binding and the modulatory influence of Fringe. *The Journal of Biological Chemistry, 280*, 30158–30165.
127. Xu, X., Choi, S. H., Hu, T., Tiyanont, K., Habets, R., Groot, A. J., Vooijs, M., Aster, J. C., Chopra, R., Fryer, C., et al. (2015). Insights into autoregulation of Notch3 from structural and functional studies of its negative regulatory region. *Structure, 23*, 1227–1235.
128. Yu, H., Takeuchi, M., LeBarron, J., Kantharia, J., London, E., Bakker, H., Haltiwanger, R. S., Li, H., & Takeuchi, H. (2015). Notch-modifying xylosyltransferase structures support an SNi-like retaining mechanism. *Nature Chemical Biology, 11*, 847–854.
129. Yuan, Z., Praxenthaler, H., Tabaja, N., Torella, R., Preiss, A., Maier, D., & Kovall, R. (2016). Structure-function of the Su(H)-Hairless repressor complex, the major antagonist of Notch signaling in D. melanogaster. *PLoS Biology, 14*, e1002509.
130. Zhang, X., Sullivan, E., Scimeca, M., Wu, X., Li, Y.-M., & Sisodia, S. S. (2016). Evidence that the "Lid" domain of nicastrin is not essential for regulating γ-secretase activity. *Journal of Biological Chemistry, 291*, 6748–6753.
131. Zhang, Y., Sandy, A. R., Wang, J., Radojcic, V., Shan, G. T., Tran, I. T., Friedman, A., Kato, K., He, S., Cui, S., et al. (2011). Notch signaling is a critical regulator of allogeneic CD4+ T-cell responses mediating graft-versus-host disease. *Blood, 117*, 299–308.
132. Zhou, S., Fujimuro, M., Hsieh, J. J., Chen, L., Miyamoto, A., Weinmaster, G., & Hayward, S. D. (2000). SKIP, a CBF1-associated protein, interacts with the ankyrin repeat domain of NotchIC to facilitate NotchIC function. *Molecular and Cellular Biology, 20*, 2400–2410.
133. Zweifel, M. E., Leahy, D. J., & Barrick, D. (2005). Structure and Notch receptor binding of the tandem WWE domain of Deltex. *Structure, 13*, 1599–1611.
134. Zweifel, M. E., Leahy, D. J., Hughson, F. M., & Barrick, D. (2003). Structure and stability of the ankyrin domain of the Drosophila Notch receptor. *Protein Science, 12*, 2622–2632.

Chapter 2
Noncanonical Notch Signaling

Jyothi Vijayaraghavan and Barbara A. Osborne

Abstract Discovered nearly a century ago, today, Notch is known to mediate several biological processes through the canonical pathway that involves ligands, RBPJ, proteases, and coactivators. However, recent studies in vertebrates and invertebrates reveal that Notch can also exert its effect independent of RBPJ, in a noncanonical fashion. These studies demonstrate that Notch can exert its noncanonical role not only through nuclear partners but also via nonnuclear or cytosolic interactions. Additionally, there now is increasing evidence that Notch signaling can be initiated in a "noncanonical" fashion, independent of ligands. In this review, we detail the different cytosolic and nuclear, noncanonical interactions of Notch and discuss how they affect signaling processes in various contexts. We also discuss the evidence for ligand-independent, noncanonical initiation of Notch signaling.

Keywords Notch signaling · Noncanonical · RBPJ-independent signaling · Noncanonical Notch · Deltex · Akt · Abl · Cell survival · β-catenin · NF-κB

2.1 Introduction

The Notch signaling pathway is ancient and conserved throughout evolution. As detailed in previous chapters, Notch signaling was first described in *Drosophila* in 1916 as a mutation that gave rise to aberrant or "notched" wings in flies [55]. With the advent of molecular biology, the genetics of Notch signaling in *Drosophila* was uncovered at the molecular level revealing a single gene encoding one Notch receptor and two genes encoding the ligands, Delta and Serrate [6]. One of the first reports of a mammalian homologue of Notch is the elegant description of an oncogenic form of Notch by Sklar and colleagues in human T lymphoblastic leukemia (T-ALL) [24]. This landmark study provides the first observation of Notch

J. Vijayaraghavan · B. A. Osborne (✉)
Department of Veterinary & Animal Sciences & Program in Molecular and Cellular Biology, University of Massachusetts, Amherst, MA, USA
e-mail: osborne@vasci.umass.edu

L. Miele, S. Artavanis-Tsakonas (eds.), *Targeting Notch in Cancer*,
https://doi.org/10.1007/978-1-4939-8859-4_2

expression in the immune system and importantly demonstrates that Notch expression can be oncogenic. Over the ensuing 25 years, it has become apparent that the Notch family of proteins are critical regulators of development in numerous vertebrate cell lineages, and, in many instances, deregulated Notch expression can be oncogenic [41].

The canonical Notch signaling pathway, observed in a wide variety of organisms, involves activation of Notch, initiated by ligand binding, followed by proteolysis through an ADAM protease and subsequent cleavage by gamma secretase. This two-step proteolysis leads to release of the intracellular domain of Notch (NICD) which rapidly translocates to the nucleus where NICD binds the DNA-binding protein, CSL/RBPJ, displacing corepressors and recruiting coactivators such as p300 and Mastermind, leading to the initiation of CSL-regulated transcription [11]. This canonical Notch signaling pathway is known to regulate many functions ascribed to Notch, and, in these instances, deletion of CSL/RBPJ usually phenocopies deletion of Notch. However, in recent years, it has become obvious that canonical Notch signaling does not account for all Notch function. We now recognize that noncanonical Notch signaling plays an important role in many Notch-driven processes. Indeed, recent evidence from *Nematostella*, the cnidarian sea anemone, suggests that the canonical Notch signaling pathway emerged after the divergence of the cnidarian-bilaterian lineages [45]. These data imply that noncanonical Notch signaling may be the ancestral signaling pathway and canonical Notch signaling evolved specifically in the bilaterian lineage.

The term noncanonical Notch signaling was originally coined to describe signaling events that are Notch dependent but do not rely on CSL/RBPJ. It was first observed in *Drosophila* using a genetic approach that examined the precise requirement of various components of the Notch signaling pathway. More recently, as our understanding of noncanonical Notch signaling has been refined, it is apparent that, at least in some instances, noncanonical Notch signaling may occur in the cytosol. We refer to this as noncanonical, cytosolic Notch signaling. Noncanonical Notch signaling can also occur in the nucleus, and we refer to this as noncanonical, nuclear Notch signaling. In the following sections, we will highlight several examples of noncanonical Notch signaling that have been observed in organisms as diverse as flies, mice, and humans and discuss the therapeutic implications of noncanonical Notch signaling.

2.2 Noncanonical, Cytosolic Notch Signaling

The notion that Notch plays a role in the cytosol is strengthened by the early observation that endogenous Notch is rarely observed in the nucleus and is mostly detected in the cytoplasm and/or cell membrane [7]. This implies that Notch may interact with various molecular partners in nonnuclear environments, affecting their function posttranslationally. Studies as early as in the 1990s have described cytoplasmic interactions of Notch that are different from the usual, previously explored, nuclear roles of Notch. However, lack of follow-up studies exploring these interactions and their biological implications prevents us from strongly categorizing these molecular factors as noncanonical partners of Notch. In this section, we illustrate the abovementioned cytosolic interactions of Notch in addition to several other studies that provide solid evidence for the nonnuclear, noncanonical pathway of Notch signaling.

2.2.1 Notch and Deltex

In the early 1990s, in an attempt to identify interacting partners of Notch, Artavanis-Tsakonas and colleagues uncovered a small number of genes called the "Notch group" [5, 91]. This group comprised the following genes – *Delta*, *Serrate*, *Enhancer of split*, *Mastermind*, *Strawberry*, *Notch*, and *Deltex* [20]. Following this, pioneering work by the Artavanis-Tsakonas lab in 1994 revealed a cytosolic interaction between Deltex and the ankyrin repeats of Notch, a first of its kind interaction for Notch [20]. The ankyrin repeats form part of the intracellular domain of the Notch receptor and constitute the most conserved region between Notch and its vertebrate counterparts [81]. These repeats have been reported to be vital for Notch-mediated signaling events by several groups [68, 69]. Deltex is a cytoplasmic protein of unknown biochemical function that is ubiquitously expressed throughout development [12]. Using three techniques – in vivo co-localization, *Drosophila* cultured cell expression assay, and yeast interaction trap assay – Diederich et al. identified Deltex as the first cytoplasmic protein known to interact with Notch ankyrin repeats, implicating Deltex in the Notch signaling pathway. Further in 1995, the same group elucidated the role of Deltex in Notch signaling using *Drosophila* as their system [52]. In this study, they described a model for the action of Deltex, wherein the Deltex-Notch interaction antagonizes the interaction between Su(H) and Notch, thus preventing the cytoplasmic retention of Su(H). [Note: Su(H) is *Drosophila* CSL.] Therefore, Artavanis-Tsakonas and colleagues were the first to uncover a cytoplasmic interaction of Notch, providing the first clue of an alternate, nonnuclear role of Notch.

Shedding more light on the Deltex-Notch interaction, a study in 1998 described E47, a protein that is essential for B lymphocyte development, as a novel target of Notch [60]. Ordentlich et al. provide convincing evidence of inhibition of full-length E47 by cytoplasmic Notch1 and Notch2. Additionally, they showed that this inhibition did not correlate with the ability of Notch to activate RBPJ/CBF1. Furthermore, E47 was also inhibited by the cytoplasmic, Notch-interacting protein, Deltex, independent of CBF1/RBPJ. Therefore, in addition to identifying E47 as a novel target of Notch, this study also showed that the pathway that connects Notch and E47 is independent of RBPJ and also involves Deltex. These data not only add to the Deltex-Notch story but also present the first indication of a cytosolic and noncanonical mode of Notch signaling.

2.2.2 An Early Description of RBPJ-Independent Notch Signaling

In the canonical pathway, Notch controls cell fate by activating expression of the transcriptional regulator RBPJ which upregulates the expression of the Hes-1 gene, a well-characterized Notch target gene [35]. One of the earliest studies providing compelling evidence of an RBPJ-independent role of Notch came almost two decades ago from Shawber and colleagues [75]. They demonstrated that constitutively active forms of Notch inhibit muscle differentiation in mouse myoblasts but do not interact with RBPJ (referred to as CBF1 in this paper) or upregulate Hes1 gene expression. The authors generated truncated, cytoplasmic forms of Notch1 that lack the Notch/RBPJ interaction sequences, and showed that, although these cytoplasmic forms cannot interact with RBPJ or upregulate Hes1, they can, nonetheless, prevent muscle cell differentiation when stably expressed in mouse myoblasts. While the mechanism by which this form of Notch prevents muscle cell differentiation was not explored in this study, it is suggestive of cytoplasmic molecular partners of Notch that propagate its signal independent of RBPJ. In addition to being one of the first reports of an RBPJ-independent role of Notch in mammals, this study also provided further proof of cytosolic functions of Notch even though these cytosolic functions were not explored in this study.

2.2.3 Notch and Abl

Another study describing a cytosolic, noncanonical function of Notch was conducted by Giniger in 1998 [30]. He showed that modest reduction in Notch levels, in the context of an Abl mutation, results in synthetic lethality and defects in *Drosophila* axon extension. Abl is a cytosolic, tyrosine kinase that is widely expressed and is involved in the development of various tissues [32, 79, 82]. It is one of the first cellular genes implicated in a common human cancer [23, 26]. More recently, a pivotal role has been established for Abl in axon patterning, particularly in *Drosophila*, where it contributes to the growth and guidance of many developing axons [29, 89]. Giniger found that Notch is present in extending axons and in growth cones of *Drosophila* and that the Abl accessory protein, Disabled, binds directly to NICD in vitro, providing the first link between the Notch and Abl pathways. These results led to speculations that Abl and its associated accessory factors might be involved in an alternate, noncanonical, Su(H)-independent signaling pathway of Notch in *Drosophila*.

Several years later in 2003, Giniger and colleagues provided additional evidence for the Notch-Abl interaction while examining the path taken by the intersegmental nerve b (ISNb) axons to approach its muscle targets [17]. The ISNb axons, which innervate body wall muscles, exit the central nervous system and reach a turning point to innervate specific target muscles in *Drosophila* [44, 84]. Crowner et al.

showed that the turning of the ISNb axons requires interaction of Notch with components of the Abl pathway and its accessory proteins. However, genetic interaction experiments failed to provide evidence for a role of the canonical, Su(H)-dependent pathway in this process. Further in 2008, Giniger and colleagues reevaluated axon guidance in *Drosophila* and provided genetic and biochemical evidence for a Su(H)-dependent Notch pathway for cell fate specification, whereas axon guidance required cytosolic interaction of Notch with Abl [27]. In this way, the Giniger group presents convincing evidence for both the canonical, Su(H)-dependent Notch pathway and the noncanonical, nonnuclear Notch pathway in the *Drosophila* nervous system.

2.2.4 Notch in Apoptosis and Cell Survival

Notch has been linked with apoptosis/cell survival for several years [18, 36, 58, 67]. Studies in the recent past attribute this anti-apoptotic role of Notch to the noncanonical, membrane-tethered or cytoplasm-localized form of Notch. Insightful studies from the Sarin laboratory have revealed the mechanisms by which Notch regulates apoptosis. In an attempt to determine if Notch mediates apoptosis in model T cell lines, Sade et al. found that ectopic expression of the intracellular domain of Notch1 confers protection against diverse apoptotic stimuli [72]. This anti-apoptotic activity results from NICD-induced increased expression of Bcl-x_L, FLIP, and IAP-2, components of three major families of anti-apoptotic proteins. Using pharmacological inhibitors and dominant-negative experiments, they showed that NICD-mediated anti-apoptotic function requires phosphatidylinositol 3-kinase (PI3K)-dependent activation of the serine/threonine kinase Akt/PKB, through the tyrosine kinase, $p56^{lck}$. They further demonstrated that endogenous Notch1 associates with PI3K and $p56^{lck}$, both of which are membrane-localized signaling complexes, lending further support to a noncanonical, cytosolic function of Notch.

In 2009, the Sarin laboratory identified a novel Notch-mediated signaling pathway that favors cell survival [64]. Here, Notch inhibits apoptosis triggered by neglect or nutrient withdrawal in mammalian cells by integrating its signal with the mTOR-Rictor signaling complex, ultimately resulting in activation of the kinase Akt/PKB. Their data reveal that, although Notch processing is required for the activation of the cascade, NICD activity did not require CSL-mediated transcription, suggesting a role for the noncanonical Notch signaling pathway. Moreover, spatial constraint experiments showed that enforced nuclear retention of NICD abrogates the anti-apoptotic activity, whereas the membrane-tethered form of NICD blocks apoptosis through mTOR-Rictor and Akt-dependent signaling. This suggests that cytoplasmic localization of NICD is required for its anti-apoptotic function. Further in 2010, Perumalsamy et al. investigated the mechanisms underlying the anti-apoptotic activity of Notch with regard to intersections with mitochondrial events [63]. They showed that Notch activity inhibits apoptosis induced by Bax, a proapoptotic protein from the Bcl2 family of proteins that determines mitochondrial involvement in apoptotic cascades. This activity of Notch required ligand-dependent processing to generate NICD but was independent of the canonical, nuclear interactions of Notch. Indeed, similar to results from previous studies from the Sarin laboratory, this anti-apoptotic activity was compromised by forced nuclear retention of NICD and recapitulated by NICD recombinants localized outside the nucleus. Experiments using siRNA and dominant-negative constructs revealed that the kinase Akt is an intermediate in the Notch-mediated anti-apoptotic pathway and that this process requires Mitofusin 1 and Mitofusin 2 (Mfn 1 and Mfn 2). Mitofusins are mitochondrial remodeling proteins that coordinately regulate mitochondrial fusion [13]. Therefore, Sarin and colleagues have identified a nonnuclear, Notch-Akt-Mfn-mediated anti-apoptotic signaling pathway, thus laying the foundation for further analysis of a noncanonical Notch pathway that regulates cell survival.

Further in 2012, Sarin and colleagues went on to identify the cellular and molecular patterns of Notch activity that govern survival outcomes of mature T cells following their activation [65]. They describe a ligand-dependent, noncanonical Notch activation pathway coupled with a spatial pattern of Notch that protects T_{regs} from apoptosis caused by cytokine withdrawal. The survival of T_{regs} was mediated by the interaction of Notch signaling with PI3K signaling and mammalian target of rapamycin complex 2 (mTORC2), wherein biochemical studies revealed a membrane-proximal complex of NICD and the mTORC2 component, Rictor. Interestingly, they found that induced Tregs (iT_{regs}) and effector T cells, where nuclear NICD is predominant, were susceptible to cytokine withdrawal-induced apoptosis. Reconstitution with the nuclear excluded forms of Notch1 protected iT_{regs} and $Notch^{-/-}$ T_{regs} from apoptosis, whereas the nuclear-localized forms failed to do so, again showing that NICD activity outside the nucleus accounts for its anti-apoptotic activity.

Liu et al. revealed another mechanism that contributes to the survival effect of Notch [49]. The X-linked inhibitor of apoptosis protein (XIAP), one of the best characterized members of caspase inhibitors, is often overexpressed in malignant cells and elevated XIAP levels increasing resistance to apoptosis [19, 74]. Liu and colleagues have shown that NICD inhibits the degradation of XIAP during apoptosis by binding directly to XIAP, thereby blocking the binding of E2 ubiquitin-conjugating enzymes and preventing the in vitro and in vivo ubiquitination of XIAP. The authors also examined whether the interaction of Notch with the cytosolic protein XIAP is possible and found that NICD is able to bind XIAP in the cytoplasm, describing another cytosolic, noncanonical interaction of Notch.

2.2.5 Notch and Akt

A number of vital biological processes such as DNA synthesis, gene expression, neurotransmission, and hormonal storage and release are regulated by discrete subcellular pools of zinc [16, 34, 48]. Previous studies have demonstrated that zinc activates both PI3K and Akt [25, 40], thereby indirectly implicating a role for zinc in Notch signaling. Based on these observations, a group in Korea investigated the crosstalk between zinc and Notch1 signaling [9]. Here, they showed that zinc acts as a negative regulator of Notch signaling by causing the cytoplasmic retention of not only NICD but also RBPJ, and this prevents their interaction both in vitro and in vivo. Their data further reveal that this cytoplasmic retention of NICD is a consequence of the activation of the PI3K-Akt signaling pathway. However, the mechanism of the zinc-mediated suppression of Notch signaling via PI3K-Akt and the biological implications of this downregulation are not understood. Nevertheless, the cytoplasmic retention of Notch and inhibition of Notch/RBPJ binding due to zinc give rise to speculation that this may be yet another instance of nonnuclear, RBPJ-independent signaling through Notch.

Another study in 2008 describing the cytoplasmic localization of Notch was conducted by the Shin group [80]. They explored the effect of Akt on NICD-mediated transcription in 293 T and Cos7 cells. Using luciferase reporter constructs, they demonstrated that constitutively active Akt downregulates NICD-dependent transcription. The CSL family protein, RBPJ/CBF1, recruits a corepressor complex involving SMRT and HDAC1 to exert its inhibitory effect on transcription after binding to DNA. Therefore, the authors further determined if this inhibition of Notch-dependent transcription by Akt is due to the effect of corepressors or HDAC activity and found that this downregulation is independent of both factors. In fact, the Akt-induced inhibition of Notch-mediated transcription was because Akt inhibited proper nuclear localization of NICD. Co-expression of the Akt isoforms resulted in cytoplasmic mislocalization of NICD. This, in turn, can lead to reduced expression of canonical Notch targets as less NICD is available in the nucleus to bind RBPJ allowing for more cytoplasmic, potential noncanonical interactions of Notch.

A hallmark of all stem cells is the maintenance of a delicate balance between differentiation and self-renewal, impairments which can lead to tumorigenesis or lineage depletion [21, 56]. In mammalian neural stem cells (NSCs) and *Drosophila* neuroblasts, the self-renewal versus differentiation decision requires Notch signaling [4, 86]; however, the mechanism by which Notch regulates these processes is not well defined. Shedding light on this aspect, a 2013 study described a new mechanism where canonical Notch signaling cooperates with a noncanonical Notch pathway to mediate Notch-directed NSC regulation [46]. In the noncanonical pathway, Notch activates the mTORC2/Akt pathway by interacting with PTEN-induced kinase 1 (PINK1) to influence mitochondrial function and enhance *Drosophila* neuroblast growth and proliferation. PINK1 is a mitochondrial serine/threonine kinase that is critical in regulating mTORC2 activity and influences mitochondrial function and dynamics [90]. Experiments exploring the mechanism by which Notch and PINK1 interact to influence mitochondrial function showed enrichment of full-length Notch at the mitochondria and the presence of increased mitochondrial Notch on PINK1 overexpression. These results demonstrate that Notch can exert effects directly at the mitochondrial membrane. Further, through co-immunoprecipitation studies, the authors showed that PINK1 and Notch physically associate in the mitochondria of human NSCs and in glioblastoma multiforme cells. These results identify a novel noncanonical role for Notch, where it regulates mTORC2/Akt activity by directly interacting with a mitochondrial kinase PINK1, thereby influencing mitochondrial function.

2.2.6 Notch and β-Catenin

In 2009, the Srivastava lab showed that Notch1 antagonizes the Wnt/β-catenin signaling pathway, which promotes the expansion of cardiac progenitor cells by reducing the levels of active β-catenin in these cells [42]. More recently, they expanded these studies to determine the mechanism by which Notch negatively regulates β-catenin and explore this interaction in other stem cell types [43]. Their data in embryonic stem cells provide evidence for the negative regulation of active β-catenin by Notch and reveal that this regulation is independent of RBPJ-mediated transcription. To further determine if this regulation involves a physical interaction between Notch and β-catenin, the authors performed co-immunoprecipitation studies and found that Notch does, indeed, physically associate with active β-catenin and that this is the membrane-tethered form of Notch. This study, therefore, highlights a different role for Notch than the known, nuclear, canonical role, where a membrane-bound form of Notch physically associates with active β-catenin and negatively regulates it through the adaptor protein, Numb.

Lending further credence to the Notch-β-catenin interaction, Acosta et al. showed that Notch interacts with β-catenin in a nonnuclear fashion in *Xenopus* blastula cells and regulates early *Xenopus* development in a CSL-independent manner [1]. Wnt signaling has been shown to be important during early development in vertebrates; however, the role of Notch at these stages is still not well understood. Therefore, the authors set out to determine if Wnt signaling and Notch interact during early stages of *Xenopus* development. Overexpression of NICD alone resulted in accumulation of Notch in both the cytoplasm and nuclei of *Xenopus* blastula cells. However, upon co-expressing NICD with β-catenin, NICD was located on cell-cell junctions and not in the nuclei, whereas β-catenin was degraded. This suggests that Notch interacts with β-catenin in a nonnuclear fashion and regulates its degradation, perhaps through endosomal trafficking. Therefore, this study contributes to another nonnuclear, CSL-independent mode of Notch signaling.

2.3 Noncanonical, Nuclear Notch Signaling

In addition to the numerous accounts of noncanonical, cytosolic Notch signaling highlighted above, there are a few examples of noncanonical, nuclear Notch signaling. A recent paper from Chiang and colleagues questions the conventional canonical Notch signaling pathway in the nucleus where a lone NICD/Mastermind/RBPJ complex regulates all Notch-responsive genes [66]. In this report, the authors demonstrate a direct physical interaction between Notch1 and Zmiz1, a member of the *p*rotein *i*nhibitor of *a*ctivated *S*TAT (PIAS) family of coactivators. The authors show that Zmiz1 and Notch interaction is important for both T cell development and leukemogenesis, but this interaction plays no role in other Notch-mediated events such as myeloid suppression or intestinal homeostasis. The data in this report suggest a previously unrecognized intricacy in the proteins that comprise the Notch/RBPJ complex. Whereas some genes are clearly regulated by canonical Notch/RBPJ complexes, others require coactivator Zmiz1. Although not directly addressed in this report, it is interesting to speculate that Zmiz1/Notch1 may regulate a unique subset of genes in the absence of RBPJ.

Additionally, a recent report from Kastner and Chan and colleagues examines the role of Ikaros in shaping the repertoire of Notch target genes in T cells [28]. In this study, DNA-binding complexes of NICD/Ikaros were identified in the absence of RBPJ. These complexes are likely repressive since the genes associated with these complexes were only expressed when cells are treated with a gamma-secretase inhibitor. Thus, another form of noncanonical Notch signaling may be a physical interaction of NICD with Ikaros that acts to repress associated genes.

2.4 Notch and NF-κB: A Player in Both Cytosolic and Nuclear Noncanonical Notch Signaling

Many investigations point to connections between NF-κB and Notch signaling pathways [61]. In some situations, NF-κB signaling can initiate Notch signaling either by direct or indirect interaction between the two pathways suggesting that NF-κB acts upstream of Notch [14]. As early as 1996, Guan and coworkers demonstrated a physical interaction between Notch1 and the p50 subunit of the NF-κB complex suggesting another level of interaction between these two pathways [88]. Following up on this observation, our group and others have observed physical interactions between Notch1 and several cytosolic proteins involved in NF-κB signaling [61, 77], and these are discussed below.

2.4.1 Notch/NF-κB Interactions in the Cytosol

A recent study investigating the effects of hyperactivated Notch signaling in breast cancer identified IL-6 as a novel target of Notch in basal breast tumor cells, where Notch upregulates IL-6 expression [37]. This Notch-induced increase in IL-6 levels further activates the JAK-STAT signaling pathway in both an autocrine and paracrine fashion and is controlled by the cellular p53 status and two proteins from the NF-κB signaling pathway – IKKα and IKKβ. Transfection of a NICD construct that lacks the CSL-binding RAM domain upregulated IL-6 expression but not the expression of the canonical target gene Hes1, suggesting a noncanonical mode of Notch action.

Furthermore, transfection of a NICD-ER fusion protein that is retained in the cytoplasm in the absence of tamoxifen upregulated IL-6 expression irrespective of the presence of tamoxifen, whereas the canonical target gene Nrarp was upregulated only in the presence of tamoxifen. This indicated that cytoplasmic localization of NICD is sufficient to upregulate IL-6, while nuclear translocation is necessary for the activation of the canonical target gene, Nrarp.

Early studies from our lab and others demonstrated that signaling through the T cell receptor (TCR) results in rapid activation of Notch1 signaling [2, 62], and these reports provided the first link of TCR signaling to Notch activation. Our data also linked TCR activation of Notch1 to triggering NF-κB activity, suggesting that Notch1 activation may drive NF-κB activity [62]. Following on this observation, we asked whether Notch1 physically interacts with NF-κB family members in lymphocytes and determined that Notch1 is found in a complex with either p50 or c-rel, two NF-κB family members, and is responsible for shuttling p50 and c-rel into the nucleus [78]. Using biochemical approaches, as well as confocal microscopy, we showed that NICD directly interacts with NF-κB and competes with IκBα, leading to retention of NF-κB in the nucleus. These data show that Notch1 plays a key role in the cytosol in escorting NF-κB into the nucleus and, in the nucleus, in promoting retention of the NF-κB complex, suggesting that Notch1/NF-κB interactions may occur in both the cytosol and the nucleus [78].

TCR-mediated signaling also induces the formation of the CBM complex (comprising CARMA1, BCL10, and MALT1) that is essential for TCR-induced NF-κB activation [70, 71, 87]. Signaling through TCR activates Notch proteins, which have also been implicated in NF-κB activation [78]. However, the molecular interactions that link Notch signaling through TCR to early events in NF-κB activation remain largely unknown. In collaboration with our colleagues, we revealed a novel cytosolic function of Notch1 where it acts as a scaffold protein and influences the formation of the CBM complex [77]. Via two distinct approaches, lipid rafts and a novel approach called biomolecular fluorescence complementation (BiFC), we demonstrated that cytosolic Notch1 physically interacts with the components of the CBM complex following stimulation through the TCR. Additionally, experiments using a luciferase reporter assay and Notch1 constructs with localization restricted to the cytoplasm or to the plasma membrane showed that nonnuclear Notch1 can enhance NF-κB transcriptional activity in stimulated T cells. Thus, this study presents a novel model where Notch1 has the ability to function in the cytoplasm to facilitate early events during T cell activation, by physically interacting with the CBM complex and initiating NF-κB signaling.

2.4.2 Notch/NF-κB Interactions in the Nucleus

A close examination of NF-κB- and CSL-consensus binding sites reveals an interesting observation. The DNA sequence recognized by CSL/RBPJ and NF-κB is quite similar and potentially overlapping. While not all CSL-binding motifs are subsets of a larger NF-κB response element, NF-κB consensus sites incorporate a nested CSL-binding site [47, 51, 85]. This observation suggests that CSL/RBPJ and NF-κB may compete for the same DNA-binding site [31].

As described above, we and others have demonstrated that TCR signaling results in rapid activation of Notch1 and blockade of Notch using various strategies, including inhibition of γ-secretase (GSI) as well as deletion of Notch1 [2, 62], result in diminished T cell activation and proliferation and reduced cytokine secretion [50, 54, 59]. To better understand how Notch1 regulates expression of various cytokine genes, we conducted ChIP analysis of promoters from a variety of cytokine genes expressed in CD4 T cells. In such studies, we identified complexes of Notch and NF-κB1 (p50), as well as Notch and c-Rel bound to DNA in the promoter region of the *IFNγ* gene [78] indicating that there may be other nuclear partners, in addition to CSL, that cooperate with Notch to regulate target genes. We followed up these observations with an examination of the promoters of several other T cell-specific genes including IL-2, granzyme B, perforin, and cyclin D3 and the transcription factors T-bet and EOMES [15, 38, 54, 78]. In all cases, we found that Notch-1 could be found in a complex with either p50 or c-rel suggesting that Notch/NF-κB complexes may regulate transcription independent of CSL/RBPJ. In some instances (EOMES, granzyme B, and perforin), we reported evidence suggesting that these complexes may form independent of CSL [38, 54, 78].

The observation that several T cell-specific genes may be regulated by Notch/NF-κB complexes led us to question whether CSL/RBPJ is required for Notch-dependent T cell function. When T cells are activated by engagement of antigen with the T cell receptor, cell division and rapid proliferation are induced. This phase of proliferation is accompanied by the production and subsequent secretion of T cell-specific cytokines such as IL-2 and interferon-γ. Additionally, if provided with appropriate signals, $CD4^+$ T cells can differentiate into one of several different effector cell subsets including T helper-1 (Th1), T helper-2 (Th2), T helper-17 (Th17), or T regulatory (Treg) cells. Notch signaling has been implicated in the activation and proliferation of T cells as well as in the production of cytokines and the differentiation of naïve T cells into various effector cell subsets [3, 8, 39, 59, 73]. We asked whether canonical Notch signaling was required for these functions [22]. In these experiments, $CD4^+$ T cells were isolated from either wild-type animals or animals in which $Notch1^{-/-}$ or $RBPJ^{-/-}$ was conditionally deleted in peripheral T cells and activated in vitro through cross-linking the T cell receptor. Surprisingly, we observed that while conditional deletion of Notch1 abrogated the ability of $CD4^+$ T cells to proliferate in response to TCR stimulation, T cells from conditional deletion of RBPJ proliferated as well and perhaps even better than wild-type T cells indicating T cell activation was not dependent upon RBPJ. We then asked if the ability to produce IL-2 and interferon-γ was dependent upon RBPJ, and again, we found that $CD4^+$ T cells from T cells lacking RBPJ expression produced as much or more IL-2 and interferon-γ than wild-type T cells. Lastly, we asked whether naïve $CD4^+$ T cells could differentiate into Th1 effector cells in the absence of RBPJ expression. Once again, we observed that $CD4^+$T cells lacking RBPJ readily differentiated into Th1 effectors. Taken together these data indicate that activation, proliferation, and differentiation of CD4+ T cells can occur in the absence of RBPJ expression and imply that these functions occur through a noncanonical Notch signaling pathway.

Based on our prior observation that localized Notch-1/NF-κB complexes on both the IL-2 and interferon-γ promoters, we asked whether Notch signaling regulates $CD4^+$ T cell activation, proliferation, and differentiation in concert with NF-κB. We used $CD4^+$ T cells from wild type mice or animals with conditional deletion of either Notch-1 or RBPJ and treated these cells with DHMEQ, an NF-κB inhibitor [83]. The results from these experiments showed that, as expected, Notch1-deleted $CD4^+$ T cells did not proliferate or produce IL-2 or interferon-γ when treated with either DMSO control or DHMEQ. However, in contrast, RBPJ-deficient $CD4^+$ T cells both proliferated and produced cytokines when treated with DMSO, but the ability to proliferate and secrete IL-2 and interferon-γ was greatly reduced by treatment with DHMEQ. These data suggest that noncanonical Notch1 signaling in $CD4^+$ T cells occurs, at least in part, through NF-κB. Whether this interaction takes place in the nucleus or cytosol remains to be determined.

2.5 Other Forms of Noncanonical Notch Signaling

Just as we recognize that Notch signaling can occur in the absence of RBPJ, it is also becoming clear that Notch signaling may be initiated in the absence of ligand binding. While this is not necessarily noncanonical as defined above, these reports indicate that Notch signaling can also be initiated in a "noncanonical" fashion. Mukherjee and colleagues found that in *Drosophila* crystal cells, a myeloid-like cell that circulates in the hemolymph, HIF-α (the *Drosophila* homologue of HIF-1α) stabilizes Notch in the endosome and enables cleavage of Notch by γ-secretase, thus releasing the active form of Notch into the cytosol [57]. Interestingly, this activation of Notch is totally independent of interaction with Notch ligands (Fig. 2.1a).

Another example of ligand-independent interaction of Notch in *Drosophila* comes from the report by Hori et al. [33] where Notch interaction in the endosomal compartment with the ESCRT protein Shrub diverts Notch from lysosomal degradation into a signaling pathway and initiates ligand-independent Notch signaling. This process is context dependent and only occurs in selected cell types during *Drosophila* development. It remains to be determined whether the ESCRT pathway or the HIF-α-dependent pathway of ligand-independent activation of Notch signaling occurs in vertebrates. However, it is tempting to speculate that because activation through the T cell receptor leads to rapid activation of HIF-1α in $CD4^+$T cells, HIF-1α may play a role in ligand-independent Notch activation in mammalian T cells as well [53].

Lastly, another example of "noncanonical" Notch signaling comes from the recent reports that Notch ligands have been found in exosomes. In particular, Sheldon et al. demonstrated that endothelial cells produce exosomes containing the Delta ligand Dll4 [76]. Exosomes are small extracellular membrane vesicles that

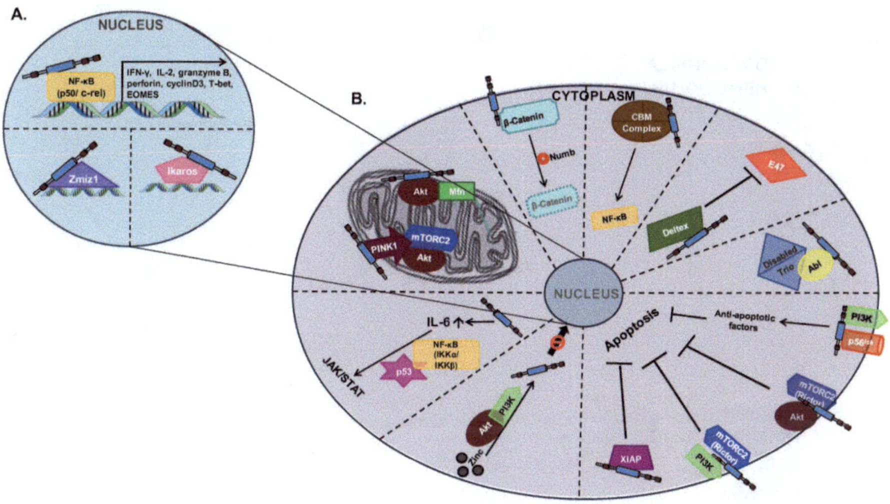

Fig. 2.1 (**a**) Noncanonical, nuclear Notch signaling. (**b**) Noncanonical, cytosolic Notch signaling

originate from endosomes. These vesicles are released from a wide variety of cell types and are postulated to influence cell signaling by interactions with cells either in the near vicinity or at more distant sites. Interestingly, DLL ligands are thought to require endocytosis to become functional [10]; therefore the incorporation of these ligands into exosomes is not surprising. One can readily see how exosomes containing Notch ligands might influence Notch signaling in a cell contact-independent fashion. In the report by Sheldon et al. [76], Dll4-containing exosomes produced by endothelial cells were shown to interact with Notch expressed in cells at a distant site. Surprisingly, rather than activating the Notch signaling pathway, these Dll4 exosomes instead inhibit Notch signaling and cause a developmental switch in the recipient cell resulting in a change in phenotype from endothelial cell to tip cell (Fig. 2.1b). During angiogenesis, a tip cell promotes the growth of new blood vessels; hence, the transfer of Dll4 exosomes to endothelial cells could promote vascularization. However, a more recent report employing Dll4 containing exosomes in a 3D microfluidic device reported a different effect and suggested that the exosomes initiate Notch signaling rather than suppressing Notch signaling. In any case, it is likely that exosomes can influence Notch signaling at distant sites.

2.6 Concluding Remarks

As highlighted above, signaling through the Notch receptor is not only complicated but also versatile, with important biological implications in several systems. The phenotype of mutations in Notch was discovered almost a century ago and the molecular components of the canonical Notch signaling pathway determined within

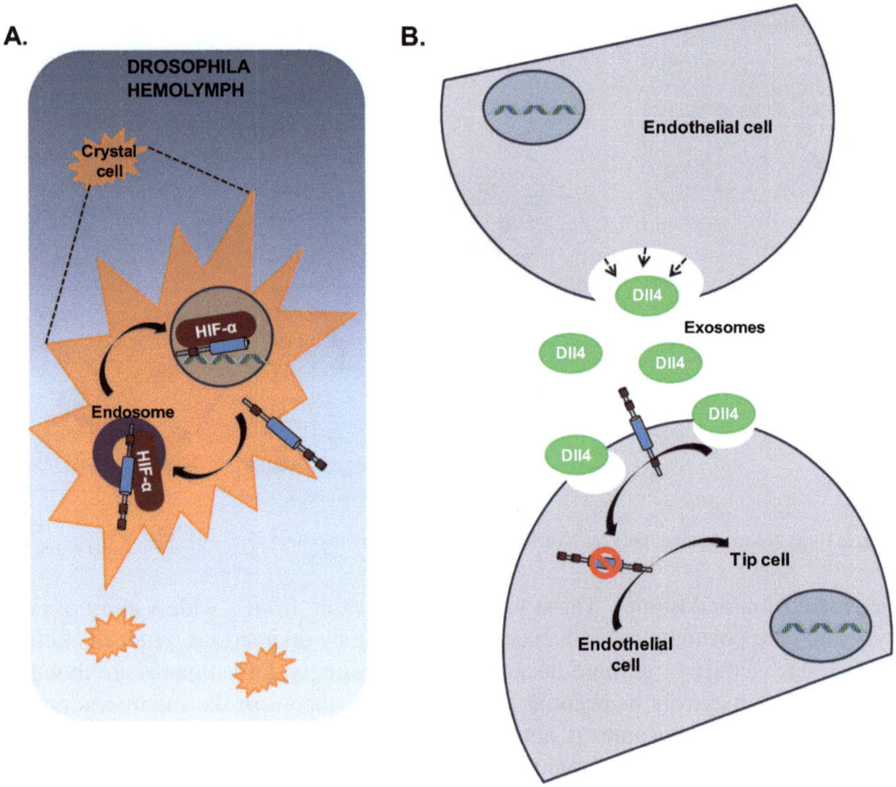

Fig. 2.2 Other forms of noncanonical Notch signaling. (**a**) Notch and HIF-1α interaction in *Drosophila* crystal cells. (**b**) Effect of Dll4 containing exosomes on Notch signaling

the past 3 decades. Canonical Notch signaling is known to impact multiple cell fate decisions. However, noncanonical Notch signaling has only recently been recognized with reports of signaling events through Notch that are RBPJ-independent. Moreover, with the growing number of studies, it is increasingly realized that noncanonical Notch signaling can occur in the nucleus as well as in nonnuclear environments. In this chapter, we have attempted to describe the various nuclear and nonnuclear interactions of Notch that contribute to its noncanonical role (summarized in Fig. 2.2). However, there is still much to be understood in terms of the molecular partners of Notch in this noncanonical pathway and the biological consequences of these interactions. Future studies in this regard will not only help reveal the multiple roles played by Notch through its noncanonical interactions but also provide a basis to explore and develop novel therapeutic strategies that influence Notch signaling in unique contexts. The ability to influence Notch signaling in situations where Notch expression drives disease (such as cancer and various autoimmune diseases) while leaving Notch signaling required for cell or tissue homeostasis (such as replacement of the epithelia in the intestine) intact could prove of great value in the clinic.

References

1. Acosta, H., López, S., Revinski, D., & Carrasco, A. (2011). Notch destabilises maternal β-catenin and restricts dorsal-anterior development in Xenopus. *Development, 138*, 2567–2579.
2. Adler, S. H., Chiffoleau, E., Xu, L., Dalton, N. M., Burg, J. M., Wells, A. D., Wolfe, M. S., Turka, L. A., & Pear, W. S. (2003). Notch signaling augments T cell responsiveness by enhancing CD25 expression. *Journal of Immunology, 171*, 2896–2903.
3. Amsen, D., Blander, J. M., Lee, G. R., Tanigaki, K., Honjo, T., & Flavell, R. A. (2004). Instruction of distinct CD4 T helper cell fates by different Notch ligands on antigen-presenting cells. *Cell, 117*, 515–526.
4. Artavanis-Tsakonas, S., & Muskavitch, M. (2010). Chapter one-notch: The past, the present, and the future. *Current Topics in Developmental Biology, 92*, 1–29.
5. Artavanis-Tsakonas, S., & Simpson, P. (1991). Choosing a cell fate: A view from the Notch locus. *Trends in Genetics, 7*, 403–408.
6. Artavanis-Tsakonas, S., Matsuno, K., & Fortini, M. (1995). Notch signaling. *Science, 268*, 225–232.
7. Artavanis-Tsakonas, S., Rand, M. D., & Lake, R. J. (1999). Notch signaling: Cell fate control and signal integration in development. *Science, 284*, 770–776.
8. Auderset, F., Schuster, S., Coutaz, M., Koch, U., Desgranges, F., Merck, E., MacDonald, H. R., Radtke, F., & Tacchini-Cottier, F. (2012). Redundant Notch1 and Notch2 signaling is necessary for IFNγ secretion by T helper 1 cells during infection with Leishmania major. *PLoS Pathogens, 8*, e1002560.
9. Baek, S., Kim, M., Mo, J., Ann, E., Lee, K., Park, J., Kim, J., Seo, M., Choi, E., & Park, H. (2007). Zinc-induced downregulation of Notch signaling is associated with cytoplasmic retention of Notch1-IC and RBP-Jk via PI3k–Akt signaling pathway. *Cancer Letters, 255*, 117–126.
10. Le Borgne, R. (2006). Regulation of Notch signalling by endocytosis and endosomal sorting. *Current Opinion in Cell Biology, 18*, 213–222.
11. Bray, S. J. (2006). Notch signalling: A simple pathway becomes complex. *Nature Reviews. Molecular Cell Biology, 7*, 678–689.
12. Busseau, I., Diederich, R., Xu, T., & Artavanis-Tsakonas, S. (1994). A member of the Notch group of interacting loci, deltex encodes a cytoplasmic basic protein. *Genetics, 136*, 585–596.
13. Cerveny, K., Tamura, Y., Zhang, Z., Jensen, R., & Sesaki, H. (2007). Regulation of mitochondrial fusion and division. *Trends in Cell Biology, 17*, 563–569.
14. Cheng, P., Zlobin, A., Volgina, V., Gottipati, S., Osborne, B., Simel, E. J., Miele, L., & Gabrilovich, D. I. (2001). Notch-1 regulates NF-kappaB activity in hemopoietic progenitor cells. *Journal of Immunology, 167*, 4458–4467.
15. Cho, O. H., Shin, H. M., Miele, L., Golde, T. E., Fauq, A., Minter, L. M., & Osborne, B. A. (2009). Notch regulates cytolytic effector function in CD8+ T cells. *Journal of Immunology, 182*, 3380–3389.
16. Cox, E., & McLendon, G. (2000). Zinc-dependent protein folding. *Current Opinion in Chemical Biology, 4*, 162–165.
17. Crowner, D., Gall, L., Gates, M., & Giniger, E. (2003). Notch steers Drosophila ISNb motor axons by regulating the Abl signaling pathway. *Current Biology, 13*, 967–972.
18. Deftos, M., He, Y., Ojala, E., & Bevan, M. (1998). Correlating notch signaling with thymocyte maturation. *Immunity, 9*, 777–786.
19. Deveraux, Q., & Reed, J. (1999). IAP family proteins—suppressors of apoptosis. *Genes and Development, 13*, 239–252.
20. Diederich, J., Matsuno, K., Hing, H., & Artavanis-Tsakonas, S. (1994). Cytosolic interaction between deltex and Notch ankyrin repeats implicates deltex in the Notch signaling pathway. *Development, 120*, 473–481.
21. Doe, C. (2008). Neural stem cells: Balancing self-renewal with differentiation. *Development, 135*, 1575–1587.

22. Dongre, A., Surampudi, L., Lawlor, R., Fauq, A., Miele, L., Golde, T., Minter, L., & Osborne, B. (2014). Non-canonical Notch signaling drives activation and differentiation of peripheral CD4+ T cells. *Frontiers in Immunology, 5*, 54.
23. Druker, B., Talpaz, M., Resta, D., Peng, B., Buchdunger, E., Ford, J., Lydon, N., Kantarjian, H., Capdeville, R., Ohno-Jones, S., & Sawyers, C. (2001). Efficacy and safety of a specific inhibitor of the BCR-ABL tyrosine kinase in chronic myeloid leukemia. *New England Journal of Medicine, 344*, 1031–1037.
24. Ellisen, L. W., Bird, J., West, D. C., Soreng, A. L., Reynolds, T. C., Smith, S. D., & Sklar, J. (1991). TAN-1, the human homolog of the Drosophila notch gene, is broken by chromosomal translocations in T lymphoblastic neoplasms. *Cell, 66*, 649–661.
25. Eom, S., Kim, E., Lee, J., Kang, H., Shim, J., Kim, S., Gwag, B., & Choi, E. (2001). Zn2+ induces stimulation of the c-Jun N-terminal kinase signaling pathway through phosphoinositide 3-kinase. *Molecular Pharmacology, 59*, 981–986.
26. Fainstein, E., Marcelle, C., Rosner, A., Canaani, E., Gale, R., Dreazen, O., Smith, S., & Croce, C. (1987). A new fused transcript in Philadelphia chromosome positive acute lymphocytic leukaemia. *Nature, 330*, 386–388.
27. Gall, L., Mattei, D., & Giniger, E. (2008). Molecular separation of two signaling pathways for the receptor, Notch. *Developmental Biology, 313*, 556–567.
28. Geimer Le Lay, A.-S. S., Oravecz, A., Mastio, J., Jung, C., Marchal, P., Ebel, C., Dembélé, D., Jost, B., Le Gras, S., Thibault, C., et al. (2014). The tumor suppressor Ikaros shapes the repertoire of notch target genes in T cells. *Science Signaling, 7*, ra28.
29. Gertler, F., Bennett, R., Clark, M., & Hoffmann, M. (1989). Drosophila abl tyrosine kinase in embryonic CNS axons: A role in axonogenesis is revealed through dosage-sensitive interactions with disabled. *Cell, 58*, 103–113.
30. Giniger, E. (1998). A role for Abl in Notch signaling. *Neuron, 20*, 667–681.
31. Heitzler, P. (2010). Biodiversity and noncanonical Notch signaling. *Current Topics in Developmental Biology, 92*, 457–481.
32. Hoffmann, M. (1991). Drosophila abl and genetic redundancy in signal transduction. *Trends in Genetics, 7*, 351–355.
33. Hori, K., Sen, A., Kirchhausen, T., & Artavanis-Tsakonas, S. (2011). Synergy between the ESCRT-III complex and Deltex defines a ligand-independent Notch signal. *The Journal of Cell Biology, 195*, 1005–1015.
34. Huang, X., Cuajungco, M., Atwood, C., Moir, R., Tanzi, R., & Bush, A. (2000). Alzheimer's disease, β-amyloid protein and zinc. *The Journal of Nutrition, 130*, 1488S–1492S.
35. Jarriault, S., Brou, C., Logeat, F., Schroeter, E., Kopan, R., & Israel, A. (1995). Signalling downstream of activated mammalian Notch. *Nature, 377*, 355–358.
36. Jehn, B., Bielke, W., Pear, W., & Osborne, B. (1999). Cutting edge: Protective effects of Notch-1 on TCR-induced apoptosis. *Journal of Immunology, 162*, 635–638.
37. Jin, S., Mutvei, A., Chivukula, I., Andersson, E., Ramsköld, D., Sandberg, R., Lee, K., Kronqvist, P., Mamaeva, V., Östling, P., Mpindi, J., Kallioniemi, O., Screpanti, I., Poellinger, L., Sahlgren, C., & Lendahl, U. (2013). Non-canonical Notch signaling activates IL-6/JAK/STAT signaling in breast tumor cells and is controlled by p53 and IKKα/IKKβ. *Oncogene, 32*, 4892–4902.
38. Joshi, I., Minter, L. M., Telfer, J., Demarest, R. M. M., Capobianco, A. J., Aster, J. C., Sicinski, P., Fauq, A., Golde, T. E., & Osborne, B. A. (2009). Notch signaling mediates G1/S cell-cycle progression in T cells via cyclin D3 and its dependent kinases. *Blood, 113*, 1689–1698.
39. Keerthivasan, S., Suleiman, R., Lawlor, R., Roderick, J., Bates, T., Minter, L., Anguita, J., Juncadella, I., Nickoloff, B. J., Le Poole, I. C., et al. (2011). Notch signaling regulates mouse and human Th17 differentiation. *Journal of Immunology, 187*, 692–701.
40. Kim, S., Jung, Y., Kim, D., Koh, H., & Chung, J. (2000). Extracellular zinc activates p70 S6 kinase through the phosphatidylinositol 3-kinase signaling pathway. *The Journal of Biological Chemistry, 275*, 25979–25984.
41. Koch, U., & Radtke, F. (2007). Haematopoietic stem cell niche in Drosophila. *BioEssays, 29*, 713–716.

42. Kwon, C., Qian, L., Cheng, P., Nigam, V., Arnold, J., & Srivastava, D. (2009). A regulatory pathway involving Notch1/β-catenin/Isl1 determines cardiac progenitor cell fate. *Nature Cell Biology, 11*, 951–957.
43. Kwon, C., Cheng, P., King, I., Andersen, P., Shenje, L., Nigam, V., & Srivastava, D. (2011). Notch post-translationally regulates [beta]-catenin protein in stem and progenitor cells. *Nature Cell Biology, 13*, 1244–1251.
44. Landgraf, M., Bossing, T., Technau, G., & Bate, M. (1997). The origin, location, and projections of the embryonic abdominal motorneurons of Drosophila. *The Journal of Neuroscience, 17*, 9642–9655.
45. Layden, M. J., & Martindale, M. Q. (2014). Non-canonical Notch signaling represents an ancestral mechanism to regulate neural differentiation. *EvoDevo, 5*, 30.
46. Lee, K., Wu, Z., Song, Y., Mitra, S., Feroze, A., Cheshier, S., & Lu, B. (2013). Roles of PINK1, mTORC2, and mitochondria in preserving brain tumor-forming stem cells in a noncanonical Notch signaling pathway. *Genes & Development, 27*, 2642–2647.
47. Lee, S. H., Wang, X., & DeJong, J. (2000). Functional interactions between an atypical NF-kappaB site from the rat CYP2B1 promoter and the transcriptional repressor RBP-Jkappa/CBF1. *Nucleic Acids Research, 28*, 2091–2098.
48. Leon, O., & Roth, M. (2000). Zinc fingers: DNA binding and protein-protein interactions. *Biological Research, 33*, 21–30. https://doi.org/10.4067/S0716-97602000000100009.
49. Liu, W., Hsiao, H., Tsou, W., & Lai, M. (2007). Notch inhibits apoptosis by direct interference with XIAP ubiquitination and degradation. *The EMBO Journal, 26*, 1660–1669.
50. Maekawa, Y., Tsukumo, S., Chiba, S., Hirai, H., Hayashi, Y., Okada, H., Kishihara, K., & Yasutomo, K. (2003). Delta1-Notch3 interactions bias the functional differentiation of activated CD4+ T cells. *Immunity, 19*, 549–559.
51. Mann, J., Oakley, F., Johnson, P. W., & Mann, D. A. (2002). CD40 induces interleukin-6 gene transcription in dendritic cells: Regulation by TRAF2, AP-1, NF-kappa B, AND CBF1. *Journal of Biological Chemistry, 277*, 17125–17138.
52. Matsuno, K., Diederich, R., Go, M., Blaumueller, C., & Artavanis-Tsakonas, S. (1995). Deltex acts as a positive regulator of Notch signaling through interactions with the Notch ankyrin repeats. *Development, 121*, 2633–2644.
53. McNamee, E. N. N., Korns Johnson, D., Homann, D., & Clambey, E. T. (2013). Hypoxia and hypoxia-inducible factors as regulators of T cell development, differentiation, and function. *Immunologic Research, 55*, 58–70.
54. Minter, L. M., Turley, D. M., Das, P., Shin, H. M., Joshi, I., Lawlor, R. G., Cho, O. H., Palaga, T., Gottipati, S., Telfer, J. C., et al. (2005). Inhibitors of gamma-secretase block in vivo and in vitro T helper type 1 polarization by preventing Notch upregulation of Tbx21. *Nature Immunology, 6*, 680–688.
55. Morgan, T. H. (1917). The theory of the gene. *The American Naturalist, 609*, 513–544.
56. Morrison, S., & Kimble, J. (2006). Asymmetric and symmetric stem-cell divisions in development and cancer. *Nature, 441*, 1068–1074.
57. Mukherjee, T., Kim, W. S., Mandal, L., & Banerjee, U. (2011). Interaction between Notch and Hif-alpha in development and survival of Drosophila blood cells. *Science, 332*, 1210–1213.
58. Nair, P., Somasundaram, K., & Krishna, S. (2003). Activated Notch1 inhibits p53-induced apoptosis and sustains transformation by human papillomavirus type 16 E6 and E7 oncogenes through a PI3K-PKB/Akt-dependent pathway. *Journal of Virology, 77*, 7106–7112.
59. Ong, C.-T. T., Sedy, J. R., Murphy, K. M., & Kopan, R. (2008). Notch and presenilin regulate cellular expansion and cytokine secretion but cannot instruct Th1/Th2 fate acquisition. *PLoS One, 3*, e2823.
60. Ordentlich, P., Lin, A., Shen, C., Blaumueller, C., Matsuno, K., Artavanis-Tsakonas, S., & Kadesch, T. (1998). Notch inhibition of E47 supports the existence of a novel signaling pathway. *Molecular and Cellular Biology, 18*, 2230–2239.
61. Osipo, C., Golde, T. E., Osborne, B. A., & Miele, L. A. (2008). Off the beaten pathway: The complex cross talk between Notch and NF-kappaB. *Laboratory Investigation, 88*, 11–17.

62. Palaga, T., Miele, L., Golde, T. E., & Osborne, B. A. (2003). TCR-mediated Notch signaling regulates proliferation and IFN-gamma production in peripheral T cells. *Journal of Immunology, 171*, 3019–3024.
63. Perumalsamy, L., Nagala, M., & Sarin, A. (2010). Notch-activated signaling cascade interacts with mitochondrial remodeling proteins to regulate cell survival. *PNAS, 107*, 6882–6887.
64. Perumalsamy, L., Nagala, M., Banerjee, P., & Sarin, A. (2009). A hierarchical cascade activated by non-canonical Notch signaling and the mTOR–Rictor complex regulates neglect-induced death in mammalian cells. *Cell Death & Differentiation, 16*, 879–889.
65. Perumalsamy, L., Marcel, N., Kulkarni, S., Radtke, F., & Sarin, A. (2012). Distinct spatial and molecular features of notch pathway assembly in regulatory T cells. *Science Signaling, 5*, ra53–ra53.
66. Pinnell, N., Yan, R., Cho, H. J., Keeley, T., Murai, M. J., Liu, Y., Alarcon, A. S., Qin, J., Wang, Q., Kuick, R., et al. (2015). The PIAS-like coactivator Zmiz1 is a direct and selective cofactor of Notch1 in T cell development and leukemia. *Immunity, 43*, 870–883.
67. Rangarajan, A., Syal, R., Selvarajah, S., Chakrabarti, O., Sarin, A., & Krishna, S. (2001). Activated Notch1 signaling cooperates with papillomavirus oncogenes in transformation and generates resistance to apoptosis on matrix withdrawal through PKB/Akt. *Virology, 286*, 23–30.
68. Rebay, I., Fehon, R., & Artavanis-Tsakonas, S. (1993). Specific truncations of Drosophila Notch define dominant activated and dominant negative forms of the receptor. *Cell, 74*, 319–329.
69. Roehl, H., & Kimble, J. (1993). Control of cell fate in C. elegans by a GLP-1 peptide consisting primarily of ankyrin repeats. *Nature, 364*, 632–635.
70. Ruland, J., Duncan, G. S., Elia, A., del Barco Barrantes, I., Nguyen, L., Plyte, S., Millar, D. G., Bouchard, D., Wakeham, A., Ohashi, P. S., et al. (2001). Bcl10 is a positive regulator of antigen receptor-induced activation of NF-kappaB and neural tube closure. *Cell, 104*, 33–42.
71. Ruland, J., Duncan, G. S., Wakeham, A., & Mak, T. W. (2003). Differential requirement for Malt1 in T and B cell antigen receptor signaling. *Immunity, 19*, 749–758.
72. Sade, H., Krishna, S., & Sarin, A. (2004). The anti-apoptotic effect of Notch-1 requires p56lck-dependent, Akt/PKB-mediated signaling in T cells. *The Journal of Biological Chemistry, 279*, 2937–2944.
73. Samon, J. B., Champhekar, A., Minter, L. M., Telfer, J. C., Miele, L., Fauq, A., Das, P., Golde, T. E., & Osborne, B. A. (2008). Notch1 and TGFbeta1 cooperatively regulate Foxp3 expression and the maintenance of peripheral regulatory T cells. *Blood, 112*, 1813–1821.
74. Schimmer, A., Dalili, S., Batey, R., & Riedl, S. (2006). Targeting XIAP for the treatment of malignancy. *Cell Death and Differentiation, 13*, 179–188.
75. Shawber, C., Nofziger, D., Hsieh, J., Lindsell, C., Bogler, O., Hayward, D., & Weinmaster, G. (1996). Notch signaling inhibits muscle cell differentiation through a CBF1-independent pathway. *Development, 122*, 3765–3773.
76. Sheldon, H., Heikamp, E., Turley, H., Dragovic, R., Thomas, P., Oon, C. E., Leek, R., Edelmann, M., Kessler, B., Sainson, R. C., et al. (2010). New mechanism for Notch signaling to endothelium at a distance by Delta-like 4 incorporation into exosomes. *Blood, 116*, 2385–2394.
77. Shin, H., Tilahun, M., Cho, O., Chandiran, K., Kuksin, C., Keerthivasan, S., Fauq, A., Golde, T., Miele, L., Thome, M., Osborne, B., & Minter, L. (2014). NOTCH1 can initiate NF-κB activation via cytosolic interactions with components of the T cell signalosome. *Frontiers in Immunology, 5*, 249. https://doi.org/10.3389/fimmu.2014.00249.
78. Shin, H. M., Minter, L. M., Cho, O. H., Gottipati, S., Fauq, A. H., Golde, T. E., Sonenshein, G. E., & Osborne, B. A. (2006). Notch1 augments NF-kappaB activity by facilitating its nuclear retention. *The EMBO Journal, 25*, 129–138.
79. Schwartzberg, P., Stall, A., Hardin, J., Bowdish, K., Humaran, T., Boast, S., Harbison, M., Robertson, E., & Goff, S. (1991). Mice homozygous for the abl m1 mutation show poor viability and depletion of selected B and T cell populations. *Cell, 65*, 1165–1175.

80. Song, J., Park, S., Kim, M., & Shin, I. (2008). Down-regulation of Notch-dependent transcription by Akt in vitro. *FEBS Letters, 582*, 1693–1699.
81. Stifani, S., Blaumueller, C., Redhead, N., Hill, R., & Artavanis-Tsakonas, S. (1992). Human homologs of a Drosophila Enhancer of split gene product define a novel family of nuclear proteins. *Nature Genetics, 2*, 119–127.
82. Tybulewicz, V., Crawford, C., Jackson, P., Bronson, R., & Mulligan, R. (1991). Neonatal lethality and lymphopenia in mice with a homozygous disruption of the c-abl proto-oncogene. *Cell, 65*, 1153–1163.
83. Ukaji, T., & Umezawa, K. (2014). Novel approaches to target NF-κB and other signaling pathways in cancer stem cells. *Advances in Biological Regulation, 56*, 108–115.
84. Vactor, V., Sink, H., Fambrough, D., Tsoo, R., & Goodman, C. (1993). Genes that control neuromuscular specificity in Drosophila. *Cell, 73*, 1137–1153.
85. Vales, L. D., & Friedl, E. M. (2002). Binding of C/EBP and RBP (CBF1) to overlapping sites regulates interleukin-6 gene expression. *The Journal of Biological Chemistry, 277*, 42438–42446.
86. Wang, H., Somers, G., Bashirullah, A., Heberlein, U., Yu, F., & Chia, W. (2006). Aurora-A acts as a tumor suppressor and regulates self-renewal of Drosophila neuroblasts. *Genes & Development, 20*, 3453–3463.
87. Wang, D., You, Y., Case, S. M., McAllister-Lucas, L. M., Wang, L., DiStefano, P. S., Nuñez, G., Bertin, J., & Lin, X. (2002). A requirement for CARMA1 in TCR-induced NF-kappa B activation. *Nature Immunology, 3*, 830–835.
88. Wang, J., Shelly, L., Miele, L., Boykins, R., Norcross, M. A., & Guan, E. (2001). Human Notch-1 inhibits NF-kappa B activity in the nucleus through a direct interaction involving a novel domain. *Journal of Immunology, 167*, 289–295.
89. Wills, Z., Bateman, J., Korey, C., Comer, A., & Vactor, V. (1999). The tyrosine kinase Abl and its substrate enabled collaborate with the receptor phosphatase Dlar to control motor axon guidance. *Neuron, 22*, 301–312.
90. Wu, Z., Sawada, T., Shiba, K., Liu, S., Kanao, T., Takahashi, R., Hattori, N., Imay, Y., & Lu, B. (2013). Tricornered/NDR kinase signaling mediates PINK1-directed mitochondrial quality control and tissue maintenance. *Genes & Development, 27*, 157–162.
91. Xu, T., & Artavanis-Tsakonas, S. (1990). Deltex, a locus interacting with the neurogenic genes, Notch, Delta and mastermind in Drosophila melanogaster. *Genetics, 126*, 665–677.

Chapter 3
Dual Function of Notch Signaling in Cancer: Oncogene and Tumor Suppressor

Ute Koch and Freddy Radtke

Abstract The Notch cascade is an evolutionarily conserved cell-to-cell signaling system that regulates many aspects of embryonic development. It regulates also self-renewal and differentiation processes as well as tissue homeostasis in several adult vertebrate organs. In the last 15 years, it has become evident that deregulated Notch signaling is associated with several human disorders, including cancer. Recently, large sequencing efforts of cancer genomes have uncovered both gain- and loss-of-function mutations in different genes involved in the Notch signaling cascade, indicating that Notch can be both oncogenic and tumor suppressive. For specific tumor types, results generated from experimental mouse models predicted and also validated such relationships, whereas for others, the conclusive findings were unanticipated. The oncogenic and tumor-suppressive functions of Notch appear to be context- and tissue-specific. In this review we will discuss the context-dependent and tissue-specific oncogenic and tumor-suppressive functions of Notch.

Keywords Notch · Cancer · Oncogene · Tumor Suppressor · Mutations

3.1 A Brief Introduction to the Notch Cascade

The Notch signaling cascade consists of membrane-bound receptors and ligands that regulate multiple functions in adult vertebrate tissues including stem cell self-renewal, cell fate specification, proliferation, and apoptosis through cell-to-cell signaling [48, 50]. Mammals possess four Notch receptors (Notch1–4), four delta-like ligands (Dll1–4), and two ligands of the Jagged family (Jag1 and 2). During maturation and transport to the cell surface, Notch receptors traffic from the endoplasmic reticulum to the Golgi where they undergo proteolytic cleavage by a furin-like protease. At the cell surface, Notch receptors exist as heterodimeric receptors consisting of an extracellular subunit (N^{EC}), which is non-covalently bound to a second

U. Koch (✉) · F. Radtke (✉)
Ecole Polytechnique Fédérale de Lausanne (EPFL), School of Life Sciences, Swiss Institute for Experimental Cancer Research (ISREC), Lausanne, Switzerland
e-mail: ute.koch@epfl.ch; Freddy.Radtke@epfl.ch

L. Miele, S. Artavanis-Tsakonas (eds.), *Targeting Notch in Cancer*,
https://doi.org/10.1007/978-1-4939-8859-4_3

subunit harboring one part of the extracellular heterodimerization (HD) domain followed by the transmembrane domain and the cytoplasmic region of the Notch receptor (N^{TM}). The extracellular subunit of Notch receptors contains between 29 and 36 epidermal growth factor-like repeats (involved in ligand binding), 3 cysteine-rich LIN12 repeats (LNR), and a hydrophobic stretch of amino acids involved in the heterodimerization of N^{EC} and N^{TM}. The LNR together with the hydrophobic stretch of amino acids constitute the negative regulatory region (NRR), which prevents ligand-independent activation of Notch receptors. The intracellular part of Notch receptors contains multiple elements including nuclear localization signals, protein-protein interaction domains, transcriptional activation domains, and a PEST sequence involved in regulating protein stability (Fig. 3.1).

Normally, Notch signaling is initiated by ligand-receptor interaction between neighboring cells. This triggers a series of proteolytic cleavage events, the first of which is mediated by metalloproteases of the ADAM family (ADAM-10 or ADAM-17), located 12–13 amino acids external to the transmembrane domain. Subsequently, the γ-secretase multi-protein complex cleaves the remaining Notch receptor within the transmembrane domain, resulting in the release of the intracellular cytoplasmic domain of Notch (NICD). NICD subsequently translocates to the nucleus where it interacts with the DNA-binding transcription factor RBP-J (also known as CSL) in order to form a short-lived transcription activation complex. The binding of NICD to RBP-J results in the recruitment of other coactivators including mastermind-like proteins (MAML1–3), p300, and many other proteins in order to induce transcription of downstream target genes [124] (for a more comprehensive description of the molecular aspects of the Notch cascade, the reader is referred to excellent reviews [11, 50]).

3.2 Notch Functions as Oncoprotein

The first evidence demonstrating that components of the Notch cascade can function as oncoproteins resulted from the finding that the NOTCH1 locus is disrupted by t(7;9) translocations in rare cases (<1%) of human T cell acute lymphoblastic leukemia (T-ALL). This translocation results in the fusion of the 3'end of the human *NOTCH1* gene to the *TCRB* promoter/enhancer region. *TCRB*-driven transcripts of this fusion gene generate a truncated, dominant active NOTCH1 protein that lacks the NRR domain [29, 86]. The oncogenic potential of this truncated form of the NOTCH1 protein was demonstrated in murine bone marrow reconstitution experiments in which expression of the truncated NOTCH1 protein was shown to be sufficient to cause T-ALL in mice [12, 70]. However, the clinical relevance of this finding appeared to be limited due to the rare number of patients that carry such translocations. In the last decade, large sequencing efforts were performed with the aim to uncover the genomic landscape of many tumor types. In the context of T-ALL, Aster and colleagues sequenced the cancer genome of multiple human T-ALL cell lines as well as of 96 primary T-ALL samples from children and

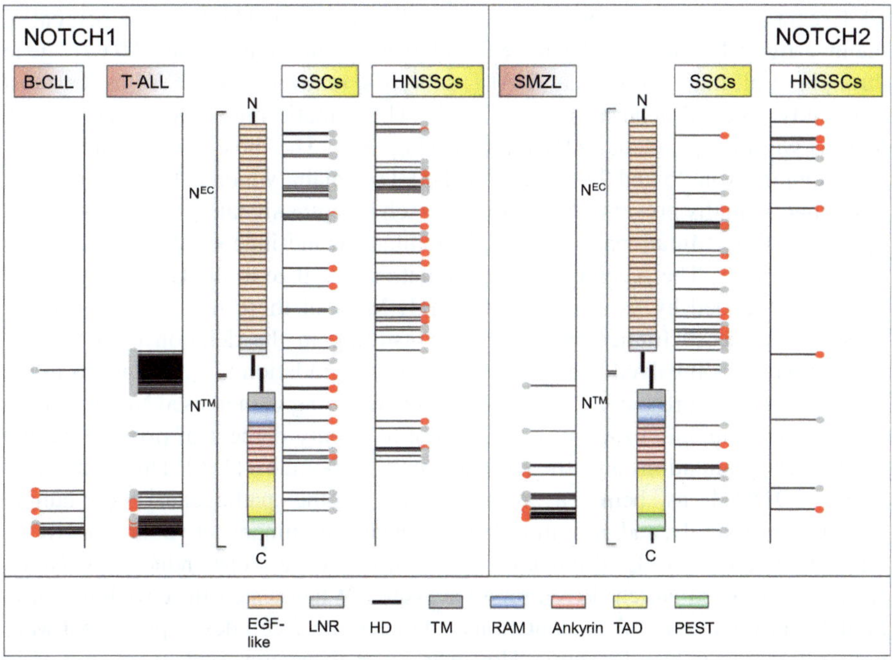

Fig. 3.1 Mutational landscape of NOTCH1 and NOTCH2 in cancers in which Notch functions as oncogene or tumor suppressor. Schematic representation of the NOTCH1 and NOTCH2 receptors with their structural distribution of missense (gray) and nonsense (red dots) mutations in indicated neoplasms. B-CLL, T-ALL, and SMZL indicated in red are neoplasms in which Notch functions as oncogene, whereas SSCS and HNSSCs indicated in yellow are cancer in which Notch exerts tumor-suppressive mutations. NOTCH1 oncogenic driver mutations in T cell acute lymphoblastic leukemia (T-ALL) [116] and B cell chronic lymphocytic leukemia (B-CLL) [24, 32, 77, 103] and Notch2 driver mutations in splenic marginal zone lymphomas (SMZL) [46, 88] [69] are displayed on the left side of the schematic Notch receptors. For NOTCH1 and T-ALL, missense mutations cluster largely to the NRR domain, while truncating mutations are mostly confined to the PEST domain. In B-CLL truncating mutations are predominant and cluster to the C-terminal PEST domain and adjacent transactivation domain. Similarly NOTCH2 mutations in SMZL are mostly confined to the PEST domain. In contrast, mutations depicted on the right side of the schematic receptors from squamous cell carcinoma (SSC) [73, 113] and head and neck squamous cell carcinoma (HNSCC) [2, 73, 106] in which Notch1 and 2 exert tumor-suppressive functions appear all over the protein, with a tendency to be more frequent in the N^{EC} domain of the receptors. Below are indicated the different protein domains of the Notch receptors. The extracellular part of the Notch receptors (N^{EC}) contains EGF-like repeats (EGF-like) followed by three cysteine-rich LIN domains (LNR) that prevent ligand-independent cleavage, the heterodimerization domain (HD) and the transmembrane domain (TM). The N^{TM} part of the receptors includes the cytoplasmic domain consisting of a RAM domain (RAM) followed by six ankyrin repeats (ankyrin) that bind to the RBP-J transcription factor, a transactivation domain (TAD) and a PEST sequence (PEST) involved in regulating protein stability

adolescents at time of diagnosis for *NOTCH1* mutations [116]. Fifty-six percent of the investigated tumor samples were found to carry mutations in the *NOTCH1* gene throughout all major molecular T-ALL subtypes, rendering *NOTCH1* as the most frequently mutated gene in human T-ALL. The somatic mutations cluster to two regions within the human *NOTCH1* gene (Fig. 3.1). The most common mutations are found in exon 26 and 27 coding for the HD domain, which is the region of the NRR that normally prevents activation of Notch receptor signaling in the absence of ligand binding. Mutations in the NRR facilitate ligand-independent activation of Notch receptors. The second cluster of mutations localize to the C-terminal PEST sequence encoded by exon 34 of NOTCH1. Most of these mutations consist of either nonsense or frame-shift mutations resulting in the deletion of the PEST domain which is involved in targeting NICD for degradation [16]. Mutations in the PEST domain are present in 20–30% of tumors resulting in increased Notch activity due to persistent stabilization of NICD. Ten to twenty percent of primary human T-ALLs carry mutations both the HD and the PEST domains [116]. This study identified NOTCH1 as being a major player in the pathogenesis of human T-ALL. Surprisingly, and in contrast to the truncated dominant active form of NICD, HD, PEST, and HD/PEST mutations were found to be weak inducers of Notch activity in in vitro Notch-driven reporter assays. When tested in retroviral mouse models, introduction of these mutations led to ectopic T cell development but were not sufficient to induce leukemia. However, when these constructs were studied in an oncogenic LSL-K-ras^{G12D} background that predisposes mice to T-ALL development, these relatively weak activating Notch mutations shortened disease latency and gave rise to T-ALL cell lines whose growth was dependent on Notch signaling [15]. These data suggest that frequently occurring *NOTCH1* mutations found in human T-ALL patients do not solely generate a sufficiently strong Notch signal to initiate leukemic development in mouse models. However these weakly leukemogenic *NOTCH1* mutations can complement and synergize with other already existing leukemogenic events. In agreement with this, other transgenic mouse models of T-ALL such as TAL1/SCL, OLIG2, and LMO1/1 have been found to develop spontaneous activating mutations in the Notch1 gene [4]. Taken together, these data suggest that the commonly found *NOTCH1* mutations in human T-ALL are likely to be secondary events that contribute to preexisting primary tumor initiating hits in order to accelerate tumor progression. Importantly, arising tumors remained sensitive to growth inhibition by pharmacological (γ-secretase inhibitor) Notch inhibitors, indicating that these tumors remained addicted to Notch. This warrants the rational to therapeutically block Notch signaling in T-ALL patients.

Activating mutations in the *NOTCH1* gene have also been identified in B cell chronic lymphocytic leukemia (B-CLL) [24, 32, 77, 103]. This was originally unanticipated due to early studies showing that overexpression of NICD antagonizes early B cell development in the bone marrow [78] and/or induces growth arrest and apoptosis in both murine and human B cell lines and in multiple B cell neoplasms [129]. On the other hand, Notch2-mediated signaling is essential for the development and maintenance of splenic marginal zone B cells [90]. Furthermore, Notch1 has been shown to synergize with B cell receptor and/or CD40 signaling to enhance

B cell activation and function [108]. Although high levels of Notch signaling are incompatible with early stages of B cell development, Notch signaling is important in more mature B cells. Therefore, retrospectively, the identification of activating Notch mutations in B cell neoplasms appears to be less of a surprise. B-CLL is among the most common types of leukemia in the Western world. Clinically, the progression of the disease is very heterogeneous. CLL patients can be subdivided in two major subgroups based on the immunoglobulin heavy chain variable (IGHV) gene status of CLL cells. Approximately 60% of CLLs carry immunoglobulin heavy chain variable genes exhibiting somatic hypermutations in their variable regions, while the remaining 40% of CLLs do not carry IGHV gene mutations. The subgroup carrying unmutated IGHV genes is associated with a more aggressive form of the disease [127]. *NOTCH1* mutations in CLL were first identified in 2009 in 2 out of 43 CLL cases analyzed. In both cases the mutations localized to exon 34 leading to predicted loss of the PEST domain [24]. A follow-up analysis of 133 CLL patients by the same group identified *NOTCH1* PEST domain mutations to occur with a frequency of approximately 5%. Neither HD domain nor NOTCH2 gene mutations were identified in this study, suggesting that mutations are restricted to the *NOTCH1* gene and in particular to exon 34 coding for the PEST sequence [103]. In 2011, two groups used next-generation sequencing to identify recurrent mutations in larger CLL cohorts. *NOTCH1* mutations were found to occur at a frequency of 8.3% and 12.2%, respectively [32, 77], all localized to the PEST domain. A more recent study reports that mutations can also occur within the noncoding region of *NOTCH1*, namely, the 3' UTR. These mutations generate a new splice acceptor site within the 3' UTR inducing aberrant splicing events that lead to deletions that include the final 158 coding bases of exon 34 [76]. Although the frequency of *NOTCH1* PEST mutations seems to vary between 5% and 10% at diagnosis, they are primarily found in samples of the more aggressive IGHV non-mutated CLL patient subgroup and often correlate with trisomy 12. Moreover, the mutation frequency appears to increase with disease progression reaching 31% in patients subsequently diagnosed with Richter transformation and 21% in chemorefractory CLL [32]. Taken together although *NOTCH1* mutations do not appear to be causative in CLL, they are associated with poor prognosis and worse outcome and are most likely acquired during disease progression.

NOTCH1 mutations clustering to the PEST sequence have also been identified in Mantle cell lymphoma (in 12% of clinical cases and 20% of cell lines) [51], an aggressive subtype of non-Hodgkin lymphoma.

Even though the identification of *NOTCH1* mutations in CLL and MCL was somewhat unanticipated, the identification of mutations in genes involved in the Notch pathway in splenic marginal zone lymphoma (SMZL) was less surprising, as NOTCH2 is a well-established master regulator of marginal zone B cell development and maintenance [42, 90]. Next-generation sequencing identified *NOTCH2* mutations in 20–25% of SMZL cases [46, 88] establishing *NOTCH2* as one of the most frequently mutated genes in SMZL. NOTCH2 mutations were also associated with adverse clinical outcomes including reduced treatment-free and overall survival [46, 69]. Surprisingly mutations in the *NOTCH1* gene were also identified in approximately 5% of the investigated cases. Mutations in both *NOTCH1* and *NOTCH2* predominantly cluster to the PEST sequence and are therefore predicted to cause sustained Notch signaling due to increased protein stability. Additional mutations in Notch signaling-associated genes such as *SPEN*, *DTX1*, and *MAML2* have also been identified, though with lower frequency to *NOTCH1/Notch2* [46, 88].

The fact that *NOTCH* mutations within B cell neoplasms are predominantly restricted to the PEST sequence, whereas the most frequent mutations in T-ALL are localized to the HD domain (Fig. 3.1), indicates that transformed B cells do not undergo selective pressure to acquire mutations that render these cells independent of Notch ligands. Thus, transformed B cells are likely to receive their Notch ligand-mediated signals through naturally occurring ligands expressed on cells located in secondary lymphoid organs. In this scenario the prediction is that circulating transformed B cells would have little or no ongoing NOTCH signaling as they migrate out from their microenvironment(s) limiting their access to Notch ligands. The correlation between PEST mutations in *NOTCH* genes in B cell neoplasms with poor patient outcome, increased chemoresistance, and disease progression is intriguing. It suggests that the Notch mutations are likely to be acquired during disease progression. However, whether these mutations are causative, how increased Notch signaling may contribute to disease progression, and whether inhibition of Notch signaling would resensitize chemoresistant B cell neoplasms to standard of care therapies is currently poorly understood and is a matter of ongoing investigation.

The first evidence that aberrant Notch signaling has oncogenic functions in solid tumors was derived from animal studies demonstrating that integration of the mouse mammary tumor virus (MMTV) into the *Notch4* gene results in the formation of mammary tumors [34]. MMTV integration into the *Notch4* locus results in the expression of long terminal repeat (LTR)-driven transcripts encoding for truncated Notch4 mRNA species named int3 [109]. Expression of this truncated dominant active form of the *Notch4/int3* gene either under the control of MMTV LTR or the whey acidic protein (WAP) promoter in transgenic mice results in the development of mammary tumors in 100% of cases [33, 44]. Similarly, transgenic female mice carrying an MMTV-N1ICD construct encoding human *NOTCH1* cDNA also developed mammary carcinomas, but only following multiple pregnancies [47]. Increased expression of *NOTCH1* and *JAGGED1* correlates with poor overall survival in women with advanced breast cancer [84], as well as reduced disease-free survival [85]. Moreover, loss of the negative Notch regulator, Numb, is observed in approximately 50% of human mammary carcinomas [71]. A recent study identified a *NOTCH4/HES/HEY* gene signature to be predictive of poor therapeutic response and prognosis in estrogen receptor-positive (ER+) patients that often acquire de novo resistance to hormonal therapy. Mechanistically, JAGGED1-mediated NOTCH4 receptor activation increases breast cancer stem cell activity and thereby drives antiestrogen resistance in human breast tumors. Combining endocrine therapy with blockage of Notch signaling was effective in overcoming resistance in ER+ human breast cancer [98].

Additional evidence for a role of Notch signaling in breast cancer is derived from transcriptomic sequencing of breast cancer cell lines and tumors. This study identified translocations within both *NOTCH1* and *NOTCH2* genes. These genetic rearrangements lead to the generation of fusion transcripts encoding truncated versions of NOTCH1 or NOTCH2 that lack most or the entire extracellular domain of corresponding receptors including the LNR domain. These translocations have been identified in approximately 10% of investigated triple-negative breast cancer samples and have been shown to correlate with high Notch signaling activity in in vitro studies [87]. This is reminiscent to observations made on rare cases of human T-ALL that express truncated dominant forms of NOTCH1 as a consequence of t(7;9) translocations. It is worth mentioning that cancers expressing these truncated dominant active forms of Notch proteins cannot be treated therapeutically with blocking Notch antibodies and are only responsive to γ-secretase inhibitors if their S3 cleavage site of their Notch receptors remains intact. In contrast, inhibitors that block Notch signaling at the level of the transcription activation complex should be effective in such cancers.

In addition to breast cancer, increased Notch signaling is also observed in approximately one third of non-small cell lung carcinomas (NSCLCs) due to the loss of Numb expression (in 30% of cases) and due to activating mutations in the *NOTCH1* gene (in 10% of cases investigated) [118]. The oncogenic role of Notch signaling in NSCLC was confirmed in a $Kras^{G12V}$-driven experimental mouse model [8]. Genetic loss-of-function (LoF) studies on RBP-J and presenilins showed that Notch signaling is essential for the formation of NSCLC. Moreover, pharmacological inhibition of Notch signaling in mice carrying autochthonous NSCLCs prevented cancer growth, characterized by increased expression of dual-specificity phosphatase1 (DUSP1), which is directly repressed by the Notch target gene *Hes1*. DUSPs are negative regulators of MAPK/ERK signaling. Accordingly, Notch inhibition results in the upregulation of DUSP1 expression and in decreased levels of phospho-Erk correlating with the inhibited growth of murine and human NSCLCs [57].

Although activating mutations in Notch genes in other solid tumors are either rare or have yet to be reported, oncogenic roles for Notch have also been linked to other solid tumors including colorectal cancer, melanoma, pancreatic cancer, cholangiocarcinoma, and medulloblastoma [49, 80, 126].

3.3 Oncogenic Notch-Driven Signaling Events: T-ALL as Paradigm

In the past decade, oncogenic Notch signaling has been associated with multiple cancers, which leads to the important question of how Notch conveys its oncogenic potential. Identification of target genes and signaling pathways that are regulated by, or cooperate, with aberrant Notch signaling is an important field of investigation. Although the Notch signaling cascade seems surprisingly simple, it is likely that certain Notch-driven oncogenic events can be tumor-specific, while others may be shared between different neoplasms. In this regard, T-ALL is in one of the best-understood Notch-driven cancers. Therefore, we will summarize the genes and signaling pathways controlled by NOTCH1 that are implicated in T cell transformation. *c-Myc* has been identified by several labs as being one of the most important direct Notch target genes [67, 94, 117]. ChIP-on-chip analysis demonstrated that c-Myc and NICD share common target genes involved in the regulation of growth, metabolism, and proliferation. This led to the generation of a model depicting a feed-forward loop through which Notch and c-Myc reinforce the expression of genes required for the growth of leukemic cells [67]. Although early ChIP analysis suggested that Notch regulates c-Myc expression via its binding to the c-Myc promoter, subsequent ChIP sequencing studies showed that Notch appears to preferentially regulate gene expression through its dynamic interactions with superenhancers [112]. Notch controls c-Myc expression in both murine and human T-ALL cells by binding to a distal enhancer located more than 1 megabase 3′ of the murine and human *C-MYC* gene. The Notch-bound enhancer complex loops and physically interacts with the c-Myc promoter [40, 123]. Similarly, NOTCH1 was first shown to regulate the expression of the interleukin 7 receptor α-chain (IL-7Rα, a receptor tyrosine kinase) by directly binding to the human *IL7R* gene promoter [38]. Subsequent studies extended these findings further and revealed that Notch1 in coordination with Runx1 regulates a superenhancer located 3′ of the *IL7R* gene [112]. IL-7 signaling is essential for proliferation and survival of T cell progenitors, and its importance in the context of T-ALL is highlighted by the identification of oncogenic *IL7R* gain-of-function mutations in 10% of T-ALL cases [74, 96, 125, 128]. Insulin-like growth factor receptor-1 (IGF1R) is another receptor tyrosine kinase that has been shown to be directly controlled by NOTCH1 and to be important for T-ALL cell growth and for leukemia-initiating activity in vivo [60]. Activation of receptor tyrosine kinases often correlates with activated PI3K/Akt and increased mTOR signaling. This has also been observed in the context of Notch-driven T-ALL. Protein microarray screens identified the mTOR pathway as being positively regulated by Notch in T-ALL cells. Pharmacological inhibition of Notch in T-ALL cell lines induced hypophosphorylation of multiple signaling proteins involved in the mTOR pathway. How Notch activates the mTOR pathway is not completely understood. The effects of pharmacological Notch inhibition on mTOR signaling could be rescued by c-Myc expression suggesting that mTOR is possibly activated via the direct Notch target gene, *c-Myc* [13]. Alternatively, as suggested by studies in *Drosophila* and human T-ALL cell lines, the basic helix-loop-helix Notch target gene Hes1 has been shown to negatively regulate the expression of the tumor suppressor *PTEN*. PTEN counteracts PI3K activity and, thereby, negatively regulates Akt/mTOR signaling [68]. This particular study also linked mutational loss of *PTEN* in T-ALL cells to the acquisition of therapeutic resistance to NOTCH inhibitors [68]. Experimentally induced loss of PTEN expression accelerated disease onset in murine T-ALL models, suggesting that Notch1 activation and PTEN deficiency collaborate in disease onset or progression [59].

The importance of the transcriptional repressor Hes1 in T-ALL, which is one of the best-known Notch target genes, has been shown through conditional LoF experiments in murine T-ALL models as well as by gene knockdown studies in human T-ALL cell lines [93, 115]. Hes1 is required for the development and the maintenance of T-ALL in both mouse and human T-ALL cells. In addition, HES1 is known to be able repress *PTEN* expression and thereby contribute to increased Akt/mTOR signaling [68]. Furthermore, a more recent study revealed that HES1 is critically required for T-ALL tumor cell survival. Mechanistically, Hes1 appears to directly downregulate the expression of the *BCL2 binding component 3* (*BBC3*) gene in T-ALL cells, which encodes for the BH3-only pro-apoptotic factor, Puma [93]. Moreover, HES1 was also implicated in transcriptionally repressing the expression of the deubiquitinase CYLD, which negatively regulates the IKK complex, consequently leading to sustained NF-κB activation in T-ALL cells [30] [21]. CYLD functions as tumor suppressor in the skin, and LoF mutations in this gene have been identified in familial cylindromatosis [9]. The fact that (i) cylindromatosis patients do not have an increased risk of developing T-ALL and that (ii) CYLD mutations in T-ALL patients have currently not been described suggest that Notch signaling must be able to maintain strong NF-κB signaling at least in part through alternative mechanisms. Strong NF-κB signaling in Notch-driven T-ALL is characterized by nuclear localization of NF-κB, which is in part mediated by nuclear retention [95] resulting in the expression of NF-κB target genes including *Bcl-2A1*, *NF-κB2*, and *ICAM1*. Importantly, repression of NF-κB signaling in T-ALL cells inhibited cell growth both in vitro and in vivo [110].

NFAT signaling is another cascade known to be activated as a result of aberrant Notch signaling in T-ALL. High levels of Notch signaling induce the expression of calcineurin, which is a calcium-activated serine/threonine phosphatase. This phosphatase is important for the activation of NFAT transcription factors and for their translocation from the cytoplasm to the nucleus. Inhibitors of calcineurin such as cyclosporin A or FK506, which are used clinically as immunosuppressants, have been shown to induce cell death in T-ALL, leading to tumor regression and prolonged survival in murine T-ALL models.

Finally, aberrant Notch signaling has also been shown to directly regulate the expression of cell cycle proteins. Expression of G1 proteins such as cyclin D3, CDK4, and CDK6 is Notch-dependent in vitro and in vivo, and *CCND3* has been identified as a direct Notch target gene [45]. Cyclin D3-deficient mice exhibit greatly reduced susceptibility to Notch-induced leukemogenesis, and knockdown of cyclin D3 in human T-ALL cells inhibited their proliferation. The results indicate that cyclin D3 may be an essential cell cycle protein through which Notch can exert its oncogenic effects [97]. In agreement with the findings that Notch directly regulates the expression of cell cycle proteins, GSI-mediated inhibition of Notch signaling has been shown to lead to the upregulated expression of cyclin-dependent kinase inhibitors CDKN2B ($p19^{INK4d}$) and *CDKN1B* ($p27^{Kip1}$) in T-ALL cell lines [82]. Consistently, increased Notch signaling induces the transcriptional expression of S phase kinase-associated protein 2 (SKP2), an F-box protein that functions as a component of the E3-ligase complex. The E3-ligase complex functions to degrade

$p27^{Kip1}$ and $p21^{Cip1}$, thereby promoting the G1-S transition [91] [26]. Notch was also shown to suppress p53 through the repression of the ARF-mdm2-p53 surveillance network in mice. Attenuation of Notch signaling led to increased p53 expression and to tumor regression by inducing apoptosis. Inhibition of the mdm2-p53 interaction by the small molecule nutlin resulted in the stabilization of p53, leading to induction of cell death even in the presence of sustained Notch signaling. These findings provide a proof of principle for p53 being a potential therapeutic target in the context of Notch-driven T-ALL.

Although many of the herein described potential mediators of oncogenic Notch signaling may be specific to T-ALL, it is interesting to note that a Notch-c-Myc axis has also been described in the context of Notch-driven breast cancers [47, 87]. Whether this is a general hallmark of oncogenic Notch signaling awaits further investigation.

3.4 Changing Metabolism Is Part of the Oncogenic Notch Program

In recent years, it has become clear that intrinsic alterations in metabolism occur as a direct consequence of aberrant oncogenic signaling in cancer cells, as opposed to a passive response of damaged mitochondria [114]. Metabolic reprogramming is now an established hallmark of cancer [39]. Cancer cells tend to rely on glycolysis for energy production and anabolic growth, even if sufficient oxygen is available for oxidative phosphorylation, a phenomenon known as the Warburg effect. One of the main reasons for cancer cells to do so is that cell growth is dependent on the biosynthesis of cellular building blocks derived from metabolic intermediates that are largely generated via the glycolytic and tricarboxylic acid pathway [114].

One of the first studies linking Notch signaling to anabolic growth is derived from work on T cell progenitors which demonstrated that Notch regulates cell size, glucose uptake, and glycolysis through PI3K/Akt activation [18]. Subsequently, gene expression analysis of T-ALL cells revealed that NOTCH1 promotes leukemic cell growth through direct transcriptional regulation of anabolic genes involved in protein translation, ribosome biosynthesis, and nucleotide and amino acid metabolism. Similarly and equally important is the regulation of anabolic gene expression by the Notch target *C-MYC*. As a result, a Notch-Myc feed-forward loop has been proposed in which Notch functions as the driver of cell growth and anabolism in T-ALL [67, 117]. A recent study by Ferrando and colleagues using murine models and xenografted primary human T-ALL shows that leukemic cells harboring *NOTCH1* mutations utilize glutamine as their predominant carbon source, which is used to generate all tricarboxylic acid cycle intermediates. Pharmacological or genetic Notch inhibition results in a dramatic reduction in glutamine usage and triggers autophagy as a compensatory mechanism to support leukemic cell metabolism. Inhibition of glutaminolysis and autophagy synergistically enhanced the efficiency of therapeutic Notch inhibition in mice harboring T-ALL. Moreover, loss of PTEN resulted in increased glycolysis in targeted cells, rescuing the metabolism of leukemic cells that were treated with Notch inhibitors [41]. This study offers a possible explanation as to why the therapeutic response of T-ALL patients to pharmacological Notch inhibitors has been rather limited so far. Furthermore, it suggests that combining Notch inhibitors with drugs that target glutaminolysis and/or autophagy could be a more effective means for treatment of T-ALL. Since the Notch-MYC-AKT/mTOR axis is also conserved in other cancers, it is possible that metabolic reprogramming by Notch signaling may be a general mechanism by which Notch exerts its oncogenic properties.

3.5 Notch Functions as Tumor Suppressor

As outlined above, a highly context-dependent role of Notch signaling has been observed in a variety of blood-borne and solid tumors. Highlighted thus far were the oncogenic properties of Notch signaling and the possible molecular modes of action involved. In the subsequent sections, we will present and discuss tumor-suppressive functions of Notch signaling in various solid tumors (skin, head and neck, lung, bladder, and brain). The general aim of the following paragraphs is to highlight the most recent findings of Notch exerting its tumor-suppressive function in a variety of pathologies. We seek to highlight general paradigms and aim to put these into more a universal context of Notch acting as a tumor suppressor.

3.5.1 Notch Tumor Suppressor in the Skin: A General Paradigm

In vitro studies performed in the Dotto laboratory revealed a crucial physiological function of Notch1 in cutaneous epithelial cells [66, 81]. Here, Notch1 signaling induces growth arrest in keratinocytes as well as promotes early stages of differentiation. Therefore, Notch1 negatively regulates the proliferation of cutaneous epithelial progenitor cells and is essential for their terminal differentiation. The first conclusive evidence, however, showing that Notch acts as a tumor suppressor came from studies in the mouse skin, in which the loss of both *Notch1* alleles was shown to lead to the development of spontaneous basal cell carcinomas (BCC) in mice [63]. Additional LoF experiments unequivocally demonstrated a tumor-suppressive function of NOTCH signaling in the skin of both mice and humans [53, 75]. Although initial studies indicated that Notch1 functions as a tumor suppressor in a cell-autonomous manner, Kopan's group has highlighted a non-cell-autonomous mechanism in mice [23], supporting the notion that the carcinogenic effect is not solely dependent on cell intrinsic mechanisms driven downstream of Notch1 deficiency. In accordance with these findings, a more recent paper from Hu et al. showed that mesenchymal loss of RBP-J in the dermis was sufficient to induce inflammation and actinic keratosis, followed by the development of squamous cell carcinoma (SCC) in the overlying epidermis in aged mice [43]. Thus, defective Notch signaling in dermal fibroblasts was sufficient to induce a pro-tumorigenic microenvironment, thereby initiating carcinogenesis in the adjacent epidermis, with possible contributions by inflammatory cells recruited to tumor sites. It was further proposed that this could be due to the role of Notch in inhibiting AP1-mediated transcription of fibroblast growth factors, cytokines, proteases, and extracellular matrix proteins in dermal fibroblasts. In summary, the nonautonomous role of Notch signaling during cutaneous carcinogenesis may be coupled to its function in regulating dermal inflammation and/or barrier function of the epidermal epithelium [23, 43]. This has been shown to be a common paradigm in several epithelial malignancies creating a protumorigenic microenvironment (reviewed in Balkwill et al. [6], Balkwill and Mantovani [7], Mantovani et al. [55], and Solinas et al. [100]).

3.6 Notch Functions as a Tumor Suppressor in SCC

NOTCH1 also functions as a tumor suppressor in human non-melanoma skin cancers. Multiple components of the Notch signaling pathway, including NOTCH1, NOTCH2, and JAGGED1, are expressed at lower levels in human BCC samples compared to normal skin samples [107]. Additional evidence strengthening the role of NOTCH in human skin cancers came from the results of clinical trials employing semagacestat, a γ-secretase inhibitor, as a treatment for Alzheimer's disease. The trial revealed that treatment with this γ-secretase inhibitor was associated with an increased risk of developing skin cancer [31] (Fig. 3.2).

The tumor-suppressive role of Notch signaling is demonstrated most clearly in SCC. SCC, which causes >900,000 deaths worldwide per year, is an epidermal malignancy that occurs in tissues normally covered with stratified epithelium. SCC can arise in many different organs such as the head and neck, skin, esophagus, and lung [122]. SCCs, other than those in the skin, commonly metastasize, and survival rates have not improved in decades [20]. A better understanding of the underlying biology of SCC is only beginning to be elucidated but should be enhanced via the characterization of the molecular alterations inherent in these cells [1]. The transcriptional downregulation of Notch [53], with concomitant p53 mutations or LoF [119], is a causative event in human epithelial malignancies. In addition to the transcriptional downregulation, Notch receptor genes were also found to acquire recurrent LoF mutations. Wang et al. were the first to identify frequent somatic Notch LoF mutations in human cutaneous and lung SCCs. However, these aberrations occurred at a greater frequency in cutaneous SCCs than in lung SCCs. The detected mutations were found to cluster mainly in the extracellular EGF-like repeat region of *NOTCH1* and *NOTCH2* [113]. Utilizing cell-based assays, it was confirmed that these mutations represent LoF mutations. They cause receptor-

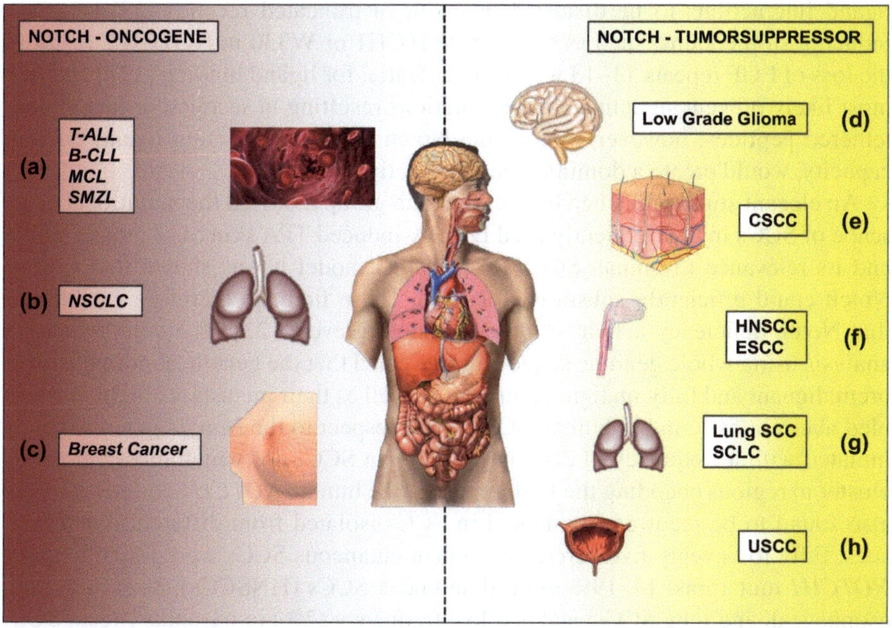

Fig. 3.2 Schematic representation of oncogenic or tumor-suppressive roles of NOTCH signaling associated with human cancers. The left side of the panel represents the major human tissues in which an *oncogenic* role for NOTCH has been described. (**a**) Weng et al. were the first to show that more than 50% of human pediatric T cell acute lymphoblastic leukemia (T-ALL) patient samples carry activating mutations in the *NOTCH1* gene [116]. Several studies [24, 32, 76, 77, 103] revealed also activating mutations in the *NOTCH1* gene in B cell chronic lymphocytic leukemia (B-CLL). *NOTCH1* mutations clustering in the PEST domain were associated with overall poor survival in mantle cell lymphoma (MCL) [51]. In splenic marginal zone lymphomas (SMZLs), next-generation sequencing identified mutations in *NOTCH2* to be more frequent than *NOTCH1*, and in both receptors, mutations clustered also mainly to the PEST domain [46, 69, 88]. (**b**) An additional oncogenic function of Notch signaling was identified in non-small cell lung carcinomas (NSCLCs) [57, 118]. (**c**) However, the first evidence that Notch signaling has an oncogenic function in solid tumors was found in breast cancer. Increased expression of NOTCH1 and JAGGED1 correlates with poor overall survival in women with advanced breast cancer, as well as reduced disease-free survival [84, 85]. On the other hand, lately several potentially *tumor-suppressive* functions of Notch signaling have been discovered in human malignancies. These are schematically highlighted on the right-side panel. (**d**) *NOTCH1* mutations have been identified in low-grade human gliomas [10], and Giachino et al. underscored the tumor-suppressive role of Notch in a mouse model [37]. (**e–g**) Notch signaling has a tumor suppressor in the skin, and its tumor-suppressive role is demonstrated most clearly in squamous cell carcinoma (SCC), and highlighted here are cutaneous (CSCC) [52, 54, 73, 102, 113], head and neck (HNSCC) [2, 106], esophageal (ESCC) [3, 35, 101], as well as lung SCC [113]. Most of these studies find potentially inactivating mutations in the *NOTCH1* and *NOTCH2* receptors, which are located predominantly in the EGF repeats (see text for details). (**g**) George et al. found, analyzing 110 human small cell lung carcinomas (SCLCs), that all four NOTCH receptors were affected with potentially inactivating mutations also clustering preferentially in the extracellular domains [36]. (**h**) NOTCH acting as a tumor suppressor in urothelial SCC (USCC), as has been shown by the groups of Real and Serrano [56] as well as by the Klinakis team [79], both using exome sequencing approaches followed by functional assays

ligand interactions to be distorted or result in truncated receptors. Truncations inducing stop codons, such as Q610 in NOTCH1 or W330 in NOTCH2, result in the loss of EGF repeats 11–13 which are essential for ligand binding [121] and will most likely prevent signaling. Other mutations resulting in secreted or membrane-tethered peptides, however, that enable Notch receptors to retain ligand-binding capacity, would create a dominant negative activity [83].

An elegant study published by the Blanpain group assessed the mutational landscape of SCCs in the frequently used DMBA-induced TPA skin SCC mouse model and its relevance to human SCCs [62]. In this model it was shown that LoF of Notch could efficiently substitute for TPA. These findings therefore established that Notch deficiency acts as a tumor-promoting event [23]. The comprehensive analysis using whole genome sequencing revealed that the genetic abnormalities in premalignant and fully malignant tumors, as well as their metastases highly resembled aberrations found in human SCCs. With respect to the *Notch1* gene, which is mutated with a frequency of 30% in mouse skin SCC – of which most mutations cluster to regions encoding the EGF repeats – the human *NOTCH1* counterpart was also found to be recurrently mutated in SCCs isolated from different human tissues. Fifty to Seventy five percent of human cutaneous SCCs were found to carry *NOTCH1* mutations, 14–19% in head and neck SCCs (HNSCCs); 8–16% in oral, esophageal, and lung SCCs; and at a low frequency (2%) in nasopharyngeal SCC. *Notch2* was found to be mutated at a low frequency of 7% in murine cutaneous SCC, whereas 31–63% of human skin SCC carried *NOTCH2* mutations. However, *NOTCH2* was mutated at much lower frequencies in HNSCC (5–9%), 6% in oral SCC, 2–4% in esophageal, and only 1% in nasopharyngeal and was absent in lung SCC. The frequently recurrent mutations detected in this study strongly correlated with previously identified NOTCH aberrations. Taken together, these findings not only validate the tumor-suppressive function of Notch in the murine skin [63] but also highlight the robust genomics approaches that will be essential to employ in order to define the mechanisms by which identified recurrently mutated genes in human cancers promote tumor initiation and/or progression.

Substantiating the study by the Cho laboratory [113], several groups recently confirmed that mutations affecting NOTCH signaling are frequently found in cutaneous SCC [52, 54, 73, 102]. A report published by South and colleagues involving whole-exome sequencing of 20 sporadic cutaneous SCC revealed an overall mean somatic mutation rate of 50 per megabase pair. The majority were C>T transitions, consistent with genetic changes found in UVR-induced DNA damage. Their findings confirm that mutations in *NOTCH1* and *NOTCH2* (frequency 82% combined) and *TP53* (63%) dominate this genetic landscape, with smaller contributions from *CDKN2A* (28%) and *RAS* family mutations (11%). Finally, the study showed that NOTCH1 expression levels were reduced in samples with Notch mutations, which is consistent with a LoF phenotype. This reduced expression pattern was even apparent in adjacent normal-appearing skin [102]. The authors concluded that NOTCH1 acts as a gatekeeper in human cutaneous SCC. The sample set was derived from a heterogeneous patient population including immunosuppressed individuals and included poorly differentiated tumors. Thus, NOTCH signaling was confirmed to be a major tumor-suppressive mechanism in this cancer, and its disruption is likely to be an early event occurring during the development of cutaneous SCC.

In addition, Pickering et al. [73] characterized somatic mutations in aggressive metastasizing cutaneous SCC and performed whole-exome sequencing on DNA from 39 patients. Six of the top mutated genes, detected in aggressive cutaneous SCC (*TP53*, *CDKN2A*, *NOTCH1*, *NOTCH2*, *HRAS*, and *FAT1*) in this study, were also reported by South and colleagues [102] in a cohort of 20 cutaneous SCCs (see above). Although two groups had previously reported high frequencies of both *NOTCH1* and *NOTCH2* mutations in cutaneous SCC [28, 102], Pickering et al. were able to demonstrate for the first time that both genes are significantly mutated in metastasizing cutaneous SCC [73]. Since conditional *Notch1* deficiency in the mouse skin predisposes animals to skin tumors [63], it is likely that Notch1 may play a similar role in cutaneous SCC. In contrast to Notch1, skin-specific deletion of *Notch2* in mice does not predispose to tumor development or any other apparent phenotype [27], suggesting that Notch2-mediated signaling is not predominant in murine skin. Loss of *Notch2* is compensated by other redundant Notch receptors in murine skin. However, the combined inactivation of *Notch1* and *Notch2* is known to lead to more severe defects in the differentiation of skin than loss of *Notch1* alone [23, 25, 27]. Thus, *NOTCH1* and *NOTCH2* signaling may both function as a barrier against carcinogenesis in some systems (human), whereas *Notch1* may be the primary barrier for other systems (mouse).

Recently, the Khavari laboratory added a study to the growing body of work on genome-level sequencing of cutaneous SCCs [52]. The authors confirmed findings that the *TP53* and *NOTCH1* genes are each mutated in approximately half of cutaneous SCCs and that *CDKN2A*, *NOTCH2*, and *HRAS* are also commonly mutated genes albeit at slightly lower frequencies. In addition, it is interesting to note that recurrent LoF mutations in NOTCH1/2 leading to a loss of tumor suppressor function occurred in the early stages of SCC carcinogenesis, in particular during actinic keratosis (precancerous stage of cutaneous SCC) and subsequently in invasive cutaneous SCC. Overall, these data sets attest to the tumor-suppressive functions of Notch signaling in normal human skin and that perturbation of the major signaling pathways in this tissue can lead to rapid expansion of preexisting tumor-initiating clonal populations, highlighting *NOTCH1* as a gatekeeper in squamous carcinogenesis of the skin.

NOTCH has also been recently attributed a tumor suppressor function in HNSCC. Agrawal et al., and Stransky et al. published two landmark studies on human HNSCC revealing inactivating mutations in *NOTCH1* and provided novel insights into the genetic basis underlying HNSCC [2, 106]. Both groups performed next-generation sequencing of the exons of all known human genes on tumor-derived DNA isolated from two distinct patient cohorts. The two groups analyzed a total of 32 [2] and 74 [106] tumor samples including tumors being either positive or negative for the human papillomavirus. Both groups independently identified *NOTCH1* mutations among other genetic aberrations previously identified as key players (*TP53, CDK2A, PIK3CA, PTEN, HRAS*) in HNSCC. In accordance with the findings from Nassar et al. [62], both studies reported inactivating mutations in

NOTCH1 in 10–15% of head and neck tumors, and it was the second most frequently mutated gene after *TP53* (mutated in 50–80% of tumors). In several tumors, both alleles harbored inactivating *NOTCH1* mutations. This finding in correlation with the observation that mice with a disrupted *Notch1* gene in the skin show a malignant phenotype [63, 75] provides strong evidence that *NOTCH1* has an important tumor suppressor function in HNSCC. Stransky et al. [106] also found mutations in other cell differentiation-related genes, such as *NOTCH2, NOTCH3*, and *TP63*, suggesting that deregulation of the terminal differentiation program of mucosal keratinocytes is critical for SCC development. *Oral* SCC is the most common subtype of HNSCC, and thus it is not surprising that mutations in *TP53, FAT1, HRAS, CASP8,* and *NOTCH1* are shared with other HNSCCs [19]. In oral SCC inactivating mutations of *NOTCH1* are also found in about 10–15% of the tumor samples analyzed (Caucasian patients) thus reflecting an equal mutational frequency found in all HNSCCs.

Whole-exome sequencing studies performed on patient cohorts from different ethnic backgrounds (Chinese and Caucasian) using *esophageal* SCC samples found *NOTCH1*, *NOTCH2*, or *NOTCH3* mutations to occur at a similar frequency in Chinese individuals (16–22%) [35, 101] as reported in US cases (28%) [3]. Thus, different ethnic populations reveal similar mutational frequencies in *NOTCH* receptor family genes in esophageal SCC.

In summary, all these observations would indicate that loss of Notch signaling activity is possibly a crucial event for the growth of tumor cells with epithelial squamous differentiation characteristics. Although high-throughput sequencing approaches can reveal many mutations in a large number of genes, this does not necessarily imply that all identified genes carry "driver mutations" causally related to the malignant transformation process. It is noteworthy though to mention here a study published by Martincorena et al. [58] that has led to a paradigm shift in the understanding of cutaneous SCC. Ultra-deep genome sequencing of normal eyelid skin was used to identify clones of cells carrying genes with attributed tumor suppressor activity. Martincorena et al. assessed 74 cancer genes in 234 biopsies isolated from the normal eyelid skin of 4 individuals. They confirmed a remarkably high frequency of somatic mutations in key genes, including *TP53*, *NOTCH1–3*, *FGFR3*, *FAT1*, and *RBM10*, and demonstrated tolerance to cancer-causing mutations in normal skin. Mutations in *NOTCH1* were especially frequent and found in up to 25% of normal keratinocytes and often occurred in conjunction with loss of heterozygosity, resulting in biallelic NOTCH1 inactivation. In 1 cm^2 of normal skin, the authors identified six clones each containing up to six driver mutations within a given cell. These findings could raise many questions about the mechanisms/gatekeepers that block progression to actinic keratosis and to invasive cutaneous SCC. It is widely assumed that driver mutations occur infrequently in long-lived lineages of rare subclones of cells [64] and that most arise in cancerous tissue that is too small to be clinically detectable. Therefore, the report by Martincorena et al. [58] overrode these assumptions and revealed that sun-exposed normal skin is already composed of a polyclonal mixture of driver mutations including NOTCH. Tumors have to be viewed as genetically unstable and acquiring many mutations including "passenger mutations" [99, 120] that occur during the progression, rather than in the initiation of the disease. Therefore scrutinizing functional studies in animal models are required to elucidate the exact role of the NOTCH receptors and other genes mutated in SCC. In conclusion, all of the abovementioned studies confirm the assumption by Nassar et al. [62] that extensive genomics studies in mice can provide a valuable resource to define genetic heterogeneity found in human cancers. However, it will be inevitable to define mechanisms by which certain genes such as *NOTCH1* and *NOTCH2* promote tumor initiation and progression. These mechanisms may be investigated in light of the Notch signaling cascade being highly context- and tissue-specific.

3.6.1 Dual Function of Notch in Lung Cancer

There are two major types of lung cancers: non-small cell lung cancers (*NSCLCs*) and small cell lung cancer (*SCLC*). *NSCLCs* account for about 85% of lung cancers, are strongly correlated with tobacco smoke, and can be further subdivided into the following three subtypes: (i) lung adenocarcinoma accounts for approximately 50% of all NSCLCs and is the most common form of lung cancer in the United States and arises predominantly in distal airways, (ii) SCC makes up 40% of NSCLCs and develops within the lining of the bronchial tubes (proximal airways), and (iii) large cell carcinomas referred to NSCLCs that are neither adenocarcinomas nor SCC [1, 22]. *SCLC* is an extremely aggressive malignancy and accounts for the remaining 15% of lung cancers in the United States. SCLC (i) occurs due to smoking at a higher frequency, (ii) grows more rapidly, and (iii) metastasizes earlier than NSCLC. However, it is also more responsive to chemotherapy. The role of the Notch signaling cascade in lung cancer is pleiotropic in terms of *tumor-suppressive* or *oncogenic* properties. Lung adenocarcinoma is the most frequent occurring NSCLC subtype, and Notch signaling has been accredited with tumor promoting effects in this malignancy although Notch-related alterations are rare (reviewed in Ntziachristos et al. [65]). The second major type of NSCLC is SCC, and the tumor-suppressive role of Notch in this malignancy has been outlined above. SCLC is a neuroendocrine subtype of lung cancer, and although it only accounts for a smaller fraction of all lung cancers (approximately 15%), it is the most malignant type of cancer. Although earlier studies have failed to identify recurrent mutations in genes of the Notch signaling cascade [72, 89], a report published by George and colleagues recently identified recurrent somatic mutations in NOTCH1, NOTCH2, NOTCH3, and NOTCH4 in tumor specimens of patients diagnosed with stage I–IV SCLC [36]. Although, previous studies already implicated a tumor-suppressive role for Notch activity in SCLC. There, it was shown that hyperactivation of Notch signaling blocks cell cycle progression of SCLC cell lines [104, 105]. It was however not until the comprehensive genomic sequencing of 110 human SCLC and additional murine samples conducted by George et al. that Notch mutations were unequivocally identified. Mutations affected Notch receptor family genes in both human (NOTCH1–4) and mouse (NOTCH3 only) SCLC, with NOTCH1 mutations occurring at a frequency of 20% in human patient tissue [36]. The mutations however did not cluster significantly in any specific domain, but a higher frequency of missense and nonsense mutations occurred in the extracellular domain. Overall, NOTCH family genes were genetically altered in 25% of human SCLC with NOTCH1 itself being most frequently affected. A functional role of Notch signaling in lung cancer was elegantly shown in a mouse model [61, 92] of lung cancer. Notch signaling may inhibit the expansion and/or differentiation of neuroendocrine cells and thereby counteracts the expansion of SCLC tumors [104, 111]. Constitutive overexpression of either Notch1 or Notch2 in a lung cancer mouse model [61, 92] led to a significant reduction in lung tumors, overall increased survival rate and seemed to block malignant progression in early tumor initiation phase. In addition, ectopic expression of N1ICD in murine and human SCLC cell lines was shown to lead to growth arrest. These studies provide the first functional analysis to identify and validate the role of Notch as a tumor suppressor in SCLC. Its function could be postulated as a key regulator of neuroendocrine differentiation.

3.7 Novel Tumor-Suppressive Roles for Notch Signaling Activity in Urothelial Cancers and Glioblastoma

As discussed above Notch signaling has a dual function acting either as an oncogene or a tumor suppressor in a highly context- and tissue-specific manner. The role of Notch signaling in other solid tumors, other than epithelial-derived, is less clear, and we would like to highlight only two other examples in which an undiscovered tumor-suppressive role was attributed to NOTCH – in *bladder cancer* and in *glioblastoma*.

Notch acts as a tumor suppressor in bladder cancer. Until recently, the role of Notch signaling in urothelial cancer (UC) remained unclear. However, lately studies were published, although with different emphasis and some divergence on the molecular and mechanistic details, and together revealed that the Notch signaling cascade is frequently inactivated in bladder cancer and exerts a tumor-suppressive role in this tissue [5, 56, 79].

The groups of Real and Serrano [56, 79], as well as the Klinakis team [79], employed exome sequencing approaches to identify somatic LoF mutations in NOTCH pathway components; in particular, *NOTCH1 and NOTCH2* genes were found to be frequently mutated. Rampias et al. [79] showed that tumors harboring NOTCH-inactivating mutations, either exclusively or in combination with *FGFR3* or *RAS* mutations, exhibited increased phosphorylation of ERK1/2, suggesting that NOTCH negatively regulates ERK1/2 activation. Consistent with this idea, activation of NOTCH signaling inhibited the proliferation of human bladder transitional carcinoma cell lines and led to reduced ERK1/2 phosphorylation via transcriptional induction of several DUSP, responsible for the dephosphorylation of ERK1/2.

Rampias et al. demonstrated that the expression of several members of the DUSP family is induced by active Notch signaling in UC cell lines [79]. Inactivation of Notch signaling results in diminished DUSP activity, thus leading to high levels of phospho-MAPK. Genetic inactivation of Notch signaling in mice promoted the development of high-grade invasive UCs characterized by high ERK1/2 phosphorylation and expression of basal cell markers, similar to the aggressive basal subtype of bladder cancer observed in humans. In contrast, the overexpression of activated NOTCH1 in UC cells reversed the cancer phenotype. Similarly, urothelium-specific loss of Notch signaling also resulted in the formation of bladder tumors exhibiting basal characteristics. These findings implicate loss of NOTCH signaling as a driver event in UC in mice and men. Although Maraver et al. [56] also concluded that the loss of tumor-suppressive activity of Notch via genetic inactivation occurs predominantly in UC with squamous features, they highlighted another consequence of LoF Notch function in UC. In a genetic LoF approach (using either tissue-specific conditional RBP-JKO or PsenKO animals), loss of Notch signaling accelerated UC tumorigenesis and promoted the formation of SCC with mesenchymal features. Notch signaling promoted the expression of the transcription factor Hes1, which prevents epithelial-mesenchymal transition (EMT). Moreover, evaluation of human bladder cancers revealed that tumors with low levels of HES1 exhibited greater EMT and invasive potential. In this context, it is interesting to note that HES1, being a transcriptional target of NOTCH, is responsible for the derepression of the EMT program in UC cells [56]. Taken together, their results also indicate that NOTCH serves as a tumor suppressor in the bladder. Therefore, inactivation of this pathway is likely to promote EMT in squamous bladder cancer cells.

A final exemplary discussion will be on the novel discovery for a role of *Notch signaling acting as a tumor suppressor in forebrain tumor subtypes* [37]. Gliomas are the most common malignancy in adult brain and have a very poor prognosis. Although Notch signaling, which is integral for neuronal stem cell (NSC) maintenance, has been suggested to play an oncogenic role in some brain tumors [14, 17], the role however of this pathway in glioma remains unclear. Giachino and colleagues [37] investigated the role of Notch signaling using mouse models of glioma. The tumor model was driven by platelet-derived growth factor (PDGF) expression and loss of *Trp53* (PDGF^{+}/*Trp53*$^{-/-}$) combined with a Hes5Cre^{ERT} mouse crossed to a Cre-inducible reporter line as a readout of activated Notch signaling. In early-stage PDGF^{+}/*Trp53*$^{-/-}$ gliomas, Hes5 was expressed in only a subpopulation of glioma cells. Targeted expression of PDGF and deletion of *Trp53* in Hes5^{+} Notch signaling cells resulted in glioma initiation. Surprisingly, loss of RBP-Jκ accelerated the growth of PDGF^{+}/*Trp53*$^{-/-}$ gliomas, which were mostly composed of HES5^{-} proliferating cells. Late-stage PDGF^{+}/*Trp53*$^{-/-}$/*Rbp-jκ*$^{-/-}$ gliomas exhibited features of poorly differentiated supratentorial primitive neuroectodermal tumors (sPNETs) and harbored proneural/mesenchymal glioblastoma gene signatures. In addition, co-deletion of *Rbp-j* and *Trp53* in quiescent NSCs induced the development of premalignant NSCs and highly penetrant sPNET-like tumors. In patients with proneural glioblastoma, *HES5* expression was inversely correlated with survival, and the expression of *HES5*, *RBP-j*, and the Notch-induced transcription factors, *HEY1* and *HEY2,* was associated with improved prognosis in grade II and III astrocytomas. In summary, these results strongly suggest that Notch signaling has a tumor suppressor function in grade II–III astrocytomas, proneural glioblastomas, and sPNETs.

It is noteworthy that NOTCH1 mutations, most likely inactivating, have been identified in low-grade human gliomas by exome sequencing [10]. Thus, the data provided by Giachino et al. [37] highlight the tumor-suppressive role of Notch in a cell-autonomous fashion in a genetic animal model and point to the feasibility of using Notch targets as biomarkers for patient prognosis and as potential treatment options.

3.8 Conclusions

Research of the last decade has emphasized the dual function of Notch in cancer. It can function as oncogene as well as tumor suppressor. The oncogenic function of Notch signaling is best understood in T-ALL, in which it is the most frequently mutated oncogene and where the availability of suitable mouse models has enabled us to gain deep insight in the molecular mechanisms underlying this disease. Next-generation sequencing has uncovered gain-of-function mutations of Notch genes in other malignancies including CLL, SMZL, Mantle cell lymphoma, and non-small cell lung cancer. Notch mutations in these malignancies often correlate with poor prognosis and occur more frequently in cases of acquired resistance to chemotherapy. This correlation infers that increased Notch signaling is involved in tumor progression or in escape to therapy. In many cases, whether these gain-of-function mutations are indeed causative and how they mechanistically contribute to tumor progression and/or to therapeutic resistance remains unknown and requires further investigation. Conversely, loss-of-function mutations have frequently been observed in cutaneous SSC, followed by head and neck SSCs, lung cancer, bladder cancer, and others indicating that Notch signaling has a tumor-suppressive function in these tissues. In agreement with this, Alzheimer patients that were treated in a phase III trial for a prolonged period of time with γ-secretase inhibitor in order to inhibit cleavage of the amyloid precursor protein and thereby the generation of the pathogenic peptides exhibited an increased incidence of skin cancer. Thus the dual function of Notch in cancer complicates the attempts to treat patients with blocking antibodies or drugs that suppress Notch signaling. It will be important to carefully select the patients as well as the indications in which blocking Notch therapeutics will be used. However, with increasing knowledge about mechanisms and the tissues in which Notch functions as an oncogene or as a tumor suppressor, combined with appropriate biomarkers, it should be possible to safely select the appropriate patients that would benefit from therapeutic Notch inhibition.

References

1. Agada, F. O., Patmore, H., Alhamarneh, O., Stafford, N. D., & Greenman, J. (2009). Genetic profile of head and neck squamous cell carcinoma: Clinical implications. *The Journal of Laryngology and Otology, 123*, 266–272.
2. Agrawal, N., Frederick, M. J., Pickering, C. R., Bettegowda, C., Chang, K., Li, R. J., Fakhry, C., Xie, T. X., Zhang, J., Wang, J., Zhang, N., El-Naggar, A. K., Jasser, S. A., Weinstein, J. N., Trevino, L., Drummond, J. A., Muzny, D. M., Wu, Y., Wood, L. D., Hruban, R. H., Westra, W. H., Koch, W. M., Califano, J. A., Gibbs, R. A., Sidransky, D., Vogelstein, B., Velculescu, V. E., Papadopoulos, N., Wheeler, D. A., Kinzler, K. W., & Myers, J. N. (2011). Exome sequencing of head and neck squamous cell carcinoma reveals inactivating mutations in NOTCH1. *Science, 333*, 1154–1157.
3. Agrawal, N., Jiao, Y., Bettegowda, C., Hutfless, S. M., Wang, Y., David, S., Cheng, Y., Twaddell, W. S., Latt, N. L., Shin, E. J., Wang, L. D., Wang, L., Yang, W., Velculescu, V. E., Vogelstein, B., Papadopoulos, N., Kinzler, K. W., & Meltzer, S. J. (2012). Comparative genomic analysis of esophageal adenocarcinoma and squamous cell carcinoma. *Cancer Discovery, 2*, 899–905.
4. Aster, J. C., Pear, W. S., & Blacklow, S. C. (2008). Notch signaling in leukemia. *Annual Review of Pathology, 3*, 587–613.
5. Balbas-Martinez, C., Sagrera, A., Carrillo-de-Santa-Pau, E., Earl, J., Marquez, M., Vazquez, M., Lapi, E., Castro-Giner, F., Beltran, S., Bayes, M., Carrato, A., Cigudosa, J. C., Dominguez, O., Gut, M., Herranz, J., Juanpere, N., Kogevinas, M., Langa, X., Lopez-Knowles, E., Lorente, J. A., Lloreta, J., Pisano, D. G., Richart, L., Rico, D., Salgado, R. N., Tardon, A., Chanock, S., Heath, S., Valencia, A., Losada, A., Gut, I., Malats, N., & Real, F. X. (2013). Recurrent inactivation of STAG2 in bladder cancer is not associated with aneuploidy. *Nature Genetics, 45*, 1464–1469.
6. Balkwill, F., Charles, K. A., & Mantovani, A. (2005). Smoldering and polarized inflammation in the initiation and promotion of malignant disease. *Cancer Cell, 7*, 211–217.
7. Balkwill, F. R., & Mantovani, A. (2012). Cancer-related inflammation: Common themes and therapeutic opportunities. *Seminars in Cancer Biology, 22*, 33–40.
8. Baumgart, A., Mazur, P. K., Anton, M., Rudelius, M., Schwamborn, K., Feuchtinger, A., Behnke, K., Walch, A., Braren, R., Peschel, C., Duyster, J., Siveke, J. T., & Dechow, T. (2015). Opposing role of Notch1 and Notch2 in a Kras(G12D)-driven murine non-small cell lung cancer model. *Oncogene, 34*, 578–588.
9. Bignell, G. R., Warren, W., Seal, S., Takahashi, M., Rapley, E., Barfoot, R., Green, H., Brown, C., Biggs, P. J., Lakhani, S. R., Jones, C., Hansen, J., Blair, E., Hofmann, B., Siebert, R., Turner, G., Evans, D. G., Schrander-Stumpel, C., Beemer, F. A., van Den Ouweland, A., Halley, D., Delpech, B., Cleveland, M. G., Leigh, I., Leisti, J., & Rasmussen, S. (2000). Identification of the familial cylindromatosis tumour-suppressor gene. *Nature Genetics, 25*, 160–165.
10. Brat, D. J., Verhaak, R. G., Aldape, K. D., Yung, W. K., Salama, S. R., Cooper, L. A., Rheinbay, E., Miller, C. R., Vitucci, M., Morozova, O., Robertson, A. G., Noushmehr, H., Laird, P. W., Cherniack, A. D., Akbani, R., Huse, J. T., Ciriello, G., Poisson, L. M., Barnholtz-Sloan, J. S., Berger, M. S., Brennan, C., Colen, R. R., Colman, H., Flanders, A. E., Giannini, C., Grifford, M., Iavarone, A., Jain, R., Joseph, I., Kim, J., Kasaian, K., Mikkelsen, T., Murray, B. A., O'Neill, B. P., Pachter, L., Parsons, D. W., Sougnez, C., Sulman, E. P., Vandenberg, S. R., Van Meir, E. G., von Deimling, A., Zhang, H., Crain, D., Lau, K., Mallery, D., Morris, S., Paulauskis, J., Penny, R., Shelton, T., Sherman, M., Yena, P., Black, A., Bowen, J., Dicostanzo, K., Gastier-Foster, J., Leraas, K. M., Lichtenberg, T. M., Pierson, C. R., Ramirez, N. C., Taylor, C., Weaver, S., Wise, L., Zmuda, E., Davidsen, T., Demchok, J. A., Eley, G., Ferguson, M. L., Hutter, C. M., Mills Shaw, K. R., Ozenberger, B. A., Sheth, M., Sofia, H. J., Tarnuzzer, R., Wang, Z., Yang, L., Zenklusen, J. C., Ayala, B., Baboud, J., Chudamani, S., Jensen, M. A., Liu, J., Pihl, T., Raman, R., Wan, Y., Wu, Y., Ally, A., Auman, J. T., Balasundaram, M., Balu,

S., Baylin, S. B., Beroukhim, R., Bootwalla, M. S., Bowlby, R., Bristow, C. A., Brooks, D., Butterfield, Y., Carlsen, R., Carter, S., Chin, L., Chu, A., Chuah, E., Cibulskis, K., Clarke, A., Coetzee, S. G., Dhalla, N., Fennell, T., Fisher, S., Gabriel, S., Getz, G., Gibbs, R., Guin, R., Hadjipanayis, A., Hayes, D. N., Hinoue, T., Hoadley, K., Holt, R. A., Hoyle, A. P., Jefferys, S. R., Jones, S., Jones, C. D., Kucherlapati, R., Lai, P. H., Lander, E., Lee, S., Lichtenstein, L., Ma, Y., Maglinte, D. T., Mahadeshwar, H. S., Marra, M. A., Mayo, M., Meng, S., Meyerson, M. L., Mieczkowski, P. A., Moore, R. A., Mose, L. E., Mungall, A. J., Pantazi, A., Parfenov, M., Park, P. J., Parker, J. S., Perou, C. M., Protopopov, A., Ren, X., Roach, J., Sabedot, T. S., Schein, J., Schumacher, S. E., Seidman, J. G., Seth, S., Shen, H., Simons, J. V., Sipahimalani, P., Soloway, M. G., Song, X., Sun, H., Tabak, B., Tam, A., Tan, D., Tang, J., Thiessen, N., Triche, T., Jr., Van Den Berg, D. J., Veluvolu, U., Waring, S., Weisenberger, D. J., Wilkerson, M. D., Wong, T., Wu, J., Xi, L., Xu, A. W., Zack, T. I., Zhang, J., Aksoy, B. A., Arachchi, H., Benz, C., Bernard, B., Carlin, D., Cho, J., DiCara, D., Frazer, S., Fuller, G. N., Gao, J., Gehlenborg, N., Haussler, D., Heiman, D. I., Iype, L., Jacobsen, A., Ju, Z., Katzman, S., Kim, H., Knijnenburg, T., Kreisberg, R. B., Lawrence, M. S., Lee, W., Leinonen, K., Lin, P., Ling, S., Liu, W., Liu, Y., Lu, Y., Mills, G., Ng, S., Noble, M. S., Paull, E., Rao, A., Reynolds, S., Saksena, G., Sanborn, Z., Sander, C., Schultz, N., Senbabaoglu, Y., Shen, R., Shmulevich, I., Sinha, R., Stuart, J., Sumer, S. O., Sun, Y., Tasman, N., Taylor, B. S., Voet, D., Weinhold, N., Weinstein, J. N., Yang, D., Yoshihara, K., Zheng, S., Zhang, W., Zou, L., Abel, T., Sadeghi, S., Cohen, M. L., Eschbacher, J., Hattab, E. M., Raghunathan, A., Schniederjan, M. J., Aziz, D., Barnett, G., Barrett, W., Bigner, D. D., Boice, L., Brewer, C., Calatozzolo, C., Campos, B., Carlotti, C. G., Jr., Chan, T. A., Cuppini, L., Curley, E., Cuzzubbo, S., Devine, K., DiMeco, F., Duell, R., Elder, J. B., Fehrenbach, A., Finocchiaro, G., Friedman, W., Fulop, J., Gardner, J., Hermes, B., Herold-Mende, C., Jungk, C., Kendler, A., Lehman, N. L., Lipp, E., Liu, O., Mandt, R., McGraw, M., McLendon, R., McPherson, C., Neder, L., Nguyen, P., Noss, A., Nunziata, R., Ostrom, Q. T., Palmer, C., Perin, A., Pollo, B., Potapov, A., Potapova, O., Rathmell, W. K., Rotin, D., Scarpace, L., Schilero, C., Senecal, K., Shimmel, K., Shurkhay, V., Sifri, S., Singh, R., Sloan, A. E., Smolenski, K., Staugaitis, S. M., Steele, R., Thorne, L., Tirapelli, D. P., Unterberg, A., Vallurupalli, M., Wang, Y., Warnick, R., Williams, F., Wolinsky, Y., Bell, S., Rosenberg, M., Stewart, C., Huang, F., Grimsby, J. L., & Radenbaugh, A. J. (2015). Comprehensive, integrative genomic analysis of diffuse lower-grade gliomas. *The New England Journal of Medicine, 372*, 2481–2498.

11. Bray, S. J. (2006). Notch signalling: A simple pathway becomes complex. *Nature Reviews. Molecular Cell Biology, 7*, 678–689.
12. Capobianco, A. J., Zagouras, P., Blaumueller, C. M., Artavanis-Tsakonas, S., & Bishop, J. M. (1997). Neoplastic transformation by truncated alleles of human NOTCH1/TAN1 and NOTCH2. *Molecular and Cellular Biology, 17*, 6265–6273.
13. Chan, S. M., Weng, A. P., Tibshirani, R., Aster, J. C., & Utz, P. J. (2007). Notch signals positively regulate activity of the mTOR pathway in T-cell acute lymphoblastic leukemia. *Blood, 110*, 278–286.
14. Charles, N., Ozawa, T., Squatrito, M., Bleau, A. M., Brennan, C. W., Hambardzumyan, D., & Holland, E. C. (2010). Perivascular nitric oxide activates notch signaling and promotes stem-like character in PDGF-induced glioma cells. *Cell Stem Cell, 6*, 141–152.
15. Chiang, M. Y., Xu, L., Shestova, O., Histen, G., L'Heureux, S., Romany, C., Childs, M. E., Gimotty, P. A., Aster, J. C., & Pear, W. S. (2008). Leukemia-associated NOTCH1 alleles are weak tumor initiators but accelerate K-ras-initiated leukemia. *The Journal of Clinical Investigation, 118*, 3181–3194.
16. Chiang, M. Y., Xu, M. L., Histen, G., Shestova, O., Roy, M., Nam, Y., Blacklow, S. C., Sacks, D. B., Pear, W. S., & Aster, J. C. (2006). Identification of a conserved negative regulatory sequence that influences the leukemogenic activity of NOTCH1. *Molecular and Cellular Biology, 26*, 6261–6271.
17. Chu, Q., Orr, B. A., Semenkow, S., Bar, E. E., & Eberhart, C. G. (2013). Prolonged inhibition of glioblastoma xenograft initiation and clonogenic growth following in vivo Notch blockade. *Clinical Cancer Research, 19*, 3224–3233.

18. Ciofani, M., & Zuniga-Pflucker, J. C. (2005). Notch promotes survival of pre-T cells at the beta-selection checkpoint by regulating cellular metabolism. *Nature Immunology, 6*, 881–888.
19. India Project Team of the International Cancer Genome Consortium. (2013). Mutational landscape of gingivo-buccal oral squamous cell carcinoma reveals new recurrently-mutated genes and molecular subgroups. *Nature Communications, 4*, 2873.
20. Czarnecki, D., Staples, M., Mar, A., Giles, G., & Meehan, C. (1994). Metastases from squamous cell carcinoma of the skin in southern Australia. *Dermatology, 189*, 52–54.
21. D'Altri, T., Gonzalez, J., Aifantis, I., Espinosa, L., & Bigas, A. (2011). Hes1 expression and CYLD repression are essential events downstream of Notch1 in T-cell leukemia. *Cell Cycle, 10*, 1031–1036.
22. Davidson, M. R., Gazdar, A. F., & Clarke, B. E. (2013). The pivotal role of pathology in the management of lung cancer. *Journal of Thoracic Disease, 5*(Suppl 5), S463–S478.
23. Demehri, S., Turkoz, A., & Kopan, R. (2009). Epidermal Notch1 loss promotes skin tumorigenesis by impacting the stromal microenvironment. *Cancer Cell, 16*, 55–66.
24. Di Ianni, M., Baldoni, S., Rosati, E., Ciurnelli, R., Cavalli, L., Martelli, M. F., Marconi, P., Screpanti, I., & Falzetti, F. (2009). A new genetic lesion in B-CLL: A NOTCH1 PEST domain mutation. *British Journal of Haematology, 146*, 689–691.
25. Di Piazza, M., Nowell, C. S., Koch, U., Durham, A. D., & Radtke, F. (2012). Loss of cutaneous TSLP-dependent immune responses skews the balance of inflammation from tumor protective to tumor promoting. *Cancer Cell, 22*, 479–493.
26. Dohda, T., Maljukova, A., Liu, L., Heyman, M., Grander, D., Brodin, D., Sangfelt, O., & Lendahl, U. (2007). Notch signaling induces SKP2 expression and promotes reduction of p27Kip1 in T-cell acute lymphoblastic leukemia cell lines. *Experimental Cell Research, 313*, 3141–3152.
27. Dumortier, A., Durham, A. D., Di Piazza, M., Vauclair, S., Koch, U., Ferrand, G., Ferrero, I., Demehri, S., Song, L. L., Farr, A. G., Leonard, W. J., Kopan, R., Miele, L., Hohl, D., Finke, D., & Radtke, F. (2010). Atopic dermatitis-like disease and associated lethal myeloproliferative disorder arise from loss of Notch signaling in the murine skin. *PLoS One, 5*, e9258.
28. Durinck, S., Ho, C., Wang, N. J., Liao, W., Jakkula, L. R., Collisson, E. A., Pons, J., Chan, S. W., Lam, E. T., Chu, C., Park, K., Hong, S. W., Hur, J. S., Huh, N., Neuhaus, I. M., Yu, S. S., Grekin, R. C., Mauro, T. M., Cleaver, J. E., Kwok, P. Y., LeBoit, P. E., Getz, G., Cibulskis, K., Aster, J. C., Huang, H., Purdom, E., Li, J., Bolund, L., Arron, S. T., Gray, J. W., Spellman, P. T., & Cho, R. J. (2011). Temporal dissection of tumorigenesis in primary cancers. *Cancer Discovery, 1*, 137–143.
29. Ellisen, L. W., Bird, J., West, D. C., Soreng, A. L., Reynolds, T. C., Smith, S. D., & Sklar, J. (1991). TAN-1, the human homolog of the Drosophila notch gene, is broken by chromosomal translocations in T lymphoblastic neoplasms. *Cell, 66*, 649–661.
30. Espinosa, L., Cathelin, S., D'Altri, T., Trimarchi, T., Statnikov, A., Guiu, J., Rodilla, V., Ingles-Esteve, J., Nomdedeu, J., Bellosillo, B., Besses, C., Abdel-Wahab, O., Kucine, N., Sun, S. C., Song, G., Mullighan, C. C., Levine, R. L., Rajewsky, K., Aifantis, I., & Bigas, A. (2010). The Notch/Hes1 pathway sustains NF-kappaB activation through CYLD repression in T cell leukemia. *Cancer Cell, 18*, 268–281.
31. Doody, R. S., Raman, R., Farlow, M., Iwatsubo, T., Vellas, B., Joffe, S., Kieburtz, K., He, F., Sun, X., Thomas, R. G., Aisen, P. S., Siemers, E., Sethuraman, G., Mohs, R., Semagacestat Study Group (2013). A phase 3 trial of semagacestat for treatment of Alzheimer's disease. *The New England Journal of Medicine, 369*(4), 341–350. https://doi.org/10.1056/NEJMoa1210951
32. Fabbri, G., Rasi, S., Rossi, D., Trifonov, V., Khiabanian, H., Ma, J., Grunn, A., Fangazio, M., Capello, D., Monti, S., Cresta, S., Gargiulo, E., Forconi, F., Guarini, A., Arcaini, L., Paulli, M., Laurenti, L., Larocca, L. M., Marasca, R., Gattei, V., Oscier, D., Bertoni, F., Mullighan, C. G., Foa, R., Pasqualucci, L., Rabadan, R., Dalla-Favera, R., & Gaidano, G. (2011). Analysis of the chronic lymphocytic leukemia coding genome: Role of NOTCH1 mutational activation. *The Journal of Experimental Medicine, 208*, 1389–1401.

33. Gallahan, D., Jhappan, C., Robinson, G., Hennighausen, L., Sharp, R., Kordon, E., Callahan, R., Merlino, G., & Smith, G. H. (1996). Expression of a truncated Int3 gene in developing secretory mammary epithelium specifically retards lobular differentiation resulting in tumorigenesis. *Cancer Research, 56*, 1775–1785.
34. Gallahan, D., Kozak, C., & Callahan, R. (1987). A new common integration region (int-3) for mouse mammary tumor virus on mouse chromosome 17. *Journal of Virology, 61*, 218–220.
35. Gao, Y. B., Chen, Z. L., Li, J. G., Hu, X. D., Shi, X. J., Sun, Z. M., Zhang, F., Zhao, Z. R., Li, Z. T., Liu, Z. Y., Zhao, Y. D., Sun, J., Zhou, C. C., Yao, R., Wang, S. Y., Wang, P., Sun, N., Zhang, B. H., Dong, J. S., Yu, Y., Luo, M., Feng, X. L., Shi, S. S., Zhou, F., Tan, F. W., Qiu, B., Li, N., Shao, K., Zhang, L. J., Xue, Q., Gao, S. G., & He, J. (2014). Genetic landscape of esophageal squamous cell carcinoma. *Nature Genetics, 46*, 1097–1102.
36. George, J., Lim, J. S., Jang, S. J., Cun, Y., Ozretic, L., Kong, G., Leenders, F., Lu, X., Fernandez-Cuesta, L., Bosco, G., Muller, C., Dahmen, I., Jahchan, N. S., Park, K. S., Yang, D., Karnezis, A. N., Vaka, D., Torres, A., Wang, M. S., Korbel, J. O., Menon, R., Chun, S. M., Kim, D., Wilkerson, M., Hayes, N., Engelmann, D., Putzer, B., Bos, M., Michels, S., Vlasic, I., Seidel, D., Pinther, B., Schaub, P., Becker, C., Altmuller, J., Yokota, J., Kohno, T., Iwakawa, R., Tsuta, K., Noguchi, M., Muley, T., Hoffmann, H., Schnabel, P. A., Petersen, I., Chen, Y., Soltermann, A., Tischler, V., Choi, C. M., Kim, Y. H., Massion, P. P., Zou, Y., Jovanovic, D., Kontic, M., Wright, G. M., Russell, P. A., Solomon, B., Koch, I., Lindner, M., Muscarella, L. A., la Torre, A., Field, J. K., Jakopovic, M., Knezevic, J., Castanos-Velez, E., Roz, L., Pastorino, U., Brustugun, O. T., Lund-Iversen, M., Thunnissen, E., Kohler, J., Schuler, M., Botling, J., Sandelin, M., Sanchez-Cespedes, M., Salvesen, H. B., Achter, V., Lang, U., Bogus, M., Schneider, P. M., Zander, T., Ansen, S., Hallek, M., Wolf, J., Vingron, M., Yatabe, Y., Travis, W. D., Nurnberg, P., Reinhardt, C., Perner, S., Heukamp, L., Buttner, R., Haas, S. A., Brambilla, E., Peifer, M., Sage, J., & Thomas, R. K. (2015). Comprehensive genomic profiles of small cell lung cancer. *Nature, 524*, 47–53.
37. Giachino, C., Boulay, J. L., Ivanek, R., Alvarado, A., Tostado, C., Lugert, S., Tchorz, J., Coban, M., Mariani, L., Bettler, B., Lathia, J., Frank, S., Pfister, S., Kool, M., & Taylor, V. (2015). A tumor suppressor function for Notch signaling in forebrain tumor subtypes. *Cancer Cell, 28*, 730–742.
38. Gonzalez-Garcia, S., Garcia-Peydro, M., Martin-Gayo, E., Ballestar, E., Esteller, M., Bornstein, R., de la Pompa, J. L., Ferrando, A. A., & Toribio, M. L. (2009). CSL-MAML-dependent Notch1 signaling controls T lineage-specific IL-7R{alpha} gene expression in early human thymopoiesis and leukemia. *The Journal of Experimental Medicine, 206*, 779–791.
39. Hanahan, D., & Weinberg, R. A. (2011). Hallmarks of cancer: The next generation. *Cell, 144*, 646–674.
40. Herranz, D., Ambesi-Impiombato, A., Palomero, T., Schnell, S. A., Belver, L., Wendorff, A. A., Xu, L., Castillo-Martin, M., Llobet-Navas, D., Cordon-Cardo, C., Clappier, E., Soulier, J., & Ferrando, A. A. (2014). A NOTCH1-driven MYC enhancer promotes T cell development, transformation and acute lymphoblastic leukemia. *Nature Medicine, 20*, 1130–1137.
41. Herranz, D., Ambesi-Impiombato, A., Sudderth, J., Sanchez-Martin, M., Belver, L., Tosello, V., Xu, L., Wendorff, A. A., Castillo, M., Haydu, J. E., Marquez, J., Mates, J. M., Kung, A. L., Rayport, S., Cordon-Cardo, C., DeBerardinis, R. J., & Ferrando, A. A. (2015). Metabolic reprogramming induces resistance to anti-NOTCH1 therapies in T cell acute lymphoblastic leukemia. *Nature Medicine, 21*, 1182–1189.
42. Hozumi, K., Negishi, N., Suzuki, D., Abe, N., Sotomaru, Y., Tamaoki, N., Mailhos, C., Ish-Horowicz, D., Habu, S., & Owen, M. J. (2004). Delta-like 1 is necessary for the generation of marginal zone B cells but not T cells in vivo. *Nature Immunology, 5*, 638–644.
43. Hu, B., Castillo, E., Harewood, L., Ostano, P., Reymond, A., Dummer, R., Raffoul, W., Hoetzenecker, W., Hofbauer, G. F., & Dotto, G. P. (2012). Multifocal epithelial tumors and field cancerization from loss of mesenchymal CSL signaling. *Cell, 149*, 1207–1220.
44. Jhappan, C., Gallahan, D., Stahle, C., Chu, E., Smith, G. H., Merlino, G., & Callahan, R. (1992). Expression of an activated Notch-related int-3 transgene interferes with cell differ-

entiation and induces neoplastic transformation in mammary and salivary glands. *Genes & Development, 6*, 345–355.
45. Joshi, I., Minter, L., Telfer, J., Demarest, R., Capobianco, A., Aster, J., Sicinski, P., Fauq, A., Golde, T., & Osborne, B. (2008). Notch signaling mediates G1/S cell cycle progression in T cells via cyclin D3 and its dependent kinases. *Blood, 113*(8), 1689–1698.
46. Kiel, M. J., Velusamy, T., Betz, B. L., Zhao, L., Weigelin, H. G., Chiang, M. Y., Huebner-Chan, D. R., Bailey, N. G., Yang, D. T., Bhagat, G., Miranda, R. N., Bahler, D. W., Medeiros, L. J., Lim, M. S., & Elenitoba-Johnson, K. S. (2012). Whole-genome sequencing identifies recurrent somatic NOTCH2 mutations in splenic marginal zone lymphoma. *The Journal of Experimental Medicine, 209*, 1553–1565.
47. Klinakis, A., Szabolcs, M., Politi, K., Kiaris, H., Artavanis-Tsakonas, S., & Efstratiadis, A. (2006). Myc is a Notch1 transcriptional target and a requisite for Notch1-induced mammary tumorigenesis in mice. *Proceedings of the National Academy of Sciences of the United States of America, 103*, 9262–9267.
48. Koch, U., Lehal, R., & Radtke, F. (2013). Stem cells living with a Notch. *Development, 140*, 689–704.
49. Koch, U., & Radtke, F. (2010). Notch signaling in solid tumors. *Current Topics in Developmental Biology, 92*, 411–455.
50. Kopan, R., & Ilagan, M. X. G. (2009). The canonical Notch signaling pathway: Unfolding the activation mechanism. *Cell, 137*, 216–233.
51. Kridel, R., Meissner, B., Rogic, S., Boyle, M., Telenius, A., Woolcock, B., Gunawardana, J., Jenkins, C., Cochrane, C., Ben-Neriah, S., Tan, K., Morin, R. D., Opat, S., Sehn, L. H., Connors, J. M., Marra, M. A., Weng, A. P., Steidl, C., & Gascoyne, R. D. (2012). Whole transcriptome sequencing reveals recurrent NOTCH1 mutations in mantle cell lymphoma. *Blood, 119*, 1963–1971.
52. Lee, C. S., Bhaduri, A., Mah, A., Johnson, W. L., Ungewickell, A., Aros, C. J., Nguyen, C. B., Rios, E. J., Siprashvili, Z., Straight, A., Kim, J., Aasi, S. Z., & Khavari, P. A. (2014). Recurrent point mutations in the kinetochore gene KNSTRN in cutaneous squamous cell carcinoma. *Nature Genetics, 46*, 1060–1062.
53. Lefort, K., Mandinova, A., Ostano, P., Kolev, V., Calpini, V., Kolfschoten, I., Devgan, V., Lieb, J., Raffoul, W., Hohl, D., Neel, V., Garlick, J., Chiorino, G., & Dotto, G. P. (2007). Notch1 is a p53 target gene involved in human keratinocyte tumor suppression through negative regulation of ROCK1/2 and MRCKalpha kinases. *Genes & Development, 21*, 562–577.
54. Li, Y. Y., Hanna, G. J., Laga, A. C., Haddad, R. I., Lorch, J. H., & Hammerman, P. S. (2015). Genomic analysis of metastatic cutaneous squamous cell carcinoma. *Clinical Cancer Research, 21*, 1447–1456.
55. Mantovani, A., Allavena, P., Sica, A., & Balkwill, F. (2008). Cancer-related inflammation. *Nature, 454*, 436–444.
56. Maraver, A., Fernandez-Marcos, P. J., Cash, T. P., Mendez-Pertuz, M., Duenas, M., Maietta, P., Martinelli, P., Munoz-Martin, M., Martinez-Fernandez, M., Canamero, M., Roncador, G., Martinez-Torrecuadrada, J. L., Grivas, D., de la Pompa, J. L., Valencia, A., Paramio, J. M., Real, F. X., & Serrano, M. (2015). NOTCH pathway inactivation promotes bladder cancer progression. *The Journal of Clinical Investigation, 125*, 824–830.
57. Maraver, A., Fernandez-Marcos, P. J., Herranz, D., Canamero, M., Munoz-Martin, M., Gomez-Lopez, G., Mulero, F., Megias, D., Sanchez-Carbayo, M., Shen, J., Sanchez-Cespedes, M., Palomero, T., Ferrando, A., & Serrano, M. (2012). Therapeutic effect of gamma-secretase inhibition in KrasG12V-driven non-small cell lung carcinoma by derepression of DUSP1 and inhibition of ERK. *Cancer Cell, 22*, 222–234.
58. Martincorena, I., Roshan, A., Gerstung, M., Ellis, P., Van Loo, P., McLaren, S., Wedge, D. C., Fullam, A., Alexandrov, L. B., Tubio, J. M., Stebbings, L., Menzies, A., Widaa, S., Stratton, M. R., Jones, P. H., & Campbell, P. J. (2015). Tumor evolution. High burden and pervasive positive selection of somatic mutations in normal human skin. *Science, 348*, 880–886.
59. Medyouf, H., Gao, X., Armstrong, F., Gusscott, S., Liu, Q., Larson Gedman, A., Matherly, L. H., Schultz, K. R., Pflumio, F., You, M. J., & Weng, A. P. (2009). Acute T-cell leukemias

remain dependent on Notch signaling despite PTEN and INK4A/ARF loss. *Blood, 115*(6), 1175–1184.

60. Medyouf, H., Gusscott, S., Wang, H., Tseng, J. C., Wai, C., Nemirovsky, O., Trumpp, A., Pflumio, F., Carboni, J., Gottardis, M., Pollak, M., Kung, A. L., Aster, J. C., Holzenberger, M., & Weng, A. P. (2011). High-level IGF1R expression is required for leukemia-initiating cell activity in T-ALL and is supported by Notch signaling. *The Journal of Experimental Medicine, 208*, 1809–1822.
61. Meuwissen, R., Linn, S. C., Linnoila, R. I., Zevenhoven, J., Mooi, W. J., & Berns, A. (2003). Induction of small cell lung cancer by somatic inactivation of both Trp53 and Rb1 in a conditional mouse model. *Cancer Cell, 4*, 181–189.
62. Nassar, D., Latil, M., Boeckx, B., Lambrechts, D., & Blanpain, C. (2015). Genomic landscape of carcinogen-induced and genetically induced mouse skin squamous cell carcinoma. *Nature Medicine, 21*, 946–954.
63. Nicolas, M., Wolfer, A., Raj, K., Kummer, J. A., Mill, P., van Noort, M., Hui, C. C., Clevers, H., Dotto, G. P., & Radtke, F. (2003). Notch1 functions as a tumor suppressor in mouse skin. *Nature Genetics, 33*, 416–421.
64. Nik-Zainal, S., Van Loo, P., Wedge, D. C., Alexandrov, L. B., Greenman, C. D., Lau, K. W., Raine, K., Jones, D., Marshall, J., Ramakrishna, M., Shlien, A., Cooke, S. L., Hinton, J., Menzies, A., Stebbings, L. A., Leroy, C., Jia, M., Rance, R., Mudie, L. J., Gamble, S. J., Stephens, P. J., McLaren, S., Tarpey, P. S., Papaemmanuil, E., Davies, H. R., Varela, I., McBride, D. J., Bignell, G. R., Leung, K., Butler, A. P., Teague, J. W., Martin, S., Jonsson, G., Mariani, O., Boyault, S., Miron, P., Fatima, A., Langerod, A., Aparicio, S. A., Tutt, A., Sieuwerts, A. M., Borg, A., Thomas, G., Salomon, A. V., Richardson, A. L., Borresen-Dale, A. L., Futreal, P. A., Stratton, M. R., & Campbell, P. J. (2012). The life history of 21 breast cancers. *Cell, 149*, 994–1007.
65. Ntziachristos, P., Lim, J. S., Sage, J., & Aifantis, I. (2014). From fly wings to targeted cancer therapies: A centennial for notch signaling. *Cancer Cell, 25*, 318–334.
66. Okuyama, R., Nguyen, B. C., Talora, C., Ogawa, E., Tommasi di Vignano, A., Lioumi, M., Chiorino, G., Tagami, H., Woo, M., & Dotto, G. P. (2004). High commitment of embryonic keratinocytes to terminal differentiation through a Notch1-caspase 3 regulatory mechanism. *Developmental Cell, 6*, 551–562.
67. Palomero, T., Lim, W. K., Odom, D. T., Sulis, M. L., Real, P. J., Margolin, A., Barnes, K. C., O'Neil, J., Neuberg, D., Weng, A. P., Aster, J. C., Sigaux, F., Soulier, J., Look, A. T., Young, R. A., Califano, A., & Ferrando, A. A. (2006). NOTCH1 directly regulates c-MYC and activates a feed-forward-loop transcriptional network promoting leukemic cell growth. *PNAS, 103*, 18261–18266.
68. Palomero, T., Sulis, M. L., Cortina, M., Real, P. J., Barnes, K., Ciofani, M., Caparros, E., Buteau, J., Brown, K., Perkins, S. L., Bhagat, G., Agarwal, A. M., Basso, G., Castillo, M., Nagase, S., Cordon-Cardo, C., Parsons, R., Zuniga-Pflucker, J. C., Dominguez, M., & Ferrando, A. A. (2007). Mutational loss of PTEN induces resistance to NOTCH1 inhibition in T-cell leukemia. *Nature Medicine, 13*, 1203–1210.
69. Parry, M., Rose-Zerilli, M. J., Ljungstrom, V., Gibson, J., Wang, J., Walewska, R., Parker, H., Parker, A., Davis, Z., Gardiner, A., McIver-Brown, N., Kalpadakis, C., Xochelli, A., Anagnostopoulos, A., Fazi, C., Gonzalez de Castro, D., Dearden, C., Pratt, G., Rosenquist, R., Ashton-Key, M., Forconi, F., Collins, A., Ghia, P., Matutes, E., Pangalis, G., Stamatopoulos, K., Oscier, D., & Strefford, J. C. (2015). Genetics and prognostication in splenic marginal zone lymphoma: Revelations from deep sequencing. *Clinical Cancer Research, 21*, 4174–4183.
70. Pear, W. S., Aster, J. C., Scott, M. L., Hasserjian, R. P., Soffer, B., Sklar, J., & Baltimore, D. (1996). Exclusive development of T cell neoplasms in mice transplanted with bone marrow expressing activated Notch alleles. *The Journal of Experimental Medicine, 183*, 2283–2291.
71. Pece, S., Serresi, M., Santolini, E., Capra, M., Hulleman, E., Galimberti, V., Zurrida, S., Maisonneuve, P., Viale, G., & Di Fiore, P. P. (2004). Loss of negative regulation by Numb

over Notch is relevant to human breast carcinogenesis. *The Journal of Cell Biology, 167*, 215–221.

72. Peifer, M., Fernandez-Cuesta, L., Sos, M. L., George, J., Seidel, D., Kasper, L. H., Plenker, D., Leenders, F., Sun, R., Zander, T., Menon, R., Koker, M., Dahmen, I., Muller, C., Di Cerbo, V., Schildhaus, H. U., Altmuller, J., Baessmann, I., Becker, C., de Wilde, B., Vandesompele, J., Bohm, D., Ansen, S., Gabler, F., Wilkening, I., Heynck, S., Heuckmann, J. M., Lu, X., Carter, S. L., Cibulskis, K., Banerji, S., Getz, G., Park, K. S., Rauh, D., Grutter, C., Fischer, M., Pasqualucci, L., Wright, G., Wainer, Z., Russell, P., Petersen, I., Chen, Y., Stoelben, E., Ludwig, C., Schnabel, P., Hoffmann, H., Muley, T., Brockmann, M., Engel-Riedel, W., Muscarella, L. A., Fazio, V. M., Groen, H., Timens, W., Sietsma, H., Thunnissen, E., Smit, E., Heideman, D. A., Snijders, P. J., Cappuzzo, F., Ligorio, C., Damiani, S., Field, J., Solberg, S., Brustugun, O. T., Lund-Iversen, M., Sanger, J., Clement, J. H., Soltermann, A., Moch, H., Weder, W., Solomon, B., Soria, J. C., Validire, P., Besse, B., Brambilla, E., Brambilla, C., Lantuejoul, S., Lorimier, P., Schneider, P. M., Hallek, M., Pao, W., Meyerson, M., Sage, J., Shendure, J., Schneider, R., Buttner, R., Wolf, J., Nurnberg, P., Perner, S., Heukamp, L. C., Brindle, P. K., Haas, S., & Thomas, R. K. (2012). Integrative genome analyses identify key somatic driver mutations of small-cell lung cancer. *Nature Genetics, 44*, 1104–1110.
73. Pickering, C. R., Zhou, J. H., Lee, J. J., Drummond, J. A., Peng, S. A., Saade, R. E., Tsai, K. Y., Curry, J. L., Tetzlaff, M. T., Lai, S. Y., Yu, J., Muzny, D. M., Doddapaneni, H., Shinbrot, E., Covington, K. R., Zhang, J., Seth, S., Caulin, C., Clayman, G. L., El-Naggar, A. K., Gibbs, R. A., Weber, R. S., Myers, J. N., Wheeler, D. A., & Frederick, M. J. (2014). Mutational landscape of aggressive cutaneous squamous cell carcinoma. *Clinical Cancer Research, 20*, 6582–6592.
74. Porcu, M., Kleppe, M., Gianfelici, V., Geerdens, E., De Keersmaecker, K., Tartaglia, M., Foa, R., Soulier, J., Cauwelier, B., Uyttebroeck, A., Macintyre, E., Vandenberghe, P., Asnafi, V., & Cools, J. (2012). Mutation of the receptor tyrosine phosphatase PTPRC (CD45) in T-cell acute lymphoblastic leukemia. *Blood, 119*, 4476–4479.
75. Proweller, A., Tu, L., Lepore, J. J., Cheng, L., Lu, M. M., Seykora, J., Millar, S. E., Pear, W. S., & Parmacek, M. S. (2006). Impaired notch signaling promotes de novo squamous cell carcinoma formation. *Cancer Research, 66*, 7438–7444.
76. Puente, X. S., Bea, S., Valdes-Mas, R., Villamor, N., Gutierrez-Abril, J., Martin-Subero, J. I., Munar, M., Rubio-Perez, C., Jares, P., Aymerich, M., Baumann, T., Beekman, R., Belver, L., Carrio, A., Castellano, G., Clot, G., Colado, E., Colomer, D., Costa, D., Delgado, J., Enjuanes, A., Estivill, X., Ferrando, A. A., Gelpi, J. L., Gonzalez, B., Gonzalez, S., Gonzalez, M., Gut, M., Hernandez-Rivas, J. M., Lopez-Guerra, M., Martin-Garcia, D., Navarro, A., Nicolas, P., Orozco, M., Payer, A. R., Pinyol, M., Pisano, D. G., Puente, D. A., Queiros, A. C., Quesada, V., Romeo-Casabona, C. M., Royo, C., Royo, R., Rozman, M., Russinol, N., Salaverria, I., Stamatopoulos, K., Stunnenberg, H. G., Tamborero, D., Terol, M. J., Valencia, A., Lopez-Bigas, N., Torrents, D., Gut, I., Lopez-Guillermo, A., Lopez-Otin, C., & Campo, E. (2015). Non-coding recurrent mutations in chronic lymphocytic leukaemia. *Nature, 526*, 519–524.
77. Puente, X. S., Pinyol, M., Quesada, V., Conde, L., Ordonez, G. R., Villamor, N., Escaramis, G., Jares, P., Bea, S., Gonzalez-Diaz, M., Bassaganyas, L., Baumann, T., Juan, M., Lopez-Guerra, M., Colomer, D., Tubio, J. M., Lopez, C., Navarro, A., Tornador, C., Aymerich, M., Rozman, M., Hernandez, J. M., Puente, D. A., Freije, J. M., Velasco, G., Gutierrez-Fernandez, A., Costa, D., Carrio, A., Guijarro, S., Enjuanes, A., Hernandez, L., Yague, J., Nicolas, P., Romeo-Casabona, C. M., Himmelbauer, H., Castillo, E., Dohm, J. C., de Sanjose, S., Piris, M. A., de Alava, E., San Miguel, J., Royo, R., Gelpi, J. L., Torrents, D., Orozco, M., Pisano, D. G., Valencia, A., Guigo, R., Bayes, M., Heath, S., Gut, M., Klatt, P., Marshall, J., Raine, K., Stebbings, L. A., Futreal, P. A., Stratton, M. R., Campbell, P. J., Gut, I., Lopez-Guillermo, A., Estivill, X., Montserrat, E., Lopez-Otin, C., & Campo, E. (2011). Whole-genome sequencing identifies recurrent mutations in chronic lymphocytic leukaemia. *Nature, 475*, 101–105.

78. Pui, J. C., Allman, D., Xu, L., DeRocco, S., Karnell, F. G., Bakkour, S., Lee, J. Y., Kadesch, T., Hardy, R. R., Aster, J. C., & Pear, W. S. (1999). Notch1 expression in early lymphopoiesis influences B versus T lineage determination. *Immunity, 11*, 299–308.
79. Rampias, T., Vgenopoulou, P., Avgeris, M., Polyzos, A., Stravodimos, K., Valavanis, C., Scorilas, A., & Klinakis, A. (2014). A new tumor suppressor role for the Notch pathway in bladder cancer. *Nature Medicine, 20*, 1199–1205.
80. Ranganathan, P., Weaver, K. L., & Capobianco, A. J. (2011). Notch signalling in solid tumours: A little bit of everything but not all the time. *Nature Reviews. Cancer, 11*, 338–351.
81. Rangarajan, A., Talora, C., Okuyama, R., Nicolas, M., Mammucari, C., Oh, H., Aster, J. C., Krishna, S., Metzger, D., Chambon, P., Miele, L., Aguet, M., Radtke, F., & Dotto, G. P. (2001). Notch signaling is a direct determinant of keratinocyte growth arrest and entry into differentiation. *The EMBO Journal, 20*, 3427–3436.
82. Rao, S. S., O'Neil, J., Liberator, C. D., Hardwick, J. S., Dai, X., Zhang, T., Tyminski, E., Yuan, J., Kohl, N. E., Richon, V. M., Van der Ploeg, L. H., Carroll, P. M., Draetta, G. F., Look, A. T., Strack, P. R., & Winter, C. G. (2009). Inhibition of NOTCH signaling by gamma secretase inhibitor engages the RB pathway and elicits cell cycle exit in T-cell acute lymphoblastic leukemia cells. *Cancer Research, 69*, 3060–3068.
83. Rebay, I., Fehon, R. G., & Artavanis-Tsakonas, S. (1993). Specific truncations of Drosophila Notch define dominant activated and dominant negative forms of the receptor. *Cell, 74*, 319–329.
84. Reedijk, M., Odorcic, S., Chang, L., Zhang, H., Miller, N., McCready, D. R., Lockwood, G., & Egan, S. E. (2005). High-level coexpression of JAG1 and NOTCH1 is observed in human breast cancer and is associated with poor overall survival. *Cancer Research, 65*, 8530–8537.
85. Reedijk, M., Pinnaduwage, D., Dickson, B. C., Mulligan, A. M., Zhang, H., Bull, S. B., O'Malley, F. P., Egan, S. E., & Andrulis, I. L. (2008). JAG1 expression is associated with a basal phenotype and recurrence in lymph node-negative breast cancer. *Breast Cancer Research and Treatment, 111*, 439–448.
86. Reynolds, T. C., Smith, S. D., & Sklar, J. (1987). Analysis of DNA surrounding the breakpoints of chromosomal translocations involving the beta T cell receptor gene in human lymphoblastic neoplasms. *Cell, 50*, 107–117.
87. Robinson, D. R., Kalyana-Sundaram, S., Wu, Y. M., Shankar, S., Cao, X., Ateeq, B., Asangani, I. A., Iyer, M., Maher, C. A., Grasso, C. S., Lonigro, R. J., Quist, M., Siddiqui, J., Mehra, R., Jing, X., Giordano, T. J., Sabel, M. S., Kleer, C. G., Palanisamy, N., Natrajan, R., Lambros, M. B., Reis-Filho, J. S., Kumar-Sinha, C., & Chinnaiyan, A. M. (2011). Functionally recurrent rearrangements of the MAST kinase and Notch gene families in breast cancer. *Nature Medicine, 17*, 1646–1651.
88. Rossi, D., Trifonov, V., Fangazio, M., Bruscaggin, A., Rasi, S., Spina, V., Monti, S., Vaisitti, T., Arruga, F., Fama, R., Ciardullo, C., Greco, M., Cresta, S., Piranda, D., Holmes, A., Fabbri, G., Messina, M., Rinaldi, A., Wang, J., Agostinelli, C., Piccaluga, P. P., Lucioni, M., Tabbo, F., Serra, R., Franceschetti, S., Deambrogi, C., Daniele, G., Gattei, V., Marasca, R., Facchetti, F., Arcaini, L., Inghirami, G., Bertoni, F., Pileri, S. A., Deaglio, S., Foa, R., Dalla-Favera, R., Pasqualucci, L., Rabadan, R., & Gaidano, G. (2012). The coding genome of splenic marginal zone lymphoma: Activation of NOTCH2 and other pathways regulating marginal zone development. *The Journal of Experimental Medicine, 209*, 1537–1551.
89. Rudin, C. M., Durinck, S., Stawiski, E. W., Poirier, J. T., Modrusan, Z., Shames, D. S., Bergbower, E. A., Guan, Y., Shin, J., Guillory, J., Rivers, C. S., Foo, C. K., Bhatt, D., Stinson, J., Gnad, F., Haverty, P. M., Gentleman, R., Chaudhuri, S., Janakiraman, V., Jaiswal, B. S., Parikh, C., Yuan, W., Zhang, Z., Koeppen, H., Wu, T. D., Stern, H. M., Yauch, R. L., Huffman, K. E., Paskulin, D. D., Illei, P. B., Varella-Garcia, M., Gazdar, A. F., de Sauvage, F. J., Bourgon, R., Minna, J. D., Brock, M. V., & Seshagiri, S. (2012). Comprehensive genomic analysis identifies SOX2 as a frequently amplified gene in small-cell lung cancer. *Nature Genetics, 44*, 1111–1116.

90. Saito, T., Chiba, S., Ichikawa, M., Kunisato, A., Asai, T., Shimizu, K., Yamaguchi, T., Yamamoto, G., Seo, S., Kumano, K., Nakagami-Yamaguchi, E., Hamada, Y., Aizawa, S., & Hirai, H. (2003). Notch2 is preferentially expressed in mature B cells and indispensable for marginal zone B lineage development. *Immunity, 18*, 675–685.
91. Sarmento, L. M., Huang, H., Limon, A., Gordon, W., Fernandes, J., Tavares, M. J., Miele, L., Cardoso, A. A., Classon, M., & Carlesso, N. (2005). Notch1 modulates timing of G1-S progression by inducing SKP2 transcription and p27 Kip1 degradation. *The Journal of Experimental Medicine, 202*, 157–168.
92. Schaffer, B. E., Park, K. S., Yiu, G., Conklin, J. F., Lin, C., Burkhart, D. L., Karnezis, A. N., Sweet-Cordero, E. A., & Sage, J. (2010). Loss of p130 accelerates tumor development in a mouse model for human small-cell lung carcinoma. *Cancer Research, 70*, 3877–3883.
93. Schnell, S. A., Ambesi-Impiombato, A., Sanchez-Martin, M., Belver, L., Xu, L., Qin, Y., Kageyama, R., & Ferrando, A. A. (2015). Therapeutic targeting of HES1 transcriptional programs in T-ALL. *Blood, 125*, 2806–2814.
94. Sharma, V. M., Calvo, J. A., Draheim, K. M., Cunningham, L. A., Hermance, N., Beverly, L., Krishnamoorthy, V., Bhasin, M., Capobianco, A. J., & Kelliher, M. A. (2006). Notch1 contributes to mouse T-Cell leukemia by directly inducing the expression of c-myc. *Molecular and Cellular Biology, 26*, 8022–8031.
95. Shin, H. M., Minter, L. M., Cho, O. H., Gottipati, S., Fauq, A. H., Golde, T. E., Sonenshein, G. E., & Osborne, B. A. (2006). Notch1 augments NF-kappaB activity by facilitating its nuclear retention. *The EMBO Journal, 25*, 129–138.
96. Shochat, C., Tal, N., Bandapalli, O. R., Palmi, C., Ganmore, I., te Kronnie, G., Cario, G., Cazzaniga, G., Kulozik, A. E., Stanulla, M., Schrappe, M., Biondi, A., Basso, G., Bercovich, D., Muckenthaler, M. U., & Izraeli, S. (2011). Gain-of-function mutations in interleukin-7 receptor-alpha (IL7R) in childhood acute lymphoblastic leukemias. *The Journal of Experimental Medicine, 208*, 901–908.
97. Sicinska, E., Aifantis, I., Le Cam, L., Swat, W., Borowski, C., Yu, Q., Ferrando, A. A., Levin, S. D., Geng, Y., von Boehmer, H., & Sicinski, P. (2003). Requirement for cyclin D3 in lymphocyte development and T cell leukemias. *Cancer Cell, 4*, 451–461.
98. Simoes, B. M., O'Brien, C. S., Eyre, R., Silva, A., Yu, L., Sarmiento-Castro, A., Alferez, D. G., Spence, K., Santiago-Gomez, A., Chemi, F., Acar, A., Gandhi, A., Howell, A., Brennan, K., Ryden, L., Catalano, S., Ando, S., Gee, J., Ucar, A., Sims, A. H., Marangoni, E., Farnie, G., Landberg, G., Howell, S. J., & Clarke, R. B. (2015). Anti-estrogen resistance in human breast tumors is driven by JAG1-NOTCH4-Dependent cancer stem cell activity. *Cell Reports, 12*, 1968–1977.
99. Sjoblom, T., Jones, S., Wood, L. D., Parsons, D. W., Lin, J., Barber, T. D., Mandelker, D., Leary, R. J., Ptak, J., Silliman, N., Szabo, S., Buckhaults, P., Farrell, C., Meeh, P., Markowitz, S. D., Willis, J., Dawson, D., Willson, J. K., Gazdar, A. F., Hartigan, J., Wu, L., Liu, C., Parmigiani, G., Park, B. H., Bachman, K. E., Papadopoulos, N., Vogelstein, B., Kinzler, K. W., & Velculescu, V. E. (2006). The consensus coding sequences of human breast and colorectal cancers. *Science, 314*, 268–274.
100. Solinas, G., Marchesi, F., Garlanda, C., Mantovani, A., & Allavena, P. (2010). Inflammation-mediated promotion of invasion and metastasis. *Cancer Metastasis Reviews, 29*, 243–248.
101. Song, Y., Li, L., Ou, Y., Gao, Z., Li, E., Li, X., Zhang, W., Wang, J., Xu, L., Zhou, Y., Ma, X., Liu, L., Zhao, Z., Huang, X., Fan, J., Dong, L., Chen, G., Ma, L., Yang, J., Chen, L., He, M., Li, M., Zhuang, X., Huang, K., Qiu, K., Yin, G., Guo, G., Feng, Q., Chen, P., Wu, Z., Wu, J., Zhao, J., Luo, L., Fu, M., Xu, B., Chen, B., Li, Y., Tong, T., Wang, M., Liu, Z., Lin, D., Zhang, X., Yang, H., & Zhan, Q. (2014). Identification of genomic alterations in oesophageal squamous cell cancer. *Nature, 509*, 91–95.
102. South, A. P., Purdie, K. J., Watt, S. A., Haldenby, S., den Breems, N. Y., Dimon, M., Arron, S. T., Kluk, M. J., Aster, J. C., McHugh, A., Xue, D. J., Dayal, J. H., Robinson, K. S., Rizvi, S. M., Proby, C. M., Harwood, C. A., & Leigh, I. M. (2014). NOTCH1 mutations occur early

during cutaneous squamous cell carcinogenesis. *The Journal of Investigative Dermatology, 134*, 2630–2638.
103. Sportoletti, P., Baldoni, S., Cavalli, L., Del Papa, B., Bonifacio, E., Ciurnelli, R., Bell, A. S., Di Tommaso, A., Rosati, E., Crescenzi, B., Mecucci, C., Screpanti, I., Marconi, P., Martelli, M. F., Di Ianni, M., & Falzetti, F. (2010). NOTCH1 PEST domain mutation is an adverse prognostic factor in B-CLL. *British Journal of Haematology, 151*, 404–406.
104. Sriuranpong, V., Borges, M. W., Ravi, R. K., Arnold, D. R., Nelkin, B. D., Baylin, S. B., & Ball, D. W. (2001). Notch signaling induces cell cycle arrest in small cell lung cancer cells. *Cancer Research, 61*, 3200–3205.
105. Sriuranpong, V., Borges, M. W., Strock, C. L., Nakakura, E. K., Watkins, D. N., Blaumueller, C. M., Nelkin, B. D., & Ball, D. W. (2002). Notch signaling induces rapid degradation of achaete-scute homolog 1. *Molecular and Cellular Biology, 22*, 3129–3139.
106. Stransky, N., Egloff, A. M., Tward, A. D., Kostic, A. D., Cibulskis, K., Sivachenko, A., Kryukov, G. V., Lawrence, M. S., Sougnez, C., McKenna, A., Shefler, E., Ramos, A. H., Stojanov, P., Carter, S. L., Voet, D., Cortes, M. L., Auclair, D., Berger, M. F., Saksena, G., Guiducci, C., Onofrio, R. C., Parkin, M., Romkes, M., Weissfeld, J. L., Seethala, R. R., Wang, L., Rangel-Escareno, C., Fernandez-Lopez, J. C., Hidalgo-Miranda, A., Melendez-Zajgla, J., Winckler, W., Ardlie, K., Gabriel, S. B., Meyerson, M., Lander, E. S., Getz, G., Golub, T. R., Garraway, L. A., & Grandis, J. R. (2011). The mutational landscape of head and neck squamous cell carcinoma. *Science, 333*, 1157–1160.
107. Thelu, J., Rossio, P., & Favier, B. (2002). Notch signalling is linked to epidermal cell differentiation level in basal cell carcinoma, psoriasis and wound healing. *BMC Dermatology, 2*, 7.
108. Thomas, M., Calamito, M., Srivastava, B., Maillard, I., Pear, W. S., & Allman, D. (2007). Notch activity synergizes with B-cell-receptor and CD40 signaling to enhance B-cell activation. *Blood, 109*, 3342–3350.
109. Uyttendaele, H., Marazzi, G., Wu, G., Yan, Q., Sassoon, D., & Kitajewski, J. (1996). Notch4/int-3, a mammary proto-oncogene, is an endothelial cell-specific mammalian Notch gene. *Development, 122*, 2251–2259.
110. Vilimas, T., Mascarenhas, J., Palomero, T., Mandal, M., Buonamici, S., Meng, F., Thompson, B., Spaulding, C., Macaroun, S., Alegre, M. L., Kee, B. L., Ferrando, A., Miele, L., & Aifantis, I. (2007). Targeting the NF-kappaB signaling pathway in Notch1-induced T-cell leukemia. *Nature Medicine, 13*, 70–77.
111. Wael, H., Yoshida, R., Kudoh, S., Hasegawa, K., Niimori-Kita, K., & Ito, T. (2014). Notch1 signaling controls cell proliferation, apoptosis and differentiation in lung carcinoma. *Lung Cancer, 85*, 131–140.
112. Wang, H., Zang, C., Taing, L., Arnett, K. L., Wong, Y. J., Pear, W. S., Blacklow, S. C., Liu, X. S., & Aster, J. C. (2014). NOTCH1-RBPJ complexes drive target gene expression through dynamic interactions with superenhancers. *Proceedings of the National Academy of Sciences of the United States of America, 111*, 705–710.
113. Wang, N. J., Sanborn, Z., Arnett, K. L., Bayston, L. J., Liao, W., Proby, C. M., Leigh, I. M., Collisson, E. A., Gordon, P. B., Jakkula, L., Pennypacker, S., Zou, Y., Sharma, M., North, J. P., Vemula, S. S., Mauro, T. M., Neuhaus, I. M., Leboit, P. E., Hur, J. S., Park, K., Huh, N., Kwok, P. Y., Arron, S. T., Massion, P. P., Bale, A. E., Haussler, D., Cleaver, J. E., Gray, J. W., Spellman, P. T., South, A. P., Aster, J. C., Blacklow, S. C., & Cho, R. J. (2011). Loss-of-function mutations in Notch receptors in cutaneous and lung squamous cell carcinoma. *Proceedings of the National Academy of Sciences of the United States of America, 108*, 17761–17766.
114. Ward, P. S., & Thompson, C. B. (2012). Metabolic reprogramming: A cancer hallmark even warburg did not anticipate. *Cancer Cell, 21*, 297–308.
115. Wendorff, A. A., Koch, U., Wunderlich, F. T., Wirth, S., Dubey, C., Bruning, J. C., MacDonald, H. R., & Radtke, F. (2010). Hes1 is a critical but context-dependent mediator of canonical Notch signaling in lymphocyte development and transformation. *Immunity, 33*, 671–684.

116. Weng, A. P., Ferrando, A. A., Lee, W., Morris, J. P. T., Silverman, L. B., Sanchez-Irizarry, C., Blacklow, S. C., Look, A. T., & Aster, J. C. (2004). Activating mutations of NOTCH1 in human T cell acute lymphoblastic leukemia. *Science, 306*, 269–271.
117. Weng, A. P., Millholland, J. M., Yashiro-Ohtani, Y., Arcangeli, M. L., Lau, A., Wai, C., Del Bianco, C., Rodriguez, C. G., Sai, H., Tobias, J., Li, Y., Wolfe, M. S., Shachaf, C., Felsher, D., Blacklow, S. C., Pear, W. S., & Aster, J. C. (2006). c-Myc is an important direct target of Notch1 in T-cell acute lymphoblastic leukemia/lymphoma. *Genes & Development, 20*, 2096–2109.
118. Westhoff, B., Colaluca, I. N., D'Ario, G., Donzelli, M., Tosoni, D., Volorio, S., Pelosi, G., Spaggiari, L., Mazzarol, G., Viale, G., Pece, S., & Di Fiore, P. P. (2009). Alterations of the Notch pathway in lung cancer. *Proceedings of the National Academy of Sciences of the United States of America, 106*, 22293–22298.
119. White, A. C., Tran, K., Khuu, J., Dang, C., Cui, Y., Binder, S. W., & Lowry, W. E. (2011). Defining the origins of Ras/p53-mediated squamous cell carcinoma. *Proceedings of the National Academy of Sciences of the United States of America, 108*, 7425–7430.
120. Wood, L. D., Parsons, D. W., Jones, S., Lin, J., Sjoblom, T., Leary, R. J., Shen, D., Boca, S. M., Barber, T., Ptak, J., Silliman, N., Szabo, S., Dezso, Z., Ustyanksky, V., Nikolskaya, T., Nikolsky, Y., Karchin, R., Wilson, P. A., Kaminker, J. S., Zhang, Z., Croshaw, R., Willis, J., Dawson, D., Shipitsin, M., Willson, J. K., Sukumar, S., Polyak, K., Park, B. H., Pethiyagoda, C. L., Pant, P. V., Ballinger, D. G., Sparks, A. B., Hartigan, J., Smith, D. R., Suh, E., Papadopoulos, N., Buckhaults, P., Markowitz, S. D., Parmigiani, G., Kinzler, K. W., Velculescu, V. E., & Vogelstein, B. (2007). The genomic landscapes of human breast and colorectal cancers. *Science, 318*, 1108–1113.
121. Xu, A., Lei, L., & Irvine, K. D. (2005). Regions of Drosophila Notch that contribute to ligand binding and the modulatory influence of Fringe. *The Journal of Biological Chemistry, 280*, 30158–30165.
122. Yan, W., Wistuba, I. I., Emmert-Buck, M. R., & Erickson, H. S. (2011). Squamous cell carcinoma - similarities and differences among anatomical sites. *American Journal of Cancer Research, 1*, 275–300.
123. Yashiro-Ohtani, Y., Wang, H., Zang, C., Arnett, K. L., Bailis, W., Ho, Y., Knoechel, B., Lanauze, C., Louis, L., Forsyth, K. S., Chen, S., Chung, Y., Schug, J., Blobel, G. A., Liebhaber, S. A., Bernstein, B. E., Blacklow, S. C., Liu, X. S., Aster, J. C., & Pear, W. S. (2014). Long-range enhancer activity determines Myc sensitivity to Notch inhibitors in T cell leukemia. *Proceedings of the National Academy of Sciences of the United States of America, 111*, E4946–E4953.
124. Yatim, A., Benne, C., Sobhian, B., Laurent-Chabalier, S., Deas, O., Judde, J. G., Lelievre, J. D., Levy, Y., & Benkirane, M. (2012). NOTCH1 nuclear interactome reveals key regulators of its transcriptional activity and oncogenic function. *Molecular Cell, 48*, 445–458.
125. Zenatti, P. P., Ribeiro, D., Li, W., Zuurbier, L., Silva, M. C., Paganin, M., Tritapoe, J., Hixon, J. A., Silveira, A. B., Cardoso, B. A., Sarmento, L. M., Correia, N., Toribio, M. L., Kobarg, J., Horstmann, M., Pieters, R., Brandalise, S. R., Ferrando, A. A., Meijerink, J. P., Durum, S. K., Yunes, J. A., & Barata, J. T. (2011). Oncogenic IL7R gain-of-function mutations in childhood T-cell acute lymphoblastic leukemia. *Nature Genetics, 43*, 932–939.
126. Zender, S., Nickeleit, I., Wuestefeld, T., Sorensen, I., Dauch, D., Bozko, P., El-Khatib, M., Geffers, R., Bektas, H., Manns, M. P., Gossler, A., Wilkens, L., Plentz, R., Zender, L., & Malek, N. P. (2013). A critical role for notch signaling in the formation of cholangiocellular carcinomas. *Cancer Cell, 23*, 784–795.
127. Zenz, T., Mertens, D., Kuppers, R., Dohner, H., & Stilgenbauer, S. (2010). From pathogenesis to treatment of chronic lymphocytic leukaemia. *Nature Reviews. Cancer, 10*, 37–50.
128. Zhang, J., Ding, L., Holmfeldt, L., Wu, G., Heatley, S. L., Payne-Turner, D., Easton, J., Chen, X., Wang, J., Rusch, M., Lu, C., Chen, S. C., Wei, L., Collins-Underwood, J. R., Ma, J., Roberts, K. G., Pounds, S. B., Ulyanov, A., Becksfort, J., Gupta, P., Huether, R., Kriwacki, R. W., Parker, M., McGoldrick, D. J., Zhao, D., Alford, D., Espy, S., Bobba, K. C., Song, G.,

Pei, D., Cheng, C., Roberts, S., Barbato, M. I., Campana, D., Coustan-Smith, E., Shurtleff, S. A., Raimondi, S. C., Kleppe, M., Cools, J., Shimano, K. A., Hermiston, M. L., Doulatov, S., Eppert, K., Laurenti, E., Notta, F., Dick, J. E., Basso, G., Hunger, S. P., Loh, M. L., Devidas, M., Wood, B., Winter, S., Dunsmore, K. P., Fulton, R. S., Fulton, L. L., Hong, X., Harris, C. C., Dooling, D. J., Ochoa, K., Johnson, K. J., Obenauer, J. C., Evans, W. E., Pui, C. H., Naeve, C. W., Ley, T. J., Mardis, E. R., Wilson, R. K., Downing, J. R., & Mullighan, C. G. (2012). The genetic basis of early T-cell precursor acute lymphoblastic leukaemia. *Nature, 481*, 157–163.

129. Zweidler-McKay, P. A., He, Y., Xu, L., Rodriguez, C. G., Karnell, F. G., Carpenter, A. C., Aster, J. C., Allman, D., & Pear, W. S. (2005). Notch signaling is a potent inducer of growth arrest and apoptosis in a wide range of B-cell malignancies. *Blood, 106*, 3898–3906.

Chapter 4
Out on the Fringe: Modulation of Notch Signaling by Glycosylation

Keli Xu and Sean E. Egan

Abstract Differential glycosylation of Notch, often as part of a feedback loop, represents a powerful mechanism by which signaling is regulated. Together with Dll (Delta) and Jagged (Serrate) ligands, Fringe, Rumi, and other sugar transferase proteins form a remarkably versatile system to coordinate Notch-dependent tissue patterning. When Fringe is induced in the same cell as Dll, it enhances signal reception through Notch, downregulates Dll through cis-inhibition, and helps to make neighboring cells distinct. When induced in a Jagged-expressing cell, it helps to create a hybrid signal sender/receiver identity with low levels of Notch signal reception, accompanied by (Jagged) signal sending activity without cis-inhibition. In this situation, Fringe can help drive neighbors to the same state. Fringe can even work together with Dll3 to inhibit Notch signaling in neighboring cells. A detailed mechanism by which Fringes control development of several tissues has begun to emerge. With time, studies on Notch glycosylation should help define how this system is used to control development in most tissues and how it can be exploited for therapeutic benefit in the fight against cancer and cardiovascular disease.

Keywords Notch · Lunatic Fringe · Manic Fringe · Radical Fringe · Rumi · Delta · Serrate · Dll · Jagged · Somitogenesis · Lymphocyte development · T-cells · Human cancer

K. Xu (✉)
Cancer Institute and Department of Neurobiology and Anatomical Sciences, University of Mississippi Medical Center, Jackson, MS, USA
e-mail: kxu@umc.edu

S. E. Egan (✉)
Program in Cell Biology, The Hospital for Sick Children and Department of Molecular Genetics, University of Toronto, Toronto, ON, Canada
e-mail: segan@sickkids.ca

L. Miele, S. Artavanis-Tsakonas (eds.), *Targeting Notch in Cancer*,
https://doi.org/10.1007/978-1-4939-8859-4_4

4.1 Introduction

In development, tissue boundaries often form "organizers" or signaling centers that help to pattern new structures, including limbs, organs, and elements of the nervous system. This is the case with a boundary formed between dorsal (D) and ventral (V) cells of the developing fly wing. In 1994, Irvine and Wieschaus described isolation and characterization of a *Drosophila* mutant with altered D/V boundary formation and loss of distal wing tisssue [1]. The mutant in question was in a gene coding for a novel secretory pathway protein, dubbed Fringe. *Fringe* is normally expressed in dorsal but not ventral cells of the developing wing imaginal disc. This gene had the remarkable property whereby a boundary between cells expressing it and those that didn't, formed a new wing margin, just like the boundary that formed between dorsal and ventral cells in the wild-type imaginal disc. Indeed, ectopic wing margins formed at the boundary between Fringe mutant clones (Fringe$^-$) in the dorsal compartment and surrounding (*Fringe*-expressing) dorsal cells. Similarly, an ectopic margin formed at the boundary between ventral cells programed to express ectopic Fringe (*Fringe*$^+$) and neighboring ventral cells that do not express. Fringe also helped to prevent the mixing of dorsal and ventral cells at the boundary [2]. Next, Irvine and colleagues tested for *Fringe*-mediated regulation of other developmental events. Indeed, they found a critical role for a *Fringe* expression boundary in specifying the D/V midline of the eye, which forms an equatorial organizer. Altered *Fringe* function or expression in this context resulted in small eyes as well as altered chirality of ommatidial units [3]. In the developing fly leg, *Fringe* is expressed in alternate segments, where an expression boundary is required for specification of joints [4]. During oogenesis, *Fringe* is expressed and dynamically regulated in somatic follicle cells, where it's required for specification of the polar cell fate [5]. Once again, as polar cells show organizer activity, a *Drosophila Fringe* expression boundary helps to control development of a major structure by coordinating formation of an organizer at a tissue boundary [6].

With description of such an unusual boundary-sensing protein, many labs began searching for vertebrate homologues. Indeed, in very short order, similar proteins were identified in frogs [7], chickens [8, 9], and mammals [10, 11]. Vertebrate *Lunatic Fringe (Lfng)*, *Manic Fringe (Mfng)*, and *Radical Fringe (Rfng)* showed remarkable expression patterns, suggestive of a conserved role in development at many tissue boundaries [10–12]. For example, *Lfng* was expressed in a striped pattern within developing somites and plays an important role in this context (see below). *Rfng* was expressed in the apical ectodermal ridge (AER), which promotes limb bud outgrowth. Functional studies in chicken suggested a role for *Rfng* in limb patterning, echoing to some extent the function identified in fruit fly wing development [8, 9] (a role for *Rfng* in AER-dependent limb outgrowth has not been seen in mice [13–15]).

Notch proteins are receptors, activated at the cell surface by Serrate and Delta family ligands. Interestingly, Notch activation at the D/V boundary of the wing imaginal disc is required for margin specification. Indeed, loss-of-function mutations in *Notch* or *Serrate* cause loss of wing tissue at the distal edge. It is this wing phenotype that led to the name, Notch. Similarly, *Serrate* mutants have a serrated

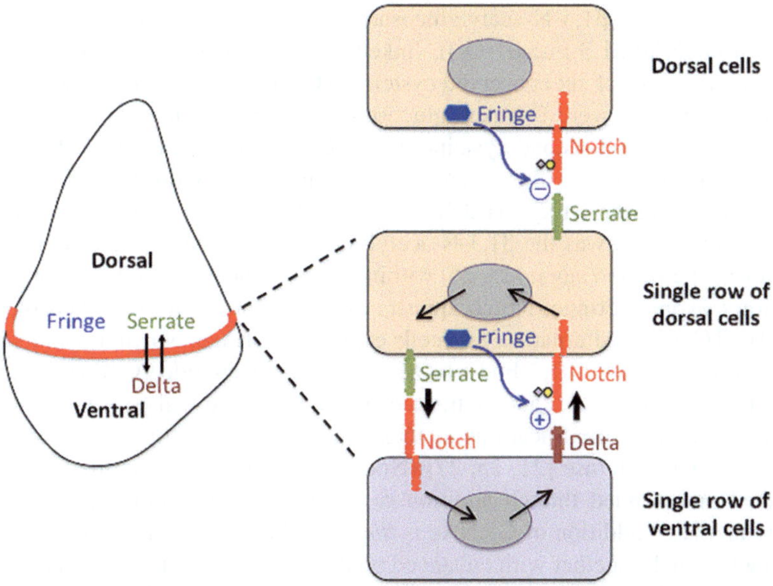

Fig. 4.1 Fringe-modulated Notch signaling in the developing *Drosophila* wing. A wing imaginal disc, which gives rise to the adult wing, is divided into dorsal and ventral compartments. Fringe and Serrate are expressed in dorsal cells, while Delta is expressed in ventral cells. Fringe potentiates Delta signaling to dorsal cells, but inhibits Serrate-mediated signaling. As a result, Notch activation occurs along the interface between both compartments (shown in red)

wing margin. As the Notch ligand/receptor system controls *Drosophila* wing margin specification and *Fringe* expression boundaries can induce ectopic margins, it seemed likely that these two systems interacted in some way. In this regard, *Drosophila* Fringe was found to block activation of Notch by Serrate in the dorsal compartment of the wing disc (but not in the single row of *ventral cells* at the D/V boundary [16, 17]). Also, Fringe promotes Delta-mediated Notch activation in the single row of *dorsal cells* at the D/V boundary and enhances Serrate expression in dorsal boundary cells [18]. Thus, the *Fringe* expression boundary limits Notch activation to a single row of ventral cells and a single row of dorsal cells, each on opposing sides of the D/V compartment boundary [17, 19] (Fig. 4.1).

4.2 Controlling Notch Activation Through Glycosylation

In 1997, Yuan et al. discovered a striking similarity between the sequence of Fringe proteins and glycosyltransferases [20]. This was a major breakthrough. Soon after, Haltiwanger and colleagues reported that Notch is glycosylated on specific serine and threonine residues within EGF-like repeats of the extracellular domain [21]. Some sugar chains were O-linked fucose tetrasaccharides (sialic acid-α2,6-galactose-β1,4-N-acetylglucosamine-β1,3-fucose-α1-O- (or Sia-α2,6-Gal-β1,4-GlcNAc-β1,3-Fuc-α1-O-)), linked to serine or threonine residues (S/T) preceding the third of six conserved cysteines ($C_2X(4)S/TC_3$) [21–23] within EGF-like repeats. Others were O-linked glucose trisaccharides linked to serine residues between the first and second cysteine ($C_1XSX(A/P)C_2$) of many EGF-like repeats [21, 23, 24]. In this case, the specific modification was Xylose-α1,3-Xylose-α1,3-Glucose-β1-O-Serine (Xyl-α1,3-Xyl-α1,3-Glc-β1-O-Ser) [21] (see below). Remarkably, Fringe was the β1,3-N-acetylglucosaminyltransferase responsible for addition of the second sugar [25, 26] within O-linked fucose moieties. Thus, in cells that don't express Fringe, Notch appears on the surface with O-linked fucose at $C_2X(4)S/TC_3$ sites. Alternatively, in cells expressing Fringe, Notch has a mixture of disaccharide (GlcNAc-β1,3-Fuc-α1-O-Ser/Thr), trisaccharide (Gal-β1,4-GlcNAc-β1,3-Fuc-α1-O-Ser/Thr), and tetrasaccharide (Sia-α2,6-Gal-β1,4-GlcNAc-β1,3-Fuc-α1-O-Ser/Thr) modifications at these sites, depending on the expression of each glycosyltransferase [21, 25, 27] (Note: in flies, the disaccharide is either not extended or extended though addition of β1–4-linked glucuronic acid [27–29]). Fringe-mediated addition of GlcNAc is *the* critical determinant of reduced Serrate binding to Notch together with enhanced binding of Delta [27]. These findings help explain how Fringe can block activation of Notch by Serrate while enhancing activation by Delta [17]. Genetic and biochemical analysis established a critical role for Golgi localization and glycosyltransferase activity of Fringe [25, 26, 30–33]. Vertebrate Lfng, Mfng, and Rfng are also fucose-specific and Notch-directed β1,3-N-acetylglucosaminyltransferases, with Lunatic being the most potent enzyme of the three [25, 31]. Like its *Drosophila* counterpart, Lfng-mediated modification of Notch1 prevents its activation by Jag1 (mammalian Serrate homologue), while enhancing activation by Dll1 (mammalian Delta homologue) [34, 35].

4.3 Preparing Notch for Fringe: The Role of Fucosylation

In 2001, a gene coding for the enzyme responsible for O-fucosylation of Notch on EGF-like repeats was identified in multiple species including human, mouse, *Drosophila*, and *C. elegans* (Note: Pofut1 and Ofut1 are the names for this protein in vertebrates and flies, respectively. *Pofut1* and *Ofut1* are the gene names) [36]. Knockdown of *Ofut1* impaired *Fringe*-dependent *and Fringe*-independent Notch activation in flies [37]. This gene was also identified as *Neurotic*, which is required for Delta/Notch signaling [38]. Shi and Stanley reported on altered somitogenesis, as well as cardiac, blood vessel, and neuronal development in *Pofut1* mutant mice, phenotypes almost indistinguishable from those seen in mice with dramatic impairment of Notch signaling (as in *Rbpjk*$^{-/-}$ mutants) [39, 40]. Interestingly, deletion of *Pofut1* within the hematopoietic compartment, or replacement of Notch1 with a mutant that cannot be fucosylated on EGF-like repeat 12 (T466A), impaired Notch1-dependent T-cell development (see below) [41, 42].

A number of studies have begun to address exactly how Pofut1/Ofut1 functions to regulate Notch. Surprisingly, this protein may control Notch through slightly different mechanisms in flies and vertebrates. This could be related to the difference in temperature at which each develops, and potentially to differences in the complex process of Notch extracellular domain folding and trafficking in each case. Alternatively, apparent differences may be a reflection of context-specific functions for Pofut1/Ofut1 and Notch fucosylation, as well as to the very challenging nature of the question being addressed: how to define biological function of a protein in the presence or absence of a modification, in this case Notch fucosylation? Indeed, fucosylation of Notch occurs on the majority of EGF-like repeats within the extracellular domain, and each of these may have different or even opposite functions. Therefore, ultimately, the function of fucosylation will have to be defined for each residue subject to this modification [43]. As a first step, however, loss-of-function mutations in the glycosyltransferase can be used to test for phenotypes caused by loss of the modification on all sites (including those on other EGF-like repeat containing proteins [44]). As noted above, this results in loss of Notch signaling in both flies and mice. Strikingly, a fucosyltransferase-defective mutant (*Ofut1*^{R254A}) could rescue aspects of this phenotype, an effect attributed to the ability of Ofut1 to chaperone Notch from the endoplasmic reticulum to the cell surface [45, 46]. Specifically, *Ofut1*^{R254A} rescued the requirement for Ofut1 during neurogenesis and resulted in phenotypes associated with loss of Fringe. Thus, while Ofut1 protein may function to enhance trafficking of Notch to the cell surface and also to facilitate regulation by Fringe, fucose addition per se is not absolutely required for activation of Notch by either ligand [46]. Based solely on this data, one might consider three scenarios in the fly: (i) Notch expressed in the absence of Ofut1 shows reduced transport or stability on the cell surface but can be activated by either Delta or Serrate once there; (ii) Notch co-expressed with Ofut1 should be efficiently trafficked to the cell surface, but once there, it functions as a Serrate (as opposed to Delta) receptor; and (iii) Notch co-expressed with Ofut1 and Fringe, in which case it will be efficiently trafficked to the cell surface and activated by Delta, but not Serrate.

Interestingly, mouse *Pofut1* is also required for Notch1 trafficking to the cell surface, or perhaps for its stabilization at the membrane of cells within developing presomitic mesoderm [47, 48]. Surprisingly, however, *Pofut1* is not required for cell surface expression of Notch in mouse embryonic stem cells (mES). Also, while ligand binding and Notch signaling is defective in mutant ES cells, both properties can be rescued, at least partially, by *Pofut1*^{R254A} [49]. These findings highlight the importance of Pofut1 chaperone activity, not necessarily for transport to the surface, but for accumulation of a ligand-activatable form of Notch. To complicate things, ectopic expression of an unrelated enzymatically inactive ER-resident glucosidase (α-Gcs1^{S440F}) was also found to rescue ligand binding and Notch signaling. Therefore, induction of the unfolded protein response is likely responsible for rescue, through increased nonspecific chaperone activity within the secretory pathway [49]. Stahl et al. have also looked at ligand binding and Notch signaling in Lec13 Chinese hamster ovary (CHO) cells, which are wild type for *Pofut1*, but have a mutation in the gene coding for GDP-mannose-4,6-dehydratase (*Gmd*). As a result, Lec13 have extremely low levels of GDP-fucose (~3% of the levels seen in parental CHO cells). This deficiency can be corrected simply by growing cells in the presence of fucose [50–53]. Lec13 cells therefore express wild-type levels of ER-resident Pofut1 but insufficient GDP-fucose to modify Notch as it is synthesized. As with

Pofut1$^{-/-}$ mES cells, Notch synthesized in Lec13 cells is expressed on the surface but shows reduced ligand binding and a dramatic loss of ligand-dependent signaling. Importantly, ligand-independent signaling was not effected. In this case, ligand binding and signaling were both rescued through addition of fucose to the media, which restores fucosylation [52]. In sum, fucosylation of Notch *and* chaperone activity of Pofut1/Ofut1 both play an important role for this enzyme in *Fringe*-dependent and *Fringe*-independent Notch-mediated development.

4.4 The Specificity of Ligand-Receptor Interaction and the Role of Specific EGF-Like Repeats

Most EGF-like repeats in Notch, whether *Drosophila* Notch or human Notch (1 through 4), have an O-fucose addition consensus sequence ($C_2X(4)S/TC_3$), and these are efficiently modified [22]. Also, many of the fucose addition sites are conserved: EGF-like repeats 2, 3, 5, 6, 8, 9, 12, 16, 17, 18, 20, 21, 23, 24, 26, 27, 30, 31, 32, 35, and 36 [22]. Notable among these are EGF-like repeat 12 (which is within a critical ligand-binding domain) and EGF-like repeats 24, 26, and 27 (which are within the Abruptex region, which is subject to mutations that impair cell-autonomous, or cis-, inhibition by ligands) [54–56]. EGF-like repeat 12 of Notch represents a particularly critical surface for binding both Delta and Serrate family ligands [57]. Luca et al. recently reported on structural analysis of a Notch1 ligand-binding fragment (EGF [11–13]) in contact with an affinity-evolved mutant fragment from Dll4 ($Dll4_{SLP}$(N-EGF2)). Their data showed binding between EGF-like repeat 11 in Notch1 and the DSL (Delta/Serrate/Lag-2) domain of Dll4, as well as between EGF-like repeat 12 in Notch1 and the Dll4 MNNL (*m*odule at the *N*-terminus of *N*otch *l*igands) domain [58]. Remarkably, addition of O-linked fucose to threonine 466 within EGF-like repeat 12 increased the affinity of interaction with Dll4 by acting as a surrogate amino acid, hydrogen bonding to tyrosine 65 within MNNL [58]. Indeed, fucosylation of T466 also increased the affinity of Notch1 EGF [11–13] for Dll1 and Jagged1, and this effect was even stronger than for Dll4 [59]. This makes sense, as Dll4 shows a higher affinity for Notch1 to start with [60]. Finally, Fringe-mediated addition of GlcNAc to T466-O-fucose further increased affinity of EGF [11–13] for Delta and Serrate family ligands [59]. These data provide a detailed molecular description for how Fringe can enhance ligand-receptor interaction. Despite this, many questions remain. For example, the mechanism by which Fringe impairs Serrate family ligand binding to Notch has yet to be determined, although other EGF-like repeats seem likely to be involved [43, 59]. The importance of further elongation at GlcNAc-β1,3-Fuc-α1-O-Ser/Thr disaccharide moieties has been described but not fully explored [61, 62]. Also, while in vitro and in vivo (see below) studies show that specific Notch receptors can respond differently to the same Fringe [34], and different Fringe proteins seem to effect individual ligands and receptors in unique ways [35, 63–65], the details underlying such complexity have yet to be defined.

4.5 Pofut1, Fringe, and Direct Modification of Ligand EGF-Like Repeats

Just like Notch, its Delta and Serrate family ligands are transmembrane proteins with multiple EGF-like repeats, and many of these have potential O-fucose acceptor sites. Indeed, *Drosophila* and vertebrate ligands are substrates for Ofut1 and for elongation of fucosylated residues by Fringe [23]. Despite this, *Ofut1* mutant clones can induce activation of Notch signaling in adjacent wild-type cells, and therefore Notch ligands maintain signaling function, even in the absence of fucosylation [37]. The importance of Dll1 fucosylation, with subsequent Fringe-mediated extension of fucose moieties through addition of GlcNAc, has been studied in vitro and in vivo. In both cases, Dll1 was found to reach the cell surface in the absence of Pofut1-mediated fucosylation [66]. In contrast, a role for fucosylation and GlcNAc addition does seem to be important for Dll3, an unusual Delta family protein in mammals that functions as a cell-autonomous mediator of Notch cis-inhibition (see below) [67–70].

4.6 Vertebrate Fringe Proteins in Paraxial Mesoderm Segmentation

In 1998, the Gridley and Johnson labs described phenotypic consequences of *Lfng* deletion in the mouse [71, 72]. These mutants were viable but small, with very short tails, as well as vertebral and rib patterning defects. All major abnormalities were traced to impaired anterior-posterior patterning of somites, transient epithelial structures that form from paraxial mesoderm during embryogenesis, which go on to generate vertebrae, ribs, and skeletal muscle. This phenotype was related to but milder than mutants for *Dll1*, *Notch1*, *Rbpjk*, *Psn1*, and *Mesp2* [73–80]. Interestingly, *Lfng* mutant mice were almost indistinguishable from *Dll3* mutants [81]. Also, congenital spondylocostal dysostosis, a vertebral disorder in humans with similarity to the phenotype seen in *Dll3* or *Lfng* mutant mice, is associated with loss-of-function mutations in *DLL3* or *LFNG*, as well as in other Notch pathway genes like *HES7*, *MESP2*, and *RIPPLY2* [82–90]. The similarity between *Lfng* and *Dll3* mutant phenotypes in mice and humans raised the possibility that Lfng and Dll3 function together during somitogenesis [70].

In *Drosophila* and related invertebrates, segmentation of the embryo takes place synchronously, along the entire anterior-posterior axis. In contrast, vertebrate segmentation occurs through sequential addition of body segments as the embryo grows at the caudal or posterior end [91]. Many events required to initiate, propagate, and precisely coordinate this process have been uncovered through studies in model systems, including mouse, chicken, zebrafish, and *Xenopus*. The number of somites, and the time taken to add a somite, can vary from one vertebrate species to another. Despite this, a related *clock-and-wavefront* model has been proposed to explain segmentation in each case [91–93]. While a detailed discussion of sequential somite addition is beyond the scope of this review, in simple terms, it involves coordination and crosstalk between FGF, Wnt, retinoic acid, and Notch signaling pathways [91, 93–98]. At the core of this system is a segmentation clock, by which each somite is generated with passage of a species-specific time window. This window can vary greatly. For example, in zebrafish, somite addition takes ~30 min, whereas in humans the somite addition cycle is 6 h long. The mouse clock takes approximately 90 min to traverse one cycle and therefore to add one somite on either side of the neural tube. Fundamentally, the clock and wavefront are both dependent on induction of delayed negative feedback loops for the above signaling pathways [99, 100]. For example, FGF signaling from caudal mesoderm induces expression of Dusp phosphatases and Sprouty, both of which suppress FGFR/Mapk signaling [101]. FGFR also activates expression of CYP26, which helps to degrade retinoic acid. This limits antagonism of FGF and Wnt signaling pathways by somite and anterior presomitic mesoderm-derived retinoic acid [102–104]. Wnt signaling induces expression of Axin2 and Dickkopf-related protein 1 (Dkk1), the former inhibiting Wnt signaling within cells and the latter inhibiting Wnt-Lrp6 interaction at the cell surface [96, 105]. Finally, Notch signaling induces expression of *Hes7*, *Nrarp*, and *Lfng*, all three of which inhibit Dll1-Notch1 signaling in this context [91, 106–108].

Interestingly, the absolute level of *Lfng* expression is important for precise coordination of somitogenesis, especially in anterior somites [109, 110]. Also, oscillation of Notch activation, rather than a Notch activation boundary per se, is *the* critical determinant of somite border formation and patterning within somites [111]. For Lfng, its fluctuation is controlled by Notch-dependent induction, followed by delays associated mostly with splicing and mRNA export from the nucleus [100, 108]. As for Lfng levels, these are limited through mir-125-5p-mediated *Lfng* mRNA destabilization [112, 113], as well as through proteolytic cleavage-mediated secretion of Lfng protein, which functions to decrease accumulation within the Golgi [114].

4.7 Cell-Autonomous and Non-cell-Autonomous Regulation of Notch and Its Ligands by Fringe Proteins

The function for *Lfng* as an inhibitor of Delta-Notch signaling in somitogenesis is striking and seems to contradict what is known about *Fringe* in *Drosophila*. Recently, an explanation for this discrepancy has begun to emerge. Indeed, recent insights on Fringe function have shown how it can be used to coordinate Notch-dependent processes quite distinct from the type of inductive signaling involved in D/V boundary formation in the fly wing. For example, unlike its positive effect on Delta-mediated Notch activation in the wing, Lfng-mediated inhibition of Notch1 signaling in presomitic mesoderm is *non-cell autonomous* [115]. This so-called transrepression activity is dependent on Dll3 and Dll1 in signaling cells and also correlates with fucosylation of Dll3 EGF-like repeats 2 and 5 at S286 and T403, respectively [115]. Fucose residues on these sites can be extended through Lfng-mediated GlcNAc addition, at least in vitro [67]. As noted, Dll3 is not a typical Delta-family ligand. Indeed, it's not even expressed on the surface of presomitic mesoderm and cannot activate Notch expressed in neighboring cells [69, 70, 84]. Thus, the most parsimonious model to explain Lfng-mediated transrepression of Notch1 in the segmentation clock involves Pofut1- and Lfng-dependent addition of fucose and GlcNAc on Dll3, which then functions either to change Dll1 into a competitive inhibitor of Notch1 activation in neighboring cells or perhaps simply to decrease the Notch activating properties of Dll1. More studies will be required to precisely determine how Lfng interacts with Dll3 (and Dll1) in somitogenesis.

While the precise mechanism by which Fringes function to coordinate Notch signaling during boundary formation in flies, the segmentation clock in vertebrates, and the myriad other developmental, homeostatic, or pathological states in which it has been implicated remains to be determined at high resolution, sophisticated cell culture techniques and mathematical modeling experiments, together with the structural studies discussed above, are beginning to shed light on cis- and trans-interactions between Notch and its ligands as well as how Fringe can effect both. For example, Sprinzak and colleagues found that mutual interaction between Delta and Notch within the same cell is used to control an ultrasensitive switch between signal sender (Delta high/Notch low) and receiver (Delta low/Notch high) states [116]. The effect of Fringe proteins on cis-interactions is very similar to its effect on trans-interactions, in that Fringe enhances (cis-inhibitory) interactions between Delta-family ligands and Notch, when all three are expressed in the same cell. Consistent with this, Fringe actually cell-autonomously reduces (cis-inhibitory) interactions between Jagged/Serrate family ligands and Notch [117]. Remarkably, the cell-autonomous and non-cell-autonomous activities of Fringe can therefore be used to precisely regulate the specific Delta/Serrate signal sender *and* Delta/Serrate signal receiver functions of neighboring cells. Indeed, Troost and Klein have teased apart two sequential Fringe-dependent events during D/V boundary formation in the wing imaginal disc, the first involving dorsally expressed Serrate activating Notch in ventral cells [19]. This causes upregulation of Delta in the ventral compartment, which subsequently activates Notch in nearby boundary cells on the dorsal side [19].

Mutsado et al. used a "synthetic biology" approach to establish a bistable system in cultured cells, whereby Lfng-mediated positive feedback facilitated propagation of a Delta-Notch signal across the population [118]. In related experiments, they went on to show that Notch-mediated induction of *Lfng* can promote lateral inhibition by partitioning a population of bipotential cells into Dll1$^+$ signal sender and Notch1$^+$ signal receiver cells [119]. In this context, Notch-induced transcriptional repression of Delta and induction of Lfng, both in receiver cells, acted redundantly to enhance the signal receiving state (at the expense of the signal sender state). This redundancy may well explain why Fringe is not considered essential with respect to lateral inhibition in vivo. Indeed, with multiple feedback systems operational, the Notch activation system can be extremely robust in some biological contexts. For example, while *Lfng* knockout or knockdown cell-autonomously reduced the number of Hes1$^+$ signal-receiving cells in the developing mouse brain, this effect did not lead to altered neuronal differentiation or patterning [119, 120].

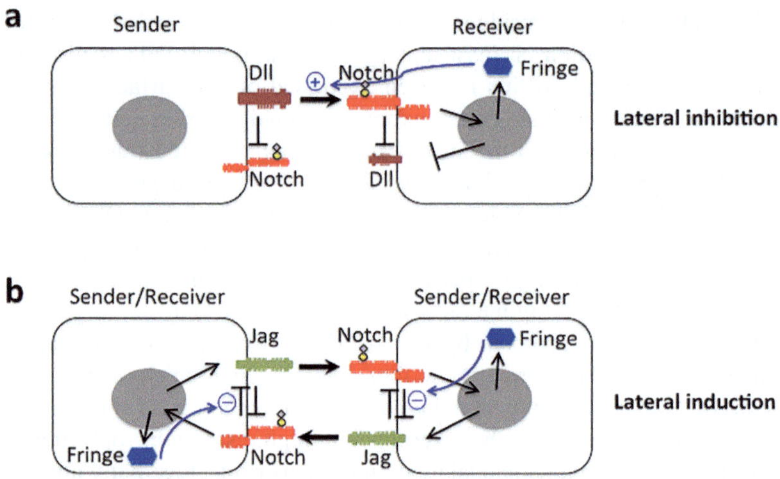

Fig. 4.2 A scheme for roles of Fringe in lateral inhibition and lateral induction. (**a**) Fringe can promote partitioning of bipotential cells into Delta^{Hi}/Notch^{Lo} signal sender and Delta^{Lo}/Notch^{Hi} signal receiver cells (lateral inhibition). In this context, Notch induces transcriptional repression of Delta and induction of Fringe both in receiver cells to enhance the signal receiving state at the expense of the signal sending state. (**b**) Fringe can facilitate formation of the hybrid Sender/Receiver state, leading to a more uniform phenotype among neighbors (lateral induction). In this regard, Notch upregulates both Serrate/Jagged and Fringe, creating a potent positive feedback loop, whereby Fringe prevents cis-inhibition of Notch in these cells

Genes coding for Delta and Jagged/Serrate family ligands are subject to distinct forms of regulation. For example, active Notch^{ICD} directly binds to and transcriptionally activates genes coding for Hes/Hey/E(spl) bHLH proteins. These, in turn, downregulate expression of *Dll1*. In contrast, Notch^{ICD} directly activates expression of *Jagged1* in some cells [121]. As noted above, Delta-Notch signaling facilitates lateral inhibition or partitioning of initially equivalent neighbors to distinct cell states: sender cells (Delta^{Hi}/Notch^{Lo}) and receiver cells (Delta^{Lo}/Notch^{Hi}). With a positive feedback loop between Notch and Jagged/Serrate, activation by ligand promotes formation of a third state: the hybrid sender/receiver state. In this hybrid state, cells can send and receive Notch signals, leading to a more uniform phenotype among neighbors (lateral induction). This idea, based to a large extent on mathematical modeling by Boareto et al., helps to explain how Fringe functions at the D/V boundary of the wing imaginal disc [122] (Fig. 4.2). In this regard, *Fringe* is upregulated by Notch^{ICD}. This creates a potent positive feedback loop, whereby Serrate and Fringe in one cell (e.g., a dorsal compartment cell) can accumulate to very high levels without cis-inhibition of Notch. The Serrate can therefore activate Notch in ventral cells. The dorsal Notch, modified by Fringe, will be very responsive to Delta, which is expressed in ventral neighbors. This model also helps to explain how Jagged and Fringe can facilitate Notch signaling between the epithelium and stroma, as well as between tumor and stromal elements [122].

4.8 Hematopoiesis and Lymphocyte Development: The Role of Lfng and Mfng

Notch signaling controls development and homeostasis within the hematopoietic system. Indeed, altered *Notch* gene function has been linked to a number of hematopoietic malignancies [123]. Once again, development of this system is complex, and roles for Notch signaling in this context are varied. We therefore refer readers to other reviews for a more exhaustive discussion [124–130]. Here we highlight a few key areas that are likely to involve Fringe or for which Fringe protein function has already been studied in detail.

Hematopoietic stem cells (HSC) derive from cells within the aorta-gonad-mesonephros (AGM) region of the embryo [131]. It is within the AGM that cells are partitioned between endothelial and hematopoietic fates on the basis of Notch1 signaling [132]. Cells exposed to a high level of Dll4 ligand are fated to become endothelium, whereas low-level Notch1 activation in response to Jagged1 induces HSC/CD45$^+$ specification [130, 133–136]. The dosage-dependent effects documented in venous vs. arterial vs. hematopoietic cell fate specification within the AGM may be paradigmatic for many Notch-dependent developmental and homeostatic events. Interestingly, Fringe genes are downregulated in AGM endothelium after exposure to Jagged1 [130]. This downregulation may well increase sensitivity to Jagged1, while reducing sensitivity to Dll4, thereby reinforcing commitment to the hematopoietic stem cell fate. Once generated, HSC migrate to the fetal liver and ultimately to the bone marrow.

The generation and diversification of T-lymphocytes proceeds through multiple Notch1-dependent steps [137]. Firstly, Dll4 expressed by Osteocalcin$^+$ cells in the bone marrow stimulates development of thymus-seeding progenitors (TSP) [138]. Upon arriving in the thymus, TSP encounters Dll4 expressed by stromal cells. Dll4-mediated Notch1 activation then stimulates differentiation of TSPs into early T-cell precursors (ETPs). This step is associated with rapid loss of B-lymphocyte developmental potential [139–141]. ETPs then respond to Dll4 on thymic stroma by differentiating into CD4$^-$CD8$^-$*d*ouble *n*egative 2 (DN2) thymocytes, which lose the ability to generate myeloid cell types [142]. DN2 cells then differentiate into DN3a cells and then into one of two alternative cell types: TCR$\gamma\delta^+$ or TCRβ^+ (DN3b). The TCRβ^+ cell requires Notch1 as it proliferates and differentiates into a CD4$^+$/CD8$^+$ double-positive (DP) cell. Notch1 expression is significantly reduced as cells differentiate into DP. Also, Dll3 is expressed in DP cells, where it functions cell-autonomously to inhibit Notch-mediated induction of *Hes5*. Biologically, inhibition of Notch by Dll3 in this context is important for positive selection of $\alpha\beta$ T-cells [143].

Lfng is highly expressed in ETP, DN2, and DN3, but not DP thymocytes. In competition experiments, *Lfng* is cell-autonomously required for Notch1-dependent T-cell development, as well as for suppression of the B-cell fate [144]. Interestingly, transgenic overexpression of *Lfng* in DN3 or DP causes them to bind so well to Dll4, that they non-cell-autonomously block wild-type TSP and ETP

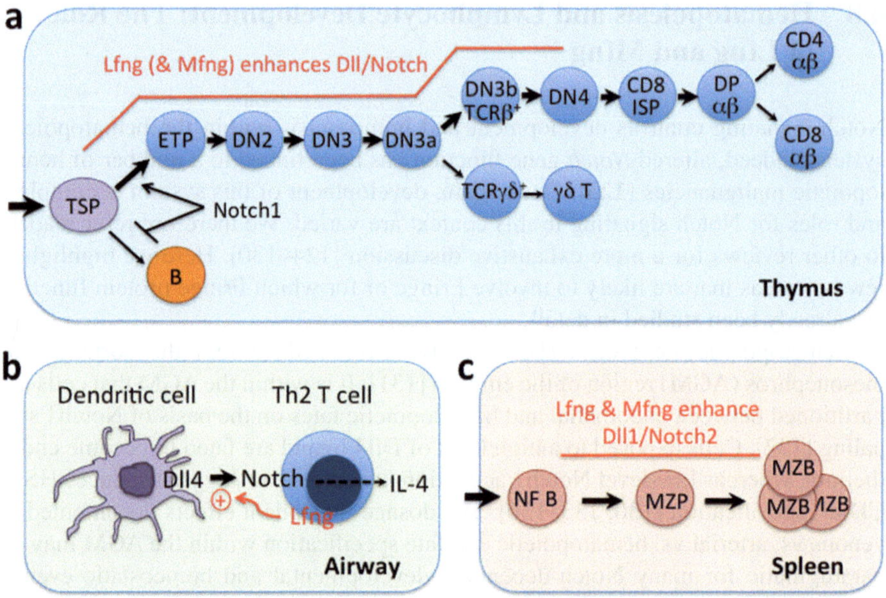

Fig. 4.3 Roles of Fringe-modulated Notch signaling in the immune system. (**a**) Lfng (and Mfng) promotes T-cell development while suppressing the B-cell fate through enhancement of Notch1 signaling. (**b**) Lfng contributes to the augmented Th2 response during viral exacerbation of existing airway allergy by enhancing Dll4-Notch activation. (**c**) Lfng and Mfng cooperatively enhance the Dll1-Notch2 interaction to promote marginal zone (MZ) B cell development in the spleen

from efficiently binding to the thymic niche, as required for Dll4-Notch1 signaling [145, 146]. As a result, transgenic cells impair T-cell specification and differentiation of immature transgenic thymocytes that have yet to activate the transgene [147] as well as wild-type immature cells that are present in chimeric mice [145]. Notch signaling also plays a role in mature effector T-cell differentiation, and this process is responsive to signaling from Jagged/Serrate *and* from Delta family ligands [148–150]; a role for Fringe proteins is to be anticipated. Indeed, *Lfng* helps control Notch-dependent T-cell differentiation in response to immunological challenge [151] (Fig. 4.3a,b).

In the thymus, Notch1 signaling promotes T-cell development at the expense of B-cells as noted above; however, Notch2 controls innate B-cell development in the spleen [152]. Dll1 expressed by fibroblasts within the splenic marginal zone (MZ) red pulp activates Notch2 in newly formed (NF) B-cells from the bone marrow [153]. Interestingly, this interaction is relatively weak [154], and hemizygous mutations in *Dll1* or *Notch2* impair innate B-cell generation [155, 156]. Indeed, this interaction is so weak that it requires Lfng- or Mfng-mediated glycosylation of Notch2 in NF B-cells [63] (Fig. 4.3c).

4.9 Role of Lfng and Mfng in Mammary Gland Development and Breast Cancer

Breast cancer is a heterogeneous disease. Most tumors express estrogen and progesterone receptors. A distinct group expresses elevated levels of the HER2/ErbB2 receptor tyrosine kinase. Another, very diverse group of tumors is defined on the basis of not expressing any of these receptors and is therefore described as "triple negative breast cancer" (TNBC) [157]. Transcriptional profiling has also been used to classify breast tumors into at least six molecular subtypes: basal-like, claudin-low, luminal A, luminal B, HER2-enriched, and normal-like. Among these, basal-like and claudin-low subtypes account for the majority of TNBCs [158–160]. Basal-like tumors expresses markers of myoepithelium/basal cells, share features with bipotent progenitors, and are thought to have originated from bipotent/luminal progenitor cells [159, 161, 162]. Claudin-low breast cancers (CLBCs) on the other hand share features with mammary stem cells (MaSCs) and cells that have undergone epithelial-to-mesenchymal transition (EMT)[158]. This has led to the suggestion that MaSCs could be the cell-of-origin for CLBC [158]. BLBC and CLBC are notoriously aggressive and prone to recurrence and metastasis. At present, no effective treatment exists for either. Understanding the unique biology of both subtypes should help provide insight into recurrence and metastasis and may identify specific targets for treatment.

It is widely believed that cancer stem cells (CSC) play an important role in tumor maintenance, tumor relapse, and metastasis. Also, EMT is known to promote metastasis in many contexts, and EMT by itself may generate cells with stem cell properties [163–166]. Notch signaling controls stem cell self-renewal, cell fate specification, and differentiation in the mammary gland [167–169]. Notch activation has also been shown to regulate EMT in developmental and pathological conditions [170]. Thus, it's not surprising that Notch plays an important role in breast cancer, especially in aggressive subtypes with features of stem cells and EMT. Indeed, high-level expression of *Jagged1* as well as *Notch1* and/or *Notch3* is associated with poor overall survival [171]. Also, functionally significant mutations, including *Notch1* and *Notch2* rearrangements, PEST domain mutations in *Notch1*, *Notch2*, and *Notch3*, and focal amplifications of *Notch2* and *Notch3*, have been linked to TNBC formation [172–174]. Recent studies have suggested many functions for Notch signaling in mammary development and cancer. For instance, Notch1 hyperactivation causes cyclin D1-dependent BLBC formation, and Notch1 signaling controls expansion of the MaSC compartment [167, 175, 176]; Notch2 genetic fate mapping reveals two previously unrecognized mammary epithelial lineages involved in branching morphogenesis and may have important implications vis-à-vis cell-of-origin for some breast tumors [177]; Notch3 marks clonogenic luminal progenitor cells, is required for luminal filling, and may induce cyclin D1-dependent luminal inflammatory breast tumors [178–180]; and Notch4 is implicated in self-renewal of breast cancer stem cells, EMT, and endocrine therapy resistance [181–183]. As a result, Notch has emerged as a potential drug target for poor prognosis breast cancer

[184–186]. However, Notch receptors, ligands, and modulators can exert complex effects on the pathogenesis of breast cancer, depending on tumor subtype, cellular context, and stage of disease progression. Therefore, it's critical to define roles for receptors, ligands, modulator, and downstream target in *each* subtype.

Within the developing mammary gland, *Lfng* is targeted to the stem cell-enriched cap cell layer of terminal end buds [187]. Consistent with this finding, human MaSC and/or bipotent progenitors express 20-fold higher levels of *Lfng* in comparison to luminally restricted progenitors [169]. Tissue-specific deletion of *Lfng* in mouse mammary epithelium (*Lfng$^{flox/flox}$;MMTV-Cre*) induced ectopic proliferation, expansion of the basal compartment, and ultimately, development of triple negative tumors. Gene expression profiling revealed that about two-thirds of these were basal-like and one-third claudin-low. Histological and immunohistochemical analyses confirmed features of both subtypes, with type I (basal-like) showing broad co-expression of markers for luminal (K8) and myoepithelial cells (K14) and type II (claudin-low) containing mostly spindle-shaped cells that were positive for EMT markers including vimentin and twist. Of note, the vast majority of human basal-like and a subset of claudin-low breast cancers show lower *Lfng* expression as compared with other subtypes or normal mammary tissue [187]. Thus *Lfng* deficiency represents a hallmark for basal-like mammary tumors in both mouse and human. Interestingly, most mammary tumors in *Lfng$^{flox/flox}$;MMTV-Cre* mice harbor Met/Caveolin gene amplification, causing elevated Met accumulation and activation. Met, a tyrosine kinase receptor, is frequently expressed at high levels in aggressive human breast cancer with EMT features, and expression of oncogenic Met (together with p53 loss) induced basal-like as well as claudin-low mammary tumors in transgenic mice [188–191]. Taken together, *Lfng* deficiency cooperates with Met/Caveolin amplification to induce BLBC (and less frequently, CLBC). Indeed, combination targeting of Met and Notch may prove beneficial for TNBC patients with Met overexpression and Notch hyperactivation [192].

It's noteworthy that very low levels of *Lfng* expression are seen in basal-like tumors, but only a small fraction of these harbor Notch-activating mutations [172–174]. Therefore downregulation of *Lfng* is more prevalent than functional mutations in Notch. The *Lfng* deletion model for TNBC will complement models that overexpress Notch intracellular domain fragments. In addition, the latter models are not good for testing most Notch-targeting agents (such as γ-secretase inhibitors), which block cleavage of the intact receptor.

While *Lfng* deficiency is a hallmark of BLBC, *Mfng* is highly expressed in CLBC, functioning as an oncogene in this context [193]. *Mfng* regulates Notch activation in human and mouse CLBC cell lines, as well as in the mouse mammary gland at puberty and during involution [193]. Knockdown of *Mfng* in CLBC cell lines reduced cell migration and tumorsphere formation associated with diminution of MaSC and/or bipotent progenitor cell populations, as well as reduced tumorigenicity. In addition, deletion of *Mfng* in the *Lfng$^{flox/flox}$;MMTV-Cre* mouse caused a tumor subtype shift away from CLBC. In this study, *Pik3cg*, which encodes PI3K catalytic subunit γ, was identified as a direct transcriptional target of *Mfng*-facilitated RBPJk-dependent Notch signaling. This finding may well shed light on why Notch pathway activation can confer resistance to PI3K inhibitors [194]. *Pik3cg* is aberrantly expressed in many invasive breast tumors, and its expression level correlates with metastatic potential of breast cancer cell lines [195]. Indeed, pharmacologic inhibition of PI3Kγ blocked migration and tumorsphere formation by CLBC cell lines [193]. Fringe-regulated Notch signaling within myeloid cells could also control response to tumor-derived chemoattractants that stimulate GPCRs coupled to PI3Kγ. In vivo studies will be required to determine precise roles for this Mfng-Notch-Pik3cg axis in CLBC pathogenesis, in particular, in the enrichment of cancer stem cells, induction of EMT, and recruitment of myeloid cells. Nonetheless, identification of Pik3cg as a Notch target prompts a new targeting strategy for treating CLBC and perhaps other poor prognosis breast cancers. As discussed above, Met was amplified in basal-like *and* claudin-low tumors from *Lfng*$^{flox/flox}$*;MMTV-Cre* mice, and Met can synergize with mutant *Trp53* to induce claudin-low like mammary tumors in the mouse [190]. Therefore, combination therapy against Met and PI3Kγ could represent an effective strategy for treatment of CLBC. *MFNG* expression in human breast cancer is highly correlated with expression of *NOTCH4*, but not with other Notch receptors. In addition, *Mfng* silencing in CLBC cell lines consistently decreased Notch4 activation/cleavage as did *Mfng* deletion in the mouse mammary gland [193]. Therefore, Mfng appears to control Notch4-mediated signaling in mammary epithelium. Given that Notch4 is enriched in MaSC, a putative cell-of-origin for CLBC, the Mfng-Notch4-Pik3cg signaling cascade may drive pathogenesis for this subtype.

The phenotypic response to Notch is often determined by the level of pathway activation, and this affects the balance between growth-stimulating and growth-suppressing effects [196]. In this context, Fringe may be used to precisely modulate signaling in distinct cell types of the mammary epithelial hierarchy. Recent studies in mice and in humans support a model whereby *Lfng* inhibits Notch activation within luminal progenitor cells to prevent BLBC, while Mfng enhances Notch4 signaling in mammary stem cells to promote CLBC initiation and progression. Of note, deletion of *Lfng and Mfng* dramatically decreased activation of multiple Notch receptors and induced adenosquamous carcinoma [193], suggesting a redundant role for these genes in MaSCs and/or multipotent progenitors of the mammary gland.

4.10 Roles of Lfng and Mfng in Lung Development and Lung Cancer

The lung is a highly specialized organ that facilitates rapid and efficient oxygenation of blood. This is achieved at the interface of alveoli and microcapillaries, each organized in a complex labyrinth of interconnected thin-walled sacs and tubules. During alveogenesis, the final stage of lung development, a multilayered structure is transformed into a thin epithelial/capillary wall composed of type II and type I alveolar cells, microcapillaries, fibroblasts, and elastic extracellular matrix. This event must occur in a highly coordinated manner under conditions where the lung is subjected to elastic forces associated with breathing. *Lfng* and other Notch pathway components are highly expressed in the developing mouse lung. At 16.5–18.5 dpc, *Lfng* is expressed in saccular cells and in cells of the distal lung mesenchyme. The highest levels of *Lfng* expression are seen in pulmonary neuroendocrine cells (PNECs), which are organized in clusters known as neuroepithelial bodies (NEBs) or as solitary cells. At P5, *Lfng* is still expressed in NEBs but now also seen in endothelial cells of large pulmonary veins. Notch1 is expressed in bronchiolar cells at 16.5 dpc, whereas *Notch2* and *3* are highly expressed in mesenchyme and airway epithelium at 17.5 dpc and beyond. *Dll1* is also expressed in PNEC throughout lung development and in vascular endothelial cells after P5. Expression of *Dll4* is localized to endothelial cells scattered throughout the mesenchyme and in PNEC at 17.5 dpc. Finally, Jagged1 is expressed in pulmonary veins and arteries throughout development and in bronchiolar epithelial cells starting at 16.5 dpc [197].

Lfng null mice exhibit a dramatic defect in lung structure, with altered patterning and reduced vascular branching. Histological analysis of lung development in these mice revealed a delay in saccule expansion starting at 16.5 dpc, followed by defective alveolar septation, which persisted in older animals. *Lfng* mutant lungs show delayed distal epithelial cell differentiation, as manifested by lower expression of integrin β6 in saccular epithelial cells and decreased level of aquaporin 5 in type I alveolar cells. Expression of the type II alveolar cell marker SP-C, the Clara cell marker CC10, and PNEC markers, Ascl1 and CGRP, are largely normal in mutant lungs. The most striking defect is that smooth muscle actin α (sma), a myofibroblast differentiation marker, is expressed in myofibroblasts of wild-type but not in *Lfng* mutant mesenchyme at 17.5 dpc. During postnatal alveolar development, sma is localized in myofibroblast cells that have migrated to branch or septation points in the developing alveoli of wild-type lungs. In contrast, sma is expressed at a low level in a small number of *Lfng* mutant mesenchymal cells, most of which are trapped within multilayered walls separating large alveoli. Myofibroblast progenitor cells in the developing distal lung require PDGFRα [198]. This receptor is expressed similarly in wild-type and mutant lungs during late embryogenesis, suggesting that differentiation but not specification or spreading of myofibroblast progenitors is affected. Myofibroblasts express and deposit elastin, which is critical for alveogenesis and lung function. Indeed, *Lfng* mutant lungs exhibit aberrant deposition of elastin, with few elastic fibers evident at P14. Despite this, elastin accumulates and is trapped within multilayered walls at 6 wk. of age. Taken together, alveolar development is impaired in Lfng mutant mice, starting in the saccule phase of fetal development, with impaired differentiation of myofibroblasts, accompanied by a modest delay of type I alveolar epithelial cell differentiation [197].

Lfng could either be enhancing or suppressing Notch activation during distal lung development.

Interestingly, *Notch2* and *3* are both highly expressed during saccular development in the distal lung, and myofibroblast differentiation is impaired in *Notch2*$^{+/-}$*Notch3*$^{-/-}$ compound mutant embryos but not in single mutants, suggesting that these receptors function redundantly to induce myofibroblast differentiation. Moreover, conditional deletion of RBPJκ caused a similar impairment of myofibroblast differentiation. A simple model to explain these findings involves a requirement for *Lfng*-mediated facilitation of Dll-induced Notch2/3 activation in myofibroblast progenitor cells. In this case, Dll4 expressed in endothelial cells of the distal lung would be the likely ligand.

Besides defective myofibroblast differentiation, *Lfng* mutant lungs exhibit a modest delay in saccule epithelial cell development that appears to correct itself by birth. This delay may be related to low-level expression of *Lfng* in saccular cells, which could affect Notch signaling in developing type II or type I cells. Previous studies suggest that Notch signaling is not required for specification of alveolar epithelial cells [199]. *Lfng* could indeed function in saccular cells to prevent Notch activation by Jagged ligands. In this case, ectopic Jagged-Notch activation would likely occur in *Lfng* mutant saccular cells and thereby block or delay alveolar epithelial differentiation [200, 201]. Alternatively, *Lfng* may not function within saccular or alveolar epithelial progenitor cells, and delayed differentiation of these cells may be secondary to impaired differentiation of myofibroblasts or other mesenchymal cell types [202].

A unique Notch expression boundary is noted at the NEB, where *Dll1*, *Dll4*, *Notch4*, and *Lfng* are expressed in PNEC cells, *Notch1*, *2*, and *3* are expressed in SSEA-1$^+$, CC10$^-$ cells surrounding the NEB, and Jagged1 is expressed in neighboring epithelial cells [197, 203, 204] (Zhang et al., unpublished data). The NEB and related bronchoalveolar junctions are thought to represent a stem cell niche [205] as well as a signaling center that controls distal lung development [206]. *Lfng* may affect stem cell differentiation kinetics in this context. Interestingly, Branchfield et al. found that PNECs are important regulators of postnatal lung function [207]. In this study, inactivation of *Robo* in the mouse lung resulted in an inability of PNECs to cluster into NEBs. This triggered increased neuropeptide production upon exposure to air, leading to an increase in immune infiltrates, which in turn remodeled the matrix and irreversibly simplified alveoli [207]. Coincidentally, *Lfng* null mice show ectopic CGRP-positive cells in the distal lung, accompanied by accumulation of macrophages and severely disrupted alveoli in postnatal life [197] (Xu and Egan, unpublished data). Thus, expression of *Lfng* in NEBs appears to prevent solitary PNECs from entering the alveolar compartment, which may impact distal lung structure and function. In future, PNEC-specific deletion of *Lfng* will be needed to probe the functional significance of these findings. Finally, PNEC is the cell-of-origin for small cell lung cancer (SCLC) [208]. A recent study identified inactivating mutations in NOTCH family genes in 25% of human SCLC [209]. Activation of Notch signaling in a preclinical SCLC mouse model strikingly reduced the number of tumors and extended the survival of mutant mice, and neuroendocrine gene expression was abrogated by Notch activity in SCLC cells [209]. In this case, although deletion of *Lfng* did not affect specification of PNEC as judged by expression of Ascl1 and CGRP, it enhanced Notch activation in these cells (Xu and Egan, unpublished data), which could influence SCLC development.

As with Notch, differential expression of Fringes suggests non-redundancy and context-dependent function. Unlike *Lfng* mutants, the *Mfng* mutant lung appeared normal (Xu et al., unpublished data) [210]. Despite this, human MFNG is located on chromosome 22q13.1, a region of homozygous deletion in many non-small cell lung cancer (NSCLC) [211, 212]. Indeed, *MFNG* expression is consistently reduced in lung cancer as compared to normal lung tissue [213]. To the contrary, *MFNG* is one of the most upregulated genes in response to antitumor B (ATB), a Chinese herbal mixture with chemopreventive activity in mouse models for lung cancer [214]. Indeed, reexpression of *MFNG* decreased expression of *HES1* and *HEYL* Notch target genes and reduced transformation-associated phenotype in vitro as well as tumorigenicity in vivo [213]. Surprisingly, these effects appear to be related to modulation of Notch3 protein stability. Indeed, Mfng enhanced degradation of Notch3, and proteasome inhibition reversed this effect [213]. A number of studies have suggested oncogenic roles of Notch3 in lung cancer. Interestingly, a recent study identified a rare population of $CD24^{+}ITGB4^{+}Notch^{hi}$ cells that drive tumor propagation in NSCLC and that require Notch3 for self-renewal [215]. This population is enriched after chemotherapy, and its gene signature correlates with poor prognosis. In agreement with this result, an investigation into inefficacy of erlotinib in advanced lung cancer found that EGFR blockade enriches for lung cancer stem-like cells through Notch3-dependent signaling [216]. Thus, Notch3 may represent an important therapeutic target for NSCLC. In this context, *Mfng*-mediated proteasome-dependent degradation of Notch3 could prove beneficial.

4.11 Tumor-Suppressive Role of Lfng in Pancreatic Cancer

Pancreatic ductal adenocarcinoma (PDAC) remains one of the most lethal malignancies owing to its diagnosis at an advanced stage and resistance to most therapies. Extensive pathological studies have established a model for initiation and progression of PDAC. The most common precursor of this disease is a microscopic pancreatic lesion associated with ducts, referred to as pancreatic intraepithelial neoplasia (PanIN). PanINs progress through defined histological and molecular stages, ultimately advancing to invasive PDAC and metastasis. Genomic analyses have identified accumulating genetic alterations associated with disease progression. In this regard, activating mutations in *KRAS* have been detected in more than 90% of the PanIN lesions, whereas mutations in tumor suppressor genes such as *TP53*, *CDKN2A*, and *SMAD4* are associated with more advanced disease [217]. Thus, *KRAS* mutations may contribute to PDAC initiation, and subsequent mutations may promote tumor progression and metastasis.

In recent years, mouse models have been designed to recapitulate pathologic changes associated with human PDAC, including activation of oncogenic *Kras* and/or inactivation of *p53*, *Ink4a/Arf*, and *Smad4*. Additional genes and signals implicated in PDAC have been identified in these models and verified in humans. Indeed, Notch pathway activation has been linked to initiation and progression [218–220]. For example, *Notch2* appears to be required for progression from PanIN to PDAC [221]. Interestingly, loss- *and* gain-of-function mutations in *Notch1* rendered acinar cells more susceptible to *Kras*-induced PanIN formation and progression [218, 222, 223]. On the other hand, deficiency of isoprenylcysteine carboxyl methyltransferase, which methylates Ras and is considered a target for cancer therapy, actually exacerbated Kras-driven PDAC via Notch suppression [224]. Thus, the importance and complexity of Notch signaling in pancreatic tumorigenesis has become increasingly evident. A dormant progenitor cell population in the adult pancreas is capable of initiating PDAC under conditions of oncogenic stimulation [225]. Acinar cells, not ductal cells, are competent to form *Kras*-induced PanIN, and active Notch signaling synergizes with *Kras* in PanIN initiation and progression [218, 226, 227]. In these studies, although nearly every pancreatic acinar cell expressed activated *Kras*, only a minority gave rise to PanIN. How the transforming activity of *Kras* is constrained, or which subset of acinar cells is preferentially targeted by *Kras*, is unknown. Notch controls cell fate specification and differentiation during pancreatic development as well as in the adult exocrine pancreas [228–231]. In this context, activation of Notch generally maintains the undifferentiated state. Thus, inappropriate Notch activation in the acinar compartment of the adult pancreas may cause accumulation of undifferentiated stem/progenitor cells, which may serve as preferred target for *Kras*-induced tumor initiation.

As noted above, *Lfng* functions to suppress tumor formation in the mammary gland, in part by preventing aberrant accumulation of stem/progenitor cells [187]. In the embryonic pancreas, *Lfng* is expressed in the same cells as Ptf1a, an exocrine cell marker [232]. In adults, *Lfng* expression is restricted to a small subset of acinar cells [233]. Given that Notch inhibits Ptf1 function, and acinar cell differentiation in the developing pancreas [234], *Lfng* could well be controlling Notch signaling to facilitate regulation of acinar cell differentiation during development and homeostasis. In the $Kras^{LSL\text{-}G12D/+}$;*Pdx1-Cre* mouse model of PDAC, deletion of *Lfng* in *Kras*-expressing cells caused increased activation of *Notch3* during tumor initiation and progression, as well as activation of Notch1 after disease onset, associated with upregulation of the Notch target gene *Hes1*. Interestingly, deletion of *Lfng* caused accumulation of Aldh1-positive stem-like cells. More importantly, loss of *Lfng* significantly accelerated PDAC development and shortened survival of these mice. Of note, *Lfng*-deficient tumors were typically poorly differentiated, with features of epithelial-to-mesenchymal transition[233]. Deletion of *Lfng* also caused Notch-mediated transcriptional repression of *Tgfb1*, *Tgfb2*, and *Tgfbr2* in otherwise wild-type mice and in the $Kras^{LSL\text{-}G12D/+}$;*Pdx1-Cre* pancreas after PDAC onset. In this regard, TGF-β might promote initiation of acinar-ductal metaplasia (ADM) and PanIN. Indeed, a recent report showed that spontaneous transition of human acinar cells toward a ductal and mesenchymal phenotype was decreased through inhibition of TGF-β signaling [235]. On the other hand, decreased TGF-β expression/signaling in animals with accelerated PDAC development suggests that TGF-β may prevent progression from PanIN to PDAC.

Although expression of *Lfng* is confined to a small subset of acinar cells, its deletion profoundly altered Notch signaling and dramatically accelerated pancreatic cancer development in the *Kras* model. Thus *Lfng*-expressing acinar cells, or their neighbors, may represent a preferential target for *Kras*-induced pancreatic cancer formation. Alternatively, *Lfng*-expressing cells may be resistant to dedifferentiation and tumor formation as compared to *Lfng*-negative cells. Since *Lfng*-expressing cells account for a small minority (~5%) of acinar cells, deletion of *Lfng* would not have such a dramatic effect on PDAC development in the latter case. However, the pancreas in this study has already lost *Lfng* expression at the embryonic stage, which may affect differentiation of most cells in the acinar compartment. Therefore, to determine whether *Lfng*-expressing cells were really targeted by *Kras* to form PanIN and PDAC, lineage tracing of *Lfng*-expressing acinar cells will be required. Interestingly, the pancreas in $Lfng^{lacZ/lacZ}$ mice contains a dramatically increased number of X-Gal-positive cells as compared with the pancreas in $Lfng^{lacZ/+}$ mice [233], suggesting that *Lfng* may negatively regulate propagation of cells in which it is expressed. Notch signaling is required for maintenance of the cancer stem cell population in pancreatic cancer [236]. Indeed, DCLK1-positive preinvasive pancreatic cancer cells have tumor-initiating properties. These cells express high levels of HES1 and HEY1, and pharmacological inhibition of γ-secretase activity reduced accumulation of these cells in murine PanIN [237]. It would be interesting to determine whether these cells derive from *Lfng*-positive cells.

Individual Notch receptors have been found to play distinct, sometimes even opposing, roles in lung and pancreatic cancers [221, 238]. As noted above, Fringe proteins can regulate activation of individual Notch receptors in unique ways, depending on the ligands presented on the surface of neighboring cells. In the adult pancreas, individual Notch receptors are expressed in distinct cell types, and all four receptors are upregulated in precancerous lesions. *Lfng* appears to differentially regulate individual Notch receptors during initiation and progression of PDAC. Indeed, deletion of *Lfng* caused sustained Notch3 activation as early as 2 months of age, long before frank neoplasia. The activation of Notch2 was largely unaffected, whereas Notch1 activation was increased only after 4 months, when PanIN are progressing toward PDAC. *LFNG* knockdown in Miapaca2 human pancreatic cancer cells also caused increased activation of Notch, mostly Notch3 [233]. These data suggest that Notch3 is a major target for *Lfng*-mediated regulation in Kras-induced PDAC. Interestingly, accumulation of nuclear $Notch3^{ICD}$ is associated with adverse clinical features in pancreatic adenocarcinoma [239, 240]. Also, expression of *Notch3* and *Jagged1* are correlated in human PDAC [241]. It therefore seems likely that *Lfng* functions to inhibit Jagged1-Notch3 signaling in the context of *Kras*-induced PDAC. Of note, antibody-mediated inhibition of Notch2/Notch3 (by tarextumab) inhibits tumor growth and decreases tumor-initiating cell frequency [186].

In summary, *Lfng* exerts a potent tumor suppressive role in *Kras*-induced PDAC. While Notch1 and Notch2 are thought to exert opposing effects on PDAC initiation and progression, studies in *Lfng* mutant mice suggests that Notch3 is a major player in pancreatic cancer. Future studies using Notch3 knockout mice could help define roles for Notch3 in pathogenesis of pancreatic cancer. Finally, *Lfng*-expressing acinar cells in the mature pancreas are likely to represent a stem-like population that is uniquely sensitive to oncogenic *Kras*-induced transformation, and self-renewal of these cells are limited by *Lfng* itself. In the future, a *Lfng*-Cre knock-in could be used to test whether *Lfng*-expressing acinar cells represent the cell-of-origin for PDAC and also whether these cells are required not only for initiation but for tumor maintenance. Ultimately, knowledge of these cells may help identify biomarkers for early detection and targeted therapies for this devastating disease.

4.12 Tumor-Suppressive Role of Lfng in Prostate Cancer Initiation

Prostate cancer is the most common malignancy in males. Despite advances in prostate cancer detection and therapy, much about this common malignancy remains unknown or controversial. Defining the cell-of-origin for prostate cancer should provide new insights into mechanism of tumor initiation, which may lead to improved prognosis and therapeutic options. Unfortunately, different approaches to this question have yielded different answers: tissue recombination assays support basal epithelial cells as the cell-of-origin, whereas genetically engineered mice coupled with lineage-tracing suggest luminal cells as the preferred target for transformation [242]. Meanwhile, it remains unclear whether tumors originating from different cell types within the prostate lead to distinct molecular subtypes, each with a distinct clinical course or outcome. In addition, how the normal prostatic epithelial hierarchy is established and maintained, and how it is subverted during oncogenic transformation, needs to be elucidated. From a clinical point of view, two important challenges are (1) the need to find new methods for distinguishing aggressive from indolent prostate cancers and (2) the need to identify effective therapeutic targets for the treatment of advanced castration-resistant prostate cancer.

Notch is a critical regulator of cell differentiation and proliferation in the prostate. Disruption of canonical Notch signaling starting from the earliest stages of prostate development through deletion of *RBPJκ* in *Nkx3.1*$^{+}$ cells resulted in decreased cell proliferation and loss of epithelial and smooth muscle progenitors. Conversely, expression of activated *Notch1*^{ICD} in *Nkx3.1*$^{+}$ cells increased cell proliferation and the number of p63^{+} progenitors in basal epithelium [243]. Interestingly, deletion of *RBPJκ* in both compartments of the adult prostate with ARR2PB-Cre caused ectopic cell proliferation in the basal compartment during regeneration [244]. When Notch is activated exclusively in K8^{+} luminal cells of the prostate, it stimulated proliferation and resistance to anoikis [245]. Thus, while Notch signaling plays complex roles during development, homeostasis, and regeneration of the prostate gland, it consistently appears to promote luminal specification and expansion of the luminal compartment.

Notch1 expression is elevated in malignant prostatic epithelial cells of primary and metastatic tumors from the TRAMP model of prostate cancer (the TRAMP mouse is a transgenic line with SV40 large T antigen expressed from the rat probasin promoter) [246]. Also, in humans, NOTCH1 and JAGGED1 are overexpressed in high-grade and metastatic prostate cancer as compared to localized prostate cancer or benign prostatic tissue [247, 248]. Interestingly, Notch2 is implicated in acquired docetaxel resistance in castration-resistant tumors [249], whereas Notch3 is activated by chronic hypoxia and contributes to progression [250]. A recent study on Notch signaling in the adult prostate and in prostatic tumor development revealed upregulation of pathway components, in particular, *Jagged1* and *2*, *Notch3*, and *Hey1* [251]. Deregulated Notch signaling in this context induces increased proliferation and expansion of the stem/progenitor compartment, thereby contributing to prostate tumorigenesis.

All three Fringe genes are expressed in the mouse prostate. Interestingly, while *Lfng* is expressed at lower level than either *Mfng* or *Rfng*, its expression is much more restricted to basal layer epithelial cells [244]. Basal cells undergo symmetric and asymmetric divisions leading to distinct cell fates. In contrast, luminal cells only divide symmetrically [252]. In fact, postnatal development of the prostate is mediated by multipotent stem cells in the basal layer that differentiate into basal, luminal, and neuroendocrine cells, as well as by unipotent basal and luminal progenitors [253]. A gene signature specific for basal cells has been identified that is enriched for expression of genes associated with late-stage metastatic prostate cancer, suggesting that aggressive tumors share a conserved transcriptional program with normal adult prostate basal stem cells [254]. Given that Notch signaling regulates basal cell proliferation and differentiation, basally expressed *Lfng* likely regulates activation. Indeed, deregulation of *Lfng*-dependent Notch signaling may promote initiation and/or progression of prostate cancer. This is somewhat reminiscent of the Lfng-modulated Notch signaling that has been shown to control basal stem/progenitor cell self-renewal and differentiation in mammary gland, where *Lfng* deficiency induces basal-like breast cancer [187].

In an attempt to define the function of *Lfng* in the prostate, Zhang et al. studied activation of different Notch receptors in the *Lfng* null prostate as well as epithelial development in this context. Deletion of *Lfng* in mice caused altered Notch activation in the prostate, associated with elevated accumulation of Notch1, Notch2, and Notch4 intracellular domains, decreased levels of the putative Notch3 intracellular fragment, as well as increased expression of Hes1, Hes5, and Hey2. Loss of *Lfng* resulted in expansion of the basal layer, increased proliferation of both luminal and basal cells, and ultimately, prostatic intraepithelial neoplasia. The *Lfng* null prostate showed downregulation of prostatic tumor suppressor gene *Nkx3.1* and increased androgen receptor expression. Interestingly, expression of LFNG and NKX3.1 were positively correlated in publically available human prostate cancer datasets. Knockdown of LFNG in DU-145 prostate cancer cells led to expansion of $CD44^{+}CD24^{-}$ and $CD49f^{+}CD24^{-}$ stem/progenitor-like cell population associated with enhanced prostatosphere-forming capacity. Taken together, these data reveal a tumor-suppressive role for *Lfng* in the prostate through differential regulation of Notch signaling [255]. *Lfng* inhibits activation of Notch1 and Notch4 in basal cells of the prostate gland, and deletion of *Lfng* resulted in accumulation of stem-like cells in the prostate basal compartment. Thus *Lfng* gene deficiency or silencing may contribute to prostate cancer initiation through Notch-mediated expansion of basal multipotent stem cells, one of the cellular origins of prostate cancer. Further, *Lfng*-modulated Notch signaling may be particularly important in the pathogenesis of aggressive prostate cancer, as these cancer cells share a molecular signature with normal adult prostate basal stem cells [254]. Finally, deletion of *Lfng* caused elevated TGF-β signaling [255], which may inhibit proliferation in early-stage lesions. However, this may promote tumor cell invasion and metastasis in advanced stages. Of note, we observed development of sarcomatoid carcinoma, a rare malignant tumor of the prostate having an aggressive clinical course and dismal prognosis, in the occasional *Lfng* null mice (Xu and Egan, unpublished data).

Future comprehensive studies using inducible deletion of *Lfng* in basal or luminal epithelial cells may help clarify the role of specific Notch receptor(s)/ligand(s) during pathogenesis of prostate cancer originated from different cell lineages, which will provide a solid basis for determining whether and how Notch should be employed as a therapeutic target for prostate cancer. Furthermore, Lfng/Notch downstream target genes in prostate cancer initiation, progression, and metastasis may well be biomarkers for the screening of aggressive prostate cancer out of many indolent ones, as well as candidate targets for effective treatment of advanced castration-resistant disease.

4.13 Notch and Rumi

As noted above, Notch is modified through addition of O-linked glucose trisaccharides (Xyl-α1,3-Xyl-α1,3-Glc-β1-O-Ser) [21] attached to serine residues between the first and second cysteine ($C_1XSX(A/P)C_2$) of many EGF-like repeats [21, 23, 24]. The glucose residue is added directly to Notch by a CAP10 domain containing glycosyltransferase, known as Rumi in *Drosophila* and Poglut1 in mammals [256, 257]. Also, in cases where two serines are present within the consensus target site ($C_1XSS(A/P)C_2$), then Rumi/Poglut1 can add glucose to the first serine or *xylose* to the second [258, 259]. Glucose addition by Rumi/Poglut1, as well as elongation of the glucose residue through xylose addition, occurs at many sites within Notch [24]. Genetic analysis in *Drosophila* reveals a temperature dependent loss of Notch signaling in *Rumi* homozygous mutant animals [256]. Similarly, deletion of *Poglut1* in mice causes a wide spectrum of Notch mutant phenotypes, not unlike deletion of *Pofut1* or *RBPJk* [257]. Interestingly, *Poglut1* mutant mice have phenotypes beyond what is expected of animals with defective Notch signaling. Indeed, other targets for Poglut1-mediated glycosylation, including Eyes Shut (Eys) and Crumbs (Crb)/Crumbs2 have been identified [260, 261].

The enzymes responsible for elongation of glucose have been identified. The first xylose is added by a glucoside xylotransferase (either *GXYLT1* or *GXYLT2*) [262]. The second xylose is added by xyloside xylosyltransferase 1 (*XXYLT1*) [263, 264]. Genetic analysis of *Drosophila* glucoside xylotransferase, known as *Shams*, strongly suggests that while glucose addition enhances Notch signaling, xylose elongation of glucose, which occurs primarily within the EGF-like repeat 14–20 region, inhibits Notch signaling by limiting cell surface expression [265]. Not surprisingly, Rumi/Poglut1 is also capable of adding glucose to $C_1XSX(A/P)C_2$ target sequences in Notch ligands. In the case of Jagged1, Rumi/Poglut1 functions to decrease accumulation of ligand in vascular smooth muscle cells (VSMC), and hemizygous deletion of *Poglut1* in VSMC suppresses Alagille syndrome like phenotypes in the liver of *Jagged1*$^{+/-}$ (C57BL/6) mice [266, 267]. Thus, at least in some contexts, *Poglut1* functions to inhibit Notch signaling when expressed in the signal-sending cell and to enhance signaling when expressed in the receiver cell.

4.14 New Frontiers

Fringes and other Notch targeted sugar transferases function to coordinate development of neighboring cells. In many cases they operate together with other Notch regulators as well as feedback loops. Therefore, any effort to define their role will require a detailed picture of which Notch ligands and receptors are expressed in which neighboring cells, which cells express fringe and/or other sugar transferases targeted to the Notch system, what biological states are being regulated by Notch, and how Notch signaling changes with time in the system. Thus far, we have a fairly good description of how fringe proteins control organizer formation at tissue boundaries in flies, as well as how Fringe proteins control somitogenesis and lymphocyte development. Below, we highlight a number of new and exciting research directions on glycosylation of Notch and its importance for development and disease.

(i) *Regulation of Notch by N-linked glycosylation and O-linked GlcNAc*: *Pofut1*-, *Fringe*-, and *Rumi*-mediated Notch modifications represent powerful mechanisms by which development/homeostasis is regulated. However, Notch and its ligands are subject to other sugar-based modifications. For example, N-linked glycosylation occurs and is likely to control folding, transport, signaling, and internalization of these proteins [22, 268–270]. Notch is also modified through direct addition of O-linked GlcNAc [29, 271, 272]. Unfortunately, the function of N-linked glycosylation or O-GlcNacylation on Notch will be very difficult to determine, unless the enzymes responsible are almost exclusively dedicated to regulation of Notch signaling. In other words, such modifications may be very important for regulating Notch, but in as much as they regulate other pathways, their function with respect to Notch will be difficult to pin down.

(ii) *Atypical Fringe proteins*: *Chondroitin sulfate synthase 1* (*CHSY1*), and related *CHSY3*, codes for type II transmembrane proteins that accumulate in the extracellular space. Both contain N-terminal fringe-related and C-terminal type-A glycosyltransferase domains. Humans with recessive mutations in *CHSY1* have preaxial brachydactyly with partial duplication of proximal phalanges [273]. In addition, patients with *CHSY1* mutations exhibit macrophthalmia. Interestingly, *Chsy1* knockdown zebrafish show many of the same phenotypes as humans with *CHSY1* mutations and show dramatically upregulated Jagged expression together with elevated Notch signaling [273]. Suppression of Morpholino-induced phenotypes and Notch hyperactivation was achieved through ectopic expression of a Morpholino-resistant wild-type *Chsy1* cDNA, but not by a cDNA with a mutation in the fringe domain [273]. Thus, Chsy1 and related chondroitin sulfate synthase genes are widely expressed Notch inhibitors, functioning either transiently in the secretory pathway or perhaps in the extracellular space where they accumulate. It remains to be determined how they control Notch activation/signaling.

(iii) *Fringe in development of the nervous system*: While neural development is grossly normal in single, double, and triple fringe mutant mice [210], a role for fringe in fine patterning or differentiation of the nervous system has yet to be explored. Indeed, Fringe expression boundaries in the developing nervous system are suggestive of a role in compartmentalization and organizer specification [274]. For example, fringe expression boundaries are found between rhombomeres of the developing hindbrain [274–276]. In the developing forebrain, a *Lfng* expression boundary corresponds to the zona limitans intrathalamica (ZFI) organizer [274, 277]. Also, *Lfng* is expressed in the developing inner ear, and a *Lfng* mutation suppresses the effect of *Jagged2* deletion in this tissue [278]. Interestingly, *Dll3* is also expressed in the developing inner ear, as is Dll1 [279]. In the neural tube, as in the inner ear, Notch-dependent lateral inhibition ensures specification and differentiation of the correct cell types in a timely manner. In both cases, *Lfng* is induced downstream of Notch signaling [280]. As multiple feedback loops are at play in lateral inhibition, the role of Fringe can be difficult to detect unless a sensitized system is established and studied. Finally, Fringe has even been implicated in control of neuron-to-glial cell signaling through Notch [281].

(iv) *Fringe-dependent regulation of the cardiovascular system*: The Notch system is a potent regulator of vascular development and homeostasis. Indeed, as discussed above, dose-dependent Notch signaling is used to differentiate hemangioblasts into venous, arterial, and hematopoietic derivative fates, as well as to pattern the vascular network [130, 282]. In this latter context, Dll4 and Jagged1 play opposing and complementary roles [283]. Vegf induces Dll4 expression in endothelial tip cells, which lead to migration and growth of vascular tubes toward the Vegf source. Dll4 then activates Notch1 in neighboring endothelial stalk cells [284]. In these cells, $Notch1^{ICD}$ induces Hey bHLH transcriptional repressors which downregulate Vegfr2 expression, preventing them from becoming tip cells [285, 286]. Jagged1 is also induced in stalk cells. In this context, Jagged1 appears to stabilize tip cell fate in the neighbor, as well as to activate Notch4 within the endothelium, thereby promoting vascular maturation [287]. Finally, Jagged1 is also thought to recruit mural cells to the growing endothelial network [284, 287]. In this system then, Dll4/Jagged1 interaction is thought to create and reinforce a boundary between tip cells and their neighboring stalk cells, which have a hybrid signal sender/receiver state [122, 288]. Fringes can stabilize the hybrid state, and all three fringes are expressed in developing vessels. Thus, in this context, fringes are thought to reinforce the tip/stalk cell-state balance, as well as to establish a dynamic system facilitating rapid cell-state transitions required for patterning [283, 287]. Very recently, *Mfng* has been implicated in coordination of Notch signaling by Dll4, Jagged1, and Jagged2 in the developing heart. Specifically, Mfng is thought to enhance Dll4-Notch1 signaling in the endocardium to promote trabeculation in the developing ventricle. Mfng is then downregulated to facilitate myocardial Jagged signaling [289]. While differential expression of fringes can help explain how tip/stalk cell balance is induced and sustained, much work remains to prove these models and to define detailed mechanisms by which fringes control Dll4 and Jagged signaling in the developing heart and vasculature.

Vascular patterning and homeostasis plays an important role in normal development and in major pathological conditions including cancer and cardiovascular disease. Indeed, much energy has been focused on developing Notch ligand- or receptor-based therapeutics [284, 290–296]. Once again, it remains to be determined what role fringes (and *Rumi/Poglut1*) play in tumor angiogenesis and cardiovascular disease, although they might well represent excellent targets for therapy directed against a limited and pathological set of Notch-controlled events, while sparing healthy vessels and other tissues.

(v) *Novel cancer therapy*: As discussed above, fringe can function as a tumor suppressor in a number of tissues. This finding is based primarily on studying fringe mutant mice, as well as on data from fringe gene expression in human tumors. However, fringe mutations are not common in the cancer genome. Also, surprisingly, fringe can actually induce transformation when overexpressed in cultured cells [297]. This complexity is almost certainly related to the tissue- and context-specific function for Notch itself, which is both an oncogene and a tumor suppressor gene. As fringe proteins are enzymes, and as they are critical regulator of Notch activation in many if not most tissues, they could represent excellent targets for cancer therapy. Before targeting fringe proteins in any pathological setting, however, it will be important to determine how Jagged and Dll ligands are functioning to activate one or other Notch in the normal and diseased tissue. In this regard, single-cell assays and mathematical modeling can help define the role of Pofut1-, Fringe-, and Rumi/Poglut1-mediated differential glycosylation in any Notch-dependent biological process.

Acknowledgments K.X. is supported by grants from the National Institutes of Health. S.E.E. is supported by grants from the Terry Fox Foundation, the Canadian Breast Cancer Foundation, the Canadian Institutes for Health Research, and the Cancer Research Society. We thank Dr. Cynthia Guidos for valuable comments on the hematopoiesis and lymphocyte development section of the manuscript.

References

1. Irvine, K. D., & Wieschaus, E. (1994). fringe, a Boundary-specific signaling molecule, mediates interactions between dorsal and ventral cells during Drosophila wing development. *Cell, 79*, 595–606.
2. Rauskolb, C., Correia, T., & Irvine, K. D. (1999). Fringe-dependent separation of dorsal and ventral cells in the Drosophila wing. *Nature, 401*, 476–480.
3. Papayannopoulos, V., Tomlinson, A., Panin, V. M., Rauskolb, C., & Irvine, K. D. (1998). Dorsal-Ventral Signaling in the Drosophila Eye. *Science, 281*, 2031–2034.
4. Rauskolb, C., & Irvine, K. D. (1999). Notch-mediated segmentation and growth control of the Drosophila leg. *Developmental Biology, 210*, 339–350.
5. Grammont, M., & Irvine, K. D. (2001). fringe and Notch specify polar cell fate during Drosophila oogenesis. *Development, 128*, 2243–2253.
6. Grammont, M., & Irvine, K. D. (2002). Organizer activity of the polar cells during Drosophila oogenesis. *Development, 129*, 5131–5140.

7. Wu, J. Y., Wen, L., Zhang, W.-J., & Rao, Y. (1996). The secreted product of Xenopus gene lunatic Fringe, a vertebrate signaling molecule. *Science, 273*, 355–358.
8. Laufer, E., et al. (1997). Expression of Radical fringe in limb-bud ectoderm regulates apical ectodermal ridge formation. *Nature, 386*, 366–373.
9. Rodriguez-Esteban, C., et al. (1997). Radical fringe positions the apical ectodermal ridge at the dorsoventral boundary of the vertebrate limb. *Nature, 386*, 360–366.
10. Cohen, B., et al. (1997). Fringe boundaries coincide with Notch-dependent patterning centres in mammals and alter Notch-dependent development in Drosophila. *Nature Genetics, 16*, 283–288.
11. Johnston, S. H., et al. (1997). A family of mammalian Fringe genes implicated in boundary determination and the Notch pathway. *Development, 124*, 2245–2254.
12. Moran, J. L., et al. (1999). Genomic structure, mapping, and expression analysis of the mammalian Lunatic, Manic, and Radical fringe genes. *Mammalian Genome, 10*, 535–541.
13. Moran, J. L., Levorse, J. M., & Vogt, T. F. (1999). Limbs move beyond the radical fringe. *Nature, 399*, 742–743.
14. Zhang, N., & Gridley, T. (1999). Reply: Limbs move beyond the Radical Fringe. *Nature, 399*, 743.
15. Zhang, N., Norton, C. R., & Gridley, T. (2002). Segmentation defects of Notch pathway mutants and absence of a synergistic phenotype in lunatic fringe/radical fringe double mutant mice. *Genesis, 33*, 21–28.
16. Fleming, R. J., Gu, Y., & Hukriede, N. A. (1997). Serrate-mediated activation of Notch is specifically blocked by the product of the gene fringe in the dorsal compartment of the Drosophila wing imaginal disc. *Development, 124*, 2973–2981.
17. Panin, V. M., Papayannopoulos, V., Wilson, R., & Irvine, K. D. (1997). Fringe modulates Notch-ligand interactions. *Nature, 387*, 908–912.
18. Kim, J., Irvine, K. D., & Carrol, S. B. (1995). Cell recognition, signal induction, and symmetrical gene activation at the Dorsal-Ventral boundary of the developing Drosophila wing. *Cell, 82*, 795–802.
19. Troost, T., & Klein, T. (2012). Sequential Notch signalling at the boundary of fringe expressing and non-expressing cells. *PLoS One, 7*, e49007.
20. Yuan, Y. P., Schultz, J., Mlodzik, M., & Bork, P. (1997). Secreted Fringe-like signaling molecules may be glycosyltransferases. *Cell, 88*, 9–11.
21. Moloney, D. J., et al. (2000). Mammalian Notch1 Is Modified with Two Unusual Forms of O-Linked Glycosylation Found on Epidermal Growth Factor-like Modules. *The Journal of Biological Chemistry, 275*, 9604–9611.
22. Shao, L., Moloney, D. J., & Haltiwanger, R. (2003). Fringe modifies O-fucose on mouse Notch1 at epidermal growth factor-like repeats within the ligand-binding site and the Abruptex region. *The Journal of Biological Chemistry, 278*, 7775–7782.
23. Panin, V. M., et al. (2002). Notch ligands are substrates for protein O-fucosyltransferase-1 and Fringe. *The Journal of Biological Chemistry, 277*, 29945–29952.
24. Rana, N. A., et al. (2011). O-glucose trisaccharide is present at high but variable stoichiometry at multiple sites on mouse Notch1. *The Journal of Biological Chemistry, 286*, 31623–31637.
25. Moloney, D. J., et al. (2000). Fringe is a glycosyltransferase that modifies Notch. *Nature, 406*, 369–375.
26. Bruckner, K., Perez, L., Clausen, H., & Cohen, S. (2000). Glycosyltransferase activity of Fringe modulates Notch-Delta interactions. *Nature, 406*, 411–415.
27. Xu, A., et al. (2007). In vitro reconstitution of the modulation of Drosophila Notch-ligand binding by Fringe. *The Journal of Biological Chemistry, 282*, 35153–35162.
28. Aoki, K., et al. (2008). The diversity of O-linked glycans expressed during Drosophila melanogaster development reflects stage- and tissue-specific requirements for cell signaling. *The Journal of Biological Chemistry, 283*, 30385–30400.
29. Rana, N. A., & Haltiwanger, R. S. (2011). Fringe benefits: functional and structural impacts of O-glycosylation on the extracellular domain of Notch receptors. *Current Opinion in Structural Biology, 21*, 583–589.

30. Correia, T., et al. (2003). Molecular genetic analysis of the glycosyltransferase Fringe in Drosophila. In *Proceedings of the National Academy of Sciences of the United States of America* (Vol. 100, pp. 6404–6409).
31. Rampal, R., et al. (2005). Lunatic fringe, manic fringe, and radical fringe recognize similar specificity determinants in O-fucosylated epidermal growth factor-like repeats. *The Journal of Biological Chemistry, 280*, 42454–42463.
32. Munro, S., & Freeman, M. (2000). The Notch signalling regulator Fringe acts in the Golgi apparatus and requires the glycosyltransferase signature motif DxD. *Current Biology, 10*, 813–820.
33. Luther, K. B., Schindelin, H., & Haltiwanger, R. S. (2009). Structural and mechanistic insights into lunatic fringe from a kinetic analysis of enzyme mutants. *The Journal of Biological Chemistry, 284*, 3294–3305.
34. Hicks, C., et al. (2000). Fringe differentially modulates Jagged1 and Delta1 signalling through Notch1 and Notch2. *Nature Cell Biology, 2*, 515–520.
35. Yang, L. T., et al. (2005). Fringe glycosyltransferases differentially modulate Notch1 proteolysis induced by Delta1 and Jagged1. *Molecular Biology of the Cell, 16*, 927–942.
36. Wang, Y., et al. (2001). Modification of epidermal growth factor-like repeats with O-fucose. Molecular cloning and expression of a novel GDP-fucose protein O-fucosyltransferase. *The Journal of Biological Chemistry, 276*, 40338–40345.
37. Okajima, T., & Irvine, K. D. (2002). Regulation of notch signaling by o-linked fucose. *Cell, 111*, 893–904.
38. Sasamura, T., et al. (2003). neurotic, a novel maternal neurogenic gene, encodes an O-fucosyltransferase that is essential for Notch-Delta interactions. *Development, 130*, 4785–4795.
39. Stanley, P., & Guidos, C. J. (2009). Regulation of Notch signaling during T- and B-cell development by O-fucose glycans. *Immunology Reviews, 230*, 201–215.
40. Shi, S., & Stanley, P. (2003). Protein O-fucosyltransferase 1 is an essential component of Notch signaling pathways. In *Proceedings of the National Academy of Sciences of the United States of America* (Vol. 100, pp. 5234–5239).
41. Yao, D., et al. (2011). Protein O-fucosyltransferase 1 (Pofut1) regulates lymphoid and myeloid homeostasis through modulation of Notch receptor ligand interactions. *Blood, 117*, 5652–5662.
42. Ge, C., & Stanley, P. (2008). The O-fucose glycan in the ligand-binding domain of Notch1 regulates embryogenesis and T cell development. In *Proceedings of the National Academy of Sciences of the United States of America 105* (pp. 1539–1544).
43. Rampal, R., Arboleda-Velasquez, J. F., Nita-Lazar, A., Kosik, K. S., & Haltiwanger, R. S. (2005). Highly conserved O-fucose sites have distinct effects on Notch1 function. *The Journal of Biological Chemistry, 280*, 32133–32140.
44. Rampal, R., Luther, K. B., & Haltiwanger, R. S. (2007). Notch signaling in normal and disease States: possible therapies related to glycosylation. *Current Molecular Medicine, 7*, 427–445.
45. Okajima, T., Xu, A., Lei, L., & Irvine, K. D. (2005). Chaperone activity of protein O-fucosyltransferase 1 promotes notch receptor folding. *Science, 307*, 1599–1603.
46. Okajima, T., Reddy, B., Matsuda, T., & Irvine, K. D. (2008). Contributions of chaperone and glycosyltransferase activities of O-fucosyltransferase 1 to Notch signaling. *BMC Biology, 6*, 1.
47. Okamura, Y., & Saga, Y. (2008). Pofut1 is required for the proper localization of the Notch receptor during mouse development. *Mechanisms of Development, 125*, 663–673.
48. Sasamura, T., et al. (2007). The O-fucosyltransferase O-fut1 is an extracellular component that is essential for the constitutive endocytic trafficking of Notch in Drosophila. *Development, 134*, 1347–1356.
49. Stahl, M., et al. (2008). Roles of Pofut1 and O-fucose in mammalian Notch signaling. *The Journal of Biological Chemistry, 283*, 13638–13651.

50. Sullivan, F. X., et al. (1998). Molecular cloning of human GDP-mannose 4,6-dehydratase and reconstitution of GDP-fucose biosynthesis in vitro. *The Journal of Biological Chemistry, 273*, 8193–8202.
51. Ohyama, C., et al. (1998). Molecular cloning and expression of GDP-D-mannose-4,6-dehydratase, a key enzyme for fucose metabolism defective in Lec13 cells. *The Journal of Biological Chemistry, 273*, 14582–14587.
52. Ripka, J., Adamany, A., & Stanley, P. (1986). Two Chinese hamster ovary glycosylation mutants affected in the conversion of GDP-mannose to GDP-fucose. *Archives of Biochemistry and Biophysics, 249*, 533–545.
53. Kanda, Y., et al. (2007). Establishment of a GDP-mannose 4,6-dehydratase (GMD) knockout host cell line: a new strategy for generating completely non-fucosylated recombinant therapeutics. *Journal of Biotechnology, 130*, 300–310.
54. Jacobsen, T. L., Brennan, K., Arias, A. M., & Muskavitch, M. A. (1998). Cis-interactions between Delta and Notch modulate neurogenic signalling in Drosophila. *Development, 125*, 4531–4540.
55. de Celis, J. F., & Bray, S. J. (2000). The Abruptex domain of Notch regulates negative interactions between Notch, its ligands and Fringe. *Development, 127*, 1291–1302.
56. Sakamoto, K., Ohara, O., Takagi, M., Takeda, S., & Katsube, K. (2002). Intracellular cell-autonomous association of Notch and its ligands: a novel mechanism of Notch signal modification. *Developmental Biology, 241*, 313–326.
57. Whiteman, P., et al. (2013). Molecular basis for Jagged-1/Serrate ligand recognition by the Notch receptor. *The Journal of Biological Chemistry, 288*, 7305–7312.
58. Luca, V. C., et al. (2015). Structural biology. Structural basis for Notch1 engagement of Delta-like 4. *Science, 347*, 847–853.
59. Taylor, P., et al. (2014). Fringe-mediated extension of O-linked fucose in the ligand-binding region of Notch1 increases binding to mammalian Notch ligands. *Proceedings of the National Academy of Sciences of the United States of America, 111*, 7290–7295.
60. Andrawes, M. B., et al. (2013). Intrinsic selectivity of Notch 1 for Delta-like 4 over Delta-like 1. *The Journal of Biological Chemistry, 288*, 25477–25489.
61. Chen, J., Moloney, D. J., & Stanley, P. (2001). Fringe modulation of Jagged1-induced Notch signaling requires the action of beta 4galactosyltransferase-1. In *Proceedings of the National Academy of Sciences of the United States of America* (Vol. 98, pp. 13716–13721).
62. Hou, X., Tashima, Y., & Stanley, P. (2012). Galactose differentially modulates lunatic and manic fringe effects on Delta1-induced NOTCH signaling. *The Journal of Biological Chemistry, 287*, 474–483.
63. Tan, J. B., et al. (2009). Lunatic and manic fringe cooperatively enhance marginal zone B cell precursor competition for delta-like 1 in splenic endothelial niches. *Immunity, 30*, 254–263.
64. Shimizu, K., et al. (2001). Manic fringe and lunatic fringe modify different sites of the Notch2 extracellular region, resulting in different signaling modulation. *The Journal of Biological Chemistry, 276*, 25753–25758.
65. Van de Walle, I., et al. (2011). Jagged2 acts as a Delta-like Notch ligand during early hematopoietic cell fate decisions. *Blood, 117*, 4449–4459.
66. Muller, J., et al. (2014). O-fucosylation of the notch ligand mDLL1 by POFUT1 is dispensable for ligand function. *PLoS One, 9*, e88571.
67. Serth, K., et al. (2015). O-fucosylation of DLL3 is required for its function during somitogenesis. *PLoS One, 10*, e0123776.
68. Heuss, S. F., Ndiaye-Lobry, D., Six, E. M., Israel, A., & Logeat, F. (2008). The intracellular region of Notch ligands Dll1 and Dll3 regulates their trafficking and signaling activity. *Proceedings of the National Academy of Sciences of the United States of America, 105*, 11212–11217.
69. Geffers, I., et al. (2007). Divergent functions and distinct localization of the Notch ligands DLL1 and DLL3 in vivo. *Journal of Cell Biology, 178*, 465–476.

70. Ladi, E., et al. (2005). The divergent DSL ligand Dll3 does not activate Notch signaling but cell autonomously attenuates signaling induced by other DSL ligands. *Journal of Cell Biology, 170*, 983–992.
71. Zhang, N., & Gridley, T. (1998). Defects in somite formation in lunatic fringe-deficient mice. *Nature, 394*, 374–377.
72. Evrard, Y. A., Lun, Y., Aulehla, A., Gan, L., & Johnson, R. L. (1998). Lunatic fringe is an essential mediator of somite segmentation and patterning. *Nature, 394*, 377–381.
73. Conlon, R. A., Reaume, A. G., & Rossant, J. (1995). Notch1 is required for the coordinate segmentation of somites. *Development, 121*, 1533–1545.
74. Barrantes, I. B., et al. (1999). Interaction between Notch signalling and Lunatic fringe during somite boundary formation in the mouse. *Current Biology, 9*, 470–480.
75. Swiatek, P. J., Lindsell, C. E., Franco del Amo, F., Weinmaster, G., & Gridley, T. (1994). Notch1 is essential for postimplantation development in mice. *Genes & Development, 8*, 707–719.
76. Oka, C., et al. (1995). Disruption of the mouse RBPJk gene results in early embryonic death. *Development, 121*, 3291–3301.
77. Hrabe de Angelis, M., McIntyre, J., 2nd, & Gossler, A. (1997). Maintenance of somite borders in mice requires the Delta homologue DII1. *Nature, 386*, 717–721.
78. Saga, Y., Hata, N., Koseki, H., & Taketo, M. M. (1997). Mesp2: a novel mouse gene expressed in the presegmented mesoderm and essential for segmentation initiation. *Genes & Development, 11*, 1827–1839.
79. Wong, P. C., et al. (1997). Presenilin 1 is required for Notch1 and DII1 expression in the paraxial mesoderm. *Nature, 387*, 288–292.
80. Shen, J., et al. (1997). Skeletal and CNS defects in Presenilin-1-deficient mice. *Cell, 89*, 629–639.
81. Kusumi, K., et al. (1998). The mouse pudgy mutation disrupts Delta homologue Dll3 and initiation of early somite boundaries. *Nature Genetics, 19*, 274–278.
82. Sparrow, D. B., et al. (2006). Mutation of the LUNATIC FRINGE gene in humans causes spondylocostal dysostosis with a severe vertebral phenotype. *American Journal of Human Genetics, 78*, 28–37.
83. Dunwoodie, S. L. (2009). The role of Notch in patterning the human vertebral column. *Current Opinion on Genetics & Development, 19*, 329–337.
84. Chapman, G., Sparrow, D. B., Kremmer, E., & Dunwoodie, S. L. (2011). Notch inhibition by the ligand DELTA-LIKE 3 defines the mechanism of abnormal vertebral segmentation in spondylocostal dysostosis. *Human Molecular Genetics, 20*, 905–916.
85. McInerney-Leo, A. M., et al. (2015). Compound heterozygous mutations in RIPPLY2 associated with vertebral segmentation defects. *Human Molecular Genetics, 24*, 1234–1242.
86. Sparrow, D. B., Guillen-Navarro, E., Fatkin, D., & Dunwoodie, S. L. (2008). Mutation of Hairy-and-Enhancer-of-Split-7 in humans causes spondylocostal dysostosis. *Human Molecular Genetics, 17*, 3761–3766.
87. Whittock, N. V., et al. (2004). Mutated MESP2 causes spondylocostal dysostosis in humans. *American journal of Human Genetics, 74*, 1249–1254.
88. Dunwoodie, S. L., et al. (2002). Axial skeletal defects caused by mutation in the spondylocostal dysplasia/pudgy gene Dll3 are associated with disruption of the segmentation clock within the presomitic mesoderm. *Development, 129*, 1795–1806.
89. Bulman, M. P., et al. (2000). Mutations in the human delta homologue, DLL3, cause axial skeletal defects in spondylocostal dysostosis. *Nature Genetics, 24*, 438–441.
90. Sparrow, D. B., Sillence, D., Wouters, M. A., Turnpenny, P. D., & Dunwoodie, S. L. (2010). Two novel missense mutations in HAIRY-AND-ENHANCER-OF-SPLIT-7 in a family with spondylocostal dysostosis. *European Journal of Human Genetics, 18*, 674–679.
91. Hubaud, A., & Pourquie, O. (2014). Signalling dynamics in vertebrate segmentation. Nature reviews. *Molecular Cell Biology, 15*, 709–721.
92. Pourquie, O. (2011). Vertebrate segmentation: from cyclic gene networks to scoliosis. *Cell, 145*, 650–663.

93. Jiang, Y. J., et al. (2000). Notch signalling and the synchronization of the somite segmentation clock. *Nature, 408*, 475–479.
94. Chalamalasetty, R. B., et al. (2011). The Wnt3a/beta-catenin target gene Mesogenin1 controls the segmentation clock by activating a Notch signalling program. *Nature Communications, 2*, 390.
95. Vilhais-Neto, G. C., et al. (2010). Rere controls retinoic acid signalling and somite bilateral symmetry. *Nature, 463*, 953–957.
96. Aulehla, A., et al. (2003). Wnt3a plays a major role in the segmentation clock controlling somitogenesis. *Developmental Cell, 4*, 395–406.
97. Dubrulle, J., McGrew, M. J., & Pourquie, O. (2001). FGF signaling controls somite boundary position and regulates segmentation clock control of spatiotemporal Hox gene activation. *Cell, 106*, 219–232.
98. Sawada, A., et al. (2001). Fgf/MAPK signalling is a crucial positional cue in somite boundary formation. *Development, 128*, 4873–4880.
99. Lewis, J. (2003). Autoinhibition with transcriptional delay: a simple mechanism for the zebrafish somitogenesis oscillator. *Current Biology, 13*, 1398–1408.
100. Hoyle, N. P., & Ish-Horowicz, D. (2013). Transcript processing and export kinetics are rate-limiting steps in expressing vertebrate segmentation clock genes. *Proceedings of the National Academy of Sciences of the United States of America, 110*, E4316–E4324.
101. Niwa, H. (2007). How is pluripotency determined and maintained? *Development, 134*, 635–646.
102. Rossant, J., Zirngibl, R., Cado, D., Shago, M., & Giguere, V. (1991). Expression of a retinoic acid response element-hsplacZ transgene defines specific domains of transcriptional activity during mouse embryogenesis. *Genes & Development, 5*, 1333–1344.
103. Shimozono, S., Iimura, T., Kitaguchi, T., Higashijima, S., & Miyawaki, A. (2013). Visualization of an endogenous retinoic acid gradient across embryonic development. *Nature, 496*, 363–366.
104. Diez del Corral, R., et al. (2003). Opposing FGF and retinoid pathways control ventral neural pattern, neuronal differentiation, and segmentation during body axis extension. *Neuron, 40*, 65–79.
105. Dequeant, M. L., et al. (2006). A complex oscillating network of signaling genes underlies the mouse segmentation clock. *Science, 314*, 1595–1598.
106. Sewell, W., et al. (2009). Cyclical expression of the Notch/Wnt regulator Nrarp requires modulation by Dll3 in somitogenesis. *Developmental Biology, 329*, 400–409.
107. Dale, J. K., et al. (2003). Periodic notch inhibition by lunatic fringe underlies the chick segmentation clock. *Nature, 421*, 275–278.
108. Cole, S. E., Levorse, J. M., Tilghman, S. M., & Vogt, T. F. (2002). Clock regulatory elements control cyclic expression of Lunatic fringe during somitogenesis. *Developmental Cell, 3*, 75–84.
109. Williams, D. R., Shifley, E. T., Lather, J. D., & Cole, S. E. (2014). Posterior skeletal development and the segmentation clock period are sensitive to Lfng dosage during somitogenesis. *Developmental Biology, 388*, 159–169.
110. Shifley, E. T., et al. (2008). Oscillatory lunatic fringe activity is crucial for segmentation of the anterior but not posterior skeleton. *Development, 135*, 899–908.
111. Oginuma, M., et al. (2010). The oscillation of Notch activation, but not its boundary, is required for somite border formation and rostral-caudal patterning within a somite. *Development, 137*, 1515–1522.
112. Riley, M. F., Bochter, M. S., Wahi, K., Nuovo, G. J., & Cole, S. E. (2013). Mir-125a-5p-mediated regulation of Lfng is essential for the avian segmentation clock. *Developmental Cell, 24*, 554–561.
113. Nitanda, Y., et al. (2014). 3'-UTR-dependent regulation of mRNA turnover is critical for differential distribution patterns of cyclic gene mRNAs. *The FEBS Journal, 281*, 146–156.
114. Shifley, E. T., & Cole, S. E. (2008). Lunatic fringe protein processing by proprotein convertases may contribute to the short protein half-life in the segmentation clock. *Biochimica et Biophysica Acta, 1783*, 2384–2390.

115. Okubo, Y., et al. (2012). Lfng regulates the synchronized oscillation of the mouse segmentation clock via trans-repression of Notch signalling. *Nature Communications, 3*, 1141.
116. Sprinzak, D., et al. (2010). Cis-interactions between Notch and Delta generate mutually exclusive signalling states. *Nature, 465*, 86–90.
117. LeBon, L., Lee, T. V., Sprinzak, D., Jafar-Nejad, H., & Elowitz, M. B. (2014). Fringe proteins modulate Notch-ligand cis and trans interactions to specify signaling states. *eLife, 3*, e02950.
118. Matsuda, M., Koga, M., Nishida, E., & Ebisuya, M. (2012). Synthetic signal propagation through direct cell-cell interaction. *Science Signaling, 5*, ra31.
119. Matsuda, M., Koga, M., Woltjen, K., Nishida, E., & Ebisuya, M. (2015). Synthetic lateral inhibition governs cell-type bifurcation with robust ratios. *Nature Communications, 6*, 6195.
120. Kato, T. M., Kawaguchi, A., Kosodo, Y., Niwa, H., & Matsuzaki, F. (2010). Lunatic fringe potentiates Notch signaling in the developing brain. *Molecular and Cellular Neurosciences, 45*, 12–25.
121. Manderfield, L. J., et al. (2012). Notch activation of Jagged1 contributes to the assembly of the arterial wall. *Circulation, 125*, 314–323.
122. Boareto, M., et al. (2015). Jagged-Delta asymmetry in Notch signaling can give rise to a Sender/Receiver hybrid phenotype. *Proceedings of the National Academy of Sciences of the United States of America, 112*, E402–E409.
123. Mullighan, C. G. (2013). Genome sequencing of lymphoid malignancies. *Blood, 122*, 3899–3907.
124. Koch, U., & Radtke, F. (2011). Mechanisms of T cell development and transformation. *Annual Review of Cell and Developmental Biology, 27*, 539–562.
125. Pajcini, K. V., Speck, N. A., & Pear, W. S. (2011). Notch signaling in mammalian hematopoietic stem cells. *Leukemia, 25*, 1525–1532.
126. Yuan, J. S., Kousis, P. C., Suliman, S., Visan, I., & Guidos, C. J. (2010). Functions of notch signaling in the immune system: consensus and controversies. *Annual Review of Immunology, 28*, 343–365.
127. Kumano, K., et al. (2003). Notch1 but not Notch2 is essential for generating hematopoietic stem cells from endothelial cells. *Immunity, 18*, 699–711.
128. Hadland, B. K., et al. (2004). A requirement for Notch1 distinguishes 2 phases of definitive hematopoiesis during development. *Blood, 104*, 3097–3105.
129. Guiu, J., et al. (2014). Identification of Cdca7 as a novel Notch transcriptional target involved in hematopoietic stem cell emergence. *The Journal of Experimental Medicine, 211*, 2411–2423.
130. Gama-Norton, L., et al. (2015). Notch signal strength controls cell fate in the haemogenic endothelium. *Nature Communications, 6*(8510), 8510.
131. Dzierzak, E., & Speck, N. A. (2008). Of lineage and legacy: the development of mammalian hematopoietic stem cells. *Nature Immunology, 9*, 129–136.
132. Bigas, A., D'Altri, T., & Espinosa, L. (2012). The Notch pathway in hematopoietic stem cells. *Current Topics in Microbiology and Immunology, 360*, 1–18.
133. Ayllon, V., et al. (2015). The Notch ligand DLL4 specifically marks human hematoendothelial progenitors and regulates their hematopoietic fate. *Leukemia, 29*, 1741–1753.
134. Jang, I. H., et al. (2015). Notch1 acts via Foxc2 to promote definitive hematopoiesis via effects on hemogenic endothelium. *Blood, 125*, 1418–1426.
135. Bigas, A., & Espinosa, L. (2012). Hematopoietic stem cells: to be or Notch to be. *Blood, 119*, 3226–3235.
136. Robert-Moreno, A., et al. (2008). Impaired embryonic haematopoiesis yet normal arterial development in the absence of the Notch ligand Jagged1. *The EMBO Journal, 27*, 1886–1895.
137. Radtke, F., et al. (1999). Deficient T cell fate specification in mice with an induced inactivation of Notch1. *Immunity, 10*, 547–558.
138. Yu, V. W., et al. (2015). Specific bone cells produce DLL4 to generate thymus-seeding progenitors from bone marrow. *The Journal of Experimental Medicine, 212*, 759–774.
139. Hozumi, K., et al. (2008). Delta-like 4 is indispensable in thymic environment specific for T cell development. *The Journal of Experimental Medicine, 205*, 2507–2513.

140. Koch, U., et al. (2008). Delta-like 4 is the essential, nonredundant ligand for Notch1 during thymic T cell lineage commitment. *The Journal of Experimental Medicine, 205*, 2515–2523.
141. Tan, J. B., Visan, I., Yuan, J. S., & Guidos, C. J. (2005). Requirement for Notch1 signals at sequential early stages of intrathymic T cell development. *Nature Immunology, 6*, 671–679.
142. Yui, M. A., & Rothenberg, E. V. (2014). Developmental gene networks: a triathlon on the course to T cell identity. *Nature Reviews. Immunology, 14*, 529–545.
143. Hoyne, G. F., Chapman, G., Sontani, Y., Pursglove, S. E., & Dunwoodie, S. L. (2011). A cell autonomous role for the Notch ligand Delta-like 3 in alphabeta T-cell development. *Immunology and Cell Biology, 89*, 696–705.
144. Visan, I., Yuan, J. S., Tan, J. B., Cretegny, K., & Guidos, C. J. (2006). Regulation of intrathymic T-cell development by Lunatic Fringe- Notch1 interactions. *Immunological Reviews, 209*, 76–94.
145. Visan, I., et al. (2006). Regulation of T lymphopoiesis by Notch1 and Lunatic fringe-mediated competition for intrathymic niches. *Nature Immunology, 7*, 634–643.
146. Visan, I., Yuan, J. S., Liu, Y., Stanley, P., & Guidos, C. J. (2010). Lunatic fringe enhances competition for delta-like Notch ligands but does not overcome defective pre-TCR signaling during thymocyte beta-selection in vivo. *Journal of Immunology, 185*, 4609–4617.
147. Koch, U., et al. (2001). Subversion of the T/B lineage decision in the thymus by lunatic fringe-mediated inhibition of Notch-1. *Immunity, 15*, 225–236.
148. Amsen, D., et al. (2007). Direct regulation of Gata3 expression determines the T helper differentiation potential of Notch. *Immunity, 27*, 89–99.
149. Amsen, D., et al. (2004). Instruction of distinct CD4 T helper cell fates by different notch ligands on antigen-presenting cells. *Cell, 117*, 515–526.
150. Backer, R. A., et al. (2014). A central role for Notch in effector CD8(+) T cell differentiation. *Nature Immunology, 15*, 1143–1151.
151. Mukherjee, S., et al. (2014). STAT5-induced lunatic fringe during Th2 development alters delta-like 4-mediated Th2 cytokine production in respiratory syncytial virus-exacerbated airway allergic disease. *Journal of Immunology, 192*, 996–1003.
152. Pillai, S., & Cariappa, A. (2009). The follicular versus marginal zone B lymphocyte cell fate decision. *Nature Reviews. Immunology, 9*, 767–777.
153. Fasnacht, N., et al. (2014). Specific fibroblastic niches in secondary lymphoid organs orchestrate distinct Notch-regulated immune responses. *The Journal of Experimental Medicine, 211*, 2265–2279.
154. Besseyrias, V., et al. (2007). Hierarchy of Notch-Delta interactions promoting T cell lineage commitment and maturation. *The Journal of Experimental Medicine, 204*, 331–343.
155. Hozumi, K., et al. (2004). Delta-like 1 is necessary for the generation of marginal zone B cells but not T cells in vivo. *Nature Immunology, 5*, 638–644.
156. Saito, T., et al. (2003). Notch2 is preferentially expressed in mature B cells and indispensable for marginal zone B lineage development. *Immunity, 18*, 675–685.
157. Perou, C. M. (2010). Molecular stratification of triple-negative breast cancers. *The Oncologist, 15*(Suppl 5), 39–48.
158. Prat, A., et al. (2010). Phenotypic and molecular characterization of the claudin-low intrinsic subtype of breast cancer. *Breast Cancer Research, 12*, R68.
159. Prat, A., & Perou, C. M. (2009). Mammary development meets cancer genomics. *Nature Medicine, 15*, 842–844.
160. Prat, A., et al. (2013). Molecular characterization of basal-like and non-basal-like triple-negative breast cancer. *The Oncologist, 18*, 123–133.
161. Visvader, J. E., & Stingl, J. (2014). Mammary stem cells and the differentiation hierarchy: current status and perspectives. *Genes & Development, 28*, 1143–1158.
162. Lim, E., et al. (2009). Aberrant luminal progenitors as the candidate target population for basal tumor development in BRCA1 mutation carriers. *Nature Medicine, 15*, 907–913.
163. Chaffer, C. L., & Weinberg, R. A. (2011). A perspective on cancer cell metastasis. *Science, 331*, 1559–1564.

164. Baccelli, I., & Trumpp, A. (2012). The evolving concept of cancer and metastasis stem cells. *The Journal of Cell Biology, 198*, 281–293.
165. Mani, S. A., et al. (2008). The epithelial-mesenchymal transition generates cells with properties of stem cells. *Cell, 133*, 704–715.
166. Creighton, C. J., Chang, J. C., & Rosen, J. M. (2010). Epithelial-mesenchymal transition (EMT) in tumor-initiating cells and its clinical implications in breast cancer. *Journal of Mammary Gland Biology and Neoplasia, 15*, 253–260.
167. Bouras, T., et al. (2008). Notch signaling regulates mammary stem cell function and luminal cell-fate commitment. *Cell Stem Cell, 3*, 429–441.
168. Buono, K. D., et al. (2006). The canonical Notch/RBP-J signaling pathway controls the balance of cell lineages in mammary epithelium during pregnancy. *Developmental Biology, 293*, 565–580.
169. Raouf, A., et al. (2008). Transcriptome analysis of the normal human mammary cell commitment and differentiation process. *Cell Stem Cell, 3*, 109–118.
170. Gonzalez, D. M., & Medici, D. (2014). Signaling mechanisms of the epithelial-mesenchymal transition. *Science Signaling, 7*, re8.
171. Reedijk, M., et al. (2005). High-level coexpression of JAG1 and NOTCH1 is observed in human breast cancer and is associated with poor overall survival. *Cancer Research, 65*, 8530–8537.
172. Stoeck, A., et al. (2014). Discovery of biomarkers predictive of GSI response in triple-negative breast cancer and adenoid cystic carcinoma. *Cancer Discovery, 4*, 1154–1167.
173. Wang, K., et al. (2015). PEST domain mutations in Notch receptors comprise an oncogenic driver segment in triple-negative breast cancer sensitive to a gamma-secretase inhibitor. *Clinical Cancer Research, 21*, 1487–1496.
174. Robinson, D. R., et al. (2011). Functionally recurrent rearrangements of the MAST kinase and Notch gene families in breast cancer. *Nature Medicine, 17*, 1646–1651.
175. Ling, H., Sylvestre, J. R., & Jolicoeur, P. (2010). Notch1-induced mammary tumor development is cyclin D1-dependent and correlates with expansion of pre-malignant multipotent duct-limited progenitors. *Oncogene, 29*, 4543–4554.
176. Gonzalez, M. E., et al. (2014). EZH2 expands breast stem cells through activation of NOTCH1 signaling. *Proceedings of the National Academy of Sciences of the United States of America, 111*, 3098–3103.
177. Sale, S., Lafkas, D., & Artavanis-Tsakonas, S. (2013). Notch2 genetic fate mapping reveals two previously unrecognized mammary epithelial lineages. *Nature Cell Biology, 15*, 451–460.
178. Lafkas, D., et al. (2013). Notch3 marks clonogenic mammary luminal progenitor cells in vivo. *The Journal of Cell Biology, 203*, 47–56.
179. Ling, H., Sylvestre, J. R., & Jolicoeur, P. (2013). Cyclin D1-dependent induction of luminal inflammatory breast tumors by activated notch3. *Cancer Research, 73*, 5963–5973.
180. Pradeep, C. R., et al. (2012). Modeling ductal carcinoma in situ: a HER2-Notch3 collaboration enables luminal filling. *Oncogene, 31*, 907–917.
181. Harrison, H., et al. (2010). Regulation of breast cancer stem cell activity by signaling through the Notch4 receptor. *Cancer Research, 70*, 709–718.
182. Simoes, B. M., et al. (2015). Anti-estrogen Resistance in Human Breast Tumors Is Driven by JAG1-NOTCH4-Dependent Cancer Stem Cell Activity. *Cell Reports, 12*, 1968–1977.
183. Lombardo, Y., et al. (2014). Nicastrin and Notch4 drive endocrine therapy resistance and epithelial to mesenchymal transition in MCF7 breast cancer cells. *Breast Cancer Research, 16*, R62.
184. Brennan, K., & Clarke, R. B. (2013). Combining Notch inhibition with current therapies for breast cancer treatment. *Therapeutic Advances in Medical Oncology, 5*, 17–24.
185. Schott, A. F., et al. (2013). Preclinical and clinical studies of gamma secretase inhibitors with docetaxel on human breast tumors. *Clinical Cancer Research, 19*, 1512–1524.
186. Yen, W. C., et al. (2015). Targeting Notch signaling with a Notch2/Notch3 antagonist (tarextumab) inhibits tumor growth and decreases tumor-initiating cell frequency. *Clinical Cancer Research, 21*, 2084–2095.

187. Xu, K., et al. (2012). Lunatic fringe deficiency cooperates with the Met/Caveolin gene amplicon to induce basal-like breast cancer. *Cancer Cell, 21*, 626–641.
188. Gastaldi, S., et al. (2013). Met signaling regulates growth, repopulating potential and basal cell-fate commitment of mammary luminal progenitors: implications for basal-like breast cancer. *Oncogene, 32*, 1428–1440.
189. Graveel, C. R., et al. (2009). Met induces diverse mammary carcinomas in mice and is associated with human basal breast cancer. *Proceedings of the National Academy of Sciences of the United States of America, 106*, 12909–12914.
190. Knight, J. F., et al. (2013). Met synergizes with p53 loss to induce mammary tumors that possess features of claudin-low breast cancer. *Proceedings of the National Academy of Sciences of the United States of America, 110*, E1301–E1310.
191. Ponzo, M. G., et al. (2009). Met induces mammary tumors with diverse histologies and is associated with poor outcome and human basal breast cancer. *Proceedings of the National Academy of Sciences of the United States of America, 106*, 12903–12908.
192. Zhang, S., Chung, W. C., Miele, L., & Xu, K. (2014). Targeting Met and Notch in the Lfng-deficient, Met-amplified triple-negative breast cancer. *Cancer Biology & Therapy, 15*, 633–642.
193. Zhang, S., et al. (2015). Manic fringe promotes a claudin-low breast cancer phenotype through notch-mediated PIK3CG induction. *Cancer Research, 75*, 1936–1943.
194. Muellner, M. K., et al. (2011). A chemical-genetic screen reveals a mechanism of resistance to PI3K inhibitors in cancer. *Nature Chemical Biology, 7*, 787–793.
195. Xie, Y., et al. (2013). Identification of upregulated phosphoinositide 3-kinase gamma as a target to suppress breast cancer cell migration and invasion. *Biochemical Pharmacology, 85*, 1454–1462.
196. Mazzone, M., et al. (2010). Dose-dependent induction of distinct phenotypic responses to Notch pathway activation in mammary epithelial cells. *Proceedings of the National Academy of Sciences of the United States of America, 107*, 5012–5017.
197. Xu, K., et al. (2010). Lunatic Fringe-mediated Notch signaling is required for lung alveogenesis. *American Journal of Physiology. Lung Cellular and Molecular Physiology, 298*, L45–L56.
198. Lindahl, P., et al. (1999). Role of platelet-derived growth factors in angiogenesis and alveogenesis. *Current Topics in Pathology, 93*, 27–33.
199. Tsao, P. N., et al. (2009). Notch signaling controls the balance of ciliated and secretory cell fates in developing airways. *Development, 136*, 2297–2307.
200. Dang, T. P., Eichenberger, S., Gonzalez, A., Olson, S., & Carbone, D. P. (2003). Constitutive activation of Notch3 inhibits terminal epithelial differentiation in lungs of transgenic mice. *Oncogene, 22*, 1988–1997.
201. Guseh, J. S., et al. (2009). Notch signaling promotes airway mucous metaplasia and inhibits alveolar development. *Development, 136*, 1751–1759.
202. Deimling, J., et al. (2007). Mesenchymal maintenance of distal epithelial cell phenotype during late fetal lung development. *American Journal of Physiology. Lung Cellular and Molecular Physiology, 292*, L725–L741.
203. Morimoto, M., Nishinakamura, R., Saga, Y., & Kopan, R. (2012). Different assemblies of Notch receptors coordinate the distribution of the major bronchial Clara, ciliated and neuroendocrine cells. *Development, 139*, 4365–4373.
204. Zhang, S., Loch, A. J., Radtke, F., Egan, S. E., & Xu, K. (2013). Jagged1 is the major regulator of Notch-dependent cell fate in proximal airways. *Developmental Dynamics, 242*, 678–686.
205. Kim, C. F., et al. (2005). Identification of bronchioalveolar stem cells in normal lung and lung cancer. *Cell, 121*, 823–835.
206. Neptune, E. R., et al. (2008). Targeted disruption of NeuroD, a proneural basic helix-loop-helix factor, impairs distal lung formation and neuroendocrine morphology in the neonatal lung. *The Journal of Biological Chemistry, 283*, 21160–21169.

207. Branchfield, K., et al. (2016). Pulmonary neuroendocrine cells function as airway sensors to control lung immune response. *Science, 351*, 707.
208. Semenova, E. A., Nagel, R., & Berns, A. (2015). Origins, genetic landscape, and emerging therapies of small cell lung cancer. *Genes & Development, 29*, 1447–1462.
209. George, J., et al. (2015). Comprehensive genomic profiles of small cell lung cancer. *Nature, 524*, 47–53.
210. Moran, J. L., et al. (2009). Manic fringe is not required for embryonic development, and fringe family members do not exhibit redundant functions in the axial skeleton, limb, or hindbrain. *Developmental Dynamics, 238*, 1803–1812.
211. Berrieman, H. K., et al. (2004). Chromosomal analysis of non-small-cell lung cancer by multicolour fluorescent in situ hybridisation. *British Journal of Cancer, 90*, 900–905.
212. Testa, J. R., et al. (1994). Cytogenetic analysis of 63 non-small cell lung carcinomas: recurrent chromosome alterations amid frequent and widespread genomic upheaval. *Genes, Chromosomes & Cancer, 11*, 178–194.
213. Yi, F., Amarasinghe, B., & Dang, T. P. (2013). Manic fringe inhibits tumor growth by suppressing Notch3 degradation in lung cancer. *American Journal of Cancer Research, 3*, 490–499.
214. Zhang, Z., et al. (2004). Cancer chemopreventive activity of a mixture of Chinese herbs (antitumor B) in mouse lung tumor models. *Oncogene, 23*, 3841–3850.
215. Zheng, Y., et al. (2013). A rare population of CD24(+)ITGB4(+)Notch(hi) cells drives tumor propagation in NSCLC and requires Notch3 for self-renewal. *Cancer Cell, 24*, 59–74.
216. Arasada, R. R., Amann, J. M., Rahman, M. A., Huppert, S. S., & Carbone, D. P. (2014). EGFR blockade enriches for lung cancer stem-like cells through Notch3-dependent signaling. *Cancer Research, 74*, 5572–5584.
217. Ryan, D. P., Hong, T. S., & Bardeesy, N. (2014). Pancreatic adenocarcinoma. *The New England Journal of Medicine, 371*, 2140–2141.
218. De La, O. J., et al. (2008). Notch and Kras reprogram pancreatic acinar cells to ductal intraepithelial neoplasia. *Proceedings of the National Academy of Sciences of the United States of America, 105*, 18907–18912.
219. Maniati, E., et al. (2011). Crosstalk between the canonical NF-kappaB and Notch signaling pathways inhibits Ppargamma expression and promotes pancreatic cancer progression in mice. *The Journal of Clinical Investigation, 121*, 4685–4699.
220. Miyamoto, Y., et al. (2003). Notch mediates TGF alpha-induced changes in epithelial differentiation during pancreatic tumorigenesis. *Cancer Cell, 3*, 565–576.
221. Mazur, P. K., et al. (2010). Notch2 is required for progression of pancreatic intraepithelial neoplasia and development of pancreatic ductal adenocarcinoma. *Proceedings of the National Academy of Sciences of the United States of America, 107*, 13438–13443.
222. Hanlon, L., et al. (2010). Notch1 functions as a tumor suppressor in a model of K-ras-induced pancreatic ductal adenocarcinoma. *Cancer Research, 70*, 4280–4286.
223. Avila, J. L., Troutman, S., Durham, A., & Kissil, J. L. (2012). Notch1 is not required for acinar-to-ductal metaplasia in a model of Kras-induced pancreatic ductal adenocarcinoma. *PLoS One, 7*, e52133.
224. Court, H., et al. (2013). Isoprenylcysteine carboxylmethyltransferase deficiency exacerbates KRAS-driven pancreatic neoplasia via Notch suppression. *The Journal of Clinical Investigation, 123*, 4681–4694.
225. Ischenko, I., Petrenko, O., & Hayman, M. J. (2014). Analysis of the tumor-initiating and metastatic capacity of PDX1-positive cells from the adult pancreas. *Proceedings of the National Academy of Sciences of the United States of America, 111*, 3466–3471.
226. Kopp, J. L., et al. (2012). Identification of Sox9-dependent acinar-to-ductal reprogramming as the principal mechanism for initiation of pancreatic ductal adenocarcinoma. *Cancer Cell, 22*, 737–750.
227. Habbe, N., et al. (2008). Spontaneous induction of murine pancreatic intraepithelial neoplasia (mPanIN) by acinar cell targeting of oncogenic Kras in adult mice. *Proceedings of the National Academy of Sciences of the United States of America, 105*, 18913–18918.

228. Apelqvist, A., et al. (1999). Notch signalling controls pancreatic cell differentiation. *Nature, 400*, 877–881.
229. Kopinke, D., et al. (2012). Ongoing Notch signaling maintains phenotypic fidelity in the adult exocrine pancreas. *Developmental Biology, 362*, 57–64.
230. Murtaugh, L. C., Stanger, B. Z., Kwan, K. M., & Melton, D. A. (2003). Notch signaling controls multiple steps of pancreatic differentiation. *Proceedings of the National Academy of Sciences of the United States of America, 100*, 14920–14925.
231. Shih, H. P., et al. (2012). A Notch-dependent molecular circuitry initiates pancreatic endocrine and ductal cell differentiation. *Development, 139*, 2488–2499.
232. Svensson, P., Bergqvist, I., Norlin, S., & Edlund, H. (2009). MFng is dispensable for mouse pancreas development and function. *Molecular and Cellular Biology, 29*, 2129–2138.
233. Zhang, S., Chung, W. C., & Xu, K. (2015). Lunatic Fringe is a potent tumor suppressor in Kras-initiated pancreatic cancer. *Oncogene*.
234. Esni, F., et al. (2004). Notch inhibits Ptf1 function and acinar cell differentiation in developing mouse and zebrafish pancreas. *Development, 131*, 4213–4224.
235. De Waele, E., Wauters, E., Ling, Z., & Bouwens, L. (2014). Conversion of human pancreatic acinar cells toward a ductal-mesenchymal phenotype and the role of transforming growth factor beta and activin signaling. *Pancreas, 43*, 1083–1092.
236. Abel, E. V., et al. (2014). The Notch pathway is important in maintaining the cancer stem cell population in pancreatic cancer. *PLoS One, 9*, e91983.
237. Bailey, J. M., et al. (2014). DCLK1 marks a morphologically distinct subpopulation of cells with stem cell properties in preinvasive pancreatic cancer. *Gastroenterology, 146*, 245–256.
238. Baumgart, A., et al. (2015). Opposing role of Notch1 and Notch2 in a Kras(G12D)-driven murine non-small cell lung cancer model. *Oncogene, 34*, 578–588.
239. Doucas, H., et al. (2008). Expression of nuclear Notch3 in pancreatic adenocarcinomas is associated with adverse clinical features, and correlates with the expression of STAT3 and phosphorylated Akt. *Journal of Surgical Oncology, 97*, 63–68.
240. Mann, C. D., et al. (2012). Notch3 and HEY-1 as prognostic biomarkers in pancreatic adenocarcinoma. *PLoS One, 7*, e51119.
241. Vo, K., et al. (2011). Targeting notch pathway enhances rapamycin antitumor activity in pancreas cancers through PTEN phosphorylation. *Molecular Cancer, 10*, 138.
242. Lee, S. H., & Shen, M. M. (2015). Cell types of origin for prostate cancer. *Current Opinion in Cell Biology, 37*, 35–41.
243. Wu, X., et al. (2011). Differentiation of the ductal epithelium and smooth muscle in the prostate gland are regulated by the Notch/PTEN-dependent mechanism. *Developmental Biology, 356*, 337–349.
244. Valdez, J. M., et al. (2012). Notch and TGFbeta form a reciprocal positive regulatory loop that suppresses murine prostate basal stem/progenitor cell activity. *Cell Stem Cell, 11*, 676–688.
245. Kwon, O. J., et al. (2014). Increased Notch signalling inhibits anoikis and stimulates proliferation of prostate luminal epithelial cells. *Nature Communications, 5*(4416), 4416.
246. Shou, J., Ross, S., Koeppen, H., de Sauvage, F. J., & Gao, W. Q. (2001). Dynamics of notch expression during murine prostate development and tumorigenesis. *Cancer Research, 61*, 7291–7297.
247. Santagata, S., et al. (2004). JAGGED1 expression is associated with prostate cancer metastasis and recurrence. *Cancer Research, 64*, 6854–6857.
248. Zhu, H., Zhou, X., Redfield, S., Lewin, J., & Miele, L. (2013). Elevated Jagged-1 and Notch-1 expression in high grade and metastatic prostate cancers. *American Journal of Translational Research, 5*, 368–378.
249. Domingo-Domenech, J., et al. (2012). Suppression of acquired docetaxel resistance in prostate cancer through depletion of notch- and hedgehog-dependent tumor-initiating cells. *Cancer Cell, 22*, 373–388.
250. Danza, G., et al. (2013). Notch3 is activated by chronic hypoxia and contributes to the progression of human prostate cancer. *International Journal of Cancer, 133*, 2577–2586.

251. Pedrosa, A. R., et al. (2015). Notch signaling dynamics in the adult healthy prostate and in prostatic tumor development. *Prostate*.
252. Wang, J., et al. (2014). Symmetrical and asymmetrical division analysis provides evidence for a hierarchy of prostate epithelial cell lineages. *Nature Communications, 5*, 4758.
253. Ousset, M., et al. (2012). Multipotent and unipotent progenitors contribute to prostate postnatal development. *Nature Cell Biology, 14*, 1131–1138.
254. Smith, B. A., et al. (2015). A basal stem cell signature identifies aggressive prostate cancer phenotypes. *Proceedings of the National Academy of Sciences of the United States of America, 112*, E6544–E6552.
255. Zhang, S., Chung, W. C., Wu, G., Egan, S. E., & Xu, K. (2014). Tumor-suppressive activity of Lunatic Fringe in prostate through differential modulation of Notch receptor activation. *Neoplasia, 16*, 158–167.
256. Acar, M., et al. (2008). Rumi is a CAP10 domain glycosyltransferase that modifies Notch and is required for Notch signaling. *Cell, 132*, 247–258.
257. Fernandez-Valdivia, R., et al. (2011). Regulation of mammalian Notch signaling and embryonic development by the protein O-glucosyltransferase Rumi. *Development, 138*, 1925–1934.
258. Takeuchi, H., et al. (2011). Rumi functions as both a protein O-glucosyltransferase and a protein O-xylosyltransferase. In *Proceedings of the National Academy of Sciences of the United States of America* (Vol. 108, pp. 16600–16605).
259. Takeuchi, H., & Haltiwanger, R. S. (2013). Enzymatic analysis of the protein O-glycosyltransferase, Rumi, acting toward epidermal growth factor-like (EGF) repeats. *Methods in Molecular Biology, 1022*, 119–128.
260. Haltom, A. R., et al. (2014). The protein O-glucosyltransferase Rumi modifies eyes shut to promote rhabdomere separation in Drosophila. *PLoS Genetics, 10*, e1004795.
261. Ramkumar, N., et al. (2015). Protein O-Glucosyltransferase 1 (POGLUT1) Promotes Mouse Gastrulation through Modification of the Apical Polarity Protein CRUMBS2. *PLoS Genetics, 11*, e1005551.
262. Sethi, M. K., et al. (2010). Identification of glycosyltransferase 8 family members as xylosyltransferases acting on O-glucosylated notch epidermal growth factor repeats. *The Journal of Biological Chemistry, 285*, 1582–1586.
263. Sethi, M. K., et al. (2012). Molecular cloning of a xylosyltransferase that transfers the second xylose to O-glucosylated epidermal growth factor repeats of notch. *The Journal of Biological Chemistry, 287*, 2739–2748.
264. Yu, H., et al. (2015). Notch-modifying xylosyltransferase structures support an SNi-like retaining mechanism. *Nature Chemical Biology, 11*, 847–854.
265. Lee, T. V., et al. (2013). Negative regulation of notch signaling by xylose. *PLoS Genetics, 9*, e1003547.
266. Huppert, S. S. (2016). A faithful JAGGED1 haploinsufficiency mouse model of arteriohepatic dysplasia (Alagille syndrome) after all. *Hepatology, 63*, 365–367.
267. Thakurdas, S. M., et al. (2016). Jagged1 heterozygosity in mice results in a congenital cholangiopathy which is reversed by concomitant deletion of one copy of Poglut1 (Rumi). *Hepatology, 63*, 550–565.
268. Johansen, K. M., Fehon, R. G., & Artavanis-Tsakonas, S. (1989). The Notch gene product is a glycoprotein expressed on the cell surface of both epidermal and neuronal precursor cells during Drosophila development. *The Journal of Cell Biology, 109*, 2427–2440.
269. Dennis, J. W., Lau, K. S., Demetriou, M., & Nabi, I. R. (2009). Adaptive regulation at the cell surface by N-glycosylation. *Traffic, 10*, 1569–1578.
270. Stanley, P., & Okajima, T. (2010). Roles of glycosylation in Notch signaling. *Current Topics in Developmental Biology, 92*, 131–164.
271. Matsuura, A., et al. (2008). O-linked N-acetylglucosamine is present on the extracellular domain of notch receptors. *The Journal of Biological Chemistry, 283*, 35486–35495.
272. Takeuchi, H., & Haltiwanger, R. S. (2014). Significance of glycosylation in Notch signaling. *Biochemical and Biophysical Research Communications, 453*, 235–242.

273. Tian, J., et al. (2010). Loss of CHSY1, a secreted FRINGE enzyme, causes syndromic brachydactyly in humans via increased NOTCH signaling. *American Journal of Human Genetics, 87*, 768–778.
274. Kiecker, C., & Lumsden, A. (2005). Compartments and their boundaries in vertebrate brain development. *Nature Reviews. Neuroscience, 6*, 553–564.
275. Tossell, K., Kiecker, C., Wizenmann, A., Lang, E., & Irving, C. (2011). Notch signalling stabilises boundary formation at the midbrain-hindbrain organiser. *Development, 138*, 3745–3757.
276. Cheng, Y. C., et al. (2004). Notch activation regulates the segregation and differentiation of rhombomere boundary cells in the zebrafish hindbrain. *Developmental Cell, 6*, 539–550.
277. Zeltser, L. M., Larsen, C. W., & Lumsden, A. (2001). A new developmental compartment in the forebrain regulated by Lunatic fringe. *Nature Neuroscience, 4*, 683–684.
278. Zhang, N., Martin, G. V., Kelley, M. W., & Gridley, T. (2000). A mutation in the Lunatic fringe gene suppresses the effects of a Jagged2 mutation on inner hair cell development in the cochlea. *Current Biology, 10*, 659–662.
279. Hartman, B. H., Hayashi, T., Nelson, B. R., Bermingham-McDonogh, O., & Reh, T. A. (2007). Dll3 is expressed in developing hair cells in the mammalian cochlea. *Developmental Dynamics, 236*, 2875–2883.
280. Nikolaou, N., et al. (2009). Lunatic fringe promotes the lateral inhibition of neurogenesis. *Development, 136*, 2523–2533.
281. Stacey, S. M., et al. (2010). Drosophila glial glutamate transporter Eaat1 is regulated by fringe-mediated notch signaling and is essential for larval locomotion. *The Journal of neuroscience : the official journal of the Society for Neuroscience, 30*, 14446–14457.
282. Benedito, R., & Hellstrom, M. (2013). Notch as a hub for signaling in angiogenesis. *Experimental Cell Research, 319*, 1281–1288.
283. Benedito, R., et al. (2009). The notch ligands Dll4 and Jagged1 have opposing effects on angiogenesis. *Cell, 137*, 1124–1135.
284. Kofler, N. M., et al. (2011). Notch signaling in developmental and tumor angiogenesis. *Genes & Cancer, 2*, 1106–1116.
285. Holderfield, M. T., et al. (2006). HESR1/CHF2 suppresses VEGFR2 transcription independent of binding to E-boxes. *Biochemical and Biophysical Research Communications, 346*, 637–648.
286. Taylor, K. L., Henderson, A. M., & Hughes, C. C. (2002). Notch activation during endothelial cell network formation in vitro targets the basic HLH transcription factor HESR-1 and downregulates VEGFR-2/KDR expression. *Microvascular Research, 64*, 372–383.
287. Pedrosa, A. R., et al. (2015). Endothelial Jagged1 antagonizes Dll4 regulation of endothelial branching and promotes vascular maturation downstream of Dll4/Notch1. *Arteriosclerosis, Thrombosis, and Vascular Biology, 35*, 1134–1146.
288. Boareto, M., Jolly, M. K., Ben-Jacob, E., & Onuchic, J. N. (2015). Jagged mediates differences in normal and tumor angiogenesis by affecting tip-stalk fate decision. *Proceedings of the National Academy of Sciences of the United States of America, 112*, E3836–E3844.
289. D'Amato, G., et al. (2016). Sequential Notch activation regulates ventricular chamber development. *Nature Cell Biology, 18*, 7–20.
290. Pedrosa, A. R., et al. (2015). Endothelial Jagged1 promotes solid tumor growth through both pro-angiogenic and angiocrine functions. *Oncotarget, 6*, 24404–24423.
291. Kangsamaksin, T., Tattersall, I. W., & Kitajewski, J. (2014). Notch functions in developmental and tumour angiogenesis by diverse mechanisms. *Biochemical Society Transactions, 42*, 1563–1568.
292. Espinoza, I., & Miele, L. (2013). Notch inhibitors for cancer treatment. *Pharmacology & Therapeutics, 139*, 95–110.
293. Wu, Y., et al. (2010). Therapeutic antibody targeting of individual Notch receptors. *Nature, 464*, 1052–1057.

294. Ridgway, J., et al. (2006). Inhibition of Dll4 signalling inhibits tumour growth by deregulating angiogenesis. *Nature, 444*, 1083–1087.
295. Yan, M., et al. (2010). Chronic DLL4 blockade induces vascular neoplasms. *Nature, 463*, E6–E7.
296. Andersson, E. R., & Lendahl, U. (2014). Therapeutic modulation of Notch signalling--are we there yet? *Nature Reviews. Drug Discovery, 13*, 357–378.
297. May, W. A., et al. (1997). EWS/FLI1-induced manic fringe renders NIH 3T3 cells tumorigenic. *Nature Genetics, 17*, 495–497.

Chapter 5
Notch Signaling: A Pivot Regulator of Adaptive and Innate Immunity

Takumi Kumai and Paulo C. Rodriguez

Abstract The coordinated activities of the innate and adaptive arms of the immune system are essential to protect individuals against infectious and neoplastic pathologies and to prevent the development of autoimmune responses. The Notch family of receptors is a highly conserved signaling pathway that controls the development, function, and differentiation of many cell types, including the immune cells. Although the effects of Notch-linked mediators in the innate and adaptive immunity are the focus of an active research field, there are still multiple unknown areas regarding how this cellular signaling pathway plays such a primary role in the regulation of immune responses. In this review, we summarize and discuss the emerging role of Notch in the regulation of adaptive and innate immunity. We postulate that a better understanding of the effects of Notch in immune cells will provide new approaches for therapies in various diseases.

Keywords Cancer · Tumor Immunity · Immune responses · T lymphocytes · Myeloid cells · Immunotherapy · Cytokines · Tolerance · Tumor growth and metastasis

5.1 Introduction

The Notch family of receptors is a highly conserved pathway that controls the development, differentiation, survival, and function of many cell types, including immune cells [1]. Mammals have four Notch receptors (Notch-1 through Notch-4) that are bound by five ligands of the Jagged (Jagged-1 and Jagged-2) and the Delta-like (DLL1, DLL3, and DLL4) families [2]. Binding of the Notch receptors to their

T. Kumai
Asahikawa Medical University, Asahikawa, Japan

Georgia Regents University (GRU) Cancer Center, Augusta, GA, USA

P. C. Rodriguez (✉)
Moffitt Cancer Center, Tampa, FL, USA
e-mail: Paulo.Rodriguez@moffitt.org

L. Miele, S. Artavanis-Tsakonas (eds.), *Targeting Notch in Cancer*,
https://doi.org/10.1007/978-1-4939-8859-4_5

ligands induces Notch proteolytic processing, including the cleavage through the ADAM metalloprotease and the γ-secretase complexes, thereby leading to the membrane release and nuclear translocation of the Notch intracellular active domain (NICD). Once there, NICD complexes with the recombination signal-binding protein-J (RBP-Jκ, also known as CSL) and the mastermind-like (MAML) coactivator, promoting the canonical induction of multiple transcripts [3]. Moreover, NICD interacts with members of the nuclear factor-κB (NF-κβ), transforming growth factor-β (TGFβ), and hypoxia-induced signaling pathways, inducing noncanonical regulation of various transcripts [4, 5]. These noncanonical signal transduction pathways also occur in the absence of Notch receptor cleavage and through the cross talk between NICD and other signaling mediators [6–8].

The fundamental role of Notch receptors and their corresponding ligands on immune cells was initially established in processes regulating the development and maturation of T cells in the thymus and during marginal zone B (MZB) cell development in the spleen [1]. More recently, Notch signaling has also emerged as a major player in the hematopoietic regulation of various subsets of myeloid cells and a key regulator of lymphocyte function [9]. In this review, we highlight recent advances pertaining to the primary role of Notch signaling in the development and the function of adaptive and innate immune cells. Especial emphasis is placed on the effect of Notch signaling in mature $CD4^+$ and $CD8^+$ T cells and in dendritic cells (DCs).

5.2 Regulation of Lymphocyte Development and Function by Notch Receptors

5.2.1 Notch Regulates the Development of T Cells

Notch signaling is instrumental in the differentiation and maturation of T cells [10]. The development of αβ or γδ T cells in the thymus is initiated after the recruitment of bone marrow-originated common lymphoid progenitors through the bloodstream. Once there, T cell precursors increase the expression of Notch-1 and Notch-3 as they start their differentiation into $CD4^-$ $CD8^-$ T cells and maintain an elevated Notch activity until they reach the double-negative 3 (DN3) stage [11]. Notch-1 and Notch-3 levels then dissipate after the progression of the cells into the β checkpoint selection phase and continue low until the mature T cells are activated in peripheral tissues [12]. As such, deletion of Notch-1 or the Notch canonical partners RBP-Jκ or MAML in bone marrow precursors results in a complete absence of T cells and instead a significant accumulation of ectopic B cells [13, 14]. In contrast, the ectopic expression of Notch-1 intracellular active domain (N1IC) beyond the DN3 phase triggers the development of acute lymphoblastic T cell leukemia (T-ALL) [15]. This effect is physiologically relevant as a high number of the patients with T-ALL carry gain-of-function mutations in Notch-1 or Notch-related genes [16]. Emerging results have also indicated the role of Notch activity in the differentiation of $CD8^+$ T cells [17]. Interestingly, T cell receptor (TCR) tickling by MHC class I is required for the Notch-induced $CD8^+$ T cell development, suggesting the key role of the interaction between Notch signaling and antigen recognition in CD8+ T cells [18]. In addition to the role of Notch receptors in T cell differentiation, recent studies have pointed on the effects of the expression of particular Notch ligands in the thymic epithelial cells as regulators of the T cell commitment. As such, expression of DLL4 or DLL1 in the thymic stroma drives Notch-1 signaling in T cell precursors [19–23]. However, T cell development is unaffected in DLL4 or DLL1 mutant mice, suggesting the potential redundancy of the expression of Notch ligands in the thymic stroma [21]. In addition to the DLL family, Jagged-2, but not Jagged-1, is capable of directing T cell lineage commitment [24]. Therefore, Notch-1 signaling after binding to DLL1, DLL4, or Jagged-2 promotes T cell development in the thymus. It is noteworthy that the high levels of DLL1 and DLL4 inhibited the development of both B cells and myeloid cells, suggesting that the differentiation of each lineage is tightly regulated by Notch signaling in a ligand-specific and a dose-dependent manner [23] (Figs. 5.1 and 5.2).

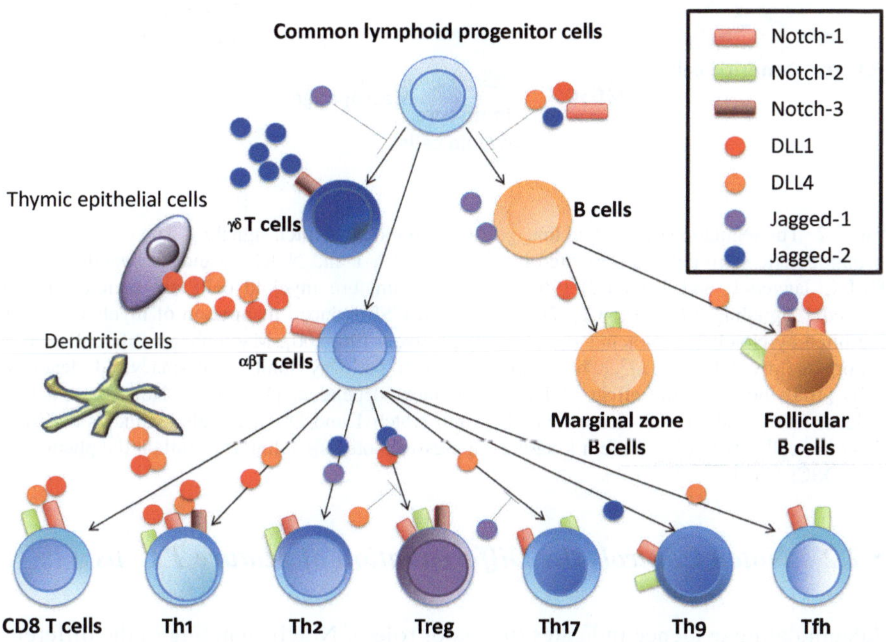

Fig. 5.1 The regulation of lymphocyte differentiation by Notch signaling. Notch-1 and Notch-3 expression and/or DLL1, DLL4, and Jagged-2 stimulation commits common lymphoid progenitor cells to T cell precursor cells [10–14]. After T cell lineage commitment, DLL1 and DLL4 from thymic epithelial cells or APCs induce αβ T cell differentiation including CD8+ T cells and Th1 subset [17, 25]. DLL1 is also capable of inducing Treg [32–34]. DLL4 induces Th17 and Tfh but inhibits Treg [35]. Although Jagged-1 is beneficial for Th2 and Treg, this ligand suppresses γδ T cells and Th17 [40]. Jagged-2 elicits the differentiation of γδ T cells, Th2, Treg, and Th9 [28, 29, 34]. After B cell lineage commitment that is suppressed by Notch-1, DLL1, DLL4, and Jagged-2 [50, 51], marginal zone B cells or follicular B cells are induced by DLL1 or DLL1, DLL4, and Jagged-1, respectively [44]

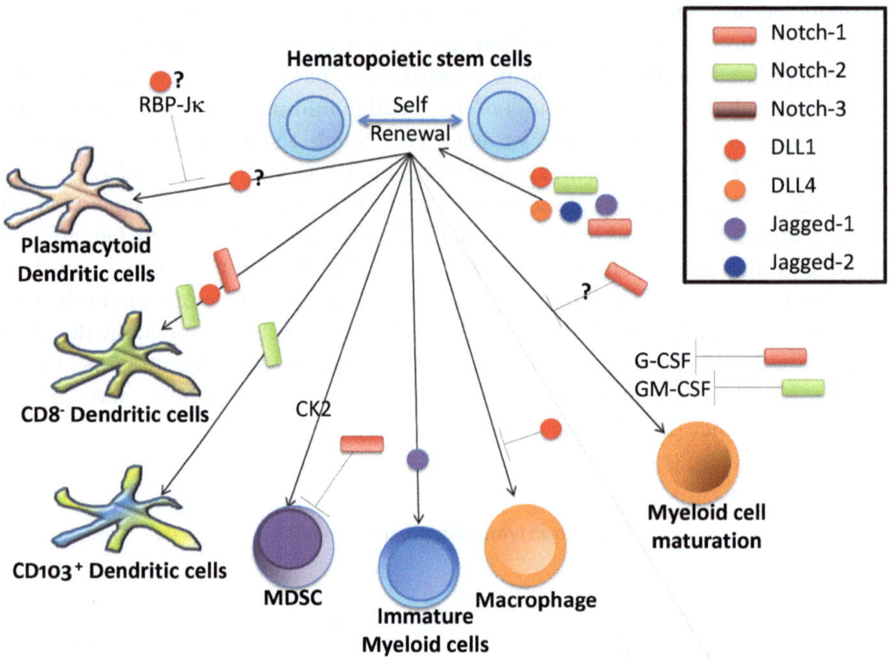

Fig. 5.2 The regulation of myeloid lineage differentiation by Notch signaling. The self-renewal of hematopoietic stem cells is promoted by Notch (Notch-1 and Notch-2) and its ligands (DLL1, DLL4, Jagged-1, and Jagged-2) [96, 100–103]. Immature myeloid cells are maintained via Jagged-1 signaling [96, 100, 101]. G-CSF- or GM-CSF-induced maturation of myeloid cells is inhibited by Notch-1 or Notch-2 signaling, respectively [96, 100]. Macrophage differentiation is suppressed by DLL1 [117]. The canonical Notch pathway inhibits plasmacytoid dendritic cells [108]; however, the effect of DLL1 is context dependent [122, 123]. Notch-2 signaling induces $CD8^-$ and $CD103^+$ dendritic cells [109]. Notch-1 and DLL1 are also inducers of $CD8^-$ dendritic cells [108, 112]. Casein kinase 2 suppresses Notch signaling to maintain the phenotype of MDSCs [113]

5.2.2 Notch Controls the Differentiation of Mature T Cells

Accumulating evidence indicates the major role of Notch signaling in the differentiation of $CD4^+$ T cells into specific T helper (Th) subsets. As such, activation of Notch-1 and Notch-2 on primed $CD4^+$ T cells by specific Notch ligands on DCs leads to their polarization into different Th subsets [25]. Interestingly, DLL1 and DLL4 promoted the development of Th1 subsets, whereas Jagged-1 and Jagged-2 induced Th2 polarization. Activation of antigen-presenting cells (APCs) with Toll-like receptor (TLR) agonists elicited the expression of Notch ligands Jagged-1, Jagged-2, DLL1, and DLL4 [25]. Expression of STAT3-induced DLL4 upon DC stimulation with LPS mediated the induction of Th1 and Th17 differentiation independent of IL-12 [26, 27]. Additional reports also showed that DLL4-carrying DCs induced Th1 polarization in an IL-12-dependent manner [28]. The induction of Th1 cells by DLL4 occurred through noncanonical pathways, adding a level of complexity on the effects of DLL/Notch in the promotion of Th subsets. Opposite to the effect induced by DLL1 and DLL4, Jagged-1 and Jagged-2 ligands triggered Th2 differentiation. In fact, Jagged-2 in the tumor microenvironment skewed T cells into Th2 cells, which promoted tumor growth [29, 30]. Moreover, the Th2 differentiation induced by Jagged/Notch signaling was significantly diminished upon deletion of RBP-Jκ, suggesting that canonical Notch activity is required for the Jagged-induced effects [31]. Thus, Th1 polarization was promoted through noncanonical Notch signaling, whereas Th2 induction depended on canonical Notch pathways. Interestingly, the levels of active Notch were similar in T cells primed in the presence of DLL or Jagged ligands, suggesting that unknown mediators are responsible for the opposite effects triggered by these ligands on Th differentiation. Because cytokines are the major determinant of the $CD4^+$ T cell fates and are major targets of Notch signaling [25], current research is exploring the role of Notch-induced cytokines in the polarization of specific Th subsets.

Notch signaling is fundamental for the generation, expansion, and suppressive function of regulatory T cells (Treg). Treg development is increased after overexpression of Notch-1 or Notch-3 in T cells, whereas Treg inhibition is induced upon treatment of T cells with γ-secretase inhibitors (GSI) [32–34]. As ligands, DLL1, Jagged-1, and Jagged-2 play a primary role to support Treg induction. DLL1 maintained the survival of natural Treg and increased Treg conversion by directly upregulating Foxp3 transcription or by cooperatively augmenting TGF-β/Smad3 signaling [34]. Jagged-1 is another ligand that induces Treg by enhancing the signaling through TGF-β/Smad3. Furthermore, $CD4^+$ T cells stimulated in the presence of Jagged-2 became Treg with a high suppressive capacity against autoimmune encephalomyelitis (EAE) [28]. Conversely, DLL4 inhibited the expansion of Treg through downregulation of JAK3 and STAT5 phosphorylation [35]. The mechanisms by which the specific Notch ligands modulate cellular signaling and trigger or inhibit Treg development remain elusive.

Th17 cells are a relatively new subset of $CD4^+$ T cells that play a fundamental role in a variety of autoimmune diseases [36]. Accumulating evidence suggests that Notch signaling regulates the differentiation of Th17 cells [37]. The induction of Th17 differentiation by TLR-activated DCs was abolished by DLL4 neutralization, suggesting that DLL4/Notch signaling is essential for Th17 development [26]. Because RBP-Jκ directly interacted with ROR-γt, the master inducer of Th17 cells, it is likely that DLL4-induced canonical Notch signaling drives Th17 differentiation [38]. Also, the production of IL-6, a well-known inducer of Th17, was decreased in Notch-1 mutant mice, suggesting that Notch signaling can indirectly impact the differentiation of Th17 by regulating IL-6 production [39]. In contrast to the role of DLL4, Jagged-1 expression on DCs had a negative effect in promoting Th17 differentiation [40]. Therefore, although the effect of Notch in Th17 cells remains unclear, it is accepted that the development of Th17 populations depends on the specific binding of Notch receptors to particular ligands on APCs in a microenvironment containing the precise levels of specific cytokines.

Th9 cells were recently identified as a subset of $CD4^+$ T cells with a potent antitumor ability [41]. Polarization of Th9 cells by TGF-β and IL-4 induced the activation of Notch-1, which controlled the Th9 expansion [28]. Moreover, Jagged-2 ligand appears to regulate the Th9 differentiation by Notch, which occurred through the phosphorylation of Smad3 [28]. While Th9 differentiation was suppressed in Notch-1 and Notch-2 knockout mice and after GSI treatment, excessive amounts of IL-4 could compensate the deficiency of Notch signaling and restore Th9 development, suggesting that Notch activity is important only under limiting amounts of IL-4.

Follicular $CD4^+$ T cells (Tfh) are essential for providing B cell help to generate high-affinity antibodies in germinal center by expressing CD40 ligand and by producing IL-4 and IL-21 [42]. The absence of Notch-1 and Notch-2 by gene ablation impaired Tfh differentiation and germinal center formation [43]. By using conditional knockout mice, it has become clear that DLL4 signaling from the stromal cell is primary for the Tfh differentiation [44]. However, the role of Notch in the development and function of Tfh cells remains unclear.

γδ T cells have a restricted TCR repertoire that recognizes phosphoantigens produced by bacteria and parasites. Because endogenous phosphoantigens are also accumulated in tumors, γδ T cells are promising cell types for the target of immunotherapy [45]. The seminal study by Washburn et al. showed that while normal Notch-1 signaling induced αβ T cells, reduced Notch-1 favored the induction of γδ T cell from $CD4^-$ $CD8^-$ progenitor cells [46]. Furthermore, Notch-3 activation by Jagged-2 or constitutive active Notch-3 promoted γδ T cell lineage differentiation [47]. This differentiation was mediated through the inhibition of TCR-β expression, which is necessary for $CD4^+$ and $CD8^+$ T cells. Collectively, the balance between DLL4/Notch-1 and Jagged-2/Notch-3 signaling appears to determine the fate of αβ T cell and γδ T cells.

NKT cells are unique subset of T cells that recognize lipid antigens presented by the CD1d molecule. There are two subsets of NKT cells, type I (invariant TCR) and type II (diverse TCR) NKT cells, whose function can be both pro-inflammatory and immunoregulatory [48]. Most of the NKT cells are either $CD4^+$ or $CD4^-$ $CD8^-$; however, it remains largely unknown the pathways that drive their development from common lymphoid progenitor cells. Recently, the importance of Notch activity in the differentiation of NKT cells has been proposed. Although deletion of Notch-1 and Notch-2 increased the number of invariant NKT cells in the thymus, these invariant NKT cells were premature ($NK1.1^-$) and sensitive to apoptosis, which thereby resulted in the decreased number of these cells in the periphery [49]. NKT cells in RBP-Jκ mutant mice showed the same increased pro-apoptotic phenotype, suggesting that canonical Notch signaling plays a primary role in NKT cell survival. However, unlike Notch-1- and Notch-2-null NKT cells, RBP-Jκ knockout NKT cells showed comparable thymic development, indicating that noncanonical Notch-1 or Notch-2 signaling is primary for the intra-thymic development and that canonical Notch signaling is essential for the periphery maturation, function, and homeostasis of NKT cells.

Although Notch-1-related activity has been extensively studied during early T cell development, the impact of Notch in the B cell compartment remains poorly understood. Initial reports showed that commitment to early B cell lineage required the inhibition of Notch-1 activity in lymphoid progenitor cells [50, 51]. The increase of B cells in Notch-1-depleted mice was not due to the compensation mechanism by the lack of normal T cell development. Moreover, B cells were increased in DLL4 knockout mice, suggesting that DLL4 is one of the responsible ligands for the inhibition of B cell commitment [22]. Expression of Notch ligands on stromal cells allowed to assess the ability of other Notch ligands in inducing B cell differentiation. In hematopoietic progenitor cells, Jagged-1 stimulation was capable of inducing B cell lineage [24]. On the contrary, DLL1, DLL4, and Jagged-2 suppressed this differentiation. Interestingly, the effect of DLL1 to modulate the fate of B cell differentiation depended on the dose and the density of its expression [52]. More recent results established the role of Notch signaling, especially Notch-2, during the development of specific subsets of B cells in the spleen. Two different populations of B cells accumulate in the spleen, namely, marginal zone B cells (MZB) and follicular B cells [53]. Follicular zone B cells represent the majority of B cells within the spleen and participate in immune responses mediated by T cells. Conversely, MZB cells are a minority of the B lymphocytes in the splenic tissue and regulate antibody responses against lipid antigens, which usually occur in a T cell-independent manner [54]. Although the number of follicular B cells is much higher than MZB, the ability to activate antigen-specific $CD4^+$ T cells of MZB is superior to that of follicular B cells [55]. B cell progenitors from the bone marrow migrate to the spleen and originate MZB cells and follicular B cells through transitional stages T1 and T2. The specification of MZB cells after T2 is highly dependent on Notch-2 signaling induced by DLL1, but not through DLL4 expression [44]. The expression of DLL1 in blood endothelial cells or DCs was dispensable during this process. This differentiation appears to be mediated through canonical pathways, as conditional deletion of RBP-Jκ and MAML resulted in a similar inhibition in the development of MZB as that induced by Notch-2 ablation [56–58]. One of the downstream targets of Notch for MZB induction is the E protein family. Downregulation of E proteins by Notch activation is necessary to drive MZB differentiation [59]. Thus, under physiological conditions, interaction of DLL1 with Notch-2 and further canonical signals induces in transitional B cells to specify MZB cells, as opposed to follicular B cells. Meanwhile, the differentiation of follicular B cells heavily relies on DLL4 on fibroblastic reticular cells [44]. In addition, DLL1 has been shown to enhance the proliferation of follicular B cells after B cell receptor or CD40 stimulation through MAPK activation, suggesting that the Notch ligand required for the differentiation and the proliferation of follicular B cells may be different [60]. For the sake of the survival, Jagged-1 in DCs rendered an anti-apoptotic feature to follicular B cells [61]. Altogether, the results suggest the key role of Notch signaling in B cell development and function.

Innate lymphoid cells (ILCs), a heterogeneous group of lymphocytes that lack T/B cell receptors and that activate in an antigen-independent manner, are emerging as major mediators in the immune responses against infectious agents and tumors and in the development of tolerance against self-antigens. Similar to CD4⁺ and CD8⁺ T cells, ILCs develop from common lymphoid progenitor cells. ILCs are divided into three major subclasses (ILC1s, ILC2s, and ILC3s). ILC1s, ILC2s, and ILC3s consist of Th1-producing T-bet⁺ cells, including natural killer (NK) cells, Th2-producing GATA3⁺ cells, and Th17-producing cells, respectively [62, 63]. While most of the studies focused on the cytokines or transcription factors mediating the induction of ICLs, Notch signaling has been shown to regulate the maturation of several subsets of ILCs, including ILC2s (nuocytes) and ILC3s (lymphoid tissue-inducer (LTi) cells) and IL-22-producing ILCs (NKp46⁺ ILCs) [64–66]. Nuocytes play an irreplaceable role in anti-helminth and allergic immunity by producing Th2-type cytokines IL-5 and IL-13. DLL1 stimulation in the presence of IL-33 and IL-7 is critical for the induction of nuocytes from progenitor cells [66]. Without nuocyte-skewed cytokines, DLL1 stimulation triggers instead CD3⁺ T cells. In ILC3s, the necessity of Notch signaling depends on its developmental stage. Notch is prerequisite for the differentiation of common lymphoid progenitor cells to RORγt⁻ fetal progenitor cells; however, this signaling blocked a successive LTi differentiation [65]. The increased expression of Notch in IL-22⁺ NKp46⁺ ILCs was mediated through the transcription factor aryl hydrocarbon receptor (AHR) and further regulated the expression of the RORγt [64]. Conditional deletion of RBP-Jκ further confirmed that canonical Notch signaling is necessary for the induction of IL-22⁺ NKp46⁺ ILCs. Because unregulated IL-22 can cause an epithelial tumorigenesis [67], Notch inhibition may indirectly suppress tumor development by eliminating IL-22⁺ NKp46⁺ ILCs. Taken together, Notch signaling controls the development and/or expansion of ILC subsets, which also depends on the specific inflammatory modulators present in the microenvironment.

5.2.3 Effects of Notch Signaling in the Function of CD4⁺ and CD8⁺ T Cells

The role of Notch signaling in the modulation of CD4⁺ T cell function is well established [68–70]. Treatment of activated mature CD4⁺ T cells with GSI impaired their activation [71], proliferation [72, 73], and survival [74], suggesting the importance of Notch signaling in CD4⁺ T cells. The CD4⁺ T cell survival effects induced by Notch appear to be mediated through the promotion of glycolysis and occurred in a Notch canonical-dependent manner [75]. Furthermore, inhibition of DLL1 and DLL4 impaired the function of activated CD4⁺ T cells, indicating the major role of these ligands in the function of CD4⁺ T cells [76]. Accordingly, DLL4 stimulation increased the sensitivity of CD4⁺ T cells to antigens by upregulating the PI3K/mTOR/GLUT1 signaling cascade [77]. As stated above, ligation of Notch to DLL1 or DLL4 ligands promoted Th1 responses, whereas their engagement to Jagged-1 or Jagged-2 induced the development of Th2 and Treg populations [31, 68, 78, 79]. Furthermore, Treg development was induced by DLL4 blockade, which resulted in the attenuation of EAE [35]. In contrast to DLL4, DLL1 not only induced Th1 but also promoted Treg differentiation. DLL1 increased the suppressive function of Treg, which was significantly inhibited upon Notch-1 blockade [33, 34]. DLL1-induced Treg cells express CD39 expression, which is a key enzyme for ATP/AMP conversion, suggesting that Notch signaling in Treg might indirectly suppress immune cells via production of adenosine. Interestingly, the development and function of Treg were significantly increased upon overexpression of Notch-1 or Notch-3 [32, 33]. Notch-3 induction in thymocytes expanded Treg that were fully competent to suppress the proliferation of bystander cells [32]. Although it is not clear if Notch-3 is solely important for the expansion of Treg, it is evident that Notch-3 acts as a pro-Treg receptor. Besides the benefit of DLL1 and Notch-3 signaling in Treg induction, the overall role of Notch-1 in Treg remains controversial [80]. The function of Th17, a prominent mediator of a variety of autoimmune diseases [36], is regulated by Notch. GSI or DLL4 blockade alleviates inflammation in asthma or EAE models by suppressing IL-17 [35, 81]. In line with this, Notch signaling supported the survival of Th17 cells by upregulating anti-apoptotic gene Bcl2 partly via HIF-1 [82]. Also, DLL3 significantly increased the number of pathogenic Th17 in collagen-induced arthritis model [83].

Although naïve $CD8^+$ T cells do not express significant levels of Notch receptors [30], they still require Notch signaling to be fully activated. Indeed, GSI treatment decreased proliferation [73], survival [74], cytokine production [73, 84], and cytotoxicity [84] of $CD8^+$ T cells. Expression of Notch-1 and Notch-2 in $CD8^+$ T cells was induced upon anti-CD3/CD28 activation and relied on mTOR and T-bet signaling [30, 85]. The role of Notch-1 and Notch-2 in the function of $CD8^+$ T cells has been demonstrated by the impaired lytic capacity found in $CD8^+$ T cells from Notch-1- and Notch-2-null mice or after the blocking of Notch-1 [30, 84, 86]. Notch signaling promoted cytotoxic activity in $CD8^+$ T cells through the induction of the effector molecules granzyme B, IFNγ, and perforin, which were upregulated through canonical signals or through the binding of NICD to Eomes or NF-κB [84, 87]. Interestingly, the induction of short-lived effector $CD8^+$ T cells (SLECs, $CD127^{low}$ $KLRG1^{high}$) was inhibited in mice lacking Notch-1 or Notch-2 after DC vaccination [85, 87]. Instead, early effector $CD8^+$ T cells ($CD127^{low}$ $KLRG1^{low}$) were increased in these mutant mice, suggesting that Notch-1 and Notch-2 are important for the conversion of early effector cells to short-lived effector cells [87]. Although Notch is dispensable for the CD8 memory generation [87], $N1IC^+$ $CD8^+$ T cells possessed a central memory phenotype ($CD44^+$ $CD62L^+$ $CD122^+$ $CD127^+$) and displayed an elevated cytotoxicity and antitumor activity after adoptive cellular transfer into tumor-bearing mice [30]. Thus, Notch signaling in $CD8^+$ T cells could represent an important immunotherapy target for cancer. With regard to Notch ligands, DLL1 overexpression increased the antitumor activity of antigen-specific $CD8^+$ T cells [88]. Indeed, Notch-2 activation on $CD8^+$ T cells by DLL1 on DCs results in a high production of granzyme B [86]. In contrast to the role of DLL1, Jagged-1 expression suppressed collagen-induced arthritis by providing negative signals in $CD8^+$ T cells [89].

The regulation of Notch signaling in T cells has emerged as a novel mechanism of tumor to escape from immunosurveillance. Myeloid-derived suppressor cells

(MDSC) suppressed the expression of full-length and cleaved Notch-1 and Notch-2 in $CD8^+$ T cells in a nitric oxide-dependent manner, suggesting that the tumor microenvironment blocks Notch signaling in $CD8^+$ T cells as a strategy to evade protective immunity [30]. Higher levels of VEGF from tumor or stromal cells would be another determinant of Notch inhibition in T cells by inhibiting the expression of DLL1 and DLL4 in the bone marrow microenvironment [88]. A recent report suggests that Notch signaling is controlled by epigenetic regulation in $CD8^+$ T cells. Enhancer of zeste homolog 2 (EZH2) stimulated Notch by the methylation of Notch repressor Numb in activated $CD8^+$ T cells [90]. $EZH2^+$ $CD8^+$ T cells were capable of producing multiple cytokines and had an anti-apoptotic feature. In ovarian cancer patients, high accumulation of $EZH2^+$ $CD8^+$ T cells correlated with good prognosis demonstrating that Notch signaling endows $CD8^+$ T cell with high antitumor activity. Notably, tumor cells dampened EZH2 expression in $CD8^+$ T cells by consuming glucose [90]. Several approaches have been reported to activate CD8 Notch signaling in the tumor microenvironment. As well as N1IC overexpression, DLL1-Fc fusion complex induced central memory $CD8^+$ T cells, which had an increased antitumor activity [30, 91]. The decreased Notch signaling in $CD8^+$ T cells of tumor-bearing mice was counteracted by a proteasome inhibitor bortezomib [92]. Collectively, decreased expression of Notch in $CD8^+$ T cells represents a key element in tumor-induced tolerance, and the restoration of Notch signaling in $CD8^+$ T cells could be a possible strategy to overcome immunosuppression in the tumors.

In addition to $CD4^+$ and $CD8^+$ T cells, the role of Notch in regulating function of γδ T cells and NKT cells has been described. Phosphoantigen stimulation by bromohydrin pyrophosphate (BrHPP) increases the expression of Notch-1 in γδ T cells. Accordingly, the γδ T cell survival, cytokine production, and cytotoxicity against tumor cells heavily rely on Notch-1 signaling [93]. The production of IL-4 by NKT cells is regulated by conserved noncoding sequences (CNS)-2 through canonical Notch signaling [94]. Moreover, Notch-1 and Notch-2 are crucial for the IFN-γ and IL-4 production in NKT cells [49]. The cytokine production of NKT cells is suppressed in RBP-Jκ knockout mice, indicating that canonical Notch signaling is indeed important for the function of NKT cells. These results suggest that the effects of Notch activity go further than those induced on classic $CD4^+$ and $CD8^+$ T cell subsets.

5.3 Notch Signaling Controls the Development and Function by Various Subsets of Myeloid Cells

5.3.1 Notch Regulates the Development of Myeloid Subsets

Myeloid cells regulate adaptive immunity through their ability to acquire and present antigens and through the expression and release of inflammatory mediators. Myeloid subsets in peripheral tissues are represented by monocytes, granulocytes, macrophages, and DCs. Additional subgroups that expand under inflammation are

MDSC, tolerogenic DCs, and suppressive plasmacytoid DCs (pDCs). Most of the myeloid populations are originated from common myeloid progenitors; however, pDCs are derived from common lymphoid progenitors. Initial reports provided compelling evidence supporting the key role of Notch in the function and differentiation of myeloid cells [95–98]. However, the exact nature of Notch-related signaling in specific subsets of myeloid cells remains unclear. Previous reports showed the role of Notch in the maintenance of myeloid progenitor cells and blockage of their terminal differentiation [99–101]; whereas others indicated the effect of Notch for the final differentiation of mature myeloid cells [16]. These differences can be explained by the stage of myeloid cell differentiation when Notch is activated, the specific Notch receptor or ligand triggering the signaling, and the inflammatory milieu present under Notch-signaling conditions.

In support of the effect of Notch as a mediator for maintaining the pool of myeloid precursors, a delayed hematopoietic cell differentiation in response to G-CSF and GM-CSF and promotion of hematopoietic precursor self-renewal were observed after specific activation of Notch-1 or Notch-2 [96, 100] or through interaction with Jagged-1 [102], Jagged-2 [101], DLL1 [103], or DLL4 [104]. Accordingly, the inhibition or deletion of Notch-1 triggered the spontaneous maturation of erythroid and myeloid precursors [105]. On the other hand, Notch activity has been shown to be required for the differentiation of mature myeloid cells. Ectopic expression of Notch-1, or its active forms, promoted the differentiation of hematopoietic progenitors and into myeloid cell [98, 106]. Furthermore, inactivation of Notch signaling by targeting γ-secretase member Nicastrin resulted in an aberrant accumulation of granulocyte/monocyte progenitors in the peripheral blood, spleen, and liver [107]. Despite the potential role of Notch signaling in the homeostatic expansion of myeloid cells, myeloid cell lineages are normal in mice deficient for Notch-1 [13] and RBP-Jκ [108], indicating that the interaction of Notch signaling and the maturation of myeloid cells are a complex process that is context dependent.

5.3.2 Notch Activity in the Development of DCs

In recent years, multiple studies based on the pharmacological inhibition of Notch activity, the overexpression of Notch receptors or ligands, and the conditional deletion of Notch receptors in DCs or hematopoietic precursors have provided conclusive evidence that Notch signaling plays an important role in the development and function of DCs. As such, conditional deletion of RBP-Jκ or Notch-2 in DCs reduced the expansion of specific DC subsets in the spleen, but not in other lymphoid tissues [108, 109]. In addition, differentiation of DCs was inhibited in mice lacking Notch-1 in hematopoietic precursors [110], as well as in embryonic stem (ES) cells mutant for Notch-1 [111]. Similar results were obtained after the conditional deletion of Notch canonical member RBP-Jκ in bone marrow cells, which induced a substantial reduction in the presence of splenic DCs, specifically the

$CD8^-$ DCs present in the marginal zone [108]. The mechanism maintaining $CD8^-$ DC expansion appears to be mediated through DLL1 [112]. Surprisingly, there was also an increased in the accumulation of pDCs in RBP-Jκ null mice, suggesting that Notch signaling controls the homeostasis of $CD8^-$ DCs and inhibits the expansion of pDCs in the spleen. In addition to splenic DCs, a subset of $CD103^+$ DCs located in the lamina propria of the intestine is strongly reduced in the absence of Notch-2 [109]. Thus, the final commitment to DC differentiation during myelopoiesis is regulated by the Notch receptor and ligand expressed through the overall microenvironment components.

In addition to the effect of Notch receptors and ligands on the differentiation of DCs, recent studies suggested the posttranslational modification of Notch in immature myeloid cells. As such, phosphorylation of Notch by casein kinase 2 (CK2) was suggested as a major mediator of the expansion of MDSC under chronic inflammation and a key inhibitor of DC differentiation. Silencing of CK2 restored Notch signaling and enabled the maturation of MDSC into DCs [113]. Furthermore, current research aims to determine the Notch ligand responsible for controlling splenic DC development. Initial studies suggested a potential distinct effect of DLL1 and Jagged-1 as mediators of Notch signaling in DCs. Incubation of bone marrow precursors with fibroblasts expressing DLL1 induced DC differentiation, whereas Jagged-1-carrying fibroblasts promoted the accumulation of immature myeloid cells [114]. The mechanisms mediating this opposite effect were mediated through the activation or inhibition of Wnt pathways by DLL1 and Jagged-1, respectively [115, 116]. Interestingly, DLL1-induced activation of Notch blocked differentiation of monocytes into macrophages but also enabled their differentiation into DCs [117]. *In addition to the interaction of Notch and Wnt pathway in DCs, there is evidence that Notch partners with* NF-κB to control the differentiation of myeloid cells. In fact, a significant decrease in the NF-κB signaling and expression is observed in bone marrow precursors from Notch-deficient mice, which was restored after reconstitution of Notch signaling [110, 118, 119]. The regulation of NF-κB by Notch is mediated by a transcriptional induction of NF-κB members and through the direct interaction of Notch active forms and NF-κB subunits [120, 121]. Recent research also established the interaction of DLL4, Notch, and NF-κB in the function of DCs [26].

pDCs are phenotypically and functionally a distinct subset of DCs. Several reports described opposite effects of Notch receptors and ligand DLL1 on the differentiation of pDCs [122, 123]. Initial studies showed that DLL1 enhanced the numbers of pDCs by promoting their differentiation rather than proliferation [123]. Conversely, stromal cells expressing DLL1 drove differentiation of thymic progenitor cells to T cells and blocked pDC development [123]. Furthermore, deletion of Notch-1 in bone marrow populations did not affect the development of pDCs in vivo [124, 125]. Opposite results were found in RBP-Jκ-deficient mice, which showed increased numbers of pDCs [108], suggesting that Notch signaling may play distinct roles in the development of pDCs. This could be explained by the redundancy in the function of Notch in different environments. In fact, an example that the effects induced by Notch signaling are highly complex and context dependent is suggested by studies showing that deletion of Notch-1 in the thymus favors the development of DCs [124, 126], without affecting pDCs.

5.3.3 Signaling Through Notch Modulates the Activity of Myeloid Cells

In recent years, an active research field has suggested the importance of the Notch signaling in the activation of myeloid cells and the subsequent effect on T cell responses. RBP-Jκ-lacking DCs had a defect in the activation, maturation, and antigen presentation in response to LPS [127]. Further studies showed that loss of RBP-Jκ in DCs impaired their ability to contain tumor growth [128]. These results demonstrated the role of canonical Notch signaling in the function of mature DCs. Additional studies have shown the important role of Jagged-1 and DLL4 in the modulation of DC-related inflammation. Activation of DCs through Jagged-1 induced the production of IL-10 and promoted the development of Treg [129]. Moreover, DLL4-dependent Notch activation in DCs triggered Th1 and Th17 responses via NF-κB activity [26, 130]. However, DLL4 also induced IL-10 production from DCs that had an ability to attenuate airway hyperresponsiveness [131]. Thus, signaling through Notch in mature DCs may result in tolerogenic or immunogenic environments, which depend on the context and the strength of the Notch activation. In fact, a switch in the Notch ligands has been observed in myeloid populations as they approach the tolerogenic tumor microenvironment [132].

Activation of Notch in myeloid populations has been reported to be mediated through TLRs and various cytokines. TLRs are widely expressed in macrophages and DCs and allow them to rapidly respond to pathogen infections. Signaling through TLR ligands leads to the induction of Notch receptors and Jagged-1, Jagged-2, DLL1, and DLL4 [25, 133, 134]. Induction of Notch receptors by TLR ligands induces synergistic effects through unknown mediators that enable the inflammatory capacity of myeloid cells. Furthermore, inflammatory cytokines such as TNF and IL-1β induce the expression of Notch-1 and Notch-4, leading to the activation of inflammatory mediators [135–138]. A common potential mediator for the induction of Notch signaling by TLRs and cytokines is the activation of NF-κB [139]. Interestingly, IFN-γ signaling blocks the induction of Notch-induced genes through unknown mechanisms adding into the complexity of Notch induction in DCs under inflammation [139].

The molecular mechanisms by which Notch regulates DC activity remain unclear. Most of the effects triggered by Notch signaling in myeloid cells are mediated through activation of NF-κB. The mechanisms by which NF-κB regulates the function of myeloid cells include cooperation with Notch transcriptional activity [140], release of the inhibitor of NF-κB (IκB) that binds to Notch targets [141], and chromatin modification of Notch target genes [141]. Moreover, Notch signaling may activate the signal transducer and activator of transcription 3 (STAT3), which then interacts with specific NF-κB subunits [142, 143]. Another group of signaling molecules implicated in mediating Notch effects is the mitogen-activated protein kinases (MAPKs) [144].

Although there are overlapping effects of Notch signaling in DCs and macrophages (TLR and Notch interaction), recent studies have delineated unique features for canonical Notch signaling during macrophage activation. Treatment of macrophages with GSI decreased the production of IL-6, iNOS, and TNFα after activation with LPS, which correlated with a lower activity of NF-κB [145]. Similar results were obtained after deletion of RBP-Jκ in macrophages [144]. Conversely, production of IL-6 and TNFα was decreased, and IL-10 was increased in macrophages carrying the active forms of Notch-1 or Notch-2 [146], suggesting a potential effect of Notch in the promotion of tolerogenic macrophages. Accordingly, depletion of RBP-Jκ in tumor-associated macrophages (TAMs) restored the infiltration of $CD8^+$ T cells into tumors [147]. These results also support the potential context-dependent effects of Notch in macrophages.

5.4 Notch Signaling in Regulation of T Cell Polarization by APCs

Although Notch activity is a clear regulator of inflammation, the interaction of Notch on DCs and T cell function remains poorly understood. Unstimulated DCs express low levels of DLL and Jagged ligands; however, TLR activation upregulates the expression of both Notch and its ligands. As mentioned above, expression of DLL1 and DLL4 on DCs appears to favor Th1-type responses, whereas Jagged-1 and Jagged-2 induce Th2-type responses [25, 148]. In agreement with this, blockade of DLL4 in RSV-infected mice reduced Th1 cell polarization and promoted Th2 responses [149]. In contrast, activation of Notch through Jagged-1 promoted the development of Th2 responses that protected mice against autoimmune encephalitis [150]. In addition, silencing of Jagged-1 in immature human DCs prevented their ability to induce Th2 polarization [151]. These results provide a strong indication that polarization of $CD4^+$ T cells indeed depends on activation of Notch signaling. Although this aspect remains highly controversial, strong evidence supports the notion that DCs direct Th2 polarization via Jagged and Th1 polarization via DLL. In addition to DCs, Notch signaling in macrophages also affects CD4 differentiation. Activated macrophages derived from Notch-1 knockout mice produced less IL-6 and have low costimulatory molecule CD80 expression that results in less induction of Th17 [39]. Collectively, the interaction between innate and acquired immunity is dynamically impacted by Notch signaling.

5.5 Future Perspectives

Despite the aforementioned fact that Notch is important for both innate and acquired immunity, the question arises whether Notch signaling is a simple ligand/receptor pathway that plays an identical role regardless of the cell types. A recent finding partially answers this question by depleting Zmiz1, a cofactor of Notch-1 signaling. Surprisingly, Zmiz1 was required for T cell development but was dispensable for Notch-dependent intestinal homeostasis or myeloid suppression [152]. Although further investigations are necessary, this result offers a novel insight that cofactors would be a cell-specific determinant of the downstream signaling of Notch in addition to the type of ligands and receptors. Also, the influence of Notch pathway in tumor or stroma cells over acquired antitumor immunity is particularly interesting. The induction of N1IC in cancer cells reduced SERPINE1 expression and inhibited granzyme H-mediated cytotoxicity, indicating that Notch activity in the malignant cells enables escape from immune surveillance [153]. Since Notch is widely accepted as an oncogene and GSI (RO4929097) has passed a phase 1 study with a manageable safety profile [154], Notch activation or inhibition could not be a simple solution for cancer therapy. Although a substantial number of studies used GSIs as Notch inhibitors, gamma secretase is not specific for Notch, and cleaves over 95 different substrates including CD44. Because γ-secretase also cleaves CD44, a marker for cancer stem cells and activated T cells [155], the results obtained from using GSI must be interpreted with caution.

There are several regulators other than GSI that have potentials to regulate Notch signaling in immune cells. Because ADAM10 is necessary for the ligand-induced Notch-1 activation and ADAM17 is required for the ligand-independent Notch-1 signaling [156], the comparison between ADAM10 inhibitors and GSIs would be useful to differentiate ligand-dependent or -independent Notch-1 signaling. Jagged-1-mimic peptide (17 amino acids) would be a cost-effective alternative for Notch stimulation [157]. Valproic acid and suberoylanilide hydroxamic acid (SBHA), both of which have been identified as histone deacetylase inhibitors [158, 159], activate Notch-1 signaling and have a potential to suppress tumor proliferation. In addition, a dietary polyphenol resveratrol activates Notch-2 and suppresses carcinoid cell growth [160]. Interestingly, treatment of tumor-bearing mice with agonistic antibodies against Notch-2 or DLL1 or DLL4-Fc fusion proteins led to antitumor responses [88, 161, 162], suggesting the potential therapeutic effect of promoting Notch signaling in cancer. Although these therapeutic approaches were systemic and did not specifically target immune cells, further understandings of Notch signaling in innate and acquired immunity will enable us to pave the way for developing powerful strategies to treat cancer and autoimmune diseases.

References

1. Radtke, F., MacDonald, H. R., & Tacchini-Cottier, F. (2013). Regulation of innate and adaptive immunity by Notch. *Nature Reviews Immunology, 13*, 427–437.
2. Guruharsha, K. G., Kankel, M. W., & rtavanis-Tsakonas, S. (2012). The Notch signalling system: Recent insights into the complexity of a conserved pathway. *Nature Reviews Genetics, 13*, 654–666.
3. Radtke, F., Fasnacht, N., & MacDonald, H. R. (2010). Notch signaling in the immune system. *Immunity, 32*, 14–27.
4. Osborne, B. A., & Minter, L. M. (2007). Notch signalling during peripheral T-cell activation and differentiation. *Nature Reviews Immunology, 7*, 64–75.
5. Minter, L. M., & Osborne, B. A. (2012). Canonical and non-canonical Notch signaling in CD4(+) T cells. *Current Topics in Microbiology and Immunology, 360*, 99–114.
6. Samon, J. B., Champhekar, A., Minter, L. M., Telfer, J. C., Miele, L., Fauq, A., Das, P., Golde, T. E., & Osborne, B. A. (2008). Notch1 and TGFbeta1 cooperatively regulate Foxp3 expression and the maintenance of peripheral regulatory T cells. *Blood, 112*, 1813–1821.
7. Poellinger, L., & Lendahl, U. (2008). Modulating Notch signaling by pathway-intrinsic and pathway-extrinsic mechanisms. *Current Opinion in Genetics & Development, 18*, 449–454.
8. Heitzler, P. (2010). Biodiversity and noncanonical Notch signaling. *Current Topics in Developmental Biology, 92*, 457–481.
9. Cheng, P., Zhou, J., & Gabrilovich, D. (2010). Regulation of dendritic cell differentiation and function by Notch and Wnt pathways. *Immunological Reviews, 234*, 105–119.
10. Tanigaki, K., & Honjo, T. (2007). Regulation of lymphocyte development by Notch signaling. *Nature Immunology, 8*, 451–456.
11. Shi, J., Fallahi, M., Luo, J. L., & Petrie, H. T. (2011). Nonoverlapping functions for Notch1 and Notch3 during murine steady-state thymic lymphopoiesis. *Blood, 118*, 2511–2519.
12. Taghon, T., Yui, M. A., Pant, R., Diamond, R. A., & Rothenberg, E. V. (2006). Developmental and molecular characterization of emerging beta- and gammadelta-selected pre-T cells in the adult mouse thymus. *Immunity, 24*, 53–64.
13. Radtke, F., Wilson, A., Stark, G., Bauer, M., van Meerwijk, J., MacDonald, H. R., & Aguet, M. (1999). Deficient T cell fate specification in mice with an induced inactivation of Notch1. *Immunity, 10*, 547–558.
14. Han, H., Tanigaki, K., Yamamoto, N., Kuroda, K., Yoshimoto, M., Nakahata, T., Ikuta, K., & Honjo, T. (2002). Inducible gene knockout of transcription factor recombination signal binding protein-J reveals its essential role in T versus B lineage decision. *International Immunology, 14*, 637–645.
15. Weng, A. P., Millholland, J. M., Yashiro-Ohtani, Y., Arcangeli, M. L., Lau, A., Wai, C., Del Bianco, C., Rodriguez, C. G., Sai, H., Tobias, J., Li, Y., Wolfe, M. S., Shachaf, C., Felsher, D., Blacklow, S. C., Pear, W. S., & Aster, J. C. (2006). c-Myc is an important direct target of Notch1 in T-cell acute lymphoblastic leukemia/lymphoma. *Genes & Development, 20*, 2096–2109.
16. Grabher, C., von Boehmer, H., & Look, A. T. (2006). Notch 1 activation in the molecular pathogenesis of T-cell acute lymphoblastic leukaemia. *Nature Reviews Cancer, 6*, 347–359.
17. Robey, E., Chang, D., Itano, A., Cado, D., Alexander, H., Lans, D., Weinmaster, G., & Salmon, P. (1996). An activated form of Notch influences the choice between CD4 and CD8 T cell lineages. *Cell, 87*, 483–492.
18. Dervovic, D. D., Liang, H. C., Cannons, J. L., Elford, A. R., Mohtashami, M., Ohashi, P. S., Schwartzberg, P. L., & Zuniga-Pflucker, J. C. (2013). Cellular and molecular requirements for the selection of in vitro-generated CD8 T cells reveal a role for Notch. *Journal of Immunology, 191*, 1704–1715.
19. Jaleco, A. C., Neves, H., Hooijberg, E., Gameiro, P., Clode, N., Haury, M., Henrique, D., & Parreira, L. (2001). Differential effects of Notch ligands Delta-1 and Jagged-1 in human lymphoid differentiation. *The Journal of Experimental Medicine, 194*, 991–1002.

20. Schmitt, T. M., & Zuniga-Pflucker, J. C. (2002). Induction of T cell development from hematopoietic progenitor cells by delta-like-1 in vitro. *Immunity, 17*, 749–756.
21. Hozumi, K., Mailhos, C., Negishi, N., Hirano, K., Yahata, T., Ando, K., Zuklys, S., Hollander, G. A., Shima, D. T., & Habu, S. (2008). Delta-like 4 is indispensable in thymic environment specific for T cell development. *The Journal of Experimental Medicine, 205*, 2507–2513.
22. Koch, U., Fiorini, E., Benedito, R., Besseyrias, V., Schuster-Gossler, K., Pierres, M., Manley, N. R., Duarte, A., Macdonald, H. R., & Radtke, F. (2008). Delta-like 4 is the essential, nonredundant ligand for Notch1 during thymic T cell lineage commitment. *The Journal of Experimental Medicine, 205*, 2515–2523.
23. Mohtashami, M., Shah, D. K., Nakase, H., Kianizad, K., Petrie, H. T., & Zuniga-Pflucker, J. C. (2010). Direct comparison of Dll1- and Dll4-mediated Notch activation levels shows differential lymphomyeloid lineage commitment outcomes. *Journal of Immunology, 185*, 867–876.
24. Van de Walle, I., De Smet, G., Gartner, M., De Smedt, M., Waegemans, E., Vandekerckhove, B., Leclercq, G., Plum, J., Aster, J. C., Bernstein, I. D., Guidos, C. J., Kyewski, B., & Taghon, T. (2011). Jagged2 acts as a Delta-like Notch ligand during early hematopoietic cell fate decisions. *Blood, 117*, 4449–4459.
25. Amsen, D., Blander, J. M., Lee, G. R., Tanigaki, K., Honjo, T., & Flavell, R. A. (2004). Instruction of distinct CD4 T helper cell fates by different notch ligands on antigen-presenting cells. *Cell, 117*, 515–526.
26. Meng, L., Bai, Z., He, S., Mochizuki, K., Liu, Y., Purushe, J., Sun, H., Wang, J., Yagita, H., Mineishi, S., Fung, H., Yanik, G. A., Caricchio, R., Fan, X., Crisalli, L. M., Hexner, E. O., Reshef, R., Zhang, Y., & Zhang, Y. (2016). The Notch ligand DLL4 defines a capability of human dendritic cells in regulating Th1 and Th17 differentiation. *Journal of Immunology, 196*, 1070–1080.
27. Skokos, D., & Nussenzweig, M. C. (2007). CD8- DCs induce IL-12-independent Th1 differentiation through Delta 4 Notch-like ligand in response to bacterial LPS. *The Journal of Experimental Medicine, 204*, 1525–1531.
28. Elyaman, W., Bassil, R., Bradshaw, E. M., Orent, W., Lahoud, Y., Zhu, B., Radtke, F., Yagita, H., & Khoury, S. J. (2012). Notch receptors and Smad3 signaling cooperate in the induction of interleukin-9-producing T cells. *Immunity, 36*, 623–634.
29. Gillgrass, A., Gill, N., Babian, A., & Ashkar, A. A. (2014). The absence or overexpression of IL-15 drastically alters breast cancer metastasis via effects on NK cells, CD4 T cells, and macrophages. *Journal of Immunology, 193*, 6184–6191.
30. Sierra, R. A., Thevenot, P., Raber, P. L., Cui, Y., Parsons, C., Ochoa, A. C., Trillo-Tinoco, J., Del Valle, L., & Rodriguez, P. C. (2014). Rescue of notch-1 signaling in antigen-specific CD8+ T cells overcomes tumor-induced T-cell suppression and enhances immunotherapy in cancer. *Cancer Immunology Research, 2*, 800–811.
31. Amsen, D., Antov, A., & Flavell, R. A. (2009). The different faces of Notch in T-helper-cell differentiation. *Nature Reviews Immunology, 9*, 116–124.
32. Barbarulo, A., Grazioli, P., Campese, A. F., Bellavia, D., Di Mario, G., Pelullo, M., Ciuffetta, A., Colantoni, S., Vacca, A., Frati, L., Gulino, A., Felli, M. P., & Screpanti, I. (2011). Notch3 and canonical NF-kappaB signaling pathways cooperatively regulate Foxp3 transcription. *Journal of Immunology, 186*, 6199–6206.
33. Asano, N., Watanabe, T., Kitani, A., Fuss, I. J., & Strober, W. (2008). Notch1 signaling and regulatory T cell function. *Journal of Immunology, 180*, 2796–2804.
34. Mota, C., Nunes-Silva, V., Pires, A. R., Matoso, P., Victorino, R. M., Sousa, A. E., & Caramalho, I. (2014). Delta-like 1-mediated Notch signaling enhances the in vitro conversion of human memory CD4 T cells into FOXP3-expressing regulatory T cells. *Journal of Immunology, 193*, 5854–5862.
35. Bassil, R., Zhu, B., Lahoud, Y., Riella, L. V., Yagita, H., Elyaman, W., & Khoury, S. J. (2011). Notch ligand delta-like 4 blockade alleviates experimental autoimmune encephalomyelitis by promoting regulatory T cell development. *Journal of Immunology, 187*, 2322–2328.

36. Crome, S. Q., Wang, A. Y., & Levings, M. K. (2010). Translational mini-review series on Th17 cells: Function and regulation of human T helper 17 cells in health and disease. *Clinical and Experimental Immunology, 159*, 109–119.
37. Keerthivasan, S., Suleiman, R., Lawlor, R., Roderick, J., Bates, T., Minter, L., Anguita, J., Juncadella, I., Nickoloff, B. J., Le Poole, I. C., Miele, L., & Osborne, B. A. (2011). Notch signaling regulates mouse and human Th17 differentiation. *Journal of Immunology, 187*, 692–701.
38. Mukherjee, S., Schaller, M. A., Neupane, R., Kunkel, S. L., & Lukacs, N. W. (2009). Regulation of T cell activation by Notch ligand, DLL4, promotes IL-17 production and Rorc activation. *Journal of Immunology, 182*, 7381–7388.
39. Wongchana, W., Lawlor, R. G., Osborne, B. A., & Palaga, T. (2015). Impact of Notch1 deletion in macrophages on proinflammatory cytokine production and the outcome of experimental autoimmune encephalomyelitis. *Journal of Immunology, 195*, 5337–5346.
40. Wang, Y., Xing, F., Ye, S., Xiao, J., Di, J., Zeng, S., & Liu, J. (2015). Jagged-1 signaling suppresses the IL-6 and TGF-beta treatment-induced Th17 cell differentiation via the reduction of RORgammat/IL-17A/IL-17F/IL-23a/IL-12rb1. *Scientific Reports, 5*, 8234.
41. Vegran, F., Apetoh, L., & Ghiringhelli, F. (2015). Th9 cells: A novel CD4 T-cell subset in the immune war against cancer. *Cancer Research, 75*, 475–479.
42. Audia, S., Rossato, M., Santegoets, K., Spijkers, S., Wichers, C., Bekker, C., Bloem, A., Boon, L., Flinsenberg, T., Compeer, E., van den Broek, T., Facy, O., Ortega-Deballon, P., Berthier, S., Leguy-Seguin, V., Martin, L., Ciudad, M., Samson, M., Trad, M., Lorcerie, B., Janikashvili, N., Saas, P., Bonnotte, B., & Radstake, T. R. (2014). Splenic TFH expansion participates in B-cell differentiation and antiplatelet-antibody production during immune thrombocytopenia. *Blood, 124*, 2858–2866.
43. Auderset, F., Schuster, S., Fasnacht, N., Coutaz, M., Charmoy, M., Koch, U., Favre, S., Wilson, A., Trottein, F., Alexander, J., Luther, S. A., MacDonald, H. R., Radtke, F., & Tacchini-Cottier, F. (2013). Notch signaling regulates follicular helper T cell differentiation. *Journal of Immunology, 191*, 2344–2350.
44. Fasnacht, N., Huang, H. Y., Koch, U., Favre, S., Auderset, F., Chai, Q., Onder, L., Kallert, S., Pinschewer, D. D., MacDonald, H. R., Tacchini-Cottier, F., Ludewig, B., Luther, S. A., & Radtke, F. (2014). Specific fibroblastic niches in secondary lymphoid organs orchestrate distinct Notch-regulated immune responses. *The Journal of Experimental Medicine, 211*, 2265–2279.
45. Parente-Pereira, A. C., Shmeeda, H., Whilding, L. M., Zambirinis, C. P., Foster, J., van der Stegen, S. J., Beatson, R., Zabinski, T., Brewig, N., Sosabowski, J. K., Mather, S., Ghaem-Maghami, S., Gabizon, A., & Maher, J. (2014). Adoptive immunotherapy of epithelial ovarian cancer with Vgamma9Vdelta2 T cells, potentiated by liposomal alendronic acid. *Journal of Immunology, 193*, 5557–5566.
46. Washburn, T., Schweighoffer, E., Gridley, T., Chang, D., Fowlkes, B. J., Cado, D., & Robey, E. (1997). Notch activity influences the alphabeta versus gammadelta T cell lineage decision. *Cell, 88*, 833–843.
47. Van de Walle, I., Waegemans, E., De Medts, J., De Smet, G., De Smedt, M., Snauwaert, S., Vandekerckhove, B., Kerre, T., Leclercq, G., Plum, J., Gridley, T., Wang, T., Koch, U., Radtke, F., & Taghon, T. (2013). Specific Notch receptor-ligand interactions control human TCR-alphabeta/gammadelta development by inducing differential Notch signal strength. *The Journal of Experimental Medicine, 210*, 683–697.
48. Terabe, M., & Berzofsky, J. A. (2014). The immunoregulatory role of type I and type II NKT cells in cancer and other diseases. *Cancer Immunology, Immunotherapy: CII, 63*, 199–213.
49. Oh, S. J., Ahn, S., Jin, Y. H., Ishifune, C., Kim, J. H., Yasutomo, K., & Chung, D. H. (2015). Notch 1 and Notch 2 synergistically regulate the differentiation and function of invariant NKT cells. *Journal of Leukocyte Biology, 98*, 781–789.
50. Wilson, A., MacDonald, H. R., & Radtke, F. (2001). Notch 1-deficient common lymphoid precursors adopt a B cell fate in the thymus. *The Journal of Experimental Medicine, 194*, 1003–1012.

51. Izon, D. J., Aster, J. C., He, Y., Weng, A., Karnell, F. G., Patriub, V., Xu, L., Bakkour, S., Rodriguez, C., Allman, D., & Pear, W. S. (2002). Deltex1 redirects lymphoid progenitors to the B cell lineage by antagonizing Notch1. *Immunity, 16*, 231–243.
52. Dallas, M. H., Varnum-Finney, B., Delaney, C., Kato, K., & Bernstein, I. D. (2005). Density of the Notch ligand Delta1 determines generation of B and T cell precursors from hematopoietic stem cells. *The Journal of Experimental Medicine, 201*, 1361–1366.
53. Schneider, P., Takatsuka, H., Wilson, A., Mackay, F., Tardivel, A., Lens, S., Cachero, T. G., Finke, D., Beermann, F., & Tschopp, J. (2001). Maturation of marginal zone and follicular B cells requires B cell activating factor of the tumor necrosis factor family and is independent of B cell maturation antigen. *The Journal of Experimental Medicine, 194*, 1691–1697.
54. Oliver, A. M., Martin, F., & Kearney, J. F. (1999). IgMhighCD21high lymphocytes enriched in the splenic marginal zone generate effector cells more rapidly than the bulk of follicular B cells. *Journal of Immunology, 162*, 7198–7207.
55. Attanavanich, K., & Kearney, J. F. (2004). Marginal zone, but not follicular B cells, are potent activators of naive CD4 T cells. *Journal of Immunology, 172*, 803–811.
56. Tanigaki, K., Han, H., Yamamoto, N., Tashiro, K., Ikegawa, M., Kuroda, K., Suzuki, A., Nakano, T., & Honjo, T. (2002). Notch-RBP-J signaling is involved in cell fate determination of marginal zone B cells. *Nature Immunology, 3*, 443–450.
57. Oyama, T., Harigaya, K., Muradil, A., Hozumi, K., Habu, S., Oguro, H., Iwama, A., Matsuno, K., Sakamoto, R., Sato, M., Yoshida, N., & Kitagawa, M. (2007). Mastermind-1 is required for Notch signal-dependent steps in lymphocyte development in vivo. *Proceedings of the National Academy of Sciences of the United States of America, 104*, 9764–9769.
58. Wu, L., Maillard, I., Nakamura, M., Pear, W. S., & Griffin, J. D. (2007). The transcriptional coactivator Maml1 is required for Notch2-mediated marginal zone B-cell development. *Blood, 110*, 3618–3623.
59. Zhang, P., Zhao, Y., & Sun, X. H. (2013). Notch-regulated periphery B cell differentiation involves suppression of E protein function. *Journal of Immunology, 191*, 726–736.
60. Thomas, M., Calamito, M., Srivastava, B., Maillard, I., Pear, W. S., & Allman, D. (2007). Notch activity synergizes with B-cell-receptor and CD40 signaling to enhance B-cell activation. *Blood, 109*, 3342–3350.
61. Yoon, S. O., Zhang, X., Berner, P., Blom, B., & Choi, Y. S. (2009). Notch ligands expressed by follicular dendritic cells protect germinal center B cells from apoptosis. *Journal of Immunology, 183*, 352–358.
62. Spits, H., & Cupedo, T. (2012). Innate lymphoid cells: Emerging insights in development, lineage relationships, and function. *Annual Review of Immunology, 30*, 647–675.
63. Spits, H., Artis, D., Colonna, M., Diefenbach, A., Di Santo, J. P., Eberl, G., Koyasu, S., Locksley, R. M., McKenzie, A. N., Mebius, R. E., Powrie, F., & Vivier, E. (2013). Innate lymphoid cells – a proposal for uniform nomenclature. *Nature Reviews Immunology, 13*, 145–149.
64. Lee, J. S., Cella, M., McDonald, K. G., Garlanda, C., Kennedy, G. D., Nukaya, M., Mantovani, A., Kopan, R., Bradfield, C. A., Newberry, R. D., & Colonna, M. (2012). AHR drives the development of gut ILC22 cells and postnatal lymphoid tissues via pathways dependent on and independent of Notch. *Nature Immunology, 13*, 144–151.
65. Cherrier, M., Sawa, S., & Eberl, G. (2012). Notch, Id2, and RORgammat sequentially orchestrate the fetal development of lymphoid tissue inducer cells. *The Journal of Experimental Medicine, 209*, 729–740.
66. Wong, S. H., Walker, J. A., Jolin, H. E., Drynan, L. F., Hams, E., Camelo, A., Barlow, J. L., Neill, D. R., Panova, V., Koch, U., Radtke, F., Hardman, C. S., Hwang, Y. Y., Fallon, P. G., & McKenzie, A. N. (2012). Transcription factor RORalpha is critical for nuocyte development. *Nature Immunology, 13*, 229–236.
67. Huber, S., Gagliani, N., Zenewicz, L. A., Huber, F. J., Bosurgi, L., Hu, B., Hedl, M., Zhang, W., O'Connor, W., Jr., Murphy, A. J., Valenzuela, D. M., Yancopoulos, G. D., Booth, C. J., Cho, J. H., Ouyang, W., Abraham, C., & Flavell, R. A. (2012). IL-22BP is regulated by the inflammasome and modulates tumorigenesis in the intestine. *Nature, 491*, 259–263.

68. Auderset, F., Schuster, S., Coutaz, M., Koch, U., Desgranges, F., Merck, E., MacDonald, H. R., Radtke, F., & Tacchini-Cottier, F. (2012). Redundant Notch1 and Notch2 signaling is necessary for IFNgamma secretion by T helper 1 cells during infection with Leishmania major. *PLoS Pathogens, 8*, e1002560.
69. Sauma, D., Ramirez, A., Alvarez, K., Rosemblatt, M., & Bono, M. R. (2012). Notch signalling regulates cytokine production by CD8+ and CD4+ T cells. *Scandinavian Journal of Immunology, 75*, 389–400.
70. Minter, L. M., & Osborne, B. A. (2012). Notch and the survival of regulatory T cells: Location is everything! *Science Signaling, 5*, e31.
71. Adler, S. H., Chiffoleau, E., Xu, L., Dalton, N. M., Burg, J. M., Wells, A. D., Wolfe, M. S., Turka, L. A., & Pear, W. S. (2003). Notch signaling augments T cell responsiveness by enhancing CD25 expression. *Journal of Immunology, 171*, 2896–2903.
72. Joshi, I., Minter, L. M., Telfer, J., Demarest, R. M., Capobianco, A. J., Aster, J. C., Sicinski, P., Fauq, A., Golde, T. E., & Osborne, B. A. (2009). Notch signaling mediates G1/S cell-cycle progression in T cells via cyclin D3 and its dependent kinases. *Blood, 113*, 1689–1698.
73. Palaga, T., Miele, L., Golde, T. E., & Osborne, B. A. (2003). TCR-mediated Notch signaling regulates proliferation and IFN-gamma production in peripheral T cells. *Journal of Immunology, 171*, 3019–3024.
74. Bheeshmachar, G., Purushotaman, D., Sade, H., Gunasekharan, V., Rangarajan, A., & Sarin, A. (2006). Evidence for a role for notch signaling in the cytokine-dependent survival of activated T cells. *Journal of Immunology, 177*, 5041–5050.
75. Maekawa, Y., Ishifune, C., Tsukumo, S., Hozumi, K., Yagita, H., & Yasutomo, K. (2015). Notch controls the survival of memory CD4+ T cells by regulating glucose uptake. *Nature Medicine, 21*, 55–61.
76. Wood, S., Feng, J., Chung, J., Radojcic, V., Sandy-Sloat, A. R., Friedman, A., Shelton, A., Yan, M., Siebel, C. W., Bishop, D. K., & Maillard, I. (2015). Transient blockade of delta-like Notch ligands prevents allograft rejection mediated by cellular and humoral mechanisms in a mouse model of heart transplantation. *Journal of Immunology, 194*, 2899–2908.
77. Laky, K., Evans, S., Perez-Diez, A., & Fowlkes, B. J. (2015). Notch signaling regulates antigen sensitivity of naive CD4+ T cells by tuning co-stimulation. *Immunity, 42*, 80–94.
78. Amsen, D., Antov, A., Jankovic, D., Sher, A., Radtke, F., Souabni, A., Busslinger, M., McCright, B., Gridley, T., & Flavell, R. A. (2007). Direct regulation of Gata3 expression determines the T helper differentiation potential of Notch. *Immunity, 27*, 89–99.
79. Tu, L., Fang, T. C., Artis, D., Shestova, O., Pross, S. E., Maillard, I., & Pear, W. S. (2005). Notch signaling is an important regulator of type 2 immunity. *Journal of Experimental Medicine, 202*, 1037–1042.
80. Charbonnier, L. M., Wang, S., Georgiev, P., Sefik, E., & Chatila, T. A. (2015). Control of peripheral tolerance by regulatory T cell-intrinsic Notch signaling. *Nature Immunology, 16*, 1162–1173.
81. Zhang, W., Zhang, X., Sheng, A., Weng, C., Zhu, T., Zhao, W., & Li, C. (2015). Gamma-secretase inhibitor alleviates acute airway inflammation of allergic asthma in mice by down-regulating Th17 cell differentiation. *Mediators of Inflammation, 2015*, 258168.
82. Kryczek, I., Zhao, E., Liu, Y., Wang, Y., Vatan, L., Szeliga, W., Moyer, J., Klimczak, A., Lange, A., & Zou, W. (2011). Human TH17 cells are long-lived effector memory cells. *Science Translational Medicine, 3*, 104ra100.
83. Jiao, Z., Wang, W., Hua, S., Liu, M., Wang, H., Wang, X., Chen, Y., Xu, H., & Lu, L. (2014). Blockade of Notch signaling ameliorates murine collagen-induced arthritis via suppressing Th1 and Th17 cell responses. *The American Journal of Pathology, 184*, 1085–1093.
84. Cho, O. H., Shin, H. M., Miele, L., Golde, T. E., Fauq, A., Minter, L. M., & Osborne, B. A. (2009). Notch regulates cytolytic effector function in CD8+ T cells. *Journal of Immunology, 182*, 3380–3389.
85. Backer, R. A., Helbig, C., Gentek, R., Kent, A., Laidlaw, B. J., Dominguez, C. X., de Souza, Y. S., van Trierum, S. E., van Beek, R., Rimmelzwaan, G. F., ten Brinke, A., Willemsen,

A. M., van Kampen, A. H., Kaech, S. M., Blander, J. M., van Gisbergen, K., & Amsen, D. (2014). A central role for Notch in effector CD8(+) T cell differentiation. *Nature Immunology, 15*, 1143–1151.
86. Maekawa, Y., Minato, Y., Ishifune, C., Kurihara, T., Kitamura, A., Kojima, H., Yagita, H., Sakata-Yanagimoto, M., Saito, T., Taniuchi, I., Chiba, S., Sone, S., & Yasutomo, K. (2008). Notch2 integrates signaling by the transcription factors RBP-J and CREB1 to promote T cell cytotoxicity. *Nature Immunology, 9*, 1140–1147.
87. Mathieu, M., Duval, F., Daudelin, J. F., & Labrecque, N. (2015). The Notch signaling pathway controls short-lived effector CD8+ T cell differentiation but is dispensable for memory generation. *Journal of Immunology, 194*, 5654–5662.
88. Huang, Y., Lin, L., Shanker, A., Malhotra, A., Yang, L., Dikov, M. M., & Carbone, D. P. (2011). Resuscitating cancer immunosurveillance: Selective stimulation of DLL1-Notch signaling in T cells rescues T-cell function and inhibits tumor growth. *Cancer Research, 71*, 6122–6131.
89. Kijima, M., Iwata, A., Maekawa, Y., Uehara, H., Izumi, K., Kitamura, A., Yagita, H., Chiba, S., Shiota, H., & Yasutomo, K. (2009). Jagged1 suppresses collagen-induced arthritis by indirectly providing a negative signal in CD8+ T cells. *Journal of Immunology, 182*, 3566–3572.
90. Zhao, E., Maj, T., Kryczek, I., Li, W., Wu, K., Zhao, L., Wei, S., Crespo, J., Wan, S., Vatan, L., Szeliga, W., Shao, I., Wang, Y., Liu, Y., Varambally, S., Chinnaiyan, A. M., Welling, T. H., Marquez, V., Kotarski, J., Wang, H., Wang, Z., Zhang, Y., Liu, R., Wang, G., & Zou, W. (2016). Cancer mediates effector T cell dysfunction by targeting microRNAs and EZH2 via glycolysis restriction. *Nature Immunology, 17*, 95–103.
91. Biktasova, A. K., Dudimah, D. F., Uzhachenko, R. V., Park, K., Akhter, A., Arasada, R. R., Evans, J. V., Novitskiy, S. V., Tchekneva, E. E., Carbone, D. P., Shanker, A., & Dikov, M. M. (2015). Multivalent forms of the Notch ligand DLL-1 enhance antitumor T-cell immunity in lung cancer and improve efficacy of EGFR-targeted therapy. *Cancer Research, 75*, 4728–4741.
92. Thounaojam, M. C., Dudimah, D. F., Pellom, S. T., Jr., Uzhachenko, R. V., Carbone, D. P., Dikov, M. M., & Shanker, A. (2015). Bortezomib enhances expression of effector molecules in anti-tumor CD8+ T lymphocytes by promoting Notch-nuclear factor-kappaB crosstalk. *Oncotarget, 6*, 32439–32455.
93. Gogoi, D., Dar, A. A., & Chiplunkar, S. V. (2014). Involvement of Notch in activation and effector functions of gammadelta T cells. *Journal of Immunology, 192*, 2054–2062.
94. Tanaka, S., Tsukada, J., Suzuki, W., Hayashi, K., Tanigaki, K., Tsuji, M., Inoue, H., Honjo, T., & Kubo, M. (2006). The interleukin-4 enhancer CNS-2 is regulated by Notch signals and controls initial expression in NKT cells and memory-type CD4 T cells. *Immunity, 24*, 689–701.
95. Milner, L. A., Bigas, A., Kopan, R., Brashem-Stein, C., Bernstein, I. D., & Martin, D. I. (1996). Inhibition of granulocytic differentiation by mNotch1. *Proceedings of the National Academy of Sciences of the United States of America, 93*, 13014–13019.
96. Bigas, A., Martin, D. I., & Milner, L. A. (1998). Notch1 and Notch2 inhibit myeloid differentiation in response to different cytokines. *Molecular and Cellular Biology, 18*, 2324–2333.
97. Schroeder, T., & Just, U. (2000). mNotch1 signaling reduces proliferation of myeloid progenitor cells by altering cell-cycle kinetics. *Experimental Hematology, 28*, 1206–1213.
98. Schroeder, T., & Just, U. (2000). Notch signalling via RBP-J promotes myeloid differentiation. *The EMBO Journal, 19*, 2558–2568.
99. Kumano, K., Chiba, S., Shimizu, K., Yamagata, T., Hosoya, N., Saito, T., Takahashi, T., Hamada, Y., & Hirai, H. (2001). Notch1 inhibits differentiation of hematopoietic cells by sustaining GATA-2 expression. *Blood, 98*, 3283–3289.
100. Tan-Pertel, H. T., Walker, L., Browning, D., Miyamoto, A., Weinmaster, G., & Gasson, J. C. (2000). Notch signaling enhances survival and alters differentiation of 32D myeloblasts. *Journal of Immunology, 165*, 4428–4436.

101. Carlesso, N., Aster, J. C., Sklar, J., & Scadden, D. T. (1999). Notch1-induced delay of human hematopoietic progenitor cell differentiation is associated with altered cell cycle kinetics. *Blood, 93*, 838–848.
102. Zhou, L., Li, L. W., Yan, Q., Petryniak, B., Man, Y., Su, C., Shim, J., Chervin, S., & Lowe, J. B. (2008). Notch-dependent control of myelopoiesis is regulated by fucosylation. *Blood, 112*, 308–319.
103. Delaney, C., Varnum-Finney, B., Aoyama, K., Brashem-Stein, C., & Bernstein, I. D. (2005). Dose-dependent effects of the Notch ligand Delta1 on ex vivo differentiation and in vivo marrow repopulating ability of cord blood cells. *Blood, 106*, 2693–2699.
104. Lauret, E., Catelain, C., Titeux, M., Poirault, S., Dando, J. S., Dorsch, M., Villeval, J. L., Groseil, A., Vainchenker, W., Sainteny, F., & Bennaceur-Griscelli, A. (2004). Membrane-bound delta-4 notch ligand reduces the proliferative activity of primitive human hematopoietic CD34+CD38low cells while maintaining their LTC-IC potential. *Leukemia, 18*, 788–797.
105. Lam, L. T., Ronchini, C., Norton, J., Capobianco, A. J., & Bresnick, E. H. (2000). Suppression of erythroid but not megakaryocytic differentiation of human K562 erythroleukemic cells by notch-1. *The Journal of Biological Chemistry, 275*, 19676–19684.
106. Henning, K., Heering, J., Schwanbeck, R., Schroeder, T., Helmbold, H., Schafer, H., Deppert, W., Kim, E., & Just, U. (2008). Notch1 activation reduces proliferation in the multipotent hematopoietic progenitor cell line FDCP-mix through a p53-dependent pathway but Notch1 effects on myeloid and erythroid differentiation are independent of p53. *Cell Death and Differentiation, 15*, 398–407.
107. Klinakis, A., Lobry, C., Abdel-Wahab, O., Oh, P., Haeno, H., Buonamici, S., van De Walle, I., Cathelin, S., Trimarchi, T., Araldi, E., Liu, C., Ibrahim, S., Beran, M., Zavadil, J., Efstratiadis, A., Taghon, T., Michor, F., Levine, R. L., & Aifantis, I. (2011). A novel tumour-suppressor function for the Notch pathway in myeloid leukaemia. *Nature, 473*, 230–233.
108. Caton, M. L., Smith-Raska, M. R., & Reizis, B. (2007). Notch-RBP-J signaling controls the homeostasis of CD8- dendritic cells in the spleen. *The Journal of Experimental Medicine, 204*, 1653–1664.
109. Lewis, K. L., Caton, M. L., Bogunovic, M., Greter, M., Grajkowska, L. T., Ng, D., Klinakis, A., Charo, I. F., Jung, S., Gommerman, J. L., Ivanov, I. I., Liu, K., Merad, M., & Reizis, B. (2011). Notch2 receptor signaling controls functional differentiation of dendritic cells in the spleen and intestine. *Immunity, 35*, 780–791.
110. Cheng, P., Zlobin, A., Volgina, V., Gottipati, S., Osborne, B., Simel, E. J., Miele, L., & Gabrilovich, D. I. (2001). Notch-1 regulates NF-kappaB activity in hemopoietic progenitor cells. *Journal of Immunology, 167*, 4458–4467.
111. Cheng, P., Nefedova, Y., Miele, L., Osborne, B. A., & Gabrilovich, D. (2003). Notch signaling is necessary but not sufficient for differentiation of dendritic cells. *Blood, 102*, 3980–3988.
112. Sekine, C., Moriyama, Y., Koyanagi, A., Koyama, N., Ogata, H., Okumura, K., & Yagita, H. (2009). Differential regulation of splenic CD8- dendritic cells and marginal zone B cells by Notch ligands. *International Immunology, 21*, 295–301.
113. Cheng, P., Kumar, V., Liu, H., Youn, J. I., Fishman, M., Sherman, S., & Gabrilovich, D. (2014). Effects of notch signaling on regulation of myeloid cell differentiation in cancer. *Cancer Research, 74*, 141–152.
114. Cheng, P., Nefedova, Y., Corzo, C. A., & Gabrilovich, D. I. (2007). Regulation of dendritic-cell differentiation by bone marrow stroma via different Notch ligands. *Blood, 109*, 507–515.
115. Liu, H., Zhou, J., Cheng, P., Ramachandran, I., Nefedova, Y., & Gabrilovich, D. I. (2013). Regulation of dendritic cell differentiation in bone marrow during emergency myelopoiesis. *Journal of Immunology, 191*, 1916–1926.
116. Zhou, J., Cheng, P., Youn, J. I., Cotter, M. J., & Gabrilovich, D. I. (2009). Notch and wingless signaling cooperate in regulation of dendritic cell differentiation. *Immunity, 30*, 845–859.
117. Ohishi, K., Varnum-Finney, B., Serda, R. E., Anasetti, C., & Bernstein, I. D. (2001). The Notch ligand, Delta-1, inhibits the differentiation of monocytes into macrophages but permits their differentiation into dendritic cells. *Blood, 98*, 1402–1407.

118. Oswald, F., Liptay, S., Adler, G., & Schmid, R. M. (1998). NF-kappaB2 is a putative target gene of activated Notch-1 via RBP-Jkappa. *Molecular and Cellular Biology, 18*, 2077–2088.
119. Bellavia, D., Campese, A. F., Alesse, E., Vacca, A., Felli, M. P., Balestri, A., Stoppacciaro, A., Tiveron, C., Tatangelo, L., Giovarelli, M., Gaetano, C., Ruco, L., Hoffman, E. S., Hayday, A. C., Lendahl, U., Frati, L., Gulino, A., & Screpanti, I. (2000). Constitutive activation of NF-kappaB and T-cell leukemia/lymphoma in Notch3 transgenic mice. *The EMBO Journal, 19*, 3337–3348.
120. Nickoloff, B. J., Qin, J. Z., Chaturvedi, V., Denning, M. F., Bonish, B., & Miele, L. (2002). Jagged-1 mediated activation of notch signaling induces complete maturation of human keratinocytes through NF-kappaB and PPARgamma. *Cell Death and Differentiation, 9*, 842–855.
121. Guan, E., Wang, J., Laborda, J., Norcross, M., Baeuerle, P. A., & Hoffman, T. (1996). T cell leukemia-associated human Notch/translocation-associated Notch homologue has I kappa B-like activity and physically interacts with nuclear factor-kappa B proteins in T cells. *The Journal of Experimental Medicine, 183*, 2025–2032.
122. Olivier, A., Lauret, E., Gonin, P., & Galy, A. (2006). The Notch ligand delta-1 is a hematopoietic development cofactor for plasmacytoid dendritic cells. *Blood, 107*, 2694–2701.
123. Dontje, W., Schotte, R., Cupedo, T., Nagasawa, M., Scheeren, F., Gimeno, R., Spits, H., & Blom, B. (2006). Delta-like1-induced Notch1 signaling regulates the human plasmacytoid dendritic cell versus T-cell lineage decision through control of GATA-3 and Spi-B. *Blood, 107*, 2446–2452.
124. Radtke, F., Ferrero, I., Wilson, A., Lees, R., Aguet, M., & MacDonald, H. R. (2000). Notch1 deficiency dissociates the intrathymic development of dendritic cells and T cells. *The Journal of Experimental Medicine, 191*, 1085–1094.
125. Ferrero, I., Held, W., Wilson, A., Tacchini-Cottier, F., Radtke, F., & MacDonald, H. R. (2002). Mouse CD11c(+) B220(+) Gr1(+) plasmacytoid dendritic cells develop independently of the T-cell lineage. *Blood, 100*, 2852–2857.
126. Feyerabend, T. B., Terszowski, G., Tietz, A., Blum, C., Luche, H., Gossler, A., Gale, N. W., Radtke, F., Fehling, H. J., & Rodewald, H. R. (2009). Deletion of Notch1 converts pro-T cells to dendritic cells and promotes thymic B cells by cell-extrinsic and cell-intrinsic mechanisms. *Immunity, 30*, 67–79.
127. Wang, Y. C., Hu, X. B., He, F., Feng, F., Wang, L., Li, W., Zhang, P., Li, D., Jia, Z. S., Liang, Y. M., & Han, H. (2009). Lipopolysaccharide-induced maturation of bone marrow-derived dendritic cells is regulated by notch signaling through the up-regulation of CXCR4. *The Journal of Biological Chemistry, 284*, 15993–16003.
128. Feng, F., Wang, Y. C., Hu, X. B., Liu, X. W., Ji, G., Chen, Y. R., Wang, L., He, F., Dou, G. R., Liang, L., Zhang, H. W., & Han, H. (2010). The transcription factor RBP-J-mediated signaling is essential for dendritic cells to evoke efficient anti-tumor immune responses in mice. *Molecular Cancer, 9*, 90.
129. Bugeon, L., Gardner, L. M., Rose, A., Gentle, M., & Dallman, M. J. (2008). Cutting edge: Notch signaling induces a distinct cytokine profile in dendritic cells that supports T cell-mediated regulation and IL-2-dependent IL-17 production. *Journal of Immunology, 181*, 8189–8193.
130. Mochizuki, K., Xie, F., He, S., Tong, Q., Liu, Y., Mochizuki, I., Guo, Y., Kato, K., Yagita, H., Mineishi, S., & Zhang, Y. (2013). Delta-like ligand 4 identifies a previously uncharacterized population of inflammatory dendritic cells that plays important roles in eliciting allogeneic T cell responses in mice. *Journal of Immunology, 190*, 3772–3782.
131. Huang, H. M., Hsiao, G., Fan, C. K., Lin, C. L., Leu, S. J., Chiang, B. L., & Lee, Y. L. (2013). Notch ligand delta-like 4-pretreated dendritic cells alleviate allergic airway responses by enhancing IL-10 production. *PLoS One, 8*, e63613.
132. Raber, P. L., Thevenot, P., Sierra, R., Wyczechowska, D., Halle, D., Ramirez, M. E., Ochoa, A. C., Fletcher, M., Velasco, C., Wilk, A., Reiss, K., & Rodriguez, P. C. (2014). Subpopulations of myeloid-derived suppressor cells impair T cell responses through independent nitric oxide-related pathways. *International Journal of Cancer, 134*, 2853–2864.

133. Fung, E., Tang, S. M., Canner, J. P., Morishige, K., Arboleda-Velasquez, J. F., Cardoso, A. A., Carlesso, N., Aster, J. C., & Aikawa, M. (2007). Delta-like 4 induces notch signaling in macrophages: Implications for inflammation. *Circulation, 115*, 2948–2956.
134. Foldi, J., Chung, A. Y., Xu, H., Zhu, J., Outtz, H. H., Kitajewski, J., Li, Y., Hu, X., & Ivashkiv, L. B. (2010). Autoamplification of Notch signaling in macrophages by TLR-induced and RBP-J-dependent induction of Jagged1. *Journal of Immunology, 185*, 5023–5031.
135. Ando, K., Kanazawa, S., Tetsuka, T., Ohta, S., Jiang, X., Tada, T., Kobayashi, M., Matsui, N., & Okamoto, T. (2003). Induction of Notch signaling by tumor necrosis factor in rheumatoid synovial fibroblasts. *Oncogene, 22*, 7796–7803.
136. Maniati, E., Bossard, M., Cook, N., Candido, J. B., Emami-Shahri, N., Nedospasov, S. A., Balkwill, F. R., Tuveson, D. A., & Hagemann, T. (2011). Crosstalk between the canonical NF-kappaB and Notch signaling pathways inhibits Ppargamma expression and promotes pancreatic cancer progression in mice. *The Journal of Clinical Investigation, 121*, 4685–4699.
137. Ottaviani, S., Tahiri, K., Frazier, A., Hassaine, Z. N., Dumontier, M. F., Baschong, W., Rannou, F., Corvol, M. T., Savouret, J. F., & Richette, P. (2010). Hes1, a new target for interleukin 1beta in chondrocytes. *Annals of the Rheumatic Diseases, 69*, 1488–1494.
138. Ostroukhova, M., Qi, Z., Oriss, T. B., Dixon-McCarthy, B., Ray, P., & Ray, A. (2006). Treg-mediated immunosuppression involves activation of the Notch-HES1 axis by membrane-bound TGF-beta. *The Journal of Clinical Investigation, 116*, 996–1004.
139. Hu, X., & Ivashkiv, L. B. (2009). Cross-regulation of signaling pathways by interferon-gamma: Implications for immune responses and autoimmune diseases. *Immunity, 31*, 539–550.
140. Osipo, C., Golde, T. E., Osborne, B. A., & Miele, L. A. (2008). Off the beaten pathway: The complex cross talk between Notch and NF-kappaB. *Laboratory Investigation, 88*, 11–17.
141. Aguilera, C., Hoya-Arias, R., Haegeman, G., Espinosa, L., & Bigas, A. (2004). Recruitment of IkappaBalpha to the hes1 promoter is associated with transcriptional repression. *Proceedings of the National Academy of Sciences of the United States of America, 101*, 16537–16542.
142. Nefedova, Y., Cheng, P., Gilkes, D., Blaskovich, M., Beg, A. A., Sebti, S. M., & Gabrilovich, D. I. (2005). Activation of dendritic cells via inhibition of Jak2/STAT3 signaling. *Journal of Immunology, 175*, 4338–4346.
143. Kusmartsev, S., Nefedova, Y., Yoder, D., & Gabrilovich, D. I. (2004). Antigen-specific inhibition of CD8+ T cell response by immature myeloid cells in cancer is mediated by reactive oxygen species. *Journal of Immunology, 172*, 989–999.
144. Hu, X., Chung, A. Y., Wu, I., Foldi, J., Chen, J., Ji, J. D., Tateya, T., Kang, Y. J., Han, J., Gessler, M., Kageyama, R., & Ivashkiv, L. B. (2008). Integrated regulation of Toll-like receptor responses by Notch and interferon-gamma pathways. *Immunity, 29*, 691–703.
145. Palaga, T., Buranaruk, C., Rengpipat, S., Fauq, A. H., Golde, T. E., Kaufmann, S. H., & Osborne, B. A. (2008). Notch signaling is activated by TLR stimulation and regulates macrophage functions. *European Journal of Immunology, 38*, 174–183.
146. Zhang, Q., Wang, C., Liu, Z., Liu, X., Han, C., Cao, X., & Li, N. (2012). Notch signal suppresses Toll-like receptor-triggered inflammatory responses in macrophages by inhibiting extracellular signal-regulated kinase 1/2-mediated nuclear factor kappaB activation. *The Journal of Biological Chemistry, 287*, 6208–6217.
147. Franklin, R. A., Liao, W., Sarkar, A., Kim, M. V., Bivona, M. R., Liu, K., Pamer, E. G., & Li, M. O. (2014). The cellular and molecular origin of tumor-associated macrophages. *Science, 344*, 921–925.
148. Maekawa, Y., Tsukumo, S., Chiba, S., Hirai, H., Hayashi, Y., Okada, H., Kishihara, K., & Yasutomo, K. (2003). Delta1-Notch3 interactions bias the functional differentiation of activated CD4+ T cells. *Immunity, 19*, 549–559.
149. Schaller, M. A., Neupane, R., Rudd, B. D., Kunkel, S. L., Kallal, L. E., Lincoln, P., Lowe, J. B., Man, Y., & Lukacs, N. W. (2007). Notch ligand Delta-like 4 regulates disease pathogenesis during respiratory viral infections by modulating Th2 cytokines. *The Journal of Experimental Medicine, 204*, 2925–2934.

150. Elyaman, W., Bradshaw, E. M., Wang, Y., Oukka, M., Kivisakk, P., Chiba, S., Yagita, H., & Khoury, S. J. (2007). JAGGED1 and delta1 differentially regulate the outcome of experimental autoimmune encephalomyelitis. *Journal of Immunology, 179*, 5990–5998.
151. Liotta, F., Frosali, F., Querci, V., Mantei, A., Fili, L., Maggi, L., Mazzinghi, B., Angeli, R., Ronconi, E., Santarlasci, V., Biagioli, T., Lasagni, L., Ballerini, C., Parronchi, P., Scheffold, A., Cosmi, L., Maggi, E., Romagnani, S., & Annunziato, F. (2008). Human immature myeloid dendritic cells trigger a TH2-polarizing program via Jagged-1/Notch interaction. *The Journal of Allergy and Clinical Immunology, 121*(1000–5), e8.
152. Pinnell, N., Yan, R., Cho, H. J., Keeley, T., Murai, M. J., Liu, Y., Alarcon, A. S., Qin, J., Wang, Q., Kuick, R., Elenitoba-Johnson, K. S., Maillard, I., Samuelson, L. C., Cierpicki, T., & Chiang, M. Y. (2015). The PIAS-like coactivator Zmiz1 is a direct and selective cofactor of Notch1 in T cell development and leukemia. *Immunity, 43*, 870–883.
153. Yu, X. M., Jaskula-Sztul, R., Georgen, M. R., Aburjania, Z., Somnay, Y. R., Leverson, G., Sippel, R. S., Lloyd, R. V., Johnson, B. P., & Chen, H. (2016). Notch1 Signaling Regulates the Aggressiveness of Differentiated Thyroid Cancer and Inhibits SERPINE1 Expression. Clinical Cancer Research.
154. Tolcher, A. W., Messersmith, W. A., Mikulski, S. M., Papadopoulos, K. P., Kwak, E. L., Gibbon, D. G., Patnaik, A., Falchook, G. S., Dasari, A., Shapiro, G. I., Boylan, J. F., Xu, Z. X., Wang, K., Koehler, A., Song, J., Middleton, S. A., Deutsch, J., Demario, M., Kurzrock, R., & Wheler, J. J. (2012). Phase I study of RO4929097, a gamma secretase inhibitor of Notch signaling, in patients with refractory metastatic or locally advanced solid tumors. *Journal of Clinical Oncology, 30*, 2348–2353.
155. Maccalli, C., & De Maria, R. (2015). Cancer stem cells: Perspectives for therapeutic targeting. *Cancer Immunology, Immunotherapy: CII, 64*, 91–97.
156. Bozkulak, E. C., & Weinmaster, G. (2009). Selective use of ADAM10 and ADAM17 in activation of Notch1 signaling. *Molecular and Cellular Biology, 29*, 5679–5695.
157. Kannan, S., Sutphin, R. M., Hall, M. G., Golfman, L. S., Fang, W., Nolo, R. M., Akers, L. J., Hammitt, R. A., McMurray, J. S., Kornblau, S. M., Melnick, A. M., Figueroa, M. E., & Zweidler-McKay, P. A. (2013). Notch activation inhibits AML growth and survival: A potential therapeutic approach. *The Journal of Experimental Medicine, 210*, 321–337.
158. Ning, L., Jaskula-Sztul, R., Kunnimalaiyaan, M., & Chen, H. (2008). Suberoyl bishydroxamic acid activates notch1 signaling and suppresses tumor progression in an animal model of medullary thyroid carcinoma. *Annals of Surgical Oncology, 15*, 2600–2605.
159. Landreville, S., Agapova, O. A., Matatall, K. A., Kneass, Z. T., Onken, M. D., Lee, R. S., Bowcock, A. M., & Harbour, J. W. (2012). Histone deacetylase inhibitors induce growth arrest and differentiation in uveal melanoma. *Clinical Cancer Research, 18*, 408–416.
160. Pinchot, S. N., Jaskula-Sztul, R., Ning, L., Peters, N. R., Cook, M. R., Kunnimalaiyaan, M., & Chen, H. (2011). Identification and validation of Notch pathway activating compounds through a novel high-throughput screening method. *Cancer, 117*, 1386–1398.
161. Sugimoto, K., Maekawa, Y., Kitamura, A., Nishida, J., Koyanagi, A., Yagita, H., Kojima, H., Chiba, S., Shimada, M., & Yasutomo, K. (2010). Notch2 signaling is required for potent antitumor immunity in vivo. *Journal of Immunology, 184*, 4673–4678.
162. Kuijk, L. M., Verstege, M. I., Rekers, N. V., Bruijns, S. C., Hooijberg, E., Roep, B. O., de Gruijl, T. D., van, K. Y., & Unger, W. W. (2013). Notch controls generation and function of human effector CD8+ T cells. *Blood, 121*, 2638–2646.

Chapter 6
Notch in Ovarian Cancer

Emily Gerry, Vivek Singh, and Tian-Li Wang

Abstract Ovarian cancers are malignancies for which improved therapeutic approaches are urgently needed. The development of chemoresistance in ovarian high-grade serous carcinoma is almost inevitable, and researchers are constantly seeking new pathways to target in order to improve the dismal survival rates of women diagnosed with this disease. The Notch pathway in ovarian cancer represents a promising subject for research into new ovarian cancer treatment modalities. Over the last 12 years, the major Notch proteins (Notch1 and NOTCH3), prominent Notch ligands (JAG1 and DLL4), and downstream proteins (Hes1 and DLGAP5) have begun to be studied in ovarian cancers. The roles of Notch in conferring chemoresistance and acting in angiogenesis have also been demonstrated. Additionally, GSI and DLL4 inhibitors as well as Notch antibodies continue to be explored in both clinical and nonclinical settings. It is clear that future studies are needed in order to translate the results from these preclinical studies into practice. Most importantly, it is crucial to demonstrate the safety and efficacy of Notch-based therapy in ovarian cancer patients. There is still much work to be done in examining the pathways and proteins with which Notch may be associated as well as in developing more specific and more effective means of inhibiting Notch pathway components.

Keywords Notch · Ovarian cancer · Chemoresistance · Platinum resistance · Cancer stem cells

---

E. Gerry · V. Singh · T.-L. Wang (✉)
Johns Hopkins University, Baltimore, MD, USA
e-mail: egerry3@jhmi.edu; vsingh14@jhu.edu; tlw@jhmi.edu

L. Miele, S. Artavanis-Tsakonas (eds.), *Targeting Notch in Cancer*,
https://doi.org/10.1007/978-1-4939-8859-4_6

6.1 Ovarian Cancer Background

Ovarian cancer is the most lethal gynecologic malignancy; fewer than 50% of women with advanced ovarian cancers will survive beyond 5 years. In the case of high-grade serous carcinoma (HGSC), which is almost always diagnosed at advanced stages (stage III or IV), only 30% of patients will survive beyond 5 years. In fact, the overall mortality of ovarian cancer has only slightly improved in the last three decades. In addition to the lack of effective detection for the disease at its early stages, one of the main reasons for the sluggish improvement in treatment outcomes is the frequent development of chemoresistance in advanced ovarian cancers. Standard chemotherapy for ovarian cancer patients is composed of a combination of platinum- and taxane-based drugs administrated by cycles of treatment. Most ovarian cancer patients initially respond to chemotherapy; however, at least 80% of those initial responders will experience recurrence, most within 18 months of initial response to chemotherapy [1]. Recurrent disease will be resistant to, or will likely become resistant to, platinum therapy. This phenomenon is the primary cause of the bleak prognosis of this deadly disease.

Although ovarian cancer is often referred to as a single disease, it is more accurately a heterogeneous group of diseases. Based on differences in morphological and clinical features, pathogenesis pathways, and unique molecular genetic alterations, epithelial ovarian cancer can broadly be divided into two groups [2]: type I, which includes low-grade serous carcinoma, clear cell carcinoma, endometrioid carcinoma, mucinous carcinoma, and malignant Brenner tumor, and type II, which mainly consists of high-grade serous carcinoma, as well as carcinosarcoma and undifferentiated carcinoma. The prevalence of the five most common subtypes is presented in Fig. 6.1, with other subtypes constituting less than 1% of the total diagnosed epithelial ovarian cancers.

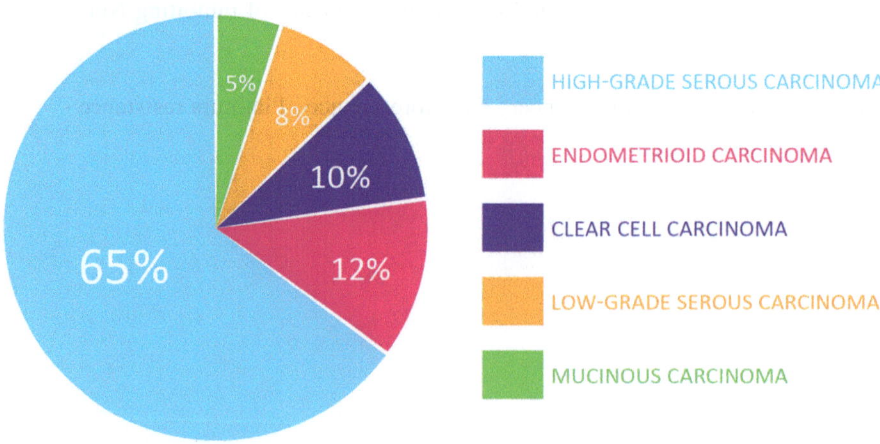

Fig. 6.1 The prevalence of the five most common ovarian cancer subtypes. High-grade serous carcinoma (including peritoneal primary, carcinosarcoma, and tubal carcinoma) is indicated in light blue, low-grade serous carcinoma in orange, clear cell carcinoma in gray, endometrioid carcinoma in yellow, and mucinous carcinoma in dark blue

Type I tumors are typically genetically stable, relatively indolent, and confined to the ovary when they present [3]. Each subtype of type I ovarian cancer presents with a distinct molecular genetic profile and morphology. Common and defining genetic alterations in type I cancers include mutations in KRAS, BRAF, and ERBB2 (low-grade serous carcinoma) [4]; PIK3CA (clear cell carcinoma) [5]; CTNNB1, PTEN, and PIK3CA (low-grade endometrioid carcinoma) [6]; KRAS (mucinous carcinoma) [7, 8]; and CDKN2A (Brenner tumors) [9]. One genetic feature that unites type I ovarian cancers is a lack of TP53 mutations [6]. Type II tumors, on the other hand, account for around 75% of epithelial ovarian cancers and are more aggressive than their type I counterparts [3]. They possess more homogenous morphologies than do type I tumors; exhibit solid, glandular, and papillary patterns; and are diagnosed based on the dominant pattern they exhibit. Type II tumors exhibit TP53 mutations in over 95% of cases as well as frequent CCNE1 amplification but rarely exhibit mutations characteristic of type I tumors [6, 10]. They are highly unstable chromosomally and present as advanced stage disease in over 75% of cases. High-grade serous carcinoma, which accounts for the vast majority of type II ovarian cancer and is highly aggressive, also exhibits BRCA inactivation (either by mutation or promoter methylation) in 40–50% of cases [11].

As a result of the major genetic and morphologic differences between type I and type II ovarian cancers, clinical presentation also differs between these two groups. Type I cancers are slow-growing and are usually confined to the ovaries when diagnosed. Patients may present with early- or late-stage disease, and the frequency of stage at diagnosis depends largely on the subtype [6]. In contrast, the vast majority of type II tumors are at advanced stages when they are diagnosed [12], and at the time of diagnosis, they have almost always spread outside of the ovaries [6]. In addition, type II tumors recur more frequently than do type I tumors [13].

The differences between type I and type II tumors also have implications for approaches to early detection and treatment. Because type I tumors are generally slower growing and are more confined to the ovary, it is typically easier to recognize these malignancies at earlier stages. Since it is so rare to observe type II tumors at stages I or II, there have been significant efforts to improve early detection strategies. Approaches have included examining fallopian tubes removed from women at risk for ovarian cancer (due to BRCA1/BRCA2 mutations) to look for evidence of ovarian cancer precursor lesions [14] and refocusing on detecting low-volume disease (as this may be the best predictor of prognosis) [15, 16]. Recently, applying a liquid Pap smear has been proposed for detection of malignant cells or DNA at early or low-volume stage in ovarian cancers [17], as a significant fraction of ovarian cancer may be derived from fallopian tube epithelial cells, which are easily dislodged and flow through the uterine cavity and cervix.

As of now, type I and type II ovarian cancers are largely treated via platinum-based chemotherapy, i.e., alternating cycles of taxane and a platinum-based agent. Identifying pathways and mutations important to specific subtypes of ovarian cancer will be important to the development of novel therapeutic agents. We must carefully examine pathways that contribute to chemoresistance and tumorigenesis and evaluate the utility of drugs that can be used to target these pathways either alone or in combination with extant therapeutic agents.

It should be clear that "ovarian cancer" is not a single, unified disease, but a collection of various subtypes with distinct genetic profiles, morphologies, and cell origins [2]. In discussing the presence and role of a specific gene or pathway in ovarian cancer, it is important to refrain from generalizing findings to all ovarian cancer subtypes. The majority of literature concentrates on high-grade serous carcinomas, the deadliest and the most common form of ovarian cancer. We will attempt to address the role of the Notch pathway in high-grade ovarian serous carcinoma and examine how targeting the Notch pathway could lead to new treatment modalities in this deadly disease.

6.2 Notch Signaling Pathway: Background

The Notch signaling pathway is evolutionally conserved and regulates a broad spectrum of functions that include cell-fate determination, cell communication, tissue patterning, and cell differentiation, proliferation, and apoptosis. While there is only one Notch receptor and two ligands in insects, four different Notch receptors, named Notch1, Notch2, Notch3, and Notch4, are present in mammals; this was likely an adaptation to deal with the complex and pleiotropic needs of mammals. Additionally, there are five different Notch ligands in mammals, including members of the Jagged family (JAG1 and JAG2), as well as members of the Delta-like family (DLL1, DLL3, and DLL4). This leads to the possibility of different ligand and receptor combinations in mammalian systems. However, when examining cancer tissues, we observed predominant forms of ligand-receptor pairs in specific types of tumor tissues. For example, of the four different Notch receptors, Notch3 is the most frequently amplified and overexpressed in ovarian cancer [18, 19]. Of the ligands, JAG1 and DLL4 have been shown in the literature to be overexpressed in ovarian cancer [20–22]. However, based on gene and transcriptome analysis of TCGA ovarian HGSC dataset, DLL3 appears to be the predominate form in this tumor type. This will be detailed in the Sects. 6.4 and 6.7.

The Notch receptors are large transmembrane proteins, each consisting of an extracellular fragment that contains many epidermal growth factor (EGF)-like repeats (e.g., 36 in Notch1), a transmembrane domain, and an intracellular cytoplasmic domain (NICD). The Notch heterodimer is auto-inhibited by a negative regulatory region (NRR), which contains a heterodimerization domain and three Lin12/Notch repeats [23]. Notch3 differs slightly from the other Notch receptors. Unlike Notch1 and Notch2, Notch3 does not have a complete transactivation domain (TAD). This may explain why the NOTCH intracellular domain (NICD) of Notch3 has weaker transactivation activity than that of Notch1 and Notch2 [24, 25]. There are further differences in the amino acid identity between Notch1 and Notch3 in several intracellular domains, such as the ankyrin repeat region, the RBP-jκ-associated molecule (RAM) domain, and the C-terminal region, as well as in the EGF repeats of the extracellular region [24, 25]. Both the JAG and DLL ligands also contain EGF-like repeats; the JAG proteins typically have 15–16, while the DLL proteins typically have 6–8 [26]. Repeats 11 and 12 are required for Notch binding [27–29]. Also required is a degenerate EGF-like repeated entitled the DSL domain shared by both the JAG and DLL ligands [30–32]. Other minor structural differences between the two include two additional DOS motifs (tandem EGF repeats) adjacent to the DSL domain and a C-rich domain adjacent to the single transmembrane domain (TMD) residue in the JAG proteins [33]. The binding of the Notch ligands to EGF-repeat region of the Notch extracellular domain is necessary to induce subsequent cleavage steps on the transmembrane domain of NOTCH [34, 35].

The basic signal transmission steps of Notch signaling are generally conserved across different Notch isoforms. The Notch receptor located at the plasma membrane binds to one of its ligands located at the plasma membrane of an adjacent juxtaposed cell. This triggers serial cleavage events on the Notch receptor. First, it is cleaved by the metalloprotease ADAM or TACE, releasing an extracellular fragment that remains bound to the ligand; the remaining cytoplasmic component is then cleaved by gamma secretase to generate the Notch intracellular domain (NICD). NICD then migrates to the nucleus, where it repels a corepressor and binds to the CBF1/Su(H)/Lag-1 (CSL) complex [36]. With the recruitment of additional coactivators (such as MAML1), the CSL complex is converted from a repressor to an activator of transcription. This in turn activates transcription of Notch target proteins [33].

The Notch pathway in ovarian cancer is unique in terms of its (1) dominant Notch receptor, (2) dominant Notch ligand(s), (3) regulatory proteins, and (4) transcriptionally activated genes. As stated above, NOTCH3 was found to be amplified and overexpressed in serous carcinomas and can thus be considered the dominant receptor [18, 19]. It is constitutively activated during tumor development. Notch1 has also been found to be active in ovarian cancer [37, 38]. There is some discussion, however, as to which Notch ligands are most dominant. One study suggests that DLL4 is overexpressed in up to 72% of carcinomas [22]. Yet, the general finding in other reports seems to be that JAG1 is the most dominant Notch ligand (although both JAG1 and DLL4, as well as JAG2, are observed ligands of Notch in ovarian cancer) [20, 21, 39]. Third, as shown in Fig. 6.2, WWP2 has been discovered to be a negative regulator of Notch3 signaling in ovarian cancer [40]. It directly interacts with and mono-ubiquinates post-secretase-cleaved Notch3 protein fragments, promoting their sorting to and degradation in lysosomes. This is thought to be one of the mechanisms by which NOTCH receptor signals are downregulated in human cancers [40].

Finally, different target genes may be transcriptionally activated by different NICD. Since the transcription cofactors are likely to be unique in different cell and tissue types, these Notch transcriptional modifiers are likely to facilitate the tissue-level complexity in the Notch transcription regulation. Based on recent genome-wide ChIP-seq studies using antibody specific to NICD1 or NICD3, Hes and Hey proteins are conserved NOTCH target genes across different cancer cell types, from T-cell lymphoblastic leukemia (T-ALL) to ovarian and breast cancers [41–45].

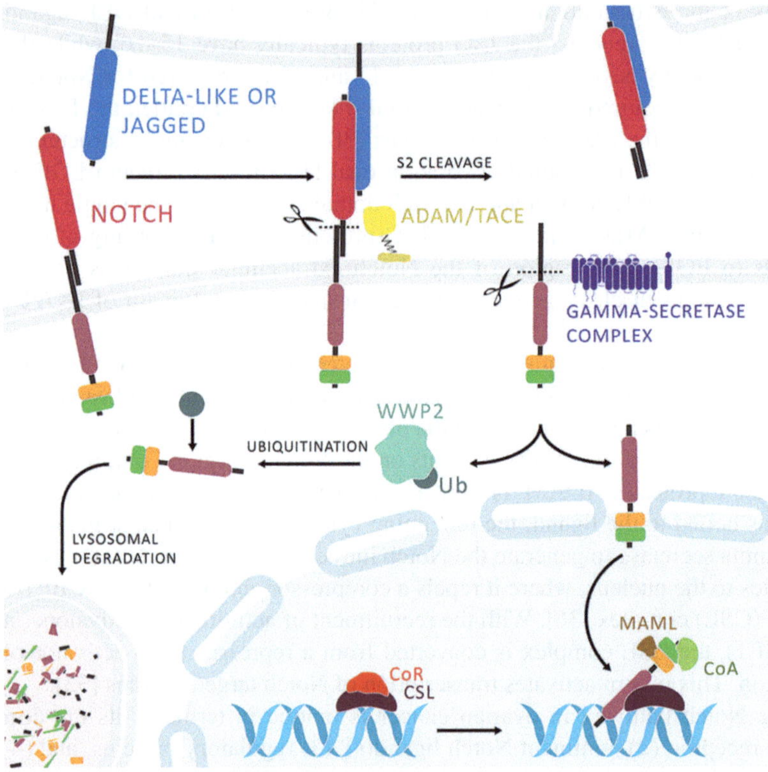

Fig. 6.2 The Notch pathway in ovarian cancer. The Notch receptor at the plasma membrane binds a ligand located on an adjacent plasma membrane. ADAM or TACE cleaves Notch3 (S2 cleavage), resulting in the separation of the extracellular Notch component. The remaining protein is then cleaved by the gamma secretase complex, resulting in the formation of the Notch3 intracellular domain (NICD3). The NICD3 fragment can then enter the nucleus, where it binds to the CSL complex, converting it to an activator of transcription with the recruitment of coactivators such as MAML1. Alternatively, the repressor WWP2 can ubiquinate Notch3, leading to its degradation in the endosome/lysosome compartments

Hes1 and Hey are both members of the helix-loop-helix (bHLH) family of transcription factors. Members of this family repress the transcription of tissue-specific transcription factors; Notch may thereby maintain stem cells through inhibiting differentiation [26, 46–48]. A variety of potential genes transcriptionally activated by Notch3 in ovarian cancer have been revealed by genome-wide chromatin immunoprecipitation (ChIP) and integrated transcriptome analyses [43]. However, the analyses are currently restricted to cancer cell lines. It will be critical to perform similar kind of experiments on tissues or at least on primary cell cultures.

6.3 NOTCH3 Signaling in Ovarian Cancer

In ovarian cancer tissues, gene amplification of chromosome 19p13.12, a locus containing the NOTCH3 gene, was first discovered using digital karyotyping and FISH techniques, and its associated overexpression was identified in ovarian high-grade serous carcinomas [18]. The discovery of NOTCH3 gene amplification in ovarian cancers was later confirmed via SNP array technique, including in experiments performed by The Cancer Genome Atlas (TCGA) [18, 19, 49]. Gene amplification of the NOTCH3 locus was found to be present in approximately 12% of serous carcinomas [18]. NOTCH3 inhibition and silencing resulted in decreased proliferation and induction of apoptosis in Notch3-expressing cell lines [18]. One of the potential Notch3 signal-initiating ligands in ovarian serous carcinoma is JAG1, which would form a juxtacrine circuit with Notch and promote proliferation of ovarian cancer cells in the intraperitoneal cavity [20]. Putative targets of NOTCH3 include Hes1 and Hes4, canonical downstream targets of the Notch1 signaling pathway, and newly identified target genes using genome-wide ChIP approaches [43]. These include DLGAP5, a mitotic apparatus organizing protein [43], ZNF155, and NRARP (unpublished data). Expression of NICD3 was shown to result in the upregulation of embryonic stem cell markers as well as ABCB1, an ATP-binding cassette family member responsible for drug efflux and multidrug resistance [50]. Various studies demonstrated that Notch3 is upregulated in chemoresistant tumors, may confer platinum resistance, and may correlate with worse disease outcome when the signaling is reactivated [50–52]. Thus, targeting Notch3 may represent a vital treatment option to overcoming chemoresistance in ovarian tumors.

Early attempts to isolate cancer stem cell-like cells (CSCs) in ovarian cancer, a special self-renewing cell population, identified Notch1 upregulation in isolated CSC spheroid cells, which also showed increased levels of CD44 and CD117 [53]. Later study demonstrated that Notch3 is expressed in ovarian CSC populations isolated from ascites [54] and that inhibition of NOTCH signaling may sensitize cells to platinum treatment [50]. Since ovarian CSCs are tightly linked to treatment failure, CSCs will be more explicitly defined, and this topic will be discussed further in the Sect. 6.5.

The role of Notch signaling in angiogenesis and vascular development has also become increasingly clear. Global knockout of NOTCH1 [55] and endothelium-specific knockout of JAG1 [56] both result in embryonic death with severe vascular defects in mice. NOTCH1 was also shown to be crucial for vascular endothelial growth factor (VEGF)-induced postnatal angiogenesis [57]. While NOTCH3 knockout does not cause the same lethality, the knockout mice show abnormalities in arterial structure and myogenic response, as well as a defect in postnatal maturation of vascular smooth muscle cells [58]. The effect of Notch3 on regulating smooth muscle is also evident when examining CADASIL, an autosomal dominant disease caused by a mutation in the NOTCH3 gene on chromosome 19 [59]. Disulfide bond formation between mutated Notch3 and other proteins is thought to lead the Notch3 extracellular domain to accumulate near vascular smooth muscle cells, leading to smooth muscle cell degeneration [60].

The role of Notch in ovarian tumor angiogenesis was first explored a decade later, when Hu et al. showed a relationship between angiogenesis regulator VEGF and Notch ligand DLL4 in ovarian tumors, reporting a link between DLL4 overexpression and poor overall survival and response to anti-VEGF therapy [22]. Thanapprapasr et al. built on this finding to propose DLL4/Notch signaling as a new approach to anti-angiogenesis therapy in ovarian cancer [61]. Over the past several years, research into anti-DLL4 and anti-JAG1 as possible anti-angiogenic Notch therapeutic strategies has also expanded. The roles of DLL4 and JAG1 in angiogenesis may explain why a number of studies have found a link between inhibition of Notch3 in ovarian cancer and reduced angiogenesis [62, 63]. The Sect. 6.6 will discuss these findings in more detail.

6.4 Genetic Alterations of Members of the Notch Signaling Pathway in Ovarian Cancer

Somatic genetic alteration is a hallmark of cancer, as it often leads to aberrant signaling pathways and disruption of cellular function, which together propel tumorigenesis. Comprehensive molecular genetic analysis of major tumor types, including ovarian HGSC, has been completed by TCGA, a US government-funded research initiative. With a publically available dataset from TCGA [19], we analyzed genetic alterations including mutation, amplification, and deletion of NOTCH1, NOTCH2, NOTCH3, and NOTCH4 and WWP2 in a number of different cancer types. NOTCH1, NOTCH2, and NOTCH4 are altered in ovarian cancer but at rates significantly lower than NOTCH3, which is altered in 12% of ovarian HGSCs, most often via gene amplifications (Fig. 6.3a). This data largely agrees with previous reports concerning NOTCH3 gene amplification in ovarian carcinomas published by our group [18, 49]. Minimal amplicon mapping has pinpointed NOTCH3 located at the core of the amplified region [18, 49]. Other co-amplified genes within this amplicon include BRD4, a BET (bromodomain and extra terminal domain) family protein that could potentially cooperate with Notch3 to promote cell dedifferentiation, repopulation, and other key steps in the tumorigenesis [18, 19].

Among the regulatory players that could fine-tune Notch3 signaling, we chose to analyze WWP2, a NEDD4-like E3 ubiquitin-protein ligase, which was found to mono-ubiquitinate NOTCH3 and target it to the lysosomal degradation pathway [40]. In ovarian cancer, WWP2, which localizes at chromosome 16q22.1, is deleted in approximately 2% of cases and downregulated in approximately 17% of tumors. Therefore, downregulation or deletion of WWP2 could, in theory, unleash the pre-programmed ubiquitination/degradation route of Notch3 and enhance its signaling activity [40].

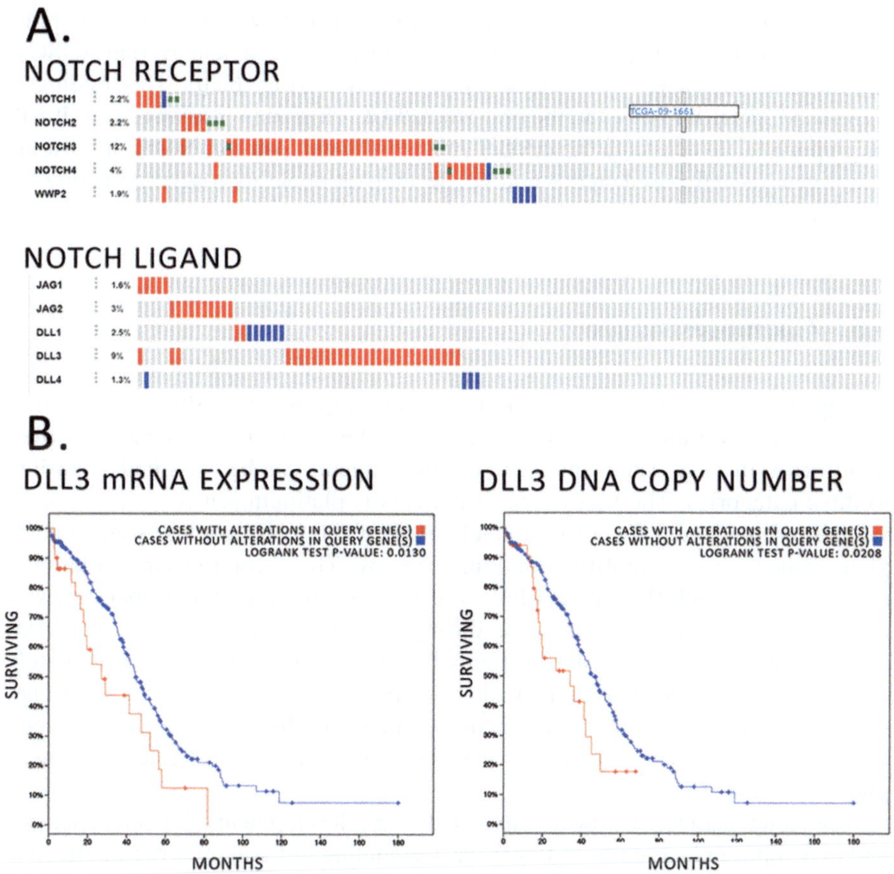

Fig. 6.3 Notch proteins, signal modifiers, and ligands are altered at different frequencies in ovarian cancer, and Notch ligand DLL3 alterations are associated with worse overall survival. (**a**) The alteration frequencies of Notch proteins Notch1, Notch2, Notch3, Notch-negative regulator WPP2, and Notch ligands JAG1, JAG2, DLL1, DLL3, and DLL4 are shown for ovarian high-grade serous carcinoma (TCGA, Nature 2011; retrieved from cBioPortal) [19]. Cases are represented with rectangles. Red rectangles indicate cases with gene amplification, blue indicate cases with gene deletion, and green indicate cases with gene mutation. Gray rectangles are cases in which the gene is unaffected. (**b**) Survival curves for high-grade serous carcinoma cases with and without alterations in DLL3 mRNA expression (left) and with and without alterations in DLL3 DNA copy number (right). Data is retrieved from cBioPortal (TCGA, Nature 2011) [19]. The y-axes denote the percentage of surviving patients, while the x-axes denote the time in months. Red curves represent cases with alterations in DLL3, and blue curves represent cases without alterations. The p-value is indicated in both plots

Notch ligands, including JAG1, JAG2, DLL1, DLL3, and DLL4, can also be altered in ovarian cancer. Based on the analysis of TCGA ovarian HGSC dataset, rare amplification events were found in the JAG1 (1.6%) and JAG2 (3%) gene loci, while rare deletion events (~2%) were observed in the DLL1 or DLL4 locus.

Contrarily, DLL3 is heavily amplified in ovarian cancers, with a 9% alteration rate (Fig. 6.3a). Furthermore, DLL3 amplification or overexpression in ovarian HGSC is significantly correlated with dismal overall survival (Fig. 6.3b). This finding is significant, as DLL4 is, by far, the best-studied DLL ligand in ovarian cancer. It will be important to delineate functional receptor-ligand pair of Notch in ovarian tumorigenesis and, based on this finding, develop rationale approaches targeting the Notch pathway.

6.5 Chemoresistance

Perhaps one of the most significant obstacles in improving the dismal survival of patients with ovarian cancer is to overcome the development of resistance to platinum-based therapy. The response to platinum agents can be classified according to three categories. The first group of patients is platinum sensitive. These individuals, who account for approximately 80% of the total patients, show a complete response to the first-line platinum therapy. The second group is platinum refractory, in which the patients fail to respond to initial platinum therapy, with either stable or progressive disease during treatment [64]. Although platinum-sensitive and platinum-resistant patients begin as distinct groups, approximately 50% of platinum-sensitive patients develop resistance during the course of chemotherapy treatment. If the tumor recurs within 6 months after the final treatment, it is considered platinum resistant, and those patients will be treated with non-platinum agents [64].

The Notch pathway has been implicated in the development of chemoresistance and may represent a promising target for overcoming this major barrier to effective treatment. The first research into the role of Notch in platinum resistance in ovarian cancer emerged in 2010, when it was found that Notch confers stem cell-like properties in ovarian HGSC [50]. Subsequent study noted NOTCH3 overexpression in platinum-resistant cells, as well as correlation of NOTCH3 overexpression with worse progression-free and overall survival in patients with advanced ovarian cancer [51]. Inhibiting Notch signaling with GSI in combination with cisplatin was found to prolong survival compared to cisplatin alone in xenograft mouse model of ovarian cancer [52].

It has been argued that one force behind the development of chemoresistance is the existence of cancer stem cell-like cells (CSCs) in the tumor microenvironment. The research on CSCs is still largely in its early stages, and thus there is still work to be done in elucidating the defining markers of CSCs and the pathways that regulate them over a variety of cancer types. These cells, which constitute only a small percentage of the bulk population of tumor cells, are refractory to primary chemotherapy. Unlike cells of the bulk population, CSCs are capable of subsequently regenerating tumor cells and repopulating the tumor microenvironment, leading to recurrence. In general, CSCs are defined according to several criteria, including self-renewal, occupation of a small percentage of the tumor population, ability to reproduce tumors in vivo, differentiation into non-tumorigenic cells, and expression of distinct cell surface markers [52]. CSCs share a number of characteristics with adult stem cells, including those that confer increased chemoresistance, such as enhanced DNA repair and increased levels of membrane efflux transporters.

The Notch signaling pathway has been shown to control survival, proliferation, maintenance, and cell fate in somatic stem cells [65], as well as to participate in regulating CSC functions over many types of cancers [66, 67]. Inhibition of Notch in ovarian cancer decreases the population of ovarian CSCs, suggesting that Notch may play a role in stem cell self-renewal and maintenance in ovarian cancer [52]. Notch1 [53] and Notch3 [52] upregulation have both been observed in the chemoresistant CSC populations. Additionally, CD44, Nanog, Oct4, drug transporters (MDR1, ABCG2, ABCB5), DNA repair genes (ATM, BRCA2), and platinum resistance-associated genes such as Connexi43/Gja1 and Cyp1a1 have been reported in ovarian CSCs [52]. Upregulation of ATP-binding cassette transporters may be a major mechanism contributing to multidrug chemoresistance [52]. In fact, overexpression of the Notch3 intracellular domain (NICD3) has been shown toconfer resistance to platinum in ovarian cancer [68] and to upregulate Nanog, Oct4, ABCB1, and other embryonic stem cell-associated genes such as Klf4, Rex1, Rif1, and Sall4 [50]. Upregulation of ABCB1, an ATP-binding cassette, may indicate increased drug efflux and thus a decrease in the accumulation of carboplatin in ovarian cancer cells, which is likely a factor in chemoresistance. The modulation of the other stem cell markers further supports the putative role of Notch signaling in CSC repopulation in ovarian cancer.

6.6 Angiogenesis

Notch also plays a key role in angiogenesis and vascular development in certain biological contexts. It was shown that both global knockout of NOTCH1 [55] and endothelium-specific knockout of JAG1 [56] result in severe vascular defects and embryonic cell death in mice, while knockout of NOTCH3 results in defects in arterial structure and myogenic response [58]. When taken together, these results indicate that the Notch signaling pathway plays an essential role in regulating embryonic vascular morphogenesis and remodeling. Interestingly, NOTCH3 knockout does not produce lethality as NOTCH1 and JAG1 knockouts do. Instead, NOTCH3 knockout mice present with deficient postnatal maturation of vascular smooth muscle cells, a phenomenon similar to that resulting from cerebral autosomal dominant arteriopathy with subcortical infarcts and leukoencephalopathy (CADASIL), a disease caused by a mutation in the NOTCH3 gene on chromosome 19 [59]. In patients with CADASIL, disulfide bonds form between mutated Notch3 and neighboring proteins, causing the Notch3 extracellular domain to accumulate near vascular smooth muscle. This, in turn, leads to smooth muscle degeneration [60].

In cancer, the Notch signaling pathway has also been implicated in angiogenesis and the development of blood vessels in ovarian tumors, including vessel maturation, pericyte recruitment, branching, and cell differentiation, proliferation, survival, and apoptosis [22]. Angiogenesis is a process that could be targeted for controlling the growth of ovarian tumors, including proteins involved in the Notch signaling pathway. As angiogenesis is necessary for tumor growth and metastasis, targeting tumor vasculature via the Notch signaling pathway holds particular therapeutic promise due to the presumed genetic stability of tumor endothelial cells [22]. Recent work has been in characterizing the effects of inhibiting Notch ligands, regulators, and modulators on angiogenesis in ovarian tumors.

The clinical promise of targeting ovarian tumor angiogenesis was initially reported using VEGF inhibitors such as bevacizumab in patients with ovarian tumors [69]. In ovarian cancers, an increased level of VEGF, which is known to play a key role in neovascularization [22, 70, 71], is inversely correlated with patient survival [72, 73]. Treatment of ovarian tumors with VEGF inhibitors in combination with paclitaxel resulted in decreased tumor burden in preclinical models [74]. While there is a demonstrable clinical benefit in using VEGF inhibitors, there are some limitations. Such therapies are not universally effective for ovarian cancers, and initially sensitive tumors often develop resistance following treatment [22]. However, the VEGF pathway is also known to participate in crosstalk with the Notch signaling pathway [75], which has led to the Notch signaling pathway being regarded as an alternate clinical target to VEGF inhibitor in ovarian cancer therapeutics. It has been shown that Notch1 is downstream of VEGF signaling and is critical for VEGF-induced postnatal angiogenesis [57]. A recent study has also demonstrated that VEGF participates in the ovarian cytokine TNF network, an autocrine malignant cell network that also includes IL6, CXCL12, and CXCR4. The Notch signaling pathway was highly enriched in association with this TNF network. Protein kinase CK2 was posited as a key signaling node of this pathway; inhibition of CK2 resulted in decreased Notch signaling and reduced angiogenesis [76].

In order to interfere with angiogenesis in tumor formation, the Notch signaling pathway can be targeted by blocking expression of Notch ligands DLL4 and JAG1, both of which are shown to be overexpressed in ovarian cancers [20–22] and both of which play a role in angiogenesis. DLL4 is induced by VEGF, and downregulates angiogenesis by decreasing VEGF receptor expression, allowing DLL4 and VEGF to form a sort of regulatory loop [22, 77, 78]. DLL4 is overexpressed in up to 72% of ovarian cancers [79], is correlated with worse patient outcome, and is a predictor of a poor response to anti-VEGF treatment [22]. Blockade of DLL4 in tumor endothelial cells with a human monoclonal antibody, REGN421, in xenograft mouse models engineered to express human DLL4 results in reduced Notch signaling in solid tumors and surrounding blood vessels, as well as the dysregulation of angiogenic processes via VEGF. This subsequently causes the formation of hyper-sprouted vessels possessing increased vascular structure but decreased vascular perfusion and leads to dose-dependent inhibition of ovarian tumor growth [80]. Chronic inhibition of DLL4 alone has been thought to foster a reversible pathological activation of endothelial cells and vascular tumorigenesis; however, the antitumor effect of DLL4 inhibition can be maintained without the consequences of chronic inhibition if used in concert with VEGF inhibition [80]. The concomitant use of a VEGF inhibitor such as bevacizumab and REGN421 results in a strong antitumor effect in xenograft ovarian tumor mouse models and demonstrates that the critical regulatory interaction between VEGF and DLL4 can be disrupted to a clinical benefit [80].

In ovarian cancer, JAG1 has been found to be upregulated in tumor and tumor-associated endothelial cells; silencing JAG1 has also been found to decrease angiogenesis [20, 81–83]. The ligand JAG1, which is predominantly upregulated in ovarian tumors, has been shown to promote angiogenesis by inhibiting the expression of anti-angiogenic VEGFR1/sFLT2. Through the use of Notch decoys that selectively block the signaling activities of DLL4 and JAG1, it was shown that the ligands have opposing effects on ovarian tumor vessel density, but inhibition of either ligand results in decreased vascular perfusion and tumor growth in vitro [32]. In the presence of the JAG1 decoy, increased levels of VEGFR1/sFLT2 and disrupted pericyte coverage reduce angiogenic sprouting and vessel perfusion, quelling tumor growth [32].

6.7 Notch-Based Antitumor Therapy

6.7.1 Gamma Secretase Inhibitors

Gamma secretase inhibitors (GSIs) have been studied in a variety of solid tumors and were at one point regarded as the most promising approach to Notch-based therapy. After ligand binding, the Notch receptor is cleaved by two sets of enzymes, an ADAM metalloprotease and gamma secretase, yielding the intracellular cytoplasmic domain fragment (NICD), which migrates to the nucleus to initiate transcription. GSI could, in principle, block the release of NICD from the plasma membrane and thus suppresses NOTCH signaling (Fig. 6.4). Single agent GSI has been found to induce cell growth inhibition, G_2-M cell-cycle arrest, and apoptosis associated with Notch1 downregulation and its downstream effectors in cell line and animal models of ovarian cancer [84]. However, Phase I studies of single agent GSIs have revealed limited to no antitumor activities [85, 86]. Unfortunately, long-term tolerability of GSIs may also be an impediment to therapy, as the vast majority of patients experience some level of adverse effects [86]. One of the most serious adverse effects is GI toxicity and diarrhea due to goblet cell metaplasia of the small intestine [87].

In ovarian cancer, a recent Phase II study of single agent gamma secretase inhibitor RO4929097 in patients with recurrent platinum-resistant ovarian cancer was largely unsuccessful, with no objective responses to the drug [88]. Combined therapy with a platinum agent, however, may prove more efficacious. Studies from several research groups have indicated that cisplatin and GSI co-therapy has a synergistic cytotoxic effect compared with monotherapies in both platinum-resistant and platinum-sensitive patients [50, 52]. This combination therapy has been shown

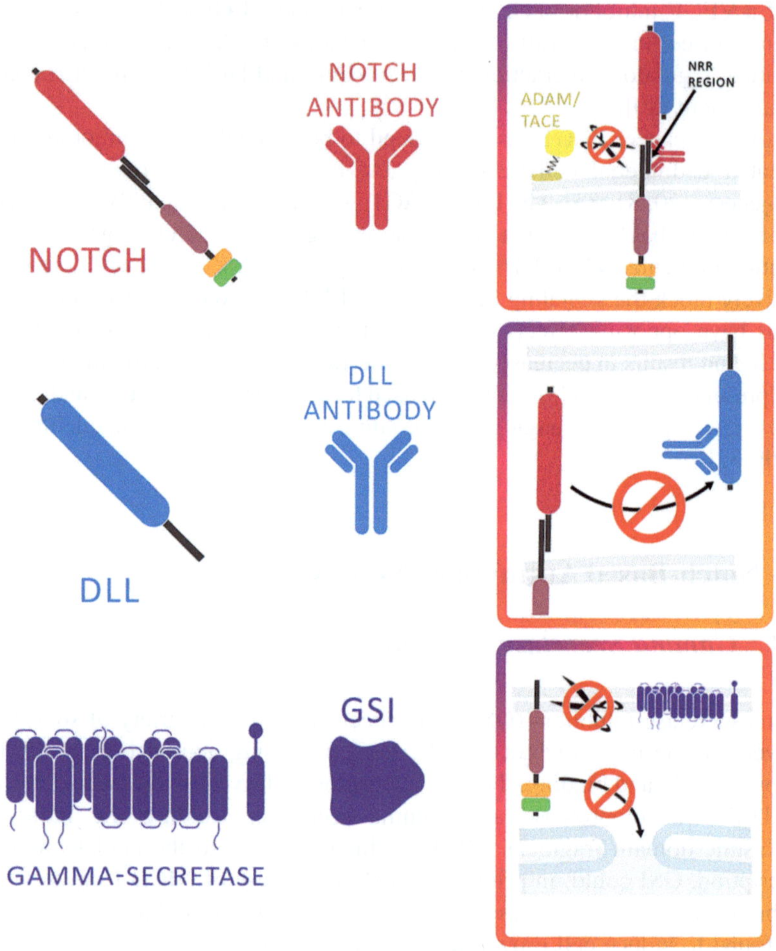

Fig. 6.4 Mechanisms of several Notch therapeutic strategies in ovarian cancer. Therapeutic approaches to treating ovarian cancer via Notch pathway inhibition include anti-Notch3 antibody, anti-DLL4 antibody, and gamma secretase inhibitor (GSI). Anti-Notch3 antibody binds to a negative regulatory (NRR) region, stabilizing it in an "off" state and thereby preventing cleavage by ADAM/TACE. DLL4 antibody binds to DLL4, preventing Notch binding and thus Notch pathway activation. GSIs bind to the gamma secretase protein, preventing the final cleavage step: generation of the Notch intracellular domain (NICD). Notch therefore fails to enter the nucleus

to eliminate both CSCs and bulk tumor cells and to increase the effects of DNA damage, G_2-M cell-cycle arrest, and apoptosis more than monotherapy. This may be because GSI sensitizes cells to cisplatin-induced DNA damage and enhances the rate of tumor cell death. Therefore, to bring GSI into clinics for cancer treatment, future research effort should focus on fine-tuning the dosages of GSI perhaps in combination therapy setting, organ site-specific drug delivery, or nanoparticle-based slow-releasing strategy to limit unwanted toxicity by monotherapy and to enhance cancer-specific targeting efficacy [86].

6.7.2 DLL Antibodies

Delta-like 4, or DLL4, is a dominant Notch ligand in tumor as well as tumor-associated blood vessels. Notch signaling mediated via DLL4 is critical for tumor angiogenesis. Therefore, DLL4 represents a valid target for tumor inhibition (Fig. 6.4). A Phase I trial of DLL4 monoclonal antibody enoticumab developed by Regeneron Pharmaceuticals was launched in year 2016 for patients with advanced solid tumors. Enoticumab treatment has led to response and stable disease in patients with ovarian cancer, not only in those with serous carcinomas but also in those with endometrioid carcinomas [89]. Anti-DLL4 therapy could also be used in combination with VEGF inhibitor, due to interactions detailed in Sect. 6.6 [80]. Progress along this research front remains to be seen. It is worth restating that anti-DLL4 antibodies result in the nonproductive proliferation of poorly differentiated blood vessels [90], which may affect our ability to effectively deliver chemotherapeutic agents through the vasculature. Anti-DLL4 antibodies raise some of the same questions as do GSIs, though there have yet to be serious adverse effects recorded.

Since DLL3 was found to be a dominant ligand in ovarian cancer (Fig. 6.3a), future research should be invested in developing therapeutic grade anti-DLL3 antibody for use in ovarian cancer. Recently, a DLL3-targeted antibody-drug conjugate (ADC) has been developed and evaluated for use in high-grade pulmonary neuroendocrine tumors, such as small cell lung cancer (SCLC) and large cell neuroendocrine carcinoma (LCNEC) [91]. A single course of the ADC SC16LD6.5 (also known as rovalpituzumab tesirine, Rova-T™) was shown to rapidly debulk tumors and lead to progression-free responses in the majority of mice bearing SCLC and LCNEC PDX tumors [91, 92]. The efficacy of this drug was highly correlated with DLL3 expression [91]. DLL3 is thought to differ from other members of the Notch family in that it is localized to the Golgi apparatus [92]. Interestingly, DLL3 is thought to interact with Notch1 and DLL1 during development in the Golgi apparatus, inhibiting them from activating Notch signaling through causing their retention in the Golgi or degradation [91, 93, 94]. Thus, future work is needed to elucidate the function of DLL3 before rationale therapeutics could be designed.

6.7.3 Notch Antibodies

Given the lack of specificity of GSIs and anti-DLL inhibitors and potential serious side effects associated with these pan-Notch inhibitors, the focus in Notch-based therapy has recently shifted to the generation of antibodies that are specific to individual Notch paralogs. A study by Wu et al. developed separate anti-Notch1 and anti-Notch2 antibodies and examined their effects both tumor cell growth and angiogenesis in preclinical T-cell acute lymphoblastic leukemia (T-ALL) models [95]. Analysis of co-crystal structure revealed that the antibodies function through stabilizing the negative regulatory regions (NRRs) of the Notch receptors; without a conformational change in receptor, ADAM protease cleavage cannot take place [95] (see Figs. 6.2 and 6.4.). Although GSI-related inhibition of both Notch1 and Notch2 receptors produces serious intestinal toxicity, targeting either Notch1 or Notch2 through its respective NRR does not produce this unwanted effect [95]. Most importantly, targeting Notch1 potently inhibited tumor growth as well as deregulation of angiogenesis associated with anti-Notch1 antibody. These results suggest that targeting NOTCH3 in a similar fashion could increase the specificity as well as limit the toxicity of Notch therapy in ovarian cancer [35].

Like Notch1 and Notch2, Notch3 also has an NRR region that locks the Notch3 receptor in an "off" state, resulting in resistance to ADAM protease cleavage [95]. A recent study of anti-Notch3 antibodies has found that the extant inhibitory anti-Notch3 antibody antagonizes Notch3 signaling through stabilizing the NRR but that it could not regress tumor xenografts in mice with NOTCH3 signaling [96]. They subsequently found that constructing an antibody-drug conjugate (ADC) by conjugating non-inhibitory or inhibitory anti-Notch3 antibody to an auristatin-based microtubule inhibitor (a type of ADC) resulted in dramatic antitumor activity and tumor regressions in breast, lung, and ovarian preclinical models. They were also able to regress OVCAR3 ovarian high-grade serous xenografts with Notch overexpression and were refractory to platinum drug or to anti-VEGF therapy. An ongoing phase I clinical trial will determine the safety and efficacy of a non-inhibitory anti-NOTCH3 ADC [96].

Recently, an anti-Notch2/anti-Notch3 antibody, OMP-59R5 (tarextumab), has yielded promising antitumorigenic effects in a xenograft study of a variety of solid tumors, including pancreatic, triple-negative breast, small cell lung, and serous ovarian tumors. In the pancreatic and ovarian models, OMP-59R5 significantly downregulated Hes1, Notch2, and Notch3 in the tumors and Hes1, Rgs5, and Notch3 in the stroma. In the pancreatic tumor model, OMP-59R5 significantly reduced CSC frequency. In the breast tumor model, it led to improved vascular stability – which, in contrast to the angiogenic effects of anti-DLL4 antibodies, would improve chemotherapeutic delivery – through downregulation of Rgs5, which regulates tumor pericytes [97]. Overall, OMP-59R5 represents a promising new treatment modality, and future clinical trials will further reveal its efficacy.

6.8 Summary

The Notch pathway is just one facet of the complex molecular landscape of ovarian cancer; however, it is ripe with potential to deepen our understanding of this deadly disease. The link between major receptors, ligands, and downstream proteins has spurred questions as to the Notch pathway's role in the development of chemoresistance as well as angiogenesis, furthering our insight into how carcinomas become viable and lethal. As for clinical applications, progress has mostly remained in its infancy, though recent advances in preclinical and phase I studies have been promising. Overall, Notch signaling constitutes an exciting avenue into the molecular landscape of ovarian cancer, and further offers a potential bevy of novel therapies.

References

1. Ledermann, J. A., Raja, F. A., Fotopoulou, C., et al. (2013). Newly diagnosed and relapsed epithelial ovarian carcinoma: ESMO Clinical Practice Guidelines for diagnosis, treatment and follow-up. *Annals of Oncology, 24*(Suppl 6), vi24–vi32.
2. Kurman, R. J., & Shih, I. (2016). Seromucinous tumors of the ovary. What's in a name? *International Journal of Gynecological Pathology, 35*(1), 78–81.
3. Kurman, R. J., & Shih, I. M. (2010). The origin and pathogenesis of epithelial ovarian cancer: A proposed unifying theory. *The American Journal of Surgical Pathology, 34*, 433–443.
4. Kuo, K. T., Guan, B., Feng, Y., et al. (2009). Analysis of DNA copy number alterations in ovarian serous tumors identifies new molecular genetic changes in low-Grade and high-grade carcinomas. *Cancer Research, 69*, 4036–4042.
5. Cho, K. R. (2009). Ovarian cancer update: Lessons from morphology, molecules, and mice. *Archives of Pathology & Laboratory Medicine, 133*(11), 1775–1781.
6. Cho, K. R., & Shih, I. M. (2009). Ovarian cancer. *Annual Review of Pathology: Mechanisms of Disease, 4*, 287–313.
7. Mok, S. C., Bell, D. A., Knapp, R. C., et al. (1993). Mutation of K-ras protooncogene in human ovarian epithelial tumors of borderline malignancy. *Cancer Research, 53*(7), 1489–1492.
8. Auner, V., Kriegshauser, G., Tong, D., et al. (2009). KRAS mutation analysis in ovarian samples using a high sensitivity biochip assay. *BMC Cancer, 9*, 111.
9. Kuhn, E., Ayhan, A., Shih, I., et al. (2014). The pathogenesis of atypical proliferative Brenner tumor: An immunohistochemical and molecular genetic analysis. *Modern Pathology, 27*(2), 231–237.
10. Ahmed, A. A., Etemadmoghadam, D., Temple, J., et al. (2010). Driver mutations in TP53 are ubiquitous in high grade serous carcinoma of the ovary. *The Journal of Pathology, 221*(1), 49–56.
11. Senturk, E., Cohen, S., Dottino, P. R., et al. (2010). A critical re-appraisal of BRCA1 methylation studies in ovarian cancer. *Gynecologic Oncology, 119*(2), 376–383.
12. Seidman, J. D., & Khedmati, F. (2008). Exploring the histogenesis of ovarian mucinous and transitional cell (Brenner) neoplasms and their relationship with Walthard cell nests: A study of 120 tumors. *Archives of Pathology & Laboratory Medicine, 132*(11), 1753–1760.
13. Skirnisdottir, I., Seidal, T., & Akerud, H. (2015). Differences in clinical and biological features between Type I and Type II tumors in FIGO stages I-II epithelial ovarian carcinoma. *International Journal of Gynecological Cancer, 25*(7), 1239–1247.
14. Rabban, J. T., Garg, K., Crawford, B., et al. (2014). Early detection of high-grade tubal serous carcinoma in women at low risk for hereditary breast and ovarian cancer syndrome by systematic examination of fallopian tubes incidentally removed during benign surgery. *The American Journal of Surgical Pathology, 38*(6), 729–742.
15. Bristow, R. E., Gossett, D. R., Shook, D. R., et al. (2002). Micropapillary serous ovarian carcinoma: Surgical management and clinical outcome. *Gynecologic Oncology, 86*(2), 163–170.
16. Jacobs, I. J., Skates, S. J., MacDonald, N., et al. (1999). Screening for ovarian cancer: A pilot randomised controlled trial. *Lancet, 353*(9160), 1207–1210.
17. Tie, J., Wang, Y., Tomasetti, C., et al. (2016). Circulating tumor DNA analysis detects minimal residual disease and predicts recurrence in patients with stage II colon cancer. *Science Translational Medicine, 8*(346), 346ra92.

18. Park, J. T., Li, M., Nakayama, K., et al. (2006). Notch3 gene amplification in ovarian cancer. *Cancer Research, 66*(12), 6312–6318.
19. Cancer Genome Atlas Research Network. (2011). Integrated genomic analyses of ovarian carcinoma. *Nature, 474*(7353), 609–615.
20. Choi, J. H., Park, J. T., Davidson, B., et al. (2008). Jagged-1 and Notch3 juxtacrine loop regulates ovarian tumor growth and adhesion. *Cancer Research, 68*(14), 5716–5723.
21. Chen, X., Stoeck, A., Lee, S. J., et al. (2010). Jagged1 expression regulated by Notch3 and Wnt/β-catenin signaling pathways in ovarian cancer. *Oncotarget, 1*(3), 210–218.
22. Hu, W., Lu, C., Dong, H. H., et al. (2011). Biological roles of the Delta family Notch ligand Dll4 in tumor and endothelial cells in ovarian cancer. *Cancer Research, 71*(18), 6030–6039.
23. Sanchez-Irizarry, C., Carpenter, A. C., Weng, A. P., et al. (2004). Notch subunit heterodimerization and prevention of ligand-independent proteolytic activation depend, respectively, on a novel domain and the LNR repeats. *Molecular and Cellular Biology, 24*(21), 9265–9273.
24. Beatus, P., Lundkvist, J., Oberg, C., et al. (2001). The origin of the ankyrin repeat region in Notch intracellular domains is critical for regulation of HES promoter activity. *Mechanisms of Development, 104*(1–2), 3–20.
25. Bellavia, D., Checquolo, S., Campese, A. F., et al. (2008). Notch3: From subtle structural differences to functional diversity. *Oncogene, 27*(38), 5092–5098.
26. Artavanis-Tsakonas, S., Rand, M. D., & Lake, R. J. (1999). Notch signaling: Cell fate control and signal integration in development. *Science, 284*(5415), 770–776.
27. Rebay, I., Fleming, R. J., Fehon, R. G., et al. (1991). Specific EGF repeats of Notch mediate interactions with Delta and Serrate: Implications for Notch as a multifunctional receptor. *Cell, 67*(4), 687–699.
28. Hambleton, S., Valeyev, N. V., Muranyi, A., et al. (2004). Structural and functional properties of the human notch-1 ligand binding region. *Structure, 12*(12), 1273–1283.
29. Cordle, J., Johnson, S., Tay, Z., et al. (2008). A conserved face of the Jagged/Serrate DSL domain is involved in Notch trans-activation and cis-inhibition. *Nature Structural & Molecular Biology, 15*(8), 849–857.
30. Henderson, S. T., Gao, D., Christensen, S., et al. (1997). Functional domains of LAG-2, a putative signaling ligand for LIN-12 and GLP-1 receptors in Caenorhabditis elegans. *Molecular Biology of the Cell, 8*(9), 1751–1762.
31. Glittenberg, M., Pitsouli, C., Garvey, C., et al. (2006). Role of conserved intracellular motifs in Serrate signalling, cis-inhibition and endocytosis. *The EMBO Journal, 25*(20), 4697–4706.
32. Kangsamaksin, T., Murtomaki, A., Kofler, N. M., et al. (2015). NOTCH decoys that selectively block DLL/NOTCH or JAG/NOTCH disrupt angiogenesis by unique mechanisms to inhibit tumor growth. *Cancer Discovery, 5*(2), 182–197.
33. Kopan, R., & Ilagan, M. X. (2009). The canonical Notch signaling pathway: Unfolding the activation mechanism. *Cell, 137*(2), 216–233.
34. Mumm, J. S., Schroeter, E. H., Saxena, M. T., et al. (2000). A ligand-induced extracellular cleavage regulates gamma-secretase-like proteolytic activation of Notch1. *Molecular Cell, 5*(2), 197–206.
35. Li, K., Li, Y., Wu, W., et al. (2008). Modulation of Notch signaling by antibodies specific for the extracellular negative regulatory region of NOTCH3. *The Journal of Biological Chemistry, 283*(12), 8046–8054.
36. Andersson, E. R., & Lendahl, U. (2014). Therapeutic modulation of Notch signalling–are we there yet? *Nature Reviews. Drug Discovery, 13*(5), 357–378.
37. Rose, S. L., Kunnimalaiyaan, M., Drenzek, J., et al. (2010). Notch 1 signaling is active in ovarian cancer. *Gynecologic Oncology, 117*(1), 130–133.
38. Hopfer, O., Zwahlen, D., Fey, M. F., et al. (2005). The Notch pathway in ovarian carcinomas and adenomas. *British Journal of Cancer, 93*(6), 709–718.
39. Euer, N. I., Kaul, S., Deissler, H., et al. (2005). Identification of L1CAM, Jagged2 and Neuromedin U as ovarian cancer-associated antigens. *Oncology Reports, 13*(3), 375–387.

40. Jung, J. G., Stoeck, A., Guan, B., et al. (2014). Notch3 interactome analysis identified WWP2 as a negative regulator of Notch3 signaling in ovarian cancer. *PLoS Genetics, 10*(10), e1004751.
41. Castel, D., Mourikis, P., Bartels, S. J., et al. (2013). Dynamic binding of RBPJ is determined by Notch signaling status. *Genes & Development, 27*(9), 1059–1071.
42. Stoeck, A., Lejnine, S., Truong, A., et al. (2014). Discovery of biomarkers predictive of GSI response in triple-negative breast cancer and adenoid cystic carcinoma. *Cancer Discovery, 4*(10), 1154–1167.
43. Chen, X., Thiaville, M. M., Chen, L., et al. (2012). Defining NOTCH3 target genes in ovarian cancer. *Cancer Research, 72*(9), 2294–2303.
44. Palomero, T., Lim, W. K., Odom, D. T., et al. (2006). NOTCH1 directly regulates c-MYC and activates a feed-forward-loop transcriptional network promoting leukemic cell growth. *Proceedings of the National Academy of Sciences of the United States of America, 103*(48), 18261–18266.
45. Wang, H., Zou, J., Zhao, B., et al. (2011). Genome-wide analysis reveals conserved and divergent features of Notch1/RBPJ binding in human and murine T-lymphoblastic leukemia cells. *Proceedings of the National Academy of Sciences of the United States of America, 108*(36), 14908–14913.
46. Radtke, F., & Raj, K. (2003). The role of Notch in tumorigenesis: Oncogene or tumour suppressor? *Nature Reviews. Cancer, 3*(10), 756–767.
47. Leong, K. G., & Karsan, A. (2006). Recent insights into the role of Notch signaling in tumorigenesis. *Blood, 107*(6), 2223–2233.
48. Katoh, M., & Katoh, M. (2007). Integrative genomic analyses on HES/HEY family: Notch-independent HES1, HES3 transcription in undifferentiated ES cells, and Notch-dependent HES1, HES5, HEY1, HEY2, HEYL transcription in fetal tissues, adult tissues, or cancer. *International Journal of Oncology, 31*(2), 461–466.
49. Nakayama, K., Nakayama, N., Jinawath, N., et al. (2007). Amplicon profiles in ovarian serous carcinomas. *International Journal of Cancer, 120*(12), 2613–2617.
50. Park, J. T., Chen, X., Trope, C. G., et al. (2010). Notch3 overexpression is related to the recurrence of ovarian cancer and confers resistance to Carboplatin. *The American Journal of Pathology, 177*(3), 1087–1094.
51. Rahman, R. T., Nakayama, K., Rahman, M., et al. (2012). Notch3 overexpression as potential therapeutic target in advanced stage chemoresistant ovarian cancer. *American Journal of Clinical Pathology, 138*(4), 535–544.
52. McAuliffe, S. M., Morgan, S. L., Wyant, G. A., et al. (2012). Targeting Notch, a key pathway for ovarian cancer stem cells, sensitizes tumors to platinum therapy. *Proceedings of the National Academy of Sciences of the United States of America, 109*(43), E2939–E2948.
53. Zhang, S., Balch, C., Chan, M. W., et al. (2008). Identification and characterization of ovarian cancer-initiating cells from primary human tumors. *Cancer Research, 68*(11), 4311–4320.
54. Vathipadiekal, V., Saxena, D., Mok, S. C., et al. (2012). Identification of a potential ovarian cancer stem cell gene expression profile from advanced stage papillary serous ovarian cancer. *PLoS One, 7*(1), e29079.
55. Krebs, L. T., Xue, Y., Norton, C. R., et al. (2000). Notch signaling is essential for vascular morphogenesis in mice. *Genes & Development, 14*(11), 1343–1352.
56. Xue, Y., Gao, X., Lindsell, C. E., et al. (1999). Embryonic lethality and vascular defects in mice lacking the Notch ligand Jagged1. *Human Molecular Genetics, 8*(5), 723–730.
57. Takeshita, K., Satoh, M., Ii, M., et al. (2007). Critical role of endothelial Notch1 signaling in postnatal angiogenesis. *Circulation Research, 100*(1), 70–78.
58. Domenga, V., Fardoux, P., Lacombe, P., et al. (2004). Notch3 is required for arterial identity and maturation of vascular smooth muscle cells. *Genes & Development, 18*(22), 2730–2735.
59. Joutel, A., Corpechot, C., Ducros, A., et al. (1996). Notch3 mutations in CADASIL, a hereditary adult-onset condition causing stroke and dementia. *Nature, 383*(6602), 707–710.
60. Opherk, C., Duering, M., Peters, N., et al. (2009). CADASIL mutations enhance spontaneous multimerization of NOTCH3. *Human Molecular Genetics, 18*(15), 2761–2767.

61. Thanapprapasr, D., Hu, W., Sood, A. K., et al. (2012). Moving beyond VEGF for anti-angiogenesis strategies in gynecologic cancer. *Current Pharmaceutical Design, 18*(19), 2713–2719.
62. Kang, H., Jeong, J. Y., Song, J. Y., et al. (2016). Notch3-specific inhibition using siRNA knockdown or GSI sensitizes paclitaxel-resistant ovarian cancer cells. *Molecular Carcinogenesis, 55*(7), 1196–1209.
63. Hu, W., Liu, T., Ivan, C., et al. (2014). Notch3 pathway alterations in ovarian cancer. *Cancer Research, 74*(12), 3282–3293.
64. Markman, M., & Bookman, M. A. (2000). Second-line treatment of ovarian cancer. *The Oncologist, 5*(1), 26–35.
65. Koch, U., Lehal, R., & Radtke, F. (2013). Stem cells living with a Notch. *Development, 140*(4), 689–704.
66. Takebe, N., Harris, P. J., Warren, R. Q., et al. (2011). Targeting cancer stem cells by inhibiting Wnt, Notch, and Hedgehog pathways. *Nature Reviews. Clinical Oncology, 8*(2), 97–106.
67. Singh, A., & Settleman, J. (2010). EMT, cancer stem cells and drug resistance: An emerging axis of evil in the war on cancer. *Oncogene, 29*(34), 4741–4751.
68. Tzeng, T. J., Cao, L., Fu, Y., et al. (2014). Methylseleninic acid sensitizes Notch3-activated OVCA429 ovarian cancer cells to carboplatin. *PLoS One, 9*(7), e101664.
69. Burger, R. A., Sill, M. W., Monk, B. J., et al. (2007). Phase II trial of bevacizumab in persistent or recurrent epithelial ovarian cancer or primary peritoneal cancer: A Gynecologic Oncology Group Study. *Journal of Clinical Oncology, 25*(33), 5165–5171.
70. Senger, D. R., Galli, S. J., Dvorak, A. M., et al. (1983). Tumor cells secrete a vascular permeability factor that promotes accumulation of ascites fluid. *Science, 219*(4587), 983–985.
71. Paley, P. J., Staskus, K. A., Gebhard, K., et al. (1997). Vascular endothelial growth factor expression in early stage ovarian carcinoma. *Cancer, 80*(1), 98–106.
72. Yamamato, S., Konishi, I., Mandai, M., et al. (1997). Expression of vascular endothelial growth factor (VEGF) in epithelial ovarian neoplasms: Correlation with clinicopathology and patient survival, and analysis of serum VEGF levels. *British Journal of Cancer, 76*(9), 1221–1227.
73. Hartenbach, E. M., Olson, T. A., Goswitz, J. J., et al. (1997). Vascular endothelial growth factor (VEGF) expression and survival in human epithelial ovarian carcinomas. *Cancer Letters, 121*(2), 169–175.
74. Hu, L., Hofmann, J., Zaloudek, C., et al. (2002). Vascular endothelial growth factor immunoneutralization plus Paclitaxel markedly reduces tumor burden and ascites in athymic mouse model of ovarian cancer. *The American Journal of Pathology, 161*(5), 1917–1924.
75. Holderfield, M. T., & Hughes, C. C. (2008). Crosstalk between vascular endothelial growth factor, notch, and transforming growth factor-beta in vascular morphogenesis. *Circulation Research, 102*(6), 637–652.
76. Kulbe, H., Iorio, F., Chakravarty, P., et al. (2016). Integrated transcriptomic and proteomic analysis identifies protein kinase CK2 as a key signaling node in an inflammatory cytokine network in ovarian cancer cells. *Oncotarget, 7*(13), 15648–15661.
77. Li, J. L., & Harris, A. L. (2009). Crosstalk of VEGF and Notch pathways in tumour angiogenesis: Therapeutic implications. *Frontiers in Bioscience (Landmark Ed), 14*, 3094–3110.
78. Thurston, G., & Kitajewski, J. (2008). VEGF and Delta-Notch: Interacting signalling pathways in tumour angiogenesis. *British Journal of Cancer, 99*(8), 1204–1209.
79. Groeneweg, J. W., Foster, R., Growdon, W. B., et al. (2014). Notch signaling in serous ovarian cancer. *Journal of Ovarian Research, 7*, 95.
80. Kuhnert, F., Chen, G., Coetzee, S., et al. (2015). Dll4 blockade in stromal cells mediates antitumor effects in preclinical models of ovarian cancer. *Cancer Research, 75*(19), 4086–4096.
81. Lu, C., Bonome, T., Li, Y., et al. (2007). Gene alterations identified by expression profiling in tumor-associated endothelial cells from invasive ovarian carcinoma. *Cancer Research, 67*(4), 1757–1768.
82. Jung, S. G., Kwon, Y. D., Song, J. A., et al. (2010). Prognostic significance of Notch 3 gene expression in ovarian serous carcinoma. *Cancer Science, 101*(9), 1977–1983.

83. Shah, M. M., Zerlin, M., Li, B. Y., et al. (2013). The role of Notch and gamma-secretase inhibition in an ovarian cancer model. *Anticancer Research, 33*(3), 801–808.
84. Chen, X., Gong, L., Ou, R., et al. (2016). Sequential combination therapy of ovarian cancer with cisplatin and γ-secretase inhibitor MK-0752. *Gynecologic Oncology, 140*(3), 537–544.
85. Krop, I., Demuth, T., Guthrie, T., et al. (2012). Phase I pharmacologic and pharmacodynamic study of the gamma secretase (Notch) inhibitor MK-0752 in adult patients with advanced solid tumors. *Journal of Clinical Oncology, 30*(19), 2307–2313.
86. Pant, S., Jones, S. F., Kurkjian, C. D., et al. (2016). A first-in-human phase I study of the oral Notch inhibitor, LY900009, in patients with advanced cancer. *European Journal of Cancer, 56*, 1–9.
87. Milano, J., McKay, J., Dagenais, C., et al. (2004). Modulation of notch processing by gamma-secretase inhibitors causes intestinal goblet cell metaplasia and induction of genes known to specify gut secretory lineage differentiation. *Toxicological Sciences, 82*(1), 341–358.
88. Diaz-Padilla, I., Wilson, M. K., Clarke, B. A., et al. (2015). A phase II study of single-agent RO4929097, a gamma-secretase inhibitor of Notch signaling, in patients with recurrent platinum-resistant epithelial ovarian cancer: A study of the Princess Margaret, Chicago and California phase II consortia. *Gynecologic Oncology, 137*(2), 216–222.
89. Chiorean, E. G., LoRusso, P., Strother, R. M., et al. (2015). A phase I first-in-human study of enoticumab (REGN421), a fully human delta-like ligand 4 (Dll4) monoclonal antibody in patients with advanced solid tumors. *Clinical Cancer Research, 21*(12), 2695–2703.
90. Noguera-Troise, I., Daly, C., Papadopolous, N. J., et al. (2006). Blockade of Dll4 inhibits tumour growth by promoting non-productive angiogenesis. *Nature, 444*(7122), 1032–1037.
91. Saunders, L. R., Bankovich, A. J., Anderson, W. C., et al. (2015). A DLL3-targeted antibody-drug conjugate eradicates high-grade pulmonary neuroendocrine tumor-initiating cells in vivo. *Science Translational Medicine, 7*(302), 302ra136.
92. Dylla, S. J. (2016). Toppling high-grade pulmonary neuroendocrine tumors with a DLL3-targeted trojan horse. *Molecular and Cellular Oncology, 3*(2), e1101515.
93. Chapman, G., Sparrow, D. B., Kremmer, E., et al. (2011). Notch inhibition by the ligand DELTA-LIKE 3 defines the mechanism of abnormal vertebral segmentation in spondylocostal dysostosis. *Human Molecular Genetics, 20*(5), 905–916.
94. Serth, K., Schuster-Gossler, K., Kremmer, E., et al. (2015). O-fucosylation of DLL3 is required for its function during somitogenesis. *PLoS One, 10*(4), e0123776.
95. Wu, Y., Cain-Hom, C., Choy, L., et al. (2010). Therapeutic antibody targeting of individual Notch receptors. *Nature, 464*(7291), 1052–1057.
96. Geles, K. G., Gao, Y., Sridharan, L., et al. (2015). Abstract 1697: Therapeutic targeting the NOTCH3 receptor with antibody drug conjugates. *Cancer Research, 75*(15), 1697.
97. Yen, W. C., Fischer, M. M., Axelrod, F., et al. (2015). Targeting Notch signaling with a Notch2/Notch3 antagonist (tarextumab) inhibits tumor growth and decreases tumor-initiating cell frequency. *Clinical Cancer Research, 21*(9), 2084–2095.

Chapter 7
Notch Signaling in Graft-Versus-Host Disease

Lisa M. Minter

Abstract Graft-versus-host disease (GVHD) refers to a constellation of adverse immune responses resulting in tissue destruction following hematopoietic stem cell or solid organ transplantation. Through a complex network of priming and activation events, immune-competent T cells residing in the transplanted tissue (the graft) become stimulated, migrate into target organs, and mediate immune destruction of the recipient's healthy tissue (the host). Paradoxically, this immune activation can also eradicate residual leukemic cells, when hematopoietic stem cell transplantation occurs in the context of hematological malignancies, resulting in a beneficial graft-versus-leukemia (GVL) effect. The Notch family of transmembrane receptors functions in many aspects of immune responses, including those that mediate GVHD. Here we will review the complex nature of GVHD and how Notch signaling may play a prominent role during the initiation and progression of the disease.

Keywords Notch · Graft-versus-host disease · GVHD · Graft-versus-leukemia · GVL · Immune destruction · Hematopoietic stem cell transplantation · Dll4 · M1 macrophages · Chemokine receptors · Toll-like receptors

7.1 Overview of Notch Signaling

Signaling mediated by Notch receptors is essential to many varied cell processes. Excellent reviews discuss Notch signaling in embryonic tissue and organ development [108], fetal hematopoiesis [13, 104], intestinal cell homeostasis [25], T cell maturation in the thymus [53, 61], and the regulation of numerous immune responses in the periphery [6, 8, 30, 80, 88]. As depicted in Fig. 7.1, in mammals the Notch family of signaling proteins is comprised of four transmembrane receptors (Notch1–4) and five signal-initiating ligands that belong to two distinct groups: Jagged ligands (Jag1,2) and Delta-like ligands (Dll1,3,4). Notch receptors undergo a series

L. M. Minter (✉)
Department of Veterinary and Animal Sciences, University of Massachusetts Amherst, Amherst, MA, USA
e-mail: lminter@vasci.umass.edu

L. Miele, S. Artavanis-Tsakonas (eds.), *Targeting Notch in Cancer*,
https://doi.org/10.1007/978-1-4939-8859-4_7

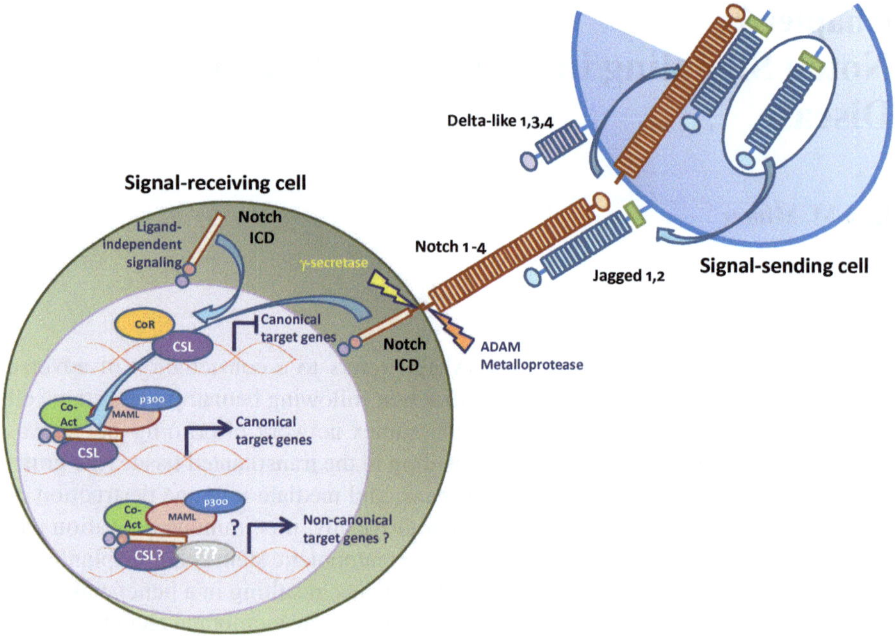

Fig. 7.1 Overview of Notch signaling. Ligand-mediated Notch signaling is initiated when a ligand of the Delta-like (Dll 1,3,4) or Jagged (Jag 1,2) family, present on the surface of a nearby signal-sending cell, binds to a Notch receptor expressed on a signal-receiving cell. Following cleavage of the extracellular domain of Notch by an ADAM protease, the Notch extracellular domain is transendocytosed by the signal-sending cell, together with the bound Notch ligand. Notch ligands can be recycled and re-expressed on the surface of the signal-sending cell. In the signal-receiving cell, following processing by ADAM protease, transmembrane-tethered Notch is cleaved just proximal to the cell membrane to release intracellular domain (ICD) of Notch, which is transcriptionally active. Notch ICD associates with its canonical DNA-binding partner, CSL, which itself resides on DNA in repressor complexes that prohibit transcription of canonical gene targets. Upon association with CSL, additional coactivators including mastermind-like (MAML) and p300 are recruited to the NotchICD-CSL complex, activating its transcriptional capabilities. Transcription of some Notch-regulated genes can proceed in the absence of CSL and is referred to as noncanonical Notch signaling

of posttranslational events that ultimately result in a mature, non-covalently linked heterodimer that is inserted in the plasma membrane of the signal-receiving cell [31]. Upon engaging a cognate ligand, often displayed on the surface of nearby signal-sending cells, Notch receptors undergo conformational change that allows membrane proximal cleavage at the S2 site by ADAM proteases [24]. The extracellular domain of Notch receptors is transendocytosed by the signal-sending cell, through a process that initiates signaling within the ligand-bearing cell [98]. Removal of the extracellular domain leaves only a short transmembrane "stub" protruding from the cell surface, generating a structural substrate for the enzymatic actions of gamma secretase. Gamma secretase, a multiprotein complex comprised of presenilins 1 and 2, APH, and nicastrin, cleaves Notch receptors at the S3 site, liberating an active, intracellular form of Notch (NIC), capable of translocating to the nucleus to regulate downstream targets [27]. Within the context of canonical signaling, NIC is recruited to preformed, DNA-bound complexes containing its canonical nuclear binding partner CSL/RBPj. Notch binding to CSL/RBPj displaces transcriptional repressors, which are subsequently replaced by transcriptional activators, and allows for gene transcription [56]. In addition to canonical signaling, noncanonical signaling (i.e., CSL/RBPj-independent) and ligand-independent signaling have also been described [10, 73, 78, 135].

7.2 Pathophysiology of GVHD

Hematopoietic stem cell transfer (HSCT) provides the means for full hematopoietic reconstitution following myeloablative therapy commonly used to treat hematologic malignancies, solid tumors, or certain immune-mediated bone marrow failure diseases, such as aplastic anemia [26, 99, 118]. Graft-versus-host disease (GVHD) refers to a constellation of adverse sequelae following HSCT, whereby immunocompetent cells present in the stem cell graft are activated and damage host tissues [109]. Studies suggest GVHD can affect greater than 40% of patients following HSCT, and, as such, it remains a significant barrier to the broader use of HSCT in the clinic. GVHD is classified as acute or chronic, based on how soon after HSCT symptoms appear. Symptoms presenting within the first 100 days post-HSCT are attributed to acute GVHD, while those occurring later than 100 days constitute chronic GVHD. Preventing acute GVHD is thought to decrease the likelihood of chronic GVHD, which also appears to have autoimmune underpinnings.

In cases of hematologic malignancy or transplant in the setting of solid tumors, conventional conditioning in preparation of HSCT is intended to reduce tumor burden and neutralize host immune responses, so as to prevent HSC rejection [67]. However, pre-transplant conditioning can also create the environment for host tissue to be targeted by HSCT-derived T cells, resulting in GVHD [121]. The pathophysiology of GVHD can be divided into three stages that represent a continuum of disease (Fig. 7.2). During the initiation phase, conditioning regimens cause the release of endogenous bacterial lipopolysaccharides (LPS) and damage host cells, resulting in inflammatory cytokine release [43]. The second, inductive phase begins when host, and possibly donor, antigen-presenting cells (APCs) are activated in response to potent LPS stimulation in the presence of pro-inflammatory cytokines, which serves to enhance their ability to present alloantigens to donor CD4 and CD8 T cells [41]. This stage progresses into the effector phase as immunocompetent T cells, resident within the stem cell graft, proliferate and differentiate after encountering major or minor histocompatibility antigens that are mismatched between donor and host. Tissue destruction is mediated during the effector phase of GVHD, which manifests when distinct subsets of differentiated T cells, directed by the chemokine receptors they express, infiltrate and damage specific host tissues [57].

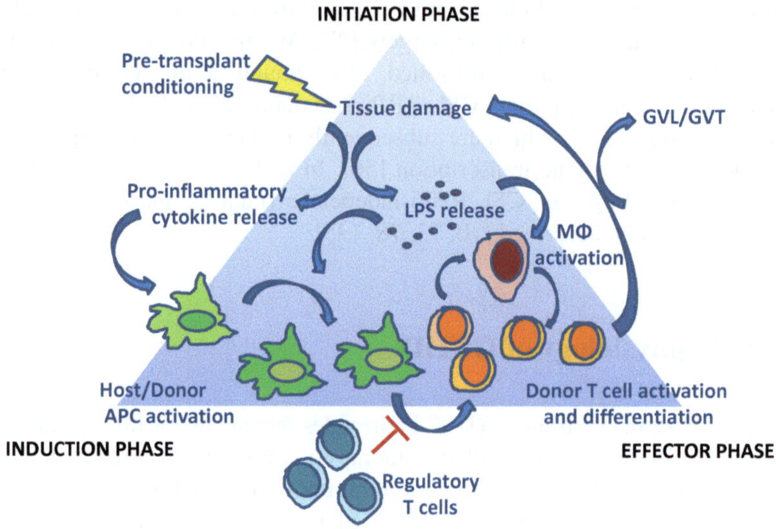

Fig. 7.2 Stages of graft-versus-host disease. Graft-versus-host disease (GVHD) is initiated as the result of host conditioning regimens, especially those that involve total body irradiation, prior to hematopoietic stem cell transplantation. Tissue damaged by pre-transplant conditioning causes the release of lipopolysaccharide (LPS) from gut bacteria, together with induction of pro-inflammatory cytokine secretion. Host/donor antigen-presenting cells (APC) and host macrophages (MΦ) are activated and primed to present alloantigen to donor T cells. Activated, differentiated donor T cells increase expression of pro-inflammatory cytokines and chemokine receptors, migrate to target tissues, and mediate tissue destruction. Regulatory T cells may negatively regulate T cell activation and differentiation, minimizing GVHD pathology

Organ involvement in GVHD can vary and may be linked to the intensity of the conditioning regimen [72, 95]. The major organs targeted for immune attack include the gut, liver, skin, and lungs. Increasingly, evidence suggests distinct populations of T helper (Th) cells mediate organ-specific destruction, likely as a combined result of the cytokines they produce together with the repertoire of chemokine receptors they express [39, 60]. To this end, Th type 1 cells (Th1) appear to be important in GVHD affecting the gut and liver, although these cells are thought to mediate, to some degree, immune attack against all of these tissues. Th2 and Th17 cells exacerbate immune-mediated damage to the skin and lungs, but Th2 cells also can contribute substantially to gut GVHD [131]. Chemokine-directed migration of Th cells has also been implicated in organ-specific trafficking. CCR9 and CCR5 are important in migration to the gut [7, 100]. CCR6 mediates targeting to the skin, while CXCR3 is critical for GVHD of the liver, gut, and skin [40, 120]. Finally, CCR2, CCR4, and CCR6 all can contribute to Th cell trafficking to the lungs [131].

For patients undergoing HSCT following myeloablative therapy for hematologic malignancies, such as leukemia or lymphoma, the allo-specific responses that result in GVHD can also provide a benefit to HSCT recipients through an immune attack directed against residual leukemic cells. This "graft-versus-leukemia" (GVL) or "graft-versus-tumor" (GVT) effect is neither well understood nor well defined, but studies do suggest it can be separated from the detrimental GVHD responses commonly observed [55, 64, 65, 133]. To preserve GVL/GVT, while selectively abrogating GVHD, is the ultimate therapeutic goal of researchers in this field.

This review will focus on the various stages of GVHD initiation and progression: activation of APCs, differentiation of the major Th subsets and secretion of their signature cytokines, as well as expression of chemokine receptors that direct tissue-specific infiltration, and how Notch signaling may be implicated in each of these.

7.3 Notch Receptors and Ligands During the Initiation and Induction Phase of GVHD

Acute GVHD occurs within 100 days in the post-transplant period and culminates in extensive tissue destruction characterized by apoptosis. Its development is absolutely dependent on the presence and function of alloreactive T cells in the donor inoculum and is closely tied to the curative GVT/GVL effect [64, 65]. However, following HSCT, tissue injury and inflammation, defined by pro-inflammatory cytokine release, are initiated by the conditioning regimen. Both the severity and the incidence of GVHD following HSCT have been associated with the intensity of the conditioning regimen, especially when total body irradiation (TBI) is included [42]. During the initiation phase of GVHD, pro-inflammatory cytokines, together with lipopolysaccharide (LPS), released as a result of conditioning-induced gut damage, converge to craft the inflammatory environment. Subsequent activation of host antigen-presenting cells (APC), including conventional dendritic cells (cDC) and macrophages, occurs during the inductive phase.

The requirement for host APCs to induce GVHD is complicated and controversial. While host APCs may not be required for GVHD to ensue [63], host DCs are sufficient to activate donor T cells [28, 64, 65] and initiate GVHD [58]. Toll receptor 4 (TLR4) is a major pattern recognition receptor capable of responding to LPS, and TLR4 expression on host cDCs exacerbates GVHD [16, 137]. Furthermore, cDC exposure to LPS also enhances expression of the Notch ligand Delta-like 4 (Dll4), likely through a TLR4-mediated process (Fig. 7.3 (1); [68, 111]). Seminal work by Flavell's group suggested engagement of specific Notch ligands can influence T helper cell differentiation, with ligands of the Delta-like family (Dll1,3,4) promoting T helper type 1 responses and those of the Jagged family (Jag1,2) facilitating T helper type 2 differentiation [3]. In the context of GVHD, Dll4 expression on host cDCs has been shown to drive allogeneic T cell responses, including increased production of IFNγ and IL-17, both in vitro and in vivo (Fig. 7.3 (2); [75, 81, 85]).This study coincided with elegant work by Maillard's group showing that administering antibodies specific for Dll1 and Dll4 in a mouse model of GVHD, early after induction, provided durable protection against disease pathology without significantly sacrificing the beneficial effects of GVL/GVT [114]. These studies not only highlight the contribution of Notch signaling to the induction of GVHD during the very

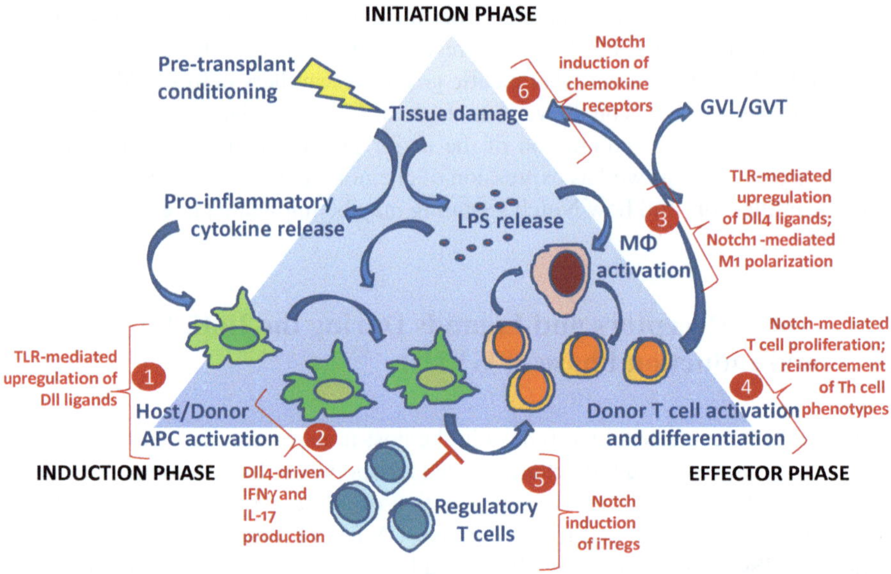

Fig. 7.3 Potential for Notch involvement in graft-versus-host disease. Notch signaling may mediate numerous aspects of GVHD. (1) Toll receptor (TLR) signaling in response to lipopolysaccharide (LPS) release following pre-transplant conditioning upregulates Dll ligands on host/donor APCs; (2) Dll4 expression on donor dendritic cells increases IFNγ and IL-17 secretion by Th1 and Th17 cells, respectively; (3) Notch1 upregulation in activated macrophages (MΦ) promotes a pro-inflammatory "M1" phenotype; (4) Notch receptors play an important role in reinforcing differentiated phenotypes of T helper (Th) CD4 cells, including Th1, Th2, and Th17 cells. (5) Notch signaling may play an important role in the development of induced regulatory T cells (iTregs); (6) Notch signaling may regulate chemokine receptor expression to direct T cell trafficking to GVHD target organs. Please refer to the text for expanded description of Notch signaling at each of these potential stages of GVHD induction and progression

early priming stages, their results suggest that inhibiting the signaling capacity of specific Notch ligands represents a viable therapeutic strategy to prevent GVHD.

The contribution of macrophages, both of host and donor origin, appears to be equally complex, especially in terms of Notch signaling. Macrophages can be polarized toward "M1" or "M2" phenotypes, and a critical involvement of Notch in this process has been described [110, 122, 129]. TLR4 signaling in macrophages increases Notch1 expression which, in turn, promotes their differentiation into pro-inflammatory M1 cells, through interaction with its canonical DNA-binding partner, CSL/RbpJ [45, 128]. Some reports show M1 macrophages exhibit increased capacity for antigen presentation, as well as increased secretion of pro-inflammatory TNF, IL-6, IL-12, and IFNγ, all through Notch1-mediated signaling cascades (Fig. 7.3 (3); [15, 82, 124, 125]). In a model of atherosclerosis, macrophage exposure to LPS was also shown to increase Dll4 expression via TLR4 signaling and promoted an M1 phenotype [34]. Thus, it is attractive to speculate that the Dll4-specific antibodies used in Maillard's studies may target M1 macrophages, as well as effectively targeting Dll4+ cDCs, although additional studies are needed to confirm this. Nonetheless, M1 macrophages can accumulate in the skin to mediate cutaneous GVHD, where the number of infiltrating M1 macrophages is directly correlated with the severity of skin pathology [86], and reducing M1 differentiation post-HSCT transfer using dexamethasone palmitate can also mitigate acute damage to the skin [87], although its effects on Notch receptors and ligands were not evaluated.

The expansion and activity of host-derived M2 macrophages can also provide protection against GVHD-mediated tissue destruction, and inhibiting Notch1 signaling in macrophages can induce an M2 cell fate [110]. CSF-1 promotes the M2 phenotype in macrophages, with reduced secretion of pro-inflammatory cytokines, suggesting an increase in M2 macrophages may provide protection from GVHD. This hypothesis was supported in a mouse model by administering CSF-1 prior to GVHD induction. CSF-1 greatly expanded the host M2 macrophage pool, decreased the expansion of donor T cells, and reduced the severity of acute GVHD [38]. Conversely, donor-derived macrophages appear to require CSF-1 to mediate chronic GVHD, since depleting macrophages using an antibody directed against the CSF-1 receptor or transferring macrophages from *csf1* deficient donors resulted in markedly reduced skin and lung GVHD, due to decreased IL-17 production [2].

Collectively, these data suggest that lingering, donor-derived M2 macrophages may contribute to tissue destruction characteristic of chronic GVHD. These confounding data underscore the complexity of temporal GVHD pathology, the diversity of cell types involved, and the potentially conflicting contributions of Notch signaling in acute vs chronic GVHD. Additional studies that specifically address Notch signaling in chronic GVHD will be imperative to clarify these discrepancies.

7.4 Notch, T Helper Cells, and the Effector Phase of GVHD

As the continuum of acute GVHD progresses into the effector phase, activated APCs are now suited to prime immunocompetent donor T cells to differentiate into various T helper (Th) subsets and expand effector CD8 T (Teff) cells. CD4 Th cells, along with CD8 cytolytic T cells (CTL), will infiltrate target organs to mediate tissue damage (Fig. 7.3 (4)).

In response to antigen stimulation, mature T cells integrate myriad external signals derived from the T cell receptor, co-stimulation, and cytokines present in the microenvironment to initiate the genetic programming that will result in their full activation, expansion, and subsequent differentiation [107]. Th type 1 (Th1), Th2, Th17, Th9, and Th22 cells have all been described based on the unique combinations of cytokines that drive their differentiation, the master transcription factor they upregulate, and the signature profile of cytokines they produce. Accumulating evidence suggests that individual Notch receptors and ligands critically influence

Th cell differentiation, both in healthy and aberrant immune responses, including in those that mediate GVHD [130].

Notch signaling in donor CD4 and CD8 T cells augments their activation and expansion and regulates expression of CD25, the high-affinity subunit of the IL-2 receptor [1, 92], supporting the notion that Notch signaling likely acts as a signal amplifier [29]. Engagement of Notch receptors on T helper cells by cognate ligands expressed on APCs was initially thought to instruct T helper cell differentiation: exposure to Dll family ligands promoted a Th1 phenotype, while binding to Jag family ligands directed a Th2 cell fate [3]. A closer examination of the conditions under which T helper cells adopt a specific, differentiated state now supports the notion that Notch signaling provides an unbiased amplification signal to helper T cells, allowing them to proliferate and reinforce a T helper phenotype (i.e., cytokine secretion) acquired as a result of response to the extracellular cytokine milieu [11, 90]. This perspective helps to reconcile the pleiotropic requirements for Notch activation in Th1, Th2, Th17, and induced regulatory T cell (iTreg) differentiation, with different ligands augmenting, rather than inducing Th signature cytokine secretion. Furthermore, redundant functions for some Notch receptors have been described, suggesting strategies aiming to target specific Notch receptors in the management of GVHD may prove ineffective [9].

7.5 Th1 Cells in GVHD

GVHD that manifests in the gut and liver is driven by a strong Th1 response [93] although IFNγ, a signature Th1 cytokine, appears to contribute to tissue damage in nearly all organs affected by GVHD. T cells that adopt a Th1 cell fate exhibit increased and sustained expression of the master transcriptional regulator, T-bet. Th1 cells secrete IFNγ which, together with IL-12, serves to reinforce the Th1 phenotype. First described by Szabo et al. in 2000, T-bet is a T cell-specific transcription factor that is absolutely required for Th1 differentiation [112]. In GVHD, T-bet is also an important determinant of disease pathology. GVHD induction using T-bet-deficient T cells resulted in significantly reduced tissue damage in the gut and liver, compared to disease induction using wild-type or IFNγ-deficient T cells, and regardless of whether the model used was mismatched for major or minor histocompatibility antigens [33]. In this study, although loss of T-bet enhanced Th17 cell differentiation, the Th17 cells were less effective at inducing GVHD. Of note, GVL/GVT effects were also compromised but could be restored following neutralization of IL-17 in hosts. By contrast, selectively inhibiting Th17 development with low-dose halofuginone in a mouse model of GVHD exacerbated Th1-mediated pathology in the liver and gut, although pulmonary GVHD was attenuated with reduced Th17 differentiation [22, 23, 93]. Moreover, in a prospective study of patients with cutaneous GVHD, an increased number of IFNγ-producing Th1, but not Th17, cells were found in skin lesions of patients with acute GVHD, compared to those without GVHD, suggesting that Th1 cells can also mediate skin-associated tissue damage [17].

The gene encoding T-bet, *Tbx21*, is a direct transcriptional target of Notch1, and inhibiting Notch signaling greatly impairs both the differentiation of Th1 cells and the production of pro-inflammatory cytokines [77, 92, 101]. Canonical Notch signaling in T cells can be compromised when a dominant negative form of a key transcriptional coactivator mastermind-like (DNMAML) is expressed [70]. In the context of GVHD, inducing disease by transferring DNMAML T cells from C57BL/6 donor mice into Balb/c recipients attenuates disease pathology and impairs IFNγ secretion, although T-bet expression remained intact [105, 136]. However, a subsequent report demonstrated that T-bet expression was independent of CSL/Rbpj signaling and, rather, was regulated via a noncanonical signaling pathway [29]. In light of these combined studies, it is likely Notch signaling contributes significantly to Th1-mediated pathology in GVHD, through its regulation of canonical and noncanonical transcriptional targets.

7.6 Th17 Cells in GVHD

Th17 cells are an additional subset of differentiated T cells capable of migrating into the gut, lung, and skin tissues where they can mediate tissue destruction [74, 133]. Th17 cells require RORγt for their terminal differentiation, and this process is facilitated by the presence of IL-6 and TGFβ [51, 71]. Plasticity between Th1 and Th17 phenotypes has been demonstrated, suggesting that within the appropriate constellation of signaling modifiers, especially those conveyed by the cytokine milieu, Th1 cells can adopt features of Th17 cells and vice versa [18, 37, 69]. Within the complex progression of GVHD, it has been shown that even when the Th1-predominant, IFNγ, and the Th17-signature, IL-17, cytokines are present, the kinetics of their accumulation in target tissues differ. In an MHC minor antigen-mismatched model of GVHD, IFNγ secretion by CD4 and CD8 T cells preceded IL-17 production in the liver and lung, as well as in the spleen and mesenteric lymph nodes. This finding suggests that, in this model of GVHD, Th1 cell differentiation occurred prior to that of Th17 cells [49]. A recent study using a mouse model of colitis suggests that, in the presence of TGFβ, Th1 cells can be converted to IFNγ+IL-17+ CD4 T cells, which exacerbate gut pathology [37]. Whether or not a similar conversion can or does occur in the context of gut GVHD remains to be examined. Th1 and Th17 cells share a common cytokine subunit: the IL-12/IL23 p40 subunit. Each of these cytokines contributes to stabilizing their respective associated Th phenotype: IL-12 will reinforce Th1 polarization, while IL-23 increases Th17 cell fate stability. Although neutralization of the common p40 subunit can attenuate GVHD in a mouse model [126], it is not known, definitively, if signaling through this common subunit influences the interconversion of these Th cell subsets in response to the complex array of cytokines in the microenvironment.

Overall, the question of how extensively Th17 cells contribute to GVHD pathology remains unanswered [47, 119]. It is clear that Th17 cells can be found in target tissues during GVHD progression, and disease severity can be attenuated when T cells lacking RORγt are used in a model of CD4 T cell-mediated GVHD. The resulting decreased levels of TNFα in the gut, liver, and lung were thought to be significant factors in the reduced pathology noted [138]. Interestingly, in a model of spontaneous type I diabetes, TNFα could be induced in a Th17-dependent manner [62, 66]. Whether or not differentiated Th17 cells act to sustain TNFα secretion produced during the induction and/or initiation phases of GVHD will require further investigation. In a separate report, in vitro-generated Th17 cells were found to be sufficient but not required to induce GVHD, and their presence also correlated with higher levels of TNFα [47]. However, RORγt-deficient CD4 T cells were also capable of inducing lethal GVHD in this model, suggesting that, although Th17 cells may contribute significantly to GVHD progression, additional subsets of Th cells also are critically important.

One important observation of the study by Iclozan et al. was that Th17 cells showed extensive expansion, in vivo, and were highly resistant to activation-induced cell death (AICD). Additional work has demonstrated that human Th17 cells constitute a long-lived memory T cell population [59]. Under various pathological conditions, these cells were shown to be highly proliferative, in vivo, resistant to AICD, and preserved their ability to further differentiate into functional Th1 and iTreg cells, although they retained their capacity for IL-17 secretion. Notably, survival of these human Th17 cells was attributed to a Notch-dependent pathway, downstream of HIF1α, since overexpression of NICD could rescue a significant percentage of Th17 cells from the apoptosis induced when HIFα signaling was blocked. These data add to our understanding of Notch signaling in Th17 cell differentiation. Dll4-Notch signaling between DCs and T cells, in the presence of the Th17-polarizing cytokines, IL-6 and TGFβ, resulted in higher percentages of Th17 cells than those polarized under identical conditions in the absence of Notch signaling [85]. Although not expressly examined in their studies, it is also possible that the robust protection from GVHD induction observed by Maillard's group during Dll4-blockade may include reduced differentiation of Th17 cells and the concomitant benefit that provides.

7.7 Th2 Cells in GVHD

A detailed study conducted by Zeng's group would suggest that some of the complexities of GVHD may be attributed to cross-regulation among Th cell subsets which, in turn, influences the severity and organ specificity of the associated pathology [131]. Using a major MHC antigen-mismatched model of GVHD (C57BL/6 donor into Balb/c recipient), they showed that transplanting IFNγ-deficient T cells augmented both Th17- and Th2-mediated tissue destruction in the lung and skin. By contrast, inducing GVHD using T cells that were doubly deficient for IFNγ and

IL-17 led to a massive upregulation and infiltration of Th2 cells into the lungs, resulting in idiopathic pneumonia syndrome (IPS). Thirteen days after GVHD induction, there was a nearly 16-fold increase in the number of CD4 Th2 cells in the lungs of mice that received doubly deficient T cells, compared to mice whose disease was induced using wild-type CD4 T cells. Mice that received IFNγ-only deficient cells had a nearly tenfold increase in Th2 and Th17 cells in the lung, compared to mice receiving wild-type T cells. This study further showed that induction of the immune-modulating ligand, B7-H1, in host lung epithelium required IFNγ for its upregulation, and absence of its expression was a compounding factor leading to IPS. In a complementary study by Yu et al. [133] that employed the same model of GVHD, transferring donor T cells that were doubly deficient for the transcription factors, T-bet and RORγt, resulted in overall decreased pathology in the gut, liver, and lung; however, significant increases in IL-4 and IL-5 expression 5 days after GVHD induction were also noted in the lungs of recipient animals [133]. These conclusions were further supported using a model of LPS inhalation-induced acute pulmonary GVHD in the context of HSCT. Transferring T-bet-deficient T cells in this model resulted in more severe lung pathology and pulmonary fibrosis, together with increased IL-13, IL-17, and Th17 cells, suggesting that, in the absence of cross regulation by IFNγ, Th17 cells can contribute significantly to lung GVHD [35].

As with other Th subsets, a role for Notch signaling in Th2 cell differentiation has also been described [4]. Using a model of *Trichuris muris* infection, Pear's group demonstrated a requirement for canonical, MAML-mediated Notch signaling to generate the protective, in vivo Th2 response necessary to clear the parasitic infection [115].

Furthermore, while TCF and β-catenin, components of the Wnt signaling pathway, initiate early, IL-4-independent GATA3 expression via their binding to the *Gata3*-1b enhancer, it would appear that Notch binding to the *Gata3*-1a enhancer leads to sustained Th2 cell differentiation by providing synergistic upregulation of IL-4 [32, 132]. Thus, as with the other Th cell subsets discussed, and which are critically important in mediating GVHD, Notch is also an important regulator of Th2 cell differentiation [5].

7.8 Regulatory T Cells in GVHD

In addition to Th cells, distinct subsets of immunosuppressive regulatory T (Treg) cells also have been identified, including naturally occurring (nTreg) and inducible (iTreg) regulatory T cells that can express either CD4 or CD8 [69, 83, 106]. To date, Tregs exhibiting a CD4+ CD25+FoxP3+ phenotype are perhaps the most well-studied. However, unlike their Th and Teff cell counterparts which drive GVHD pathology, Treg cells have been shown to attenuate the severity of acute GVHD, mitigate the extent of tissue involvement, and prevent chronic GVHD altogether [76, 116].

Naïve T cells will adopt a Treg phenotype when they differentiate in the presence of TGFβ and IL-2 and are characterized by increased expression of the master transcriptional regulator FoxP3. In vivo, the Treg phenotype is considered to be unstable, with reports of interconversion of Tregs to effector T cells in the presence of high levels of inflammatory cytokines, especially IL-6 and IL-17 [54, 127].

Extensive and impressive progress has been made in defining the protective effects of Tregs and their mechanisms of action, both in murine and human studies. Functional Treg suppression has been reported to be faulty in patients with acute GVHD [14]. This may be due to the observed lower surface expression of CCR5 and CXCR3 on donor Tregs, resulting in impaired trafficking to target organs [117]. Studies also suggest that donor-derived, or third-party, Tregs provide far more potent immunosuppression than host Tregs when used as an immunotherapy [94]. Human trials using ex vivo-expanded nTregs as a potential prophylaxis for GVHD were recently concluded [19].

The encouraging results showed that, when administered at the time of HSCT, only 9% of patients who received expanded Tregs exhibited grade II–IV acute GVHD at 100 days post-transplant, compared to a control cohort in which 45% showed symptoms of GVHD, grade II or higher.

Patients in both cohorts received identical conditioning regimens prior to HSCT. Furthermore, while approximately 14% of the non-Treg-treated patients showed signs of chronic GVHD at 1 year post-HSCT, none of the patients who received the ex vivo-expanded Tregs exhibited chronic GVHD. The impressive results of this trial may be due to the co-administration of Tregs at the time of HSC transfer. In complementary studies, Negrin's group utilized a minor antigen MHC-mismatched model to show that the immunosuppressive capacity of transferred Tregs, both donor-derived and third party, is most effective early after their transplantation and suggests that the timing of administering Tregs is a critical factor to be considered [97]. A small study using donor-derived or third-party expanded Tregs in the treatment of established cases of chronic and acute GVHD were less positive [113], lending support to Negrin's findings.

There is a preponderance of evidence supporting a positive role for Notch signaling in iTreg differentiation and which further support the influence of specific Notch ligands in this process (Fig. 7.3 (5)). Notch signaling may generate Tregs through both direct and indirect mechanisms. In an early report, APCs engineered to overexpress Jag1 (serrate1) could induce a regulatory phenotype in co-cultured CD4 T cells, and these cells maintained antigen-specific suppressive activity when transferred into naïve hosts prior to immune challenge [44]. Two subsequent studies revealed Notch1 and TGFβ can cooperate to induce FoxP3 expression, and this process may involve canonical Notch signaling via CSL/Rbpj binding to the *FOXP3* promoter [89, 91, 103]. Notch3 has also been implicated in *Foxp3* transcription during nTreg generation, and this has been shown to proceed through an NF-κB-dependent pathway [12, 20]. Furthermore, it was demonstrated that human memory CD4 T cells could adopt a Treg phenotype, including expression of FoxP3 and upregulation of TGFβ, when exposed to Dll1 during in vitro culture [84].

Indirect involvement of Notch signaling in Treg-mediated immunosuppression has also been demonstrated. Co-incubating CD4+CD25- T cells with Dll4 or Jag1 increased their responsiveness to Treg-mediated suppression by upregulating

TGFβRII expression [46]. Additionally, Notch signaling is also important for production of the immunosuppressive cytokine, IL-10, in T cells, and this is enhanced when CD4 T cells are co-cultured with Dll4-expressing plasmacytoid DCs [50, 102]. Elegant work by Sarin's group showed that differential localization of Notch1 mediated Treg survival through a membrane-associated NICD/Rictor complex, which was stabilized by interactions with Dll1. This protection was lost when NICD was targeted to the nucleus [96]. Recent work, however, challenges the notion that Notch signaling positively regulates Treg induction [21]. The results of this study showed that when NICD was overexpressed in FoxP3+ Tregs, the Treg phenotype was destabilized, resulting in an autoimmune lymphoproliferative manifestation. Canonical Notch signaling mediated this phenomenon, since loss of *Rbpj* restored the number and frequency of Tregs and protected them from apoptosis in a model of GVHD generated by major histocompatibility antigen mismatch. Reconciling these seemingly disparate data will be important to informing therapeutic strategies aimed at limiting Notch signaling in GVHD.

7.9 Concluding Remarks and Future Directions

Much has been learned about the constellation of alloimmune responses that can be generated after HSCT and that result in the complex pathology of GVHD. However, much less is known about the mechanisms of the beneficial GVT responses that may also come into play following HSCT. Indeed, details regarding this phenomenon are only recently emerging and suggest that factors responsible for mediating this effect will be as complex as those that drive GVHD. It is also likely that multiple cellular subsets contribute to GVT; therefore, approaches that target multiple cell populations may ultimately prove to be the most successful.

Effective ex vivo expansion and delivery of donor-derived nTregs or in vivo generation of donor-derived iTregs represent viable approaches to attenuating GVDII, although the effect of increased numbers of Tregs on GVT has not been well-characterized. One caveat to this approach is the demonstrated capacity for Tregs to be converted to Th1 or Th17 cells in the context of a robust pro-inflammatory environment and will need to be considered when designing Treg-based therapies. As discussed above, the degree to which Notch signaling positively or negatively regulates Treg development also has not been fully elucidated. Thus, approaches that aim to attenuate GVHD by manipulating Notch signaling may need to be precise and acutely applied.

Manipulating chemokine receptors, which play a vital role in T cell trafficking, may be one means of achieving selective organ targeting to reduce Teff cell infiltration or to increase trafficking of Tregs to specific organs. CXCR3, CCR5, and CCR9 have been identified as chemokine receptors that facilitate T cell migration, and gut infiltration of CCR9+ CD4 T cells is associated with tissue destruction [7, 134]. CXCR3 has been shown to be a transcriptional target of T-bet [48, 52], which itself is regulated by Notch1 [77, 101]. Furthermore, CCR5 and CCR9 have both been demonstrated to be regulated by Notch1 in T-ALL [79]; however, whether Notch also primes Teff cells for gut infiltration in GVHD is not yet known (Fig. 7.3 (6)). Interestingly, CCR9 also mediates the migration of plasmacytoid DCs (pDC) to the intestines [123], and CCR9+ pDCs show an immature phenotype with a high capacity for suppressing GVHD by reducing the number of IL-17 producing cells and increasing the number of FoxP3+ Treg cells [36]. Further investigation is needed to determine if Notch signaling regulates CCR9 expression in pDC, as it does in CD4+ T cells.

Therapeutic modalities for the treatment and prevention GVHD that aim to limit Notch signaling represent an exciting and active area of investigation. Very early reports suggest that, at least in animal models, this is a promising approach that may serve both to attenuate tissue damage and preserve beneficial GVT effects. Current research in therapies that range from delivering ligand-specific neutralizing antibodies to developing γ-secretase inhibitors designed to selectively modulate Notch signaling, to expanded use of Treg cells as immune modulators, makes for an impressive, and hopefully successful, array of approaches to tackle a complex and complicated disease.

References

1. Adler, S. H., Chiffoleau, E., Xu, L., Dalton, N. M., Burg, J. M., Wells, A. D., Wolfe, M. S., Turka, L. A., & Pear, W. S. (2003). Notch signaling augments T cell responsiveness by enhancing CD25 expression. *Journal of Immunology, 171*, 2896–2903.
2. Alexander, K. A., Flynn, R., Lineburg, K. E., Kuns, R. D., Teal, B. E., Olver, S. D., Lor, M., Raffelt, N. C., Koyama, M., Leveque, L., Le Texier, L., Melino, M., Markey, K. A., Varelias, A., Engwerda, C., Serody, J. S., Janela, B., Ginhoux, F., Clouston, A. D., Blazar, B. R., Hill, G. R., & MacDonald, K. P. (2014). CSF-1- dependant donor-derived macrophages mediate chronic graft-versus-host disease. *The Journal of Clinical Investigation, 124*, 4266–4280. https://doi.org/10.1172/JCI75935.
3. Amsen, D., Blander, J. M., Lee, G. R., Tanigaki, K., Honjo, T., & Flavell, R. A. (2004). Instruction of distinct CD4 T helper cell fates by different notch ligands on antigen-presenting cells. *Cell, 117*, 515–526.
4. Amsen, D., Antov, A., Jankovic, D., Sher, A., Radtke, F., Souabni, A., Busslinger, M., McCright, B., Gridley, T., & Flavell, R. A. (2007). Direct regulation of Gata3 expression determines the T helper differentiation potential of Notch. *Immunity, 27*, 89–99.
5. Amsen, D., Spilianakis, C. G., & Flavell, R. A. (2009). How are T(H)1 and T(H)2 effector cells made? *Current Opinion in Immunology, 21*, 153–160. https://doi.org/10.1016/j.coi.2009.03.010.
6. Amsen, D., Helbig, C., & Backer, R. A. (2015). Notch in T cell differentiation: All things considered. *Trends in Immunology, 36*, 802–814. https://doi.org/10.1016/j.it.2015.10.007.
7. Aoyama, K., Saha, A., Tolar, J., Riddle, M. J., Veenstra, R. G., Taylor, P. A., Blomhoff, R., Panoskaltsis Mortari, A., Klebanoff, C. A., Socié, G., Munn, D. H., Murphy, W. J., Serody, J. S., Fulton, L. M., Teshima, T., Chandraratna, R. A., Dmitrovsky, E., Guo, Y., Noelle, R. J., & Blazar, B. R. (2013). Inhibiting retinoic acid signaling ameliorates graft-versus-host disease by modifying T-cell differentiation and intestinal migration. *Blood, 122*, 2125–2134. https://doi.org/10.1182/blood-2012-11-470252.

8. Aster, J. C. (2014). In brief: Notch signalling in health and disease. *The Journal of Pathology, 232*, 1–3. https://doi.org/10.1002/path.4291.
9. Auderset, F., Schuster, S., Coutaz, M., Koch, U., Desgranges, F., Merck, E., MacDonald, H. R., Radtke, F., & Tacchini-Cottier, F. (2012). Redundant Notch1 and Notch2 signaling is necessary for IFNγ secretion by T helper 1 cells during infection with Leishmania major. *PLoS Pathogens, 8*, e1002560. https://doi.org/10.1371/journal.ppat.1002560.
10. Ayaz, F., & Osborne, B. A. (2014). Non-canonical notch signaling in cancer and immunity. *Frontiers in Oncology, 4*, 345. https://doi.org/10.3389/fonc.2014.00345.
11. Bailis, W., Yashiro-Ohtani, Y., Fang, T. C., Hatton, R. D., Weaver, C. T., Artis, D., & Pear, W. S. (2013). Notch simultaneously orchestrates multiple helper T cell programs independently of cytokine signals. *Immunity, 39*, 148–159. https://doi.org/10.1016/j.immuni.2013.07.006.
12. Barbarulo, A., Grazioli, P., Campese, A. F., Bellavia, D., Di Mario, G., Pelullo, M., Ciuffetta, A., Colantoni, S., Vacca, A., Frati, L., Gulino, A., Felli, M. P., & Screpanti, I. (2011). Notch3 and canonical NF- kappaB signaling pathways cooperatively regulate Foxp3 transcription. *Journal of Immunology, 186*, 6199–6206. https://doi.org/10.4049/jimmunol.1002136.
13. Bigas, A., Guiu, J., & Gama-Norton, L. (2013). Notch and Wnt signaling in the emergence of hematopoietic stem cells. *Blood Cells, Molecules & Diseases, 51*, 264–270. https://doi.org/10.1016/j.bcmd.2013.07.005.
14. Beres, A., Komorowski, R., Mihara, M., & Drobyski, W. R. (2011). Instability of FOXP3 expression limits the ability of induced regulatory T cells to mitigate graft versus host disease. *Clinical Cancer Research, 17*, 3969–3983. https://doi.org/10.1158/1078-0432.CCR-10-3347.
15. Boonyatecha, N., Sangphech, N., Wongchana, W., Kueanjinda, P., & Palaga, T. (2012). Involvement of Notch signaling pathway in regulating IL-12 expression via c-Rel in activated macrophages. *Molecular Immunology, 51*, 255–262. https://doi.org/10.1016/j.molimm.2012.03.017.
16. Brennan, T. V., Lin, L., Huang, X., Cardona, D. M., Li, Z., Dredge, K., Chao, N. J., & Yang, Y. (2012). Heparan sulfate, an endogenous TLR4 agonist, promotes acute GVHD after allogeneic stem cell transplantation. *Blood, 120*, 2899–2908. https://doi.org/10.1182/blood-2011-07-368720.
17. Broady, R., Yu, J., Chow, V., Tantiworawit, A., Kang, C., Berg, K., Martinka, M., Ghoreishi, M., Dutz, J., & Levings, M. K. (2010). Cutaneous GVHD is associated with the expansion of tissue-localized Th1 and not Th17 cells. *Blood, 116*, 5748–5751. https://doi.org/10.1182/blood-2010-07-295436.
18. Brown, C. C., Esterhazy, D., Sarde, A., London, M., Pullabhatla, V., Osma-Garcia, I., Al-Bader, R., Ortiz, C., Elgueta, R., Arno, M., de Rinaldis, E., Mucida, D., Lord, G. M., & Noelle, R. J. (2015). Retinoic acid is essential for Th1 cell lineage stability and prevents transition to a Th17 cell program. *Immunity, 42*, 499–511. https://doi.org/10.1016/j.immuni.2015.02.003.
19. Brunstein, C. G., Miller, J. S., McKenna, D. H., Hippen, K. L., DeFor, T. E., Sumstad, D., Curtsinger, J., Verneris, M. R., ML, M. M., Levine, B. L., Riley, J. I., June, C. H., Le, C., Weisdorf, D., McGlave, P. B., Blazar, B. R., & Wagner, J. E. (2015). Umbilical cord blood-derived T regulatory cells to prevent GVHD: kinetics, toxicity profile and clinical effect. *Journal of Immunology, 195*, 347–355. https://doi.org/10.4049/jimmunol.1402861.
20. Campese, A. F., Grazioli, P., Colantoni, S., Anastasi, E., Mecarozzi, M., Checquolo, S., De Luca, G., Bellavia, D., Frati, L., Gulino, A., & Screpanti, I. (2009). Notch3 and pTalpha/pre-TCR sustain the in vivo function of naturally occurring regulatory T cells. *International Immunology, 21*, 727–743. https://doi.org/10.1093/intimm/dxp042.
21. Charbonnier, L. M., Wang, S., Georgiev, P., Sefik, E., & Chatila, T. A. (2015). Control of peripheral tolerance by regulatory T cell-intrinsic Notch signaling. *Nature Immunology, 16*, 1162–1173. https://doi.org/10.1038/ni.3288.

22. Cheng, H., Tian, J., Li, Z., Zeng, L., Pan, B., Song, G., Chen, W., & Xu, K. (2012). TH17 cells are critical for skin-specific pathological injury in acute graft-versus-host disease. *Transplantation Proceedings, 44*, 1412–1418. https://doi.org/10.1016/j.transproceed.2011.12.078.
23. Cheng, H., Tian, J., Zeng, L., Pan, B., Li, Z., Song, G., Chen, W., & Xu, K. (2012). Halofugine prevents cutaneous graft versus host disease by suppression of Th17 differentiation. *Hematology, 17*, 261–267. https://doi.org/10.1179/1607845412Y.0000000016.
24. Christian, L. M. (2012). The ADAM family: Insights into Notch proteolysis. *Fly (Austin)., 6*, 30–34. https://doi.org/10.4161/fly.18823.
25. Demitrack, E. S., & Samuelson, L. C. (2016). Notch regulation of gastrointestinal stem cells. *The Journal of Physiology, 594*, 4791–4803. https://doi.org/10.1113/JP271667.
26. Dietz, A. C., Lucchini, G., Samarasinghe, S., & Pulsipher, M. A. (2016). Evolving hematopoietic stem cell transplantation strategies in severe aplastic anemia. *Current Opinion in Pediatrics, 28*, 3–11. https://doi.org/10.1097/MOP.0000000000000299.
27. Duggan, S. P., & McCarthy, J. V. (2016). Beyond γ-secretase activity: The multifunctional nature of presenilins in cell signalling pathways. *Cellular Signalling, 28*, 1–11. https://doi.org/10.1016/j.cellsig.2015.10.006.
28. Duffner, U. A., Maeda, Y., Cooke, K. R., Reddy, P., Ordemann, R., Liu, C., Ferrara, J. L., & Teshima, T. (2004). Host dendritic cells alone are sufficient to initiate acute graft-versus-host disease. *Journal of Immunology, 172*, 7393–7398.
29. Dongre, A., Surampudi, L., Lawlor, R. G., Fauq, A. H., Miele, L., Golde, T. E., Minter, L. M., & Osborne, B. A. (2014). Non-canonical Notch signaling drives activation and differentiation of peripheral CD4(+) T cells. *Frontiers in Immunology, 5*, 54. https://doi.org/10.3389/fimmu.2014.00054.
30. Ebens, C. L., & Maillard, I. (2013). Notch signaling in hematopoietic cell transplantation and T cell alloimmunity. *Blood Reviews, 27*, 269–277. https://doi.org/10.1016/j.blre.2013.08.001.
31. Ehebauer, M., Hayward, P., & Martinez-Arias, A. (2006). Notch signaling pathway. *Science's STKE, 2006*(364), cm7.
32. Fang, T. C., Yashiro-Ohtani, Y., Del Bianco, C., Knoblock, D. M., Blacklow, S. C., & Pear, W. S. (2007). Notch directly regulates Gata3 expression during T helper 2 cell differentiation. *Immunity, 27*, 100–110.
33. Fu, J., Wang, D., Yu, Y., Heinrichs, J., Wu, Y., Schutt, S., Kaosaard, K., Liu, C., Haarberg, K., Bastian, D., McDonald, D. G., Anasetti, C., & Yu, X. Z. (2015). T-bet is critical for the development of acute graft- versus-host disease through controlling T cell differentiation and function. *Journal of Immunology, 194*, 388–397. https://doi.org/10.4049/jimmunol.1401618.
34. Fung, E., Tang, S. M., Canner, J. P., Morishige, K., Arboleda-Velasquez, J. F., Cardoso, A. A., Carlesso, N., Aster, J. C., & Aikawa, M. (2007). Delta-like 4 induces notch signaling in macrophages: Implications for inflammation. *Circulation, 115*, 2948–2956.
35. Gowdy, K. M., Nugent, J. L., Martinu, T., Potts, E., Snyder, L. D., Foster, W. M., & Palmer, S. M. (2011). Protective role of T-bet and Th1 cytokines in pulmonary graft-versus-host disease and peribronchiolar fibrosis. *American Journal of Respiratory Cell and Molecular Biology, 46*, 249–256. https://doi.org/10.1165/rcmb.2011-0131OC.
36. Hadeiba, H., Sato, T., Habtezion, A., Oderup, C., Pan, J., & Butcher, E. C. (2008). CCR9 expression defines tolerogenic plasmacytoid dendritic cells able to suppress acute graft-versus-host disease. *Nature Immunology, 9*, 1253–1260. https://doi.org/10.1038/ni.1658.
37. Harbour, S. N., Maynard, C. L., Zindl, C. L., Schoeb, T. R., & Weaver, C. T. (2015). Th17 cells give rise to Th1 cells that are required for the pathogenesis of colitis. *Proceedings of the National Academy of Sciences of the United States of America, 112*, 7061–7066. https://doi.org/10.1073/pnas.1415675112.
38. Hashimoto, D., Chow, A., Greter, M., Saenger, Y., Kwan, W. H., Leboeuf, M., Ginhoux, F., Ochando, J. C., Kunisaki, Y., van Rooijen, N., Liu, C., Teshima, T., Heeger, P. S., Stanley, E. R., Frenette, P. S., & Merad, M. (2011). Pretransplant CSF-1 therapy expands recipient macrophages and ameliorates GVHD after allogeneic hematopoietic cell transplantation. *The Journal of Experimental Medicine, 208*, 1069–1082. https://doi.org/10.1084/jem.20101709.

39. Hayashida, J. N., Nakamura, S., Toyoshima, T., Moriyama, M., Sasaki, M., Kawamura, E., Ohyama, Y., Kumamaru, W., & Shirasuna, K. (2013). Possible involvement of cytokines, chemokines and chemokine receptors in the initiation and progression of chronic GVHD. *Bone Marrow Transplantation, 48*, 115–123. https://doi.org/10.1038/bmt.2012.100.
40. He, S., Cao, Q., Qiu, Y., Mi, J., Zhang, J. Z., Jin, M., Ge, H., Emerson, S. G., Zhang, Y., & Zhang, Y. (2008). A new approach to the blocking of alloreactive T cell-mediated graft-versus-host disease by in vivo administration of anti-CXCR3 neutralizing antibody. *Journal of Immunology, 181*, 7581–7592.
41. Heidegger, S., van den Brink, M. R., Haas, T., & Poeck, H. (2014). The role of pattern-recognition receptors in graft-versus-host disease and graft-versus-leukemia after allogeneic stem cell transplantation. *Frontiers in Immunology, 5*, 337. https://doi.org/10.3389/fimmu.2014.00337.
42. Hill, G. R., Crawford, J. M., Cooke, K. R., Brinson, Y. S., Pan, L., & Ferrara, J. L. (1997). Total body irradiation and acute graft-versus-host disease: The role of gastrointestinal damage and inflammatory cytokines. *Blood, 90*, 3204–3213.
43. Holler, E., Landfried, K., Meier, J., Hausmann, M., & Rogler, G. (2013). The role of bacteria and pattern recognition receptors in GVHD. *International Journal of Inflammation, 2010*, 814326. https://doi.org/10.4061/2010/814326.
44. Hoyne, G. F., Le Roux, I., Corsin-Jimenez, M., Tan, K., Dunne, J., Forsyth, L. M., Dallman, M. J., Owen, M. J., Ish-Horowicz, D., & Lamb, J. R. (2000). Serrate1-induced notch signalling regulates the decision between immunity and tolerance made by peripheral CD4(+) T cells. *International Immunology, 12*, 177–185.
45. Hu, X., Chung, A. Y., Wu, I., Foldi, J., Chen, J., Ji, J. D., Tateya, T., Kang, Y. J., Han, J., Gessler, M., Kageyama, R., & Ivashkiv, L. B. (2008). Integrated regulation of Toll-like receptor responses by Notch and interferon-gamma pathways. *Immunity, 29*, 691–703. https://doi.org/10.1016/j.immuni.2008.08.016.
46. Hue, S., Kared, H., Mehwish, Y., Mouhamad, S., Balbo, M., & Levy, Y. (2012). Notch activation on effector T cells increases their sensitivity to Treg cell-mediated suppression through upregulation of TGF-βRII expression. *European Journal of Immunology, 42*, 1796–1803. https://doi.org/10.1002/eji.201142330.
47. Iclozan, C., Yu, Y., Liu, C., Liang, Y., Yi, T., Anasetti, C., & Yu, X. Z. (2009). T helper17 cells are sufficient but not necessary to induce acute graft-versus-host disease. *Biology of Blood and Marrow Transplantation, 16*, 170–178. https://doi.org/10.1016/j.bbmt.2009.09.023.
48. Imanguli, M. M., Swaim, W. D., League, S. C., Gress, R. E., Pavletic, S. Z., & Hakim, F. T. (2009). Increased T- bet+ cytotoxic effectors and type I interferon-mediated processes in chronic graft-versus-host disease of the oral mucosa. *Blood, 113*, 3620–3630. https://doi.org/10.1182/blood-2008-07-168351.
49. Ju, J. M., Lee, H., Oh, K., Lee, D. S., & Choi, E. Y. (2014). Kinetics of IFN-γ and IL-17 production by CD4 and CD8 T cells during acute graft-versus-host disease. *Immune Network, 14*, 89–99. https://doi.org/10.4110/in.2014.14.2.89.
50. Kassner, N., Krueger, M., Yagita, H., Dzionek, A., Hutloff, A., Kroczek, R., Scheffold, A., & Rutz, S. (2010). Cutting edge: Plasmacytoid dendritic cells induce IL-10 production in T cells via the Delta-like-4/Notch axis. *Journal of Immunology, 184*, 550–554. https://doi.org/10.4049/jimmunol.0903152.
51. Kimura, A., Naka, T., & Kishimoto, T. (2007). IL-6-dependent and -independent pathways in the development of interleukin 17-producing T helper cells. *Proceedings of the National Academy of Sciences of the United States of America, 104*, 12099–12104.
52. Koch, M. A., Tucker-Heard, G., Perdue, N. R., Killebrew, J. R., Urdahl, K. B., & Campbell, D. J. (2009). The transcription factor T-bet controls regulatory T cell homeostasis and function during type 1 inflammation. *Nature Immunology, 10*, 595–602. https://doi.org/10.1038/ni.1731.

53. Koch, U., & Radtke, F. (2011). Mechanisms of T cell development and transformation. *Annual Review of Cell and Developmental Biology, 27*, 539–562. https://doi.org/10.1146/annurev-cellbio-092910-154008.
54. Komatsu, N., Okamoto, K., Sawa, S., Nakashima, T., Oh-hora, M., Kodama, T., Tanaka, S., Bluestone, J. A., & Takayanagi, H. (2014). Pathogenic conversion of Foxp3+ T cells into TH17 cells in autoimmune arthritis. *Nature Medicine, 20*, 62–68. https://doi.org/10.1038/nm.3432.
55. Kotsiou, E., & Davies, J. K. (2013). New ways to separate graft-versus-host disease and graft-versus- tumour effects after allogeneic haematopoietic stem cell transplantation. *British Journal of Haematology, 160*, 133–145. https://doi.org/10.1111/bjh.12115.
56. Kovall, R. A. (2007). Structures of CSL, Notch and Mastermind proteins: Piecing together an active transcription complex. *Current Opinion in Structural Biology, 17*, 117–127.
57. Koyama, M., Cheong, M., Markey, K. A., Gartlan, K. H., Kuns, R. D., Locke, K. R., Lineburg, K. E., Teal, B. E., Leveque-El Mouttie, L., Bunting, M. D., Vuckovic, S., Zhang, P., Teng, M. W., Varelias, A., Tey, S. K., Wockner, L. F., Engwerda, C. R., Smyth, M. J., Belz, G. T., McColl, S. R., MacDonald, K. P., & Hill, G. R. (2015). Donor colonic CD103+ dendritic cells determine the severity of acute graft-versus-host disease. *The Journal of Experimental Medicine, 212*, 1303–1321. https://doi.org/10.1084/jem.20150329.
58. Koyama, M., Hashimoto, D., Aoyama, K., Matsuoka, K., Karube, K., Niiro, H., Harada, M., Tanimoto, M., Akashi, K., & Teshima, T. (2009). Plasmacytoid dendritic cells prime alloreactive T cells to mediate graft-versus-host disease as antigen-presenting cells. *Blood, 113*, 2088–2095. https://doi.org/10.1182/blood-2008-07-168609.
59. Kryczek, I., Zhao, E., Liu, Y., Wang, Y., Vatan, L., Szeliga, W., Moyer, J., Klimczak, A., Lange, A., & Zou, W. (2011). Human TH17 cells are long-lived effector memory cells. *Science Translational Medicine, 3*, 104ra100. https://doi.org/10.1126/scitranslmed.3002949.
60. Lai, H. Y., Chou, T. Y., Tzeng, C. H., & Lee, O. K. (2012). Cytokine profiles in various graft-versus- host disease target organs following hematopoietic stem cell transplantation. *Cell Transplantation, 21*, 2033–2045. https://doi.org/10.3727/096368912X653110.
61. Laky, K., & Fowlkes, B. J. (2008). Notch signaling in CD4 and CD8 T cell development. *Current Opinion in Immunology, 20*, 197–202. https://doi.org/10.1016/j.coi.2008.03.004.
62. Li, C. R., Mueller, E. E., & Bradley, L. M. (2014). Islet antigen-specific Th17 cells can induce TNF-α- dependent autoimmune diabetes. *Journal of Immunology, 192*, 1425–1432. https://doi.org/10.4049/jimmunol.1301742.
63. Li, H., Demetris, A. J., McNiff, J., Matte-Martone, C., Tan, H. S., Rothstein, D. M., & Lakkis, F. G. (2012). Shlomchik WD (2012) Profound depletion of host conventional dendritic cells, plasmacytoid dendritic cells, and B cells does not prevent graft-versus-host disease induction. *Journal of Immunology, 188*(8), 3804–3811. https://doi.org/10.4049/jimmunol.1102795.
64. Li, J. M., Giver, C. R., Lu, Y., Hossain, M. S., Akhtari, M., & Waller, E. K. (2009). Separating graft-versus- leukemia from graft-versus-host disease in allogeneic hematopoietic stem cell transplantation. *Immunotherapy, 1*, 599–621.
65. Li, N., Chen, Y., He, W., Yi, T., Zhao, D., Zhang, C., Lin, C. L., Todorov, I., Kandeel, F., Forman, S., & Zeng, D. (2009). Anti-CD3 preconditioning separates GVL from GVHD via modulating host dendritic cell and donor T-cell migration in recipients conditioned with TBI. *Blood, 113*, 953–962. https://doi.org/10.1182/blood-2008-06-165522.
66. Li, S., Xie, Q., Zeng, Y., Zou, C., Liu, X., Wu, S., Deng, H., Xu, Y., Li, X. C., & Dai, Z. (2014). A naturally occurring CD8(+)CD122(+) T-cell subset as a memory-like Treg family. *Cellular & Molecular Immunology, 11*, 326–331. https://doi.org/10.1038/cmi.2014.25.
67. Lin, X., Lu, Z. G., Song, C. Y., Huang, Y. X., Guo, K. Y., Deng, L., Tu, S. F., He, Y. Z., Xu, J. H., Long, H., & Wu, B. Y. (2015). Long-term outcome of HLA-haploidentical hematopoietic stem cell transplantation without in vitro T-cell depletion based on an FBCA conditioning regimen for hematologic malignancies. *Bone Marrow Transplantation, 50*, 1092–1097. https://doi.org/10.1038/bmt.2015.108.

68. Liotta, F., Frosali, F., Querci, V., Mantei, A., Filì, L., Maggi, L., Mazzinghi, B., Angeli, R., Ronconi, E., Santarlasci, V., Biagioli, T., Lasagni, L., Ballerini, C., Parronchi, P., Scheffold, A., Cosmi, L., Maggi, E., Romagnani, S., & Annunziato, F. (2008). Human immature myeloid dendritic cells trigger a TH2- polarizing program via Jagged-1/Notch interaction. *The Journal of Allergy and Clinical Immunology, 121*, 1000–1005.e8. https://doi.org/10.1016/j.jaci.2008.01.004.
69. Liu, H. P., Cao, A. T., Feng, T., Li, Q., Zhang, W., Yao, S., Dann, S. M., Elson, C. O., & Cong, Y. (2015). TGF-β converts Th1 cells into Th17 cells through stimulation of Runx1 expression. *European Journal of Immunology, 45*, 1010–1018. https://doi.org/10.1002/eji.201444726.
70. Maillard, I., Weng, A. P., Carpenter, A. C., Rodriguez, C. G., Sai, H., Xu, L., Allman, D., Aster, J. C., & Pear, W. S. (2004). Mastermind critically regulates Notch-mediated lymphoid cell fate decisions. *Blood, 104*, 1696–1702.
71. Mangan, P. R., Harrington, L. E., O'Quinn, D. B., Helms, W. S., Bullard, D. C., Elson, C. O., Hatton, R. D., Wahl, S. M., Schoeb, T. R., & Weaver, C. T. (2006). Transforming growth factor-beta induces development of the T(H)17 lineage. *Nature, 441*, 231–234.
72. Mapara, M. Y., Leng, C., Kim, Y. M., Bronson, R., Lokshin, A., Luster, A., & Sykes, M. (2006). Expression of chemokines in GVHD target organs is influenced by conditioning and genetic factors and amplified by GVHR. *Biology of Blood and Marrow Transplantation, 12*, 623–634.
73. Martinez Arias, A., Zecchini, V., & Brennan, K. (2002). CSL-independent Notch signalling: A checkpoint in cell fate decisions during development? *Current Opinion in Genetics & Development, 12*, 524–533.
74. Mauermann, N., Burian, J., von Garnier, C., Dirnhofer, S., Germano, D., Schuett, C., Tamm, M., Bingisser, R., Eriksson, U., & Hunziker, L. (2008). Interferon-gamma regulates idiopathic pneumonia syndrome, a Th17+CD4+ T-cell-mediated graft-versus-host disease. *American Journal of Respiratory and Critical Care Medicine, 178*, 379–388. https://doi.org/10.1164/rccm.200711-1648OC.
75. Meng, L., Bai, Z., He, S., Mochizuki, K., Liu, Y., Purushe, J., Sun, H., Wang, J., Yagita, H., Mineishi, S., Fung, H., Yanik, G. A., Caricchio, R., Fan, X., Crisalli, L. M., Hexner, E. O., Reshef, R., Zhang, Y., & Zhang, Y. (2016). The Notch ligand DLL4 defines a capability of human dendritic cells in regulating Th1 and Th17 differentiation. *Journal of Immunology, 196*(3), 1070–1080. https://doi.org/10.4049/jimmunol.1501310. Epub 2015 Dec 28.
76. Michael, M., Shimoni, A., & Nagler, A. (2013). Regulatory T cells in allogeneic stem cell transplantation. *Clinical & Developmental Immunology, 2013*, 608951. https://doi.org/10.1155/2013/608951.
77. Minter, L. M., Turley, D. M., Das, P., Shin, H. M., Joshi, I., Lawlor, R. G., Cho, O. H., Palaga, T., Gottipati, S., Telfer, J. C., Kostura, L., Fauq, A. H., Simpson, K., Such, K. A., Miele, L., Golde, T. E., Miller, S. D., & Osborne, B. A. (2005). Inhibitors of gamma-secretase block in vivo and in vitro T helper type 1 polarization by preventing Notch upregulation of Tbx21. *Nature Immunology, 6*, 680–688.
78. Minter, L. M., & Osborne, B. A. (2012). Canonical and non-canonical Notch signaling in $CD4^+$ T cells. *Current Topics in Microbiology and Immunology, 360*, 99–114. https://doi.org/10.1007/82_2012_233.
79. Mirandola, L., Chiriva-Internati, M., Montagna, D., Locatelli, F., Zecca, M., Ranzani, M., Basile, A., Locati, M., Cobos, E., Kast, W. M., Asselta, R., Paraboschi, E. M., Comi, P., & Chiaramonte, R. (2012). Notch1 regulates chemotaxis and proliferation by controlling the CC-chemokine receptors 5 and 9 in T cell acute lymphoblastic leukaemia. *The Journal of Pathology, 226*, 713–722. https://doi.org/10.1002/path.3015.
80. Mochizuki, K., He, S., & Zhang, Y. (2011). Notch and inflammatory T-cell response: New developments and challenges. *Immunotherapy, 3*, 1353–1366. https://doi.org/10.2217/imt.11.126.
81. Mochizuki, K., Xie, F., He, S., Tong, Q., Liu, Y., Mochizuki, I., Guo, Y., Kato, K., Yagita, H., Mineishi, S., & Zhang, Y. (2013). Delta-like ligand 4 identifies a previously uncharacterized

population of inflammatory dendritic cells that plays important roles in eliciting allogeneic T cell responses in mice. *Journal of Immunology, 190*, 3772–3782. https://doi.org/10.4049/jimmunol.1202820.
82. Monsalve, E., Pérez, M. A., Rubio, A., Ruiz-Hidalgo, M. J., Baladrón, V., García-Ramírez, J. J., Gómez, J. C., Laborda, J., & Díaz-Guerra, M. J. (2006). Notch-1 up-regulation and signaling following macrophage activation modulates gene expression patterns known to affect antigen-presenting capacity and cytotoxic activity. *Journal of Immunology, 176*, 5362–5373.
83. Morikawa, H., & Sakaguchi, S. (2014). Genetic and epigenetic basis of Treg cell development and function: From a FoxP3-centered view to an epigenome-defined view of natural Treg cells. *Immunological Reviews, 259*, 192–205. https://doi.org/10.1111/imr.12174.
84. Mota, C., Nunes-Silva, V., Pires, A. R., Matoso, P., Victorino, R. M., Sousa, A. E., & Caramalho, I. (2014). Delta-like 1-mediated Notch signaling enhances the in vitro conversion of human memory CD4 T cells intoFOXP3-expressing regulatory T cells. *Journal of Immunology, 193*, 5854–5862. https://doi.org/10.4049/jimmunol.1400198.
85. Mukherjee, S., Schaller, M. A., Neupane, R., Kunkel, S. L., & Lukacs, N. W. (2009). Regulation of T cell activation by Notch ligand, DLL4, promotes IL-17 production and Rorc activation. *Journal of Immunology, 182*, 7381–7388. https://doi.org/10.4049/jimmunol.0804322.
86. Nishiwaki, S., Terakura, S., Ito, M., Goto, T., Seto, A., Watanabe, K., Yanagisawa, M., Imahashi, N., Tsukamoto, S., Shimba, M., Ozawa, Y., & Miyamura, K. (2009). Impact of macrophage infiltration of skin lesions on survival after allogeneic stem cell transplantation: A clue to refractory graft- versus-host disease. *Blood, 114*, 3113–3116. https://doi.org/10.1182/blood-2009-03-209635.
87. Nishiwaki, S., Nakayama, T., Murata, M., Nishida, T., Terakura, S., Saito, S., Kato, T., Mizuno, H., Imahashi, N., Seto, A., Ozawa, Y., Miyamura, K., Ito, M., Takeshita, K., Kato, H., Toyokuni, S., Nagao, K., Ueda, R., & Naoe, T. (2014). Dexamethasone palmitate ameliorates macrophages-rich graft-versus- host disease by inhibiting macrophage functions. *PLoS One, 9*, e96252. https://doi.org/10.1371/journal.pone.0096252.
88. Osborne, B. A., & Minter, L. M. (2007). Notch signalling during peripheral T-cell activation and differentiation. *Nature Reviews. Immunology, 7*, 64–75.
89. Ostroukhova, M., Qi, Z., Oriss, T. B., Dixon-McCarthy, B., Ray, P., & Ray, A. (2006). Treg-mediated immunosuppression involves activation of the Notch-HES1 axis by membrane-bound TGF-beta. *The Journal of Clinical Investigation, 116*, 996–1004.
90. Ong, C. T., Sedy, J. R., Murphy, K. M., & Kopan, R. (2008). Notch and presenilin regulate cellular expansion and cytokine secretion but cannot instruct Th1/Th2 fate acquisition. *PLoS One, 3*, e2823. https://doi.org/10.1371/journal.pone.0002823.
91. Ou-Yang, H. F., Zhang, H. W., Wu, C. G., Zhang, P., Zhang, J., Li, J. C., Hou, L. H., He, F., Ti, X. Y., Song, L. Q., Zhang, S. Z., Feng, L., Qi, H. W., & Han, H. (2009). Notch signaling regulates the FOXP3 promoter through RBP-J- and Hes1-dependent mechanisms. *Molecular and Cellular Biochemistry, 320*, 109–114. https://doi.org/10.1007/s11010-008-9912-4.
92. Palaga, T., Miele, L., Golde, T. E., & Osborne, B. A. (2003). TCR-mediated Notch signaling regulates proliferation and IFN-gamma production in peripheral T cells. *Journal of Immunology, 171*, 3019–3024.
93. Pan, B., Zhang, Y., Sun, Y., Cheng, H., Wu, Y., Song, G., Chen, W., Zeng, L., & Xu, K. (2014). Deviated balance between Th1 and Th17 cells exacerbates acute graft-versus-host disease in mice. *Cytokine, 68*, 69–75. https://doi.org/10.1016/j.cyto.2014.04.002.
94. Parmar, S., Liu, X., Tung, S. S., Robinson, S. N., Rodriguez, G., Cooper, L. J., Yang, H., Shah, N., Yang, H., Konopleva, M., Molldrem, J. J., Garcia-Manero, G., Najjar, A., Yvon, E., McNiece, I., Rezvani, K., Savoldo, B., Bollard, C. M., & Shpall, E. J. (2015). Third-party umbilical cord blood-derived regulatory T cells prevent xenogenic graft-versus-host disease. Blood. pii: blood-2015-06-653667. [Epub ahead of print].
95. Pasquini, M. C. (2008). Impact of graft-versus-host disease on survival. *Best Practice & Research. Clinical Haematology, 21*, 193–204. https://doi.org/10.1016/j.beha.2008.02.011

96. Perumalsamy, L. R., Marcel, N., Kulkarni, S., Radtke, F., & Sarin, A. (2012). Distinct spatial and molecular features of notch pathway assembly in regulatory T cells. *Science Signaling, 5*, ra53. https://doi.org/10.1126/scisignal.2002859.
97. Pierini, A., Colonna, L., Alvarez, M., Schneidawind, D., Nishikii, H., Baker, J., Pan, Y., Florek, M., Kim, B. S., & Negrin, R. S. (2014). Donor requirements for regulatory T cell suppression of murine graft- versus-host disease. *Cytotherapy, 16*, 90–100. https://doi.org/10.1016/j.jcyt.2013.07.009.
98. Pratt, E. B., Wentzell, J. S., Maxson, J. E., Courter, L., Hazelett, D., & Christian, J. L. (2011). The cell giveth and the cell taketh away: An overview of Notch pathway activation by endocytic trafficking of ligands and receptors. *Acta Histochemica, 113*, 248–255. https://doi.org/10.1016/j.acthis.2010.01.006.
99. Ratajczak, M. Z., & Suszynska, M. (2016). Emerging strategies to enhance homing and engraftment of hematopoietic stem cells. *Stem Cell Reviews, 12*, 121–128. https://doi.org/10.1007/s12015-015-9625-5.
100. Reshef, R., Luger, S. M., Hexner, E. O., Loren, A. W., Frey, N. V., Nasta, S. D., Goldstein, S. C., Stadtmauer, E. A., Smith, J., Bailey, S., Mick, R., Heitjan, D. F., Emerson, S. G., Hoxie, J. A., Vonderheide, R. H., & Porter, D. L. (2012). Blockade of lymphocyte chemotaxis in visceral graft-versus-host disease. *The New England Journal of Medicine, 367*, 135–145. https://doi.org/10.1056/NEJMoa1201248.
101. Roderick, J. E., Gonzalez-Perez, G., Kuksin, C. A., Dongre, A., Roberts, E. R., Srinivasan, J., Andrzejewski, C., Jr., Fauq, A. H., Golde, T. E., Miele, L., & Minter, L. M. (2013). Therapeutic targeting of NOTCH signaling ameliorates immune-mediated bone marrow failure of aplastic anemia. *The Journal of Experimental Medicine, 210*, 1311–1329. https://doi.org/10.1084/jem.20112615.
102. Rutz, S., Janke, M., Kassner, N., Hohnstein, T., Krueger, M., & Scheffold, A. (2008). Notch regulates IL- 10 production by T helper 1 cells. *Proceedings of the National Academy of Sciences of the United States of America, 105*, 3497–3502. https://doi.org/10.1073/pnas.0712102105.
103. Samon, J. B., Champhekar, A., Minter, L. M., Telfer, J. C., Miele, L., Fauq, A., Das, P., Golde, T. E., & Osborne, B. A. (2008). Notch1 and TGFbeta1 cooperatively regulate Foxp3 expression and the maintenance of peripheral regulatory T cells. *Blood, 112*, 1813–1821. https://doi.org/10.1182/blood-2008-03-144980.
104. Sandy, A. R., Jones, M., & Maillard, I. (2012). Notch signaling and development of the hematopoietic system. *Advances in Experimental Medicine and Biology, 727*, 71–88. https://doi.org/10.1007/978-1-4614-0899-4_6.
105. Sandy, A. R., Chung, J., Toubai, T., Shan, G. T., Tran, I. T., Friedman, A., Blackwell, T. S., Reddy, P., King, P. D., & Maillard, I. (2013). T cell-specific notch inhibition blocks graft-versus-host disease by inducing a hyporesponsive program in alloreactive CD4+ and CD8+ T cells. *Journal of Immunology, 190*, 5818–5828. https://doi.org/10.4049/jimmunol.1203452.
106. Schmitt, E. G., & Williams, C. B. (2013). Generation and function of induced regulatory T cells. *Frontiers in Immunology, 4*, 152. https://doi.org/10.3389/fimmu.2013.00152. eCollection 2013.
107. Schmitt, N., & Ueno, H. (2015). Regulation of human helper T cell subset differentiation by cytokines. *Current Opinion in Immunology, 34*, 130–136. https://doi.org/10.1016/j.coi.2015.03.007.
108. Schwanbeck, R. (2015). The role of epigenetic mechanisms in Notch signaling during development. *Journal of Cellular Physiology, 230*, 969–981. https://doi.org/10.1002/jcp.24851.
109. Shlomchik, W. D. (2007). Graft-versus-host disease. *Nature Reviews. Immunology, 7*, 340–352.
110. Singla, R. D., Wang, J., & Singla, D. K. (2014). Regulation of Notch 1 signaling in THP-1 cells enhances M2 macrophage differentiation. *American Journal of Physiology. Heart and Circulatory Physiology, 307*, H1634–H1642. https://doi.org/10.1152/ajpheart.00896.2013.

111. Skokos, D., & Nussenzweig, M. C. (2007). CD8− DCs induce IL-12–independent Th1 differentiation through Delta 4 Notch-like ligand in response to bacterial LPS. *The Journal of Experimental Medicine, 204*, 1525–1531. https://doi.org/10.1084/jem.20062305.
112. Szabo, S. J., Kim, S. T., Costa, G. L., Zhang, X., Fathman, C. G., & Glimcher, L. H. (2000). A novel transcription factor, T-bet, directs Th1 lineage commitment. *Cell, 100*, 655–669.
113. Theil, A., Tuve, S., Oelschlägel, U., Maiwald, A., Döhler, D., Oßmann, D., Zenkel, A., Wilhelm, C., Middeke, J. M., Shayegi, N., Trautmann-Grill, K., von Bonin, M., Platzbecker, U., Ehninger, G., Bonifacio, E., & Bornhäuser, M. (2015). Adoptive transfer of allogeneic regulatory T cells into patients with chronic graft-versus-host disease. *Cytotherapy, 17*, 473–486. https://doi.org/10.1016/j.jcyt.2014.11.005.
114. Tran, I. T., Sandy, A. R., Carulli, A. J., Ebens, C., Chung, J., Shan, G. T., Radojcic, V., Friedman, A., Gridley, T., Shelton, A., Reddy, P., Samuelson, L. C., Yan, M., Siebel, C. W., & Maillard, I. (2013). Blockade of individual Notch ligands and receptors controls graft-versus-host disease. *The Journal of Clinical Investigation, 123*, 1590–1604.
115. Tu, L., Fang, T. C., Artis, D., Shestova, O., Pross, S. E., Maillard, I., & Pear, W. S. (2005). Notch signaling is an important regulator of type 2 immunity. *The Journal of Experimental Medicine, 202*, 1037–1042.
116. Ukena, S. N., Grosse, J., Mischak-Weissinger, E., Buchholz, S., Stadler, M., Ganser, A., & Franzke, A. (2011). Acute but not chronic graft-versus-host disease is associated with a reduction of circulating CD4(+)CD25 (high)CD127 (low/-) regulatory T cells. *Annals of Hematology, 90*, 213–218. https://doi.org/10.1007/s00277-010-1068-0. (a).
117. Ukena, S. N., Velaga, S., Geffers, R., Grosse, J., Baron, U., Buchholz, S., Stadler, M., Bruder, D., Ganser, A., & Franzke, A. (2012). Human regulatory T cells in allogeneic stem cell transplantation. *Blood, 118*, e82–e92. https://doi.org/10.1182/blood-2011-05-352708. (b).
118. van den Brink, M. R., Velardi, E., & Perales, M. A. (2015). Immune reconstitution following stem cell transplantation. *Hematology. American Society of Hematology. Education Program, 2015*, 215–219. https://doi.org/10.1182/asheducation-2015.1.215.
119. van der Waart, A. B., van der Velden, W. J., Blijlevens, N. M., & Dolstra, H. (2014). Targeting the IL17 pathway for the prevention of graft-versus-host disease. *Biology of Blood and Marrow Transplantation, 20*, 752–759. https://doi.org/10.1016/j.bbmt.2014.02.007.
120. Varona, R., Cadenas, V., Gómez, L., Martínez-A, C., & Márquez, G. (2005). CCR6 regulates CD4+ T- cell-mediated graft-versus-host disease responses. *Blood, 106*, 18–26.
121. Vianello, F., Cannella, L., Coe, D., Chai, J. G., Golshayan, D., Marelli-Berg, F. M., & Dazzi, F. (2013). Enhanced and aberrant T cell trafficking following total body irradiation: a gateway to graft- versus-host disease? *British Journal of Haematology, 162*, 808–818. https://doi.org/10.1111/bjh.12472.
122. Wang, Y. C., He, F., Feng, F., Liu, X. W., Dong, G. Y., Qin, H. Y., Hu, X. B., Zheng, M. H., Liang, L., Feng, L., Liang, Y. M., & Han, H. (2010). Notch signaling determines the M1 versus M2 polarization of macrophages in antitumor immune responses. *Cancer Research, 70*, 4840–4849. https://doi.org/10.1158/0008-5472.CAN-10-0269.
123. Wendland, M., Czeloth, N., Mach, N., Malissen, B., Kremmer, E., Pabst, O., & Förster, R. (2007). CCR9 is a homing receptor for plasmacytoid dendritic cells to the small intestine. *Proceedings of the National Academy of Sciences of the United States of America, 104*, 6347–6352.
124. Wongchana, W., & Palaga, T. (2012). Direct regulation of interleukin-6 expression by Notch signaling in macrophages. *Cellular & Molecular Immunology, 9*, 155–162. https://doi.org/10.1038/cmi.2011.36.
125. Wongchana, W., Lawlor, R. G., Osborne, B. A., & Palaga, T. (2015). Impact of Notch1 deletion in macrophages on proinflammatory cytokine production and the outcome of experimental autoimmune encephalomyelitis. *Journal of Immunology, 195*, 5337–5346. https://doi.org/10.4049/jimmunol.1401770.
126. Wu, Y., Bastian, D., Schutt, S., Nguyen, H., Fu, J., Heinrichs, J., Xia, C., & Yu, X. Z. (2015). Essential role of interleukin-12/23p40 in the development of graft-versus-host disease in mice.

Biology of Blood and Marrow Transplantation, 21, 1195–1204. https://doi.org/10.1016/j.bbmt.2015.03.016.

127. Xiao, S., Jin, H., Korn, T., Liu, S. M., Oukka, M., Lim, B., & Kuchroo, V. K. (2008). Retinoic acid increases Foxp3+ regulatory T cells and inhibits development of Th17 cells by enhancing TGF-beta-driven Smad3 signaling and inhibiting IL-6 and IL-23 receptor expression. *Journal of Immunology, 181*, 2277–2284.
128. Xu, H., Zhu, J., Smith, S., Foldi, J., Zhao, B., Chung, A. Y., Outtz, H., Kitajewski, J., Shi, C., Weber, S., Saftig, P., Li, Y., Ozato, K., Blobel, C. P., Ivashkiv, L. B., & Hu, X. (2012). Notch-RBP-J signaling regulates the transcription factor IRF8 to promote inflammatory macrophage polarization. *Nature Immunology, 13*, 642–650. https://doi.org/10.1038/ni.2304.
129. Xu, J., Chi, F., Guo, T., Punj, V., Lee, W. N., French, S. W., & Tsukamoto, H. (2015). NOTCH reprograms mitochondrial metabolism for proinflammatory macrophage activation. *The Journal of Clinical Investigation, 125*, 1579–1590. https://doi.org/10.1172/JCI76468.
130. Yamane, H., & Paul, W. E. (2013). Early signaling events that underlie fate decisions of naive CD4(+) T cells toward distinct T-helper cell subsets. *Immunological Reviews, 252*, 12–23. https://doi.org/10.1111/imr.12032.
131. Yi, T., Chen, Y., Wang, L., Du, G., Huang, D., Zhao, D., Johnston, H., Young, J., Todorov, I., Umetsu, D. T., Chen, L., Iwakura, Y., Kandeel, F., Forman, S., & Zeng, D. (2009). Reciprocal differentiation and tissue- specific pathogenesis of Th1, Th2, and Th17 cells in graft-versus-host disease. *Blood, 114*, 3101–3112. https://doi.org/10.1182/blood-2009-05-219402.
132. Yu, Q., Sharma, A., Oh, S. Y., Moon, H. G., Hossain, M. Z., Salay, T. M., Leeds, K. E., Du, H., Wu, B., Waterman, M. L., Zhu, Z., & Sen, J. M. (2009). T cell factor 1 initiates the T helper type 2 fate by inducing the transcription factor GATA-3 and repressing interferon-gamma. *Nature Immunology, 10*, 992–999. https://doi.org/10.1038/ni.1762.
133. Yu, Y., Wang, D., Liu, C., Kaosaard, K., Semple, K., Anasetti, C., & Yu, X. Z. (2011). Prevention of GVHD while sparing GVL effect by targeting Th1 and Th17 transcription factor T-bet and RORγt in mice. *Blood, 118*, 5011–5020. https://doi.org/10.1182/blood-2011-03-340315.
134. Yuan, J., Ren, H. Y., Shi, Y. J., & Liu, W. (2015). Prophylaxis of acute graft-versus-host disease by CCR5 blockade combined with cyclosporine A in a murine model. *Inflammation Research, 64*, 137–144. https://doi.org/10.1007/s00011-014-0793-6.
135. Zeng, C., Xing, R., Liu, J., & Xing, F. (2016). Role of CSL-dependent and independent Notch signaling pathways in cell apoptosis. *Apoptosis, 21*, 1–12. [Epub ahead of print].
136. Zhang, Y., Sandy, A. R., Wang, J., Radojcic, V., Shan, G. T., Tran, I. T., Friedman, A., Kato, K., He, S., Cui, S., Hexner, E., Frank, D. M., Emerson, S. G., Pear, W. S., & Maillard, I. (2011). Notch signaling is a critical regulator of allogeneic CD4+ T-cell responses mediating graft-versus-host disease. *Blood, 117*, 299–308. https://doi.org/10.1182/blood-2010-03-271940.
137. Zhao, Y., Liu, Q., Yang, L., He, D., Wang, L., Tian, J., Li, Y., Zi, F., Bao, H., Yang, Y., Zheng, Y., Shi, J., Xue, X., & Cai, Z. (2013). TLR4 inactivation protects from graft-versus-host disease after allogeneic hematopoietic stem cell transplantation. *Cellular & Molecular Immunology, 10*, 165–175. https://doi.org/10.1038/cmi.2012.58.
138. Fulton, L. M., Carlson, M. J., Coghill, J. M., Ott, L. E., West, M. L., Panoskaltsis-Mortari, A., Littman, D. R., Blazar, B. R., & Serody, J. S. (2012). Attenuation of Acute Graft-versus-Host Disease in the Absence of the Transcription Factor RORÂ t. *The Journal of Immunology, 189*(4):1765–1772. https://doi.org/10.4049/jimmunol.1200858. Epub 2012 Jul 9.

Chapter 8
Notch Signaling in T-Cell Acute Lymphoblastic Leukemia and Other Hematologic Malignancies

Catherine Hoofd, Vincenzo Giambra, and Andrew P. Weng

Abstract Notch is a highly conserved signaling pathway that is crucial for development and homeostasis of many normal tissues and cell types. Deregulated Notch signaling is associated with human disease in several different tissue contexts but is perhaps best characterized in T-cell acute lymphoblastic leukemia/lymphoma (T-ALL). Activating mutations in the *NOTCH1* gene and other elements of the Notch signaling pathway such as *FBW7* result in increased Notch signaling intensity and/or duration and are acquired spontaneously at high frequency in primary human T-ALL and in experimentally derived mouse models of T-ALL. As well, enforced expression of activated NOTCH1 in normal hematopoietic progenitors promotes cellular transformation and leads to development of T-ALL-like disease in mice. Recent work has highlighted a role for the Notch pathway in other hematologic malignancies as well. While gain-of-function mutations in NOTCH receptors occur frequently in mature B-cell malignancies such as chronic lymphocytic leukemia (CLL), mantle cell lymphoma (MCL), and splenic marginal zone lymphoma (SMZL), activation of the Notch pathway can also block tumor progression in myeloid malignancies, highlighting its highly versatile and context-dependent nature. In this chapter, we summarize the most recent findings regarding the pathogenic role of Notch signaling in various hematologic malignancies and current strategies to inhibit it therapeutically.

Keywords Notch · Leukemia · Lymphoma · T-ALL · Signal transduction · Gene mutation · γ-secretase inhibitor · Mouse model

---

*Catherine Hoofd and Vincenzo Giambra contributed equally to this work.

C. Hoofd · V. Giambra · A. P. Weng (✉)
Terry Fox Laboratory, BC Cancer Agency, Vancouver, BC, Canada
e-mail: choofd@bccrc.ca; vgiambra@bccrc.ca; aweng@bccrc.ca

L. Miele, S. Artavanis-Tsakonas (eds.), *Targeting Notch in Cancer*,
https://doi.org/10.1007/978-1-4939-8859-4_8

8.1 Notch Signaling Pathway

8.1.1 Notch Receptors and Ligands

The Notch signaling pathway is highly evolutionarily conserved and provides for communication between neighboring cells that is important for normal tissue development and homeostasis. In mammals, there are four Notch receptors (NOTCH1–4) and multiple ligands of the Delta/Serrate/Lag-1 (DSL) family including Delta-like (DLL)-1, DLL-3, and DLL-4 and Jagged (JAG)1 and JAG2. All four Notch receptors are single-pass transmembrane proteins that include multimerized epidermal growth factor (EGF) repeats within the extracellular domain which mediate interaction with DSL ligands. Glycosyltransferase homologs of the Fringe family including Lunatic, Manic, and Radical Fringe [1, 2] can modify specific EGF repeats that provide for ligand selectivity [3–5].

Notch receptors are initially translated as a single polypeptide but are cleaved at the S1 site by a furin-like protease in the trans-Golgi [6] into two subunits that noncovalently reassociate before trafficking to the cell surface. The extracellular domain consists of EGF repeats that mediate interactions with ligand, three tandem Lin-12/Notch repeats (LNR), and the N-terminal portion of the heterodimerization domain (HD^N). HD^N associates with its partner C-terminal HD domain (HD^C) which resides at the N-terminus of the transmembrane subunit and holds the two subunits together [7, 8]. The LNR portion "drapes" over the HD domain to shield it from cleavage by intramembrane proteases [9, 10] (Fig. 8.1).

Ligand binding and subsequent bilateral endocytosis (ligand endocytosis by the signal-"sending" cell and receptor endocytosis by the signal-"receiving" cell) is thought to exert a physical pull that displaces the LNR domain, thus exposing the S2 site within the HD^C domain to proteolytic cleavage by an intramembrane ADAM metalloprotease [11–13]. This reveals yet another proteolytic cleavage site S3 near the inner leaflet of the plasma membrane that is acted upon by γ-secretase, a multisubunit intramembrane protease complex consisting of presenilin 1 or 2, PEN-2, APH-1, and nicastrin. Cleavage at the S3 site releases the intracellular domain (ICN) from its membrane tether, and ICN is then free to translocate to the nucleus by virtue of its two nuclear localization signals (Fig. 8.2).

ICN itself contains an Rbp-associated molecule (RAM) domain which mediates association with the DNA-binding factor CSL (CBF1, Suppressor of Hairless, Lag-2; also known as RBPJ), an ankyrin repeat domain (ANK) which mediates protein-protein interactions, a transactivation domain (TAD), and negative regulatory proline/glutamic acid/serine/threonine-rich (PEST) domain at the C-terminus [3, 14] (Fig. 8.1). CSL can interact with various cofactors to build either repressor complexes containing histone deacetylases such as SMRT/NCoR [15, 16] or activator complexes with ICN and Mastermind-like (MAML) proteins which recruit chromatin-modifier proteins such as histone acetyltransferases p300 and pCAF [17, 18]. CSL/ICN/MAML transcriptional complexes also recruit kinases such as CDK8

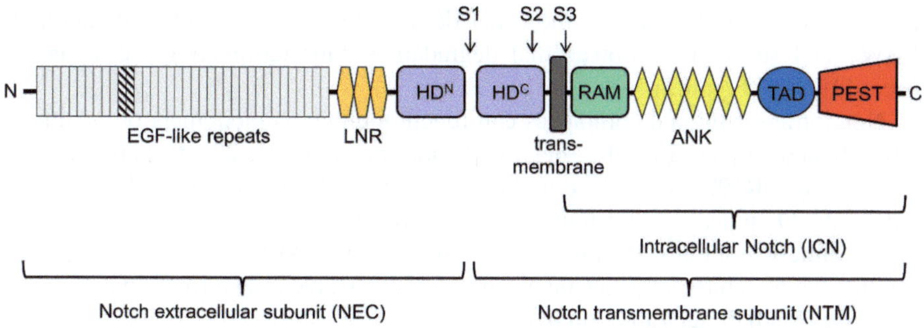

Fig. 8.1 Structure of human NOTCH1. *NOTCH1* is translated as a single polypeptide that is cleaved by a furin-like protease at the S1 site, yielding two subunits that non-covalently reassociate prior to trafficking to the cell surface. The extracellular subunit (NEC) includes epidermal growth factor (EGF) repeats 11–12 (cross-hatched bars) involved in ligand binding, three tandem Lin-12/Notch repeats (LNR), and the N-terminal portion of the heterodimerization domain (HD^N). The transmembrane subunit (NTM) includes the C-terminal portion of the HD (HD^C), a transmembrane domain, the Rbp-associated molecule (RAM) domain which binds CSL, ankyrin repeats (ANK), a transactivation domain (TAD), and a C-terminal negative regulatory proline/glutamic acid/serine/threonine-rich (PEST) domain. Ligand binding produces an allosteric structural change affecting the HD domain, exposing the S2 site to proteolytic cleavage by an ADAM metalloprotease. This reveals the S3 site, which is cleaved in turn by γ-secretase, releasing intracellular Notch (ICN) from the plasma membrane

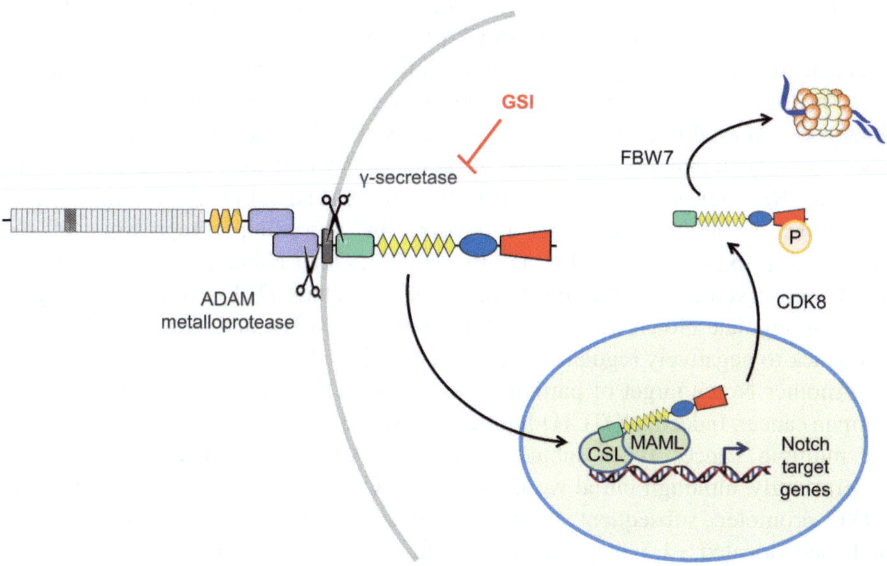

Fig. 8.2 The canonical Notch signaling pathway. Ligand binding induces sequential proteolytic cleavages by ADAM metalloprotease and γ-secretase, releasing ICN from the membrane. ICN then translocates to the nucleus where it forms a transcriptional complex with the DNA-binding factor CBF1/Suppressor of hairless/Lag-1 (CSL; also known as RBPJ) and the co-activator Mastermind-like (MAML) to drive expression of downstream target genes. Signaling is terminated by phosphorylation, ubiquitination, and ultimately proteasomal degradation of ICN. GSI γ-secretase inhibitor, CDK8 cyclin-dependent kinase 8, FBW7 F-box and WD repeat domain-containing 7

that phosphorylate ICN within the PEST domain, targeting it for ubiquitination by FBW7 and subsequent proteasomal degradation, thus terminating the signaling event [19, 20] (Fig. 8.2).

Notch transcriptional complexes can function either as monomers or as dimers when bound to paired head-to-head CSL-binding sites [21, 22]. In particular the ICN1 residue R1985 is involved in the interaction of ANK domains of ICN1 molecule [23]. Of note, specific mutations (e.g., R1985A) abrogate the formation of Notch dimeric complex and prevent the induction of T-ALL in mice [24], suggesting that the Notch target genes involved in leukemogenic transformation are modulated via Notch dimerization on paired sites.

8.1.2 Notch Target Genes

One recurring theme in Notch signaling is that the precise outcome of signaling is highly dependent on cellular and developmental context. Accordingly, Notch signaling may alternatively promote self-renewal or differentiation, proliferation or cell cycle arrest, and survival or apoptosis. These disparate cellular outcomes are presumably mediated in part by different complements of target genes activated, directly or indirectly, downstream of Notch. For instance, *CD25* [25], *PTCRA* [26], and *GATA3* [27] represent cell type-specific Notch targets and manifest developmental stage-specific cellular outcomes [28]. Despite this, some target genes are consistently downstream of Notch in multiple tissue contexts. Most notably, members of the Hairy/Enhancer of Split (*HES*) gene family are induced directly by Notch in several different tissue contexts besides T-ALL such as neural cells where they control cell fate and muscle and intestinal cells where they guide normal development. *HES* genes encode basic helix-loop-helix (bHLH) DNA-binding proteins that function as transcriptional repressors by recruiting corepressors of the transducing-like enhancer (TLE) family [29, 30]. Other Notch targets that are relatively conserved across different tissue contexts include *DTX1*, an ubiquitin ligase that can regulate Notch trafficking at the membrane [31], and *NRARP*, which can feedback to negatively regulate Notch signaling [32–34].

Another Notch target of particular interest is *MYC* due to its important role in human cancer. Indeed, NOTCH1 has been shown to induce *MYC* expression directly in multiple cancer types including T-ALL [35–38] and breast cancer [39]. Interestingly, although initial work focused on CSL-binding sites residing near the *MYC* promoter, subsequent studies revealed a critical Notch-dependent distal enhancer located ~1.5 megabases downstream of the human *MYC* gene that is broadly conserved between mammals, birds, and reptiles [35, 40, 41]. This enhancer was shown to loop back to the *MYC* promoter by chromatin conformation capture (3C) assay; however, the topology was stable despite γ-secretase inhibitor (GSI) treatment, implying that NOTCH1 occupancy is not required to maintain the chromatin loop. Other cancer-relevant Notch targets include *CCND1* [42] and the tumor suppressor *CDKN1A* [43].

8.2 Notch and Early Hematopoiesis

Notch plays important roles throughout hematopoietic development. Notch1 signaling is required very early in embryonic hematopoiesis including during development of the first definitive hematopoietic stem cells (HSC) [44, 45]. Subsequent fetal HSC development has also been shown to be dependent on NOTCH1 through the use of transactivation domain (TAD) mutant mice [46]. Initial gain-of-function experiments showed that NOTCH1 supported expansion of adult HSC [47, 48]; however, subsequent loss-of-function experiments showed Notch signaling to be dispensable for adult HSC maintenance [49], suggesting HSC expansion may represent an artifact of supraphysiological levels of signaling.

8.3 Notch and T-Cells

8.3.1 NOTCH1 Signaling in Normal T-Cell Development

Perhaps the greatest amount of work has focused on the role of Notch signaling in normal T-cell development. Both gain- and loss-of-function experiments have highlighted that NOTCH1 critically directs lymphoid progenitors in a binary fate decision between B and T lineages. In particular, inducible deletion of *Notch1* or *Rbpj* in hematopoietic progenitors suppresses T-cell development, resulting in accumulation of ectopic B-cells in the thymus, whereas constitutively activated NOTCH1 promotes T-cell differentiation within the marrow and at the expense of B-cells [50–52]. While both DLL1 [53] and DLL4 ligands [54] are capable of supporting T-cell development in vitro, stromal cues guiding NOTCH1 activation during normal intrathymic T-cell development are provided by the ligand DLL4 as expressed on thymic epithelial cells [55, 56], whereas DLL1 has been shown to be dispensable for this process [57]. NOTCH1 signaling can also influence binary cell fate decisions at later stages of T-cell development including between αβ and γδ lineages [58] and between CD4 and CD8 [59, 60] or Th1 and Th2 differentiation [61].

8.3.2 NOTCH1 Signaling in T-Cell Acute Lymphoblastic Leukemia (T-ALL)

The first evidence of an oncogenic role for Notch was the discovery of balanced t(7;9) translocations involving the T-cell receptor β (TRB) locus on chromosome 7 and the *NOTCH1* gene on chromosome 9 in rare cases of human T-ALL by Jeff Sklar's group [62]. This translocation resulted in expression of 5' truncated *NOTCH1* transcripts in developing T-cells which encoded constitutively active forms of the receptor [62]. As well, retroviral insertional mutagenesis screens in mice have reported that common proviral insertions occur near or within the extracellular negative regulatory region (NRR) of *Notch1* that presumably result in viral LTR-driven expression of similarly truncated forms of the receptor [63–66]. Subsequent work by Warren Pear and others demonstrated that enforced expression of similar N-terminally truncated forms of human NOTCH1 in mouse bone marrow-derived hematopoietic stem progenitor cells (HSPC) by retroviral transduction followed by transplantation into syngeneic recipients resulted in short-latency, high-penetrance T-ALL-like disease in mice [67–69]. The potency of activated NOTCH1 in producing T-ALL was also confirmed by distinct but similar experimental approaches including transgenic mice [70, 71] and transgenic zebrafish [72] and more recently by our own group, using human cord blood progenitors (Kusakabe et al., manuscript in preparation). Of note, less potently activated forms of NOTCH1 arrest T-cell development at the CD4+CD8+, or "double-positive" (DP) stage, but do not produce T-ALL disease, suggesting that increasing thresholds of NOTCH1 signaling are required for effects on T-cell development and transformation [73–75]. Importantly, inhibition of NOTCH1 in each of these settings results in reduced growth and/or apoptosis of T-ALL cells and can be accomplished either genetically with reagents like dominant-negative MAML1 (dnMAML1) [76] or pharmacologically with γ-secretase inhibitors (GSI) [76] or anti-NOTCH1 antibodies [77].

8.3.3 NOTCH1 Mutations in T-ALL

Despite work in mouse models, *NOTCH1* was generally regarded as a "boutique" oncogene in human T-ALL whose involvement was limited to those rare cases harboring the classic (7;9) chromosomal translocation. This view was revised following the discovery of point mutations and small indels in *NOTCH1* leading to gain-of-function in ~60% of human T-ALL by Jon Aster's group [78]. This discovery came as a result of screening human T-ALL cell lines for sensitivity to gamma-secretase inhibition as we had recently shown this was effective against mouse T-ALL generated with activated NOTCH1 [76]. As well, our motivation to look within the HD domain for mutations was critically informed by structural studies in Steve Blacklow's lab that suggested it played an important role in maintaining structural integrity of the receptor and restraining its activation [8]. Others have subsequently confirmed these findings in larger and varied cohorts using targeted or whole genome/exome sequencing [79–88] (Table 8.1).

Activating mutations in *NOTCH1* are distributed predominantly within the two regions, the heterodimerization (HD) domain and the C-terminal PEST domain. HD mutations occur in 40–45% of human T-ALL cases and can be divided in two distinct structural classes [99]. The more common class I mutations consist of small deletions involving at most a few amino acids, short in-frame insertions, or single amino acid substitutions within exons 26 and 27 that encode N- and C-terminal halves of the HD domain, respectively. These class I alterations maintain the reading frame and destabilize or completely disrupt physical association between the

Table 8.1 Frequencies of *NOTCH* mutations in hematologic malignancies

Disease	NOTCH receptor (domain)	Frequency of mutation	References
T-ALL	NOTCH1 (HD)	40–45%	[78–88]
	NOTCH1 (PEST)	20–25%	
CLL	NOTCH1 (PEST)	10–30% (mostly delCT)	[89–93]
MCL	NOTCH1 (PEST)	5–10%	[94, 95]
	NOTCH2 (PEST)	5%	
SMZL	NOTCH1 (PEST)	5%	[96, 97]
	NOTCH2 (PEST)	20–25% (mostly delCT)	
DLBCL	NOTCH2 (PEST)	8%	[98]

two HD subunits, thereby reducing the threshold for ligand-mediated activation or spontaneously activating the receptor outright, respectively [99]. Conversely, class II mutations are rare and consist of tandem insertions of 12–15 amino acids which duplicate the S2 cleavage site in the C-terminal portion of the HD domain. The presumed mechanism for activation by class II mutations is informed by structural studies of the extracellular negative regulatory region (NRR), which would predict that the duplicated HD region places an extra S2 cleavage site beyond the protection of the NRR [9, 10]. Yet a third but again rare type of activating *NOTCH1* mutation, so-called juxtamembrane expansion (JME), introduces additional in-frame amino acids just external to the cell membrane and proximal to the HD domain which render the receptor more susceptible to S2 cleavage, possibly by destabilizing interaction of the otherwise intact NRR/HD complex with integral membrane proteins or allowing intramembrane proteases illegitimate access to the base of the receptor stalk [100].

Genetic alterations within the C-terminal PEST domain occur in 20–25% of T-ALL cases and consist of nonsense and frameshift mutations that lead to premature stop codons [78]. These truncated polypeptides lack critical portions of the PEST domain required for ubiquitination and proteolytic turnover of intracellular NOTCH1 (ICN1) [101, 102]. The deleted region of the PEST domain consistently includes a highly conserved sequence, ^{2521}WSSSSP^{2526}, which contains important phosphorylation site(s) that are required for subsequent ubiquitination [103]. Other common deletions fall between the ^{2482}FLTPPSQ^{2488} and ^{2510}FLTPSPE^{2516} sequences, each of which are recognized by E3 ligase complexes containing the F-box protein FBW7 and are similar to the ^{55}LLPTPPLSP^{63} sequence present in MYC that regulates its proteolytic turnover [104]. The ultimate result of these alterations is reduced proteolytic turnover of ICN1 and prolonged duration of signaling following receptor activation.

It remains unresolved which kinases modulate activity and turnover of ICN1. It has been reported that the cyclin-dependent kinase 8 (CDK8) interacts physically with the Notch transcriptional complex (ICN1, Mastermind-like-1 (MAML1), and CSL) and phosphorylates specific serine residues on ICN1 including S2514, S2517, and S2539 [19]. These phosphorylation events are then thought to target ICN1 for subsequent ubiquitination and proteasomal degradation. Accordingly, mutations affecting these residues could lead to reduced ICN1 turnover and prolonged duration of signaling that could contribute to T-ALL pathogenesis.

Akin to NOTCH1 PEST deletion, there is also biological selection in T-ALL for inactivating mutations in *FBW7*, the ubiquitin ligase that is responsible for targeting ICN1 for proteasomal degradation. Inactivating *FBW7* mutations occur in 10–20% of T-ALL and are mutually exclusive to *NOTCH1* PEST mutations [79, 101, 102, 105, 106]. Of course, FBW7 is responsible for the degradation of other proteins in the cell, among which include MYC [107, 108], and thus inactivation of FBW7 may support T-ALL pathogenesis in multiple, potentially synergistic ways. About 15% of T-ALL cases harbor both HD and PEST *NOTCH1* mutations in *cis* [78], and 5–10% harbor a *NOTCH1* HD mutation along with an *FBW7* mutation [79, 101, 102], both of which presumably lead to synergistic hyperactivation of NOTCH1 signaling.

Similar *Notch1* mutations involving the PEST domain also occur with high frequency in nearly all mouse models of T-ALL [109–115]. The paucity of spontaneous HD mutations in mouse models is presumably due to the prevalence of illegitimate RAG-dependent recombination within the mouse *Notch1* locus that deletes 5′ exons and results in expression of truncated peptides similar to those created by the t(7;9) in human disease [116]. Of note, irradiated SCID or $ATM^{-/-}$ mice also develop T-cell leukemias that also show frequent deletions in the proximal promoter and express similar N-terminally truncated NOTCH1 polypeptides [115]. These data reinforce the notion that there is strong selective pressure for activation of NOTCH1 signaling in T-cell transformation and support its prominent role in T-ALL pathogenesis, even in other organisms.

8.3.4 Clinical Significance of NOTCH1 Mutations in T-ALL

The presence of recurrent activating mutations in NOTCH1 raises the question whether these have any biologic or prognostic significance. Early studies showed that the activating mutations in *NOTCH1* correlated with improved clinical outcome, but subsequent studies suggest that this association is dependent on the therapeutic protocol [80, 83, 84]. More recent efforts to resolve this issue showed that *NOTCH1* and *FBW7* mutations were indeed associated with improved response to chemotherapy and in particular to glucocorticoids; however, this early benefit did not consistently translate into improvement in survival [117–119]. Moreover, *NOTCH1/FBW7* mutations were either not prognostic or possibly portended a worse outcome among high-risk patients. Of note, the association between activating *NOTCH1* mutations and improved response to glucocorticoid therapy did not affirm prior work that showed Notch inhibition with GSI could reverse glucocorticoid resistance [120], implying that such relationships are likely highly dependent upon genetic context.

8.3.5 Genes and Pathways Downstream of NOTCH1 in T-ALL

Several groups have contributed to defining the complement of genes and pathways which are ultimately activated downstream of NOTCH1 and that are functionally relevant to T-ALL pathogenesis (Fig. 8.3). Besides those already mentioned above, expression of *NOTCH3* is also induced by NOTCH1 in T-ALL [35, 38]. As there is substantial homology between ICN1 and ICN3, it is notable that ICN3 generates T-cell leukemia in mice similarly to ICN1 [70, 75, 121, 122]; however, deletion of *Notch3* has no effect on leukemia induction in the hypomorphic Ikaros-driven mouse T-ALL model, whereas deletion of *Rbpj* introduces a substantial delay [123], and spontaneous mutations in *NOTCH3* are conspicuously lacking in human T-ALL.

Activated NOTCH1 can potentiate PI3K/AKT/mTOR signaling by several means including repression of *PTEN* through HES1 [124] or upregulation of receptor tyrosine kinases (RTK) such as IL7 receptor (*IL7R*) [125, 126] and insulin-like growth factor 1 receptor (*IGF1R*) [127] (Fig. 8.3). Importantly, inhibiting PI3K/AKT/mTOR or upstream RTKs results in reduced growth and/or survival of T-ALL cells both in vitro and in vivo. Of note, PTEN loss, either by mutation [111, 124], silencing [128], or inactivation [129], can contribute to Notch-independent T-ALL cell growth by compensating for reduced Notch-dependent glutaminolysis with enhanced aerobic glycolysis [130]. This mechanism is indeed operative in many, but

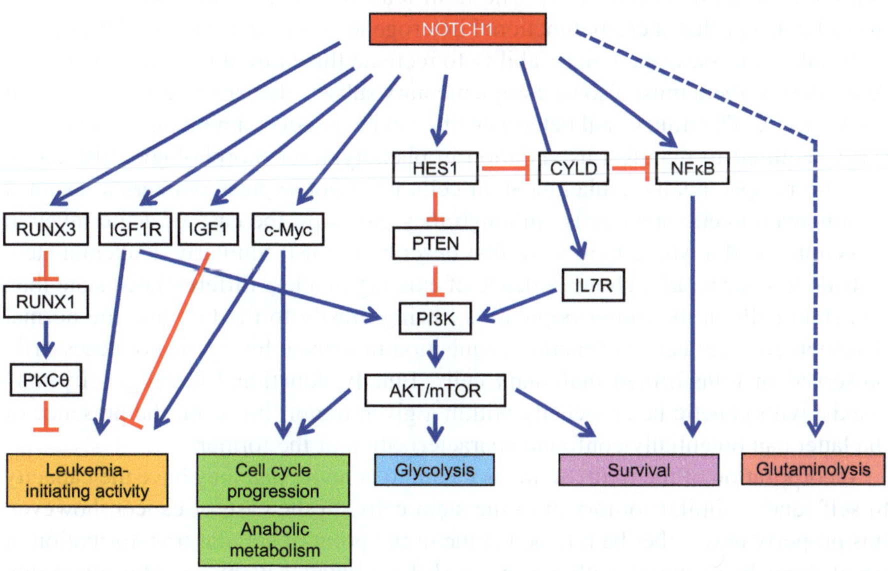

Fig. 8.3 Genes and pathways downstream of NOTCH1 in T-ALL. See text for details. RUNX3 runt-related transcription factor 3, RUNX1 runt-related transcription factor 1, PKCθ protein kinase C theta, IGF1R insulin-like growth factor 1 receptor, IGF1 insulin-like growth factor 1, c-Myc myelocytomatosis, HES1 hairy/enhancer of split 1, PTEN phosphatase and tensin homolog, PI3K phosphoinositide 3-kinase, mTOR mammalian target of rapamycin, CYLD cylindromatosis, NFκB nuclear factor kappa-light-chain-enhancer of activated B-cells, IL7R interleukin-7 receptor

not all contexts [131]. As well, the observation that PTEN loss accelerates NOTCH1-induced leukemogenesis [131] would support the notion that NOTCH1 and PI3K/AKT pathways function collaboratively and provide nonredundant contributions to T-ALL pathogenesis.

Other work has revealed interaction between NFκB and Notch pathways in T-ALL. Indeed, mouse T-cell leukemias, induced by activated NOTCH1 or NOTCH3, show high levels of NFκB activity [70, 132]. NOTCH1 induces NFκB activity directly by upregulating transcription of *Relb* and *Nfkb2* [133, 134], enhancing NFκB nuclear retention [135], and interacting physically with the IKK complex [134]. NOTCH1 also promotes NFκB activity indirectly by HES1-dependent repression of *CYLD*, a deubiquitinase that negatively regulates the IKK complex [136] (Fig. 8.3). Importantly, inhibition of NFκB activity antagonizes T-ALL cell growth/survival in vitro and in vivo [70, 134, 136].

8.3.6 NOTCH1 and Leukemia Stem Cells

Leukemia stem cells (and cancer stem cells more generally) have had a murky history, fraught with confusing and inconsistent use of terminology and misconceptions regarding what are core aspects of the concept versus what are related but non-requisite associations [137]. The term leukemia stem cells encompasses the overall concept that there is functional heterogeneity within a tumor whereby discrete subsets possess the unique ability to recreate the entire tumor in a naïve host. Accordingly, there must also be complementary subsets that are relatively devoid of such activity. This functional heterogeneity can be associated with but is not necessarily required to manifest as variation in phenotypic or morphologic differentiation. More specifically, leukemia stem cells need not express markers associated with hematopoietic stem cells, although they can as in the case of acute myeloid leukemia (AML) where they were first described [138]. Similarly, leukemia stem cells do not necessarily show evidence of existing in a less differentiated state than non-stem cells in the tumor population, owing mostly to the fact that the normal developmental sequence of marker acquisition in a given lineage is not necessarily preserved in transformed malignant cells. Finally, functional heterogeneity may coexist with genetic heterogeneity within a given tumor; however, the presence of the latter can potentially confound characterization of the former.

Incorporation of the term "stem" is meant to connote that they have the capacity to self-renew, similar to normal tissue stem cells. In the case of cancer, however, this property may either be retained at the initial point of cellular transformation or spontaneously acquired within a more differentiated cell by genetic alteration. Literally, this translates to the notion that leukemia stem cells are cancer cells that have stemlike properties and are not necessarily cancerous versions of normal tissue stem cells. As an experimental approach, serial transplantation (often performed at limiting dilution) into a naïve host is the gold standard for documenting that leukemia stem cells are indeed present within a given test population; however, the assay itself actually measures so-called leukemia-initiating cell, or LIC, activity which is read out solely by the presence or absence of disease in the transplanted recipient [137].

In human T-ALL, several groups have demonstrated asymmetric localization of LIC activity within tumor subpopulations defined by surface markers including CD7, CD1a, and CD34 [139–141]. As well, LIC have been characterized within various mouse models of T-ALL [107, 142–147]. Signaling through NOTCH1 has been shown both in human and mouse T-ALL to sustain LIC activity [145, 148–150]. Work from our own group and others has identified *IGF1R*, *IGF1*, *PKCθ*, and *MYC* as relevant downstream targets of NOTCH1 that mediate its effects in supporting LIC [127, 149, 151] (Fig. 8.3). Implication of *MYC* has also prompted studies involving selective BET bromodomain inhibitors (e.g., JQ-1) that can potently silence *MYC* expression by epigenetic means and thus may represent a viable therapeutic strategy whose target range specifically includes LIC [107, 152]. Our work highlighting the transcriptional circuit linking NOTCH1 to repression of *PKCθ* and reactive oxygen species (ROS) via *RUNX3* and *RUNX1* also raises the possibility of targeting these other elements to specifically antagonize LIC [149].

8.4 Notch and B-Cells

8.4.1 Notch Signaling in Normal B-Cell Development

Although NOTCH1 signaling favors commitment of lymphoid progenitors to the T-cell lineage at the expense of B-cells, NOTCH2 has been shown to play a role later in B-cell development where it guides binary cell fate decisions between marginal zone (MZ) and follicular B-cells in the mouse spleen. Expression of *Notch2* increases with B-cell maturation, and deletion of either *Notch2* itself or *Rbpj* results in a complete failure of MZ B-cell development [153, 154]. This role of Notch signaling in MZ B-cell development was further confirmed in studies that knocked out other elements of the Notch signaling apparatus including MAML1 [155], DLL1 [57, 156], MIB1 [157], and ADAM10 [158], but interestingly does not require HES1 [159].

8.4.2 Notch Signaling in B-Cell Acute Lymphoblastic Leukemia (B-ALL)

Given the trophic effect of Notch activation on T-cell fate and leukemogenesis, yet suppressive role on early B-cell differentiation, it is notable that enforced expression of active forms of all four Notch receptors (ICN1-4) induced growth arrest and apoptosis in immature B-ALL cell lines which could be recapitulated by HES1 alone [3, 160]. Similar effects were seen in myeloma and Hodgkin cell lines. Subsequent work has shown that Notch/HES pathway elements are epigenetically silenced in B-ALL cell lines and patient samples as compared to T-ALL [161], supporting that signaling through Notch/HES is incompatible with the generation and/or maintenance of early B-cell malignancies.

8.4.3 Notch Signaling in Chronic Lymphocytic Leukemia (CLL)

CLL is a very common, low-grade malignancy of mature B-cells characterized by infrequently dividing but long-lived cells. The more aggressive form is thought to arise from naïve CD5+ B-cells with unmutated *IGHV* genes, whereas the less aggressive form shows *IGHV* mutations consistent with derivation from post-germinal center B-cells [162]. Early work showed NOTCH2 was responsible for driving expression of *CD23* [163], and aberrant activation of NOTCH1 and/or NOTCH2 supported survival/resistance to apoptosis via increased NFκB activity [164]. Mutations involving *NOTCH1* were first reported among 2 of 43 patients in 2009, and subsequent larger studies demonstrated *NOTCH1* mutations in about 10% of CLL cases at diagnosis, with higher incidence ~20% among patients with chemorefractory disease and ~30% in cases that had progressed/undergone Richter transformation [89–91]. While *NOTCH1* mutations in T-ALL target both HD and PEST domains, mutations in CLL are restricted to the PEST domain, and strikingly, over 80% of these are represented by the exact same 2bp deletion (ΔCT75447545, P2515fs) that results in frameshift and premature stop codon to delete the PEST degron. With more sensitive, allele-specific PCR-based methodologies, the *NOTCH1* c.7544_7545delCT PEST mutational frequency has been reported as high as 20% among unselected patients [93] and even higher at ~74% among trisomy 21 patients (C. Hoofd et al., manuscript in preparation) [165, 166]. Though *NOTCH1* PEST mutations are associated with unmutated *IGHV* genes and wild-type *TP53*, they represent an unfavorable prognostic factor independent of both *IGHV* and *TP53* status [91, 167, 168]. Mutations within the noncoding region of NOTCH1 have also been reported to occur in CLL that cause aberrant splicing and result in expression of truncated forms lacking the C-terminal PEST domain [169].

Immunohistochemical studies that are able to detect activated ICN1 in the nucleus of CLL cells have revealed the pathway to be activated in nearly 90% cases, occurring similarly in *NOTCH1* mutated and non-mutated groups [170, 171]. NOTCH1 activation is lost rapidly in vitro, irrespective of mutational status [172], suggesting that signaling relies upon stroma-derived ligand within the tumor microenvironment.

8.4.4 Notch Signaling in Mantle Cell Lymphoma (MCL)

Mantle cell lymphoma (MCL) is a less common but more aggressive type of mature B-cell non-Hodgkin lymphoma that is molecularly defined by the t(11;14)(q13;q32) chromosomal translocation which results in overexpression of cyclin D1 (CCND1) [173]. Our group identified gain-of-function *NOTCH1* mutations, nearly exclusively by PEST deletion, to occur in 12% of MCL cases ($n = 108$) and to be associated with poor prognosis [94]. Half of these were represented by the c.7544_7545delCT mutation seen in CLL. A subsequent study found *NOTCH1* and *NOTCH2* mutations each to occur at ~5% among a cohort of 172 MCL cases, were restricted to the PEST domain, and tended not to co-occur within the same tumor [95]. *NOTCH1/2* mutations in this cohort were also associated with poor clinical outcome. In contrast to CLL, immunohistochemical staining for ICN1 failed to reveal evidence for widespread activation of NOTCH1 in MCL tissues [170, 171].

8.4.5 Notch Signaling in Splenic Marginal Zone Lymphoma (SMZL)

Splenic marginal zone lymphoma (SMZL) is another uncommon but indolent mature B-cell non-Hodgkin lymphoma with recurrent chromosome 7q deletions [174] and activation of the NFκB pathway [175]. SMZL has been associated with hepatitis C virus (HCV) infection [176], and interestingly, some patients show responses to antiviral therapy [177]. The role of NOTCH2 in MZ B-cell development in mice perhaps portended the finding by two groups of recurrent *NOTCH2* mutations in ~20–25% of SMZL cases, again with a preponderance resulting in deletion of the C-terminal PEST domain, but a rare activating HD mutation was also observed [96, 97]. The clinical significance of *NOTCH2* mutations in SMZL remains unclear, however, as the two studies reported opposite results for their respective patient cohorts (longer overall survival, $n = 94$ vs. shorter relapse-free survival, $n = 46$). Of note, one of the studies also identified the *NOTCH1* c.7544_7545delCT mutation to occur at ~5% within their SMZL cohort [96, 97]. As in MCL, identified *NOTCH1* and *NOTCH2* mutations in SMZL were mutually exclusive.

8.4.6 Notch Signaling in Other Non-Hodgkin Lymphomas

Follicular lymphoma (FL) is one of the most common nodal non-Hodgkin lymphomas, second only to diffuse large B-cell lymphoma (DLBCL). While many cases of FL are indolent and slow-growing, approximately 2–3% of FL patients per year will undergo histologic transformation to a more aggressive lymphoma, often DLBCL [178]. As reported in abstract form, mutations in *NOTCH1* and *NOTCH2* were identified in FL to occur at a combined frequency of ~6% (five mutations in *NOTCH1* and two mutations in *NOTCH2* among a cohort of 114 FL cases) [179]. These mutations were all predicted to encode truncated proteins lacking the C-terminal PEST domain. Formal publication of this study, however, remains pending.

Recurrent mutations in *NOTCH2* were reported to occur in ~8% of DLBCL cases ($n = 63$) and were represented mostly as causing deletion of the PEST domain [98]. Mutations in both *NOTCH1* and *NOTCH2* have also been identified in DLBCL associated with HCV infection, occurring at frequencies of 4% and 26%, respectively, among of cohort of 46 cases [180]. These mutations were also exclusively of the PEST deletion variety and were associated with poor clinical outcome in this small cohort. Given the association between HCV and SMZL and the similarities in *NOTCH1/2* mutation frequency and pattern with that observed in SMZL, it remains possible that these cases of HCV-associated DLBCL may have arisen by transformation from a preexistent but unrecognized SMZL clone.

Multiple myeloma (MM) is a malignancy of terminally differentiated plasma cells that typically affects older adults. While recurrent gene mutations affecting the Notch pathway have not been reported in this disease, several studies have shown upregulation of Notch receptors and/or ligands including NOTCH1, NOTCH2, JAG1, and JAG2 [181, 182]. Moreover, pharmacologic inhibition of Notch signaling has been shown to prevent localization of MM cells to the bone marrow [183] and enhance their sensitivity to chemotherapy [184].

8.4.7 Notch Signaling in Classical Hodgkin Lymphoma

Classical Hodgkin lymphoma is characterized by a relatively minor proportion of malignant Hodgkin and Reed-Sternberg (HRS) cells that are thought to derive from "crippled" germinal center B-cells [185] and which secrete abundant cytokines, resulting in the bulk of the tumor mass being composed of infiltrating reactive immune cells. Immunohistochemical studies have revealed that HRS cells within patient tumors express both NOTCH1 and JAG1 highly, and that nearby stromal cells also express JAG1 [184, 186, 187], suggesting that ligand-dependent activation of Notch signaling in HRS cells may occur by homo- and heterotypic cell interactions. Cultured HRS cell lines express both NOTCH1 and NOTCH2 and respond to JAG1 ligand with increased proliferation and reduced apoptosis. Additional cell line studies from the same group have suggested that Notch signaling supports cell survival through activation of the alternative NFκB pathway [188].

8.5 Notch and Myeloid Cells

8.5.1 Notch Signaling in Normal Myeloid Development

The role of Notch signaling in myeloid development is ambiguous as several reports have suggested that Notch activation may alternately promote or inhibit various aspects of granulocyte/monocyte differentiation [189–192], yet conditional knock-out of *Rbpj* and enforced expression of dominant-negative MAML1 both showed no impairment of myeloid lineage commitment or differentiation [49, 51]. As well, there are conflicting reports that Notch signaling either promotes or antagonizes megakaryocyte differentiation [193, 194]. Taken together, these studies suggest that Notch plays a complex role in myeloid cell fate decisions that will require further study to resolve.

8.5.2 Notch Signaling in Myeloid Leukemia

Early studies have found that despite high expression of NOTCH1 receptors in acute myelogenous leukemia (AML) patients, activation of the pathway was limited [195, 196]. Moreover, exposure to DLL1 and JAG1 ligands produced variable outcomes in terms of short-term growth of primary patient AML blasts [197] which echoed prior findings with established AML cell lines [198, 199]. More recently, a pair of studies examined gene expression profile data from large cohorts of AML patients and confirmed the expression of multiple Notch receptors; however, pathway activation was again found to be limited compared to normal hematopoietic cells [200, 201]. Interestingly, enforced expression of activated NOTCH1 (ICN1) blocked proliferation and induced apoptosis in AML cell lines and patient samples and antagonized LIC activity in an MLL-AF9-induced mouse model of AML. As well, enforced expression of HES1, a transcriptional repressor immediately downstream of Notch, led to growth arrest both in vitro and in a xenograft mouse model [200, 202], an effect that may be mediated through repression of *FLT3* [203].

Mice doubly deleted for *Notch1/Notch2* or just nicastrin (*Ncstn*), a component of the γ-secretase complex responsible for activation of Notch receptors, leads to the development of a myeloproliferative disorder in mice [204]. Additional studies showed that loss of nicastrin in multipotent hematopoietic progenitors was associated with induction of a broad myeloid transcriptional program, an effect that was reversed in part by enforced expression of HES1. These findings led the investigators to search for evidence of loss of Notch signaling function in human myeloproliferative disorders, and indeed they found 6 somatic loss-of-function mutations involving *NCSTN*, *APH1*, *MAML1*, and *NOTCH2* within 5 of 42 samples (12%) from patients with chronic myelomonocytic leukemia (CMML). Taken together, these studies support the notion that Notch signaling may act as a tumor suppressor in the myeloid cell context and that therapies that activate Notch signaling may have clinical utility in myeloproliferative disease.

8.6 Therapeutic Approaches to Target the Notch Pathway

The relevance of Notch signaling in T-ALL and other hematologic malignancies has created interest in the development of various pharmacologic modulators of the pathway. The first volley of agents were small molecule inhibitors of γ-secretase, which is required for proteolytic cleavage of all four Notch receptors and liberation of their respective ICN subunits from the plasma membrane. γ-Secretase inhibitors, or GSIs, were ripe for plucking as these drugs were already in clinical development to prevent processing and accumulation of β-amyloid from amyloid precursor protein (APP), a candidate etiology in Alzheimer's disease progression [205]. The antitumoral activity of several GSIs (e.g., MRK-003, MRK-0752, and RO4929097) has been already tested in mouse models of T-ALL in phase I clinical trials for patients with relapsed T-ALL [206–209]. These efforts were stymied, however, by dose-limiting toxicities primarily affecting the gut where pan-Notch inhibition leads to goblet cell hyperplasia and resultant severe diarrhea. Subsequent work revealed that this effect required inhibition of both NOTCH1 and NOTCH2 in intestinal crypt progenitors [210, 211] but could be ameliorated either by intermittent dosing [208] or rescue with glucocorticoids [120].

Another strategy proposed the use of chemically stapled α-helical peptides [212] similar to dnMAML1 [76, 213] to render the Notch transcriptional complex functionally inert; however, this approach has remained in the research literature thus far.

Antibodies have also been designed against specific regions of Notch receptors, specifically the negative regulatory region (NRR), on the premise that these would help to stabilize the receptor heterodimer and restrict ADAM protease-mediated receptor cleavage and activation, induced either by ligand binding or mutations involving the HD domain [77, 214–217]. One issue that has arisen, however, is lower activity of NRR-directed antibodies as compared to GSI, possibly due to incomplete allosteric inhibition of the ligand-induced conformational change [214]. Other targets for therapeutic antibodies include the ligand-binding EGF repeats of Notch receptors, or alternatively, the ligands themselves [218, 219]. Identification of additional targets, including those effectors downstream of Notch signaling that contribute ultimately to enacting cellular phenotypes, as well as further development of specific pharmacologic agents will be required to capitalize upon our knowledge of the role Notch signaling plays in human disease.

References

1. Wang, Y., Shao, L., Shi, S., et al. (2001). Modification of epidermal growth factor-like repeats with O-fucose. Molecular cloning and expression of a novel GDP-fucose protein O-fucosyltransferase. *The Journal of Biological Chemistry, 276*, 40338–40345.
2. Ju, B. G., Jeong, S., Bae, E., et al. (2000). Fringe forms a complex with Notch. *Nature, 405*, 191–195.
3. Lubman, O. Y., Ilagan, M. X., Kopan, R., et al. (2007). Quantitative dissection of the Notch:CSL interaction: Insights into the Notch-mediated transcriptional switch. *Journal of Molecular Biology, 365*, 577–589.
4. Shimizu, K., Chiba, S., Kumano, K., et al. (1999). Mouse jagged1 physically interacts with notch2 and other notch receptors. Assessment by quantitative methods. *The Journal of Biological Chemistry, 274*, 32961–32969.
5. Ohishi, K., Katayama, N., Shiku, H., et al. (2003). Notch signalling in hematopoiesis. *Seminars in Cell & Developmental Biology, 14*, 143–150.
6. Logeat, F., Bessia, C., Brou, C., et al. (1998). The Notch1 receptor is cleaved constitutively by a furin-like convertase. *Proceedings of the National Academy of Sciences of the United States of America, 95*, 8108–8112.
7. Rand, M. D., Grimm, L. M., Artavanis-Tsakonas, S., et al. (2000). Calcium depletion dissociates and activates heterodimeric notch receptors. *Molecular and Cellular Biology, 20*, 1825–1835.
8. Sanchez-Irizarry, C., Carpenter, A. C., Weng, A. P., et al. (2004). Notch subunit heterodimerization and prevention of ligand-independent proteolytic activation depend, respectively, on a novel domain and the LNR repeats. *Molecular and Cellular Biology, 24*, 9265–9273.
9. Gordon, W. R., Vardar-Ulu, D., Histen, G., et al. (2007). Structural basis for autoinhibition of Notch. *Nature Structural & Molecular Biology, 14*, 295–300.
10. Gordon, W. R., Roy, M., Vardar-Ulu, D., et al. (2009). Structure of the Notch1-negative regulatory region: Implications for normal activation and pathogenic signaling in T-ALL. *Blood, 113*, 4381–4390.
11. van Tetering, G., van Diest, P., Verlaan, I., et al. (2009). Metalloprotease ADAM10 is required for Notch1 site 2 cleavage. *The Journal of Biological Chemistry, 284*, 31018–31027.
12. Bozkulak, E. C., & Weinmaster, G. (2009). Selective use of ADAM10 and ADAM17 in activation of Notch1 signaling. *Molecular and Cellular Biology, 29*, 5679–5695.
13. Gordon Wendy, R., Zimmerman, B., He, L., et al. (2015). Mechanical allostery: Evidence for a force requirement in the proteolytic activation of Notch. *Developmental Cell, 33*, 729–736.
14. Rechsteiner, M., & Rogers, S. W. (1996). PEST sequences and regulation by proteolysis. *Trends in Biochemical Sciences, 21*, 267–271.
15. Lai, E. C. (2002). Keeping a good pathway down: Transcriptional repression of Notch pathway target genes by CSL proteins. *EMBO Reports, 3*, 840–845.
16. Liefke, R., Oswald, F., Alvarado, C., et al. (2010). Histone demethylase KDM5A is an integral part of the core Notch-RBP-J repressor complex. *Genes & Development, 24*, 590–601.
17. Oswald, F., Tauber, B., Dobner, T., et al. (2001). p300 acts as a transcriptional coactivator for mammalian notch-1. *Molecular and Cellular Biology, 21*, 7761–7774.
18. Wallberg, A. E., Pedersen, K., Lendahl, U., et al. (2002). p300 and PCAF act cooperatively to mediate transcriptional activation from chromatin templates by notch intracellular domains in vitro. *Molecular and Cellular Biology, 22*, 7812–7819.
19. Fryer, C. J., White, J. B., & Jones, K. A. (2004). Mastermind recruits CycC:CDK8 to phosphorylate the Notch ICD and coordinate activation with turnover. *Molecular Cell, 16*, 509–520.
20. Oberg, C., Li, J., Pauley, A., et al. (2001). The notch intracellular domain is ubiquitinated and negatively regulated by the mammalian sel-10 homolog. *The Journal of Biological Chemistry, 276*, 35847–35853.

21. Ehebauer, M. T., Chirgadze, D. Y., Hayward, P., et al. (2005). High-resolution crystal structure of the human Notch 1 ankyrin domain. *The Biochemical Journal, 392*, 13–20.
22. Nam, Y., Sliz, P., Song, L., et al. (2006). Structural basis for cooperativity in recruitment of MAML coactivators to Notch transcription complexes. *Cell, 124*, 973–983.
23. Nam, Y., Sliz, P., Pear, W. S., et al. (2007). Cooperative assembly of higher-order Notch complexes functions as a switch to induce transcription. *Proceedings of the National Academy of Sciences of the United States of America, 104*, 2103–2108.
24. Liu, H., Chi, A. W., Arnett, K. L., et al. (2010). Notch dimerization is required for leukemogenesis and T-cell development. *Genes & Development, 24*, 2395–2407.
25. Adler, S. H., Chiffoleau, E., Xu, L., et al. (2003). Notch signaling augments T cell responsiveness by enhancing CD25 expression. *Journal of Immunology, 171*, 2896–2903.
26. Reizis, B., & Leder, P. (2002). Direct induction of T lymphocyte-specific gene expression by the mammalian Notch signaling pathway. *Genes & Development, 16*, 295–300.
27. Ho, I. C., Tai, T. S., & Pai, S. Y. (2009). GATA3 and the T-cell lineage: Essential functions before and after T-helper-2-cell differentiation. *Nature Reviews. Immunology, 9*, 125–135.
28. Borggrefe, T., & Oswald, F. (2009). The Notch signaling pathway: Transcriptional regulation at Notch target genes. *Cellular and Molecular Life Sciences, 66*, 1631–1646.
29. Grbavec, D., & Stifani, S. (1996). Molecular interaction between TLE1 and the carboxyl-terminal domain of HES-1 containing the WRPW motif. *Biochemical and Biophysical Research Communications, 223*, 701–705.
30. Fischer, A., & Gessler, M. (2007). Delta-Notch–and then? Protein interactions and proposed modes of repression by Hes and Hey bHLH factors. *Nucleic Acids Research, 35*, 4583–4596.
31. Mukherjee, A., Veraksa, A., Bauer, A., et al. (2005). Regulation of Notch signalling by non-visual beta-arrestin. *Nature Cell Biology, 7*, 1191–1201.
32. Matsuno, K., Diederich, R. J., Go, M. J., et al. (1995). Deltex acts as a positive regulator of Notch signaling through interactions with the Notch ankyrin repeats. *Development, 121*, 2633–2644.
33. Lamar, E., Deblandre, G., Wettstein, D., et al. (2001). Nrarp is a novel intracellular component of the Notch signaling pathway. *Genes & Development, 15*, 1885–1899.
34. Yun, T. J., & Bevan, M. J. (2003). Notch-regulated ankyrin-repeat protein inhibits Notch1 signaling: Multiple Notch1 signaling pathways involved in T cell development. *Journal of Immunology, 170*, 5834–5841.
35. Weng, A. P., Millholland, J. M., Yashiro-Ohtani, Y., et al. (2006). c-Myc is an important direct target of Notch1 in T-cell acute lymphoblastic leukemia/lymphoma. *Genes & Development, 20*, 2096–2109.
36. Sharma, V. M., Calvo, J. A., Draheim, K. M., et al. (2006). Notch1 contributes to mouse T-cell leukemia by directly inducing the expression of c-myc. *Molecular and Cellular Biology, 26*, 8022–8031.
37. Li, X., Gounari, F., Protopopov, A., et al. (2008a). Oncogenesis of T-ALL and nonmalignant consequences of overexpressing intracellular NOTCH1. *The Journal of Experimental Medicine, 205*, 2851–2861.
38. Palomero, T., Lim, W. K., Odom, D. T., et al. (2006). NOTCH1 directly regulates c-MYC and activates a feed-forward-loop transcriptional network promoting leukemic cell growth. *Proceedings of the National Academy of Sciences of the United States of America, 103*, 18261–18266.
39. Klinakis, A., Szabolcs, M., Politi, K., et al. (2006). Myc is a Notch1 transcriptional target and a requisite for Notch1-induced mammary tumorigenesis in mice. *Proceedings of the National Academy of Sciences of the United States of America, 103*, 9262–9267.
40. Yashiro-Ohtani, Y., Wang, H., Zang, C., et al. (2014). Long-range enhancer activity determines Myc sensitivity to Notch inhibitors in T cell leukemia. *Proceedings of the National Academy of Sciences of the United States of America, 111*, E4946–E4953.

41. Herranz, D., Ambesi-Impiombato, A., Palomero, T., et al. (2014). A NOTCH1-driven MYC enhancer promotes T cell development, transformation and acute lymphoblastic leukemia. *Nature Medicine, 20*, 1130–1137.
42. Cohen, B., Shimizu, M., Izrailit, J., et al. (2010). Cyclin D1 is a direct target of JAG1-mediated Notch signaling in breast cancer. *Breast Cancer Research and Treatment, 123*, 113–124.
43. Rangarajan, A., Talora, C., Okuyama, R., et al. (2001). Notch signaling is a direct determinant of keratinocyte growth arrest and entry into differentiation. *The EMBO Journal, 20*, 3427–3436.
44. Kumano, K., Chiba, S., Kunisato, A., et al. (2003). Notch1 but not Notch2 is essential for generating hematopoietic stem cells from endothelial cells. *Immunity, 18*, 699–711.
45. Hadland, B. K., Huppert, S. S., Kanungo, J., et al. (2004). A requirement for Notch1 distinguishes 2 phases of definitive hematopoiesis during development. *Blood, 104*, 3097–3105.
46. Gerhardt, D. M., Pajcini, K. V., D'Altri, T., et al. (2014). The Notch1 transcriptional activation domain is required for development and reveals a novel role for Notch1 signaling in fetal hematopoietic stem cells. *Genes & Development, 28*, 576–593.
47. Stier, S., Cheng, T., Dombkowski, D., et al. (2002). Notch1 activation increases hematopoietic stem cell self-renewal in vivo and favors lymphoid over myeloid lineage outcome. *Blood, 99*, 2369–2378.
48. Varnum-Finney, B., Wu, L., Yu, M., et al. (2000). Immobilization of Notch ligand, Delta-1, is required for induction of notch signaling. *Journal of Cell Science, 113*(Pt 23), 4313–4318.
49. Maillard, I., Koch, U., Dumortier, A., et al. (2008a). Canonical notch signaling is dispensable for the maintenance of adult hematopoietic stem cells. *Cell Stem Cell, 2*, 356–366.
50. Radtke, F., Wilson, A., Stark, G., et al. (1999). Deficient T cell fate specification in mice with an induced inactivation of Notch1. *Immunity, 10*, 547–558.
51. Han, H., Tanigaki, K., Yamamoto, N., et al. (2002). Inducible gene knockout of transcription factor recombination signal binding protein-J reveals its essential role in T versus B lineage decision. *International Immunology, 14*, 637–645.
52. Pui, J. C., Allman, D., Xu, L., et al. (1999). Notch1 expression in early lymphopoiesis influences B versus T lineage determination. *Immunity, 11*, 299–308.
53. Schmitt, T. M., & Zuniga-Pflucker, J. C. (2002). Induction of T cell development from hematopoietic progenitor cells by delta-like-1 in vitro. *Immunity, 17*, 749–756.
54. Mohtashami, M., Shah, D. K., Nakase, H., et al. (2010). Direct comparison of Dll1- and Dll4-mediated Notch activation levels shows differential lymphomyeloid lineage commitment outcomes. *Journal of Immunology, 185*, 867–876.
55. Hozumi, K., Mailhos, C., Negishi, N., et al. (2008). Delta-like 4 is indispensable in thymic environment specific for T cell development. *The Journal of Experimental Medicine, 205*, 2507–2513.
56. Koch, U., Fiorini, E., Benedito, R., et al. (2008). Delta-like 4 is the essential, nonredundant ligand for Notch1 during thymic T cell lineage commitment. *The Journal of Experimental Medicine, 205*, 2515–2523.
57. Hozumi, K., Negishi, N., Suzuki, D., et al. (2004). Delta-like 1 is necessary for the generation of marginal zone B cells but not T cells in vivo. *Nature Immunology, 5*, 638–644.
58. Wolfer, A., Wilson, A., Nemir, M., et al. (2002). Inactivation of Notch1 impairs VDJbeta rearrangement and allows pre-TCR-independent survival of early alpha beta Lineage Thymocytes. *Immunity, 16*, 869–879.
59. Wolfer, A., Bakker, T., Wilson, A., et al. (2001). Inactivation of Notch 1 in immature thymocytes does not perturb CD4 or CD8T cell development. *Nature Immunology, 2*, 235–241.
60. Robey, E., Chang, D., Itano, A., et al. (1996). An activated form of Notch influences the choice between CD4 and CD8 T cell lineages. *Cell, 87*, 483–492.
61. Tu, L., Fang, T. C., Artis, D., et al. (2005). Notch signaling is an important regulator of type 2 immunity. *The Journal of Experimental Medicine, 202*, 1037–1042.

62. Ellisen, L. W., Bird, J., West, D. C., et al. (1991). TAN-1, the human homolog of the Drosophila notch gene, is broken by chromosomal translocations in T lymphoblastic neoplasms. *Cell, 66*, 649–661.
63. Girard, L., Hanna, Z., Beaulieu, N., et al. (1996). Frequent provirus insertional mutagenesis of Notch1 in thymomas of MMTVD/myc transgenic mice suggests a collaboration of c-myc and Notch1 for oncogenesis. *Genes & Development, 10*, 1930–1944.
64. Shen, H., Suzuki, T., Munroe, D. J., et al. (2003). Common sites of retroviral integration in mouse hematopoietic tumors identified by high-throughput, single nucleotide polymorphism-based mapping and bacterial artificial chromosome hybridization. *Journal of Virology, 77*, 1584–1588.
65. Howard, G., Eiges, R., Gaudet, F., et al. (2008). Activation and transposition of endogenous retroviral elements in hypomethylation induced tumors in mice. *Oncogene, 27*, 404–408.
66. Hoemann, C. D., Beaulieu, N., Girard, L., et al. (2000). Two distinct Notch1 mutant alleles are involved in the induction of T-cell leukemia in c-myc transgenic mice. *Molecular and Cellular Biology, 20*, 3831–3842.
67. Aster, J., Pear, W., Hasserjian, R., et al. (1994). Functional analysis of the TAN-1 gene, a human homolog of Drosophila notch. *Cold Spring Harbor Symposia on Quantitative Biology, 59*, 125–136.
68. Pear, W. S., Aster, J. C., Scott, M. L., et al. (1996). Exclusive development of T cell neoplasms in mice transplanted with bone marrow expressing activated Notch alleles. *The Journal of Experimental Medicine, 183*, 2283–2291.
69. Campese, A. F., Garbe, A. I., Zhang, F., et al. (2006). Notch1-dependent lymphomagenesis is assisted by but does not essentially require pre-TCR signaling. *Blood, 108*, 305–310.
70. Bellavia, D., Campese, A. F., Alesse, E., et al. (2000). Constitutive activation of NF-kappaB and T-cell leukemia/lymphoma in Notch3 transgenic mice. *The EMBO Journal, 19*, 3337–3348.
71. Beverly, L. J., & Capobianco, A. J. (2003). Perturbation of Ikaros isoform selection by MLV integration is a cooperative event in Notch(IC)-induced T cell leukemogenesis. *Cancer Cell, 3*, 551–564.
72. Chen, J., Jette, C., Kanki, J. P., et al. (2007). NOTCH1-induced T-cell leukemia in transgenic zebrafish. *Leukemia, 21*, 462–471.
73. Chiang, M. Y., Xu, L., Shestova, O., et al. (2008). Leukemia-associated NOTCH1 alleles are weak tumor initiators but accelerate K-ras-initiated leukemia. *The Journal of Clinical Investigation, 118*, 3181–3194.
74. Aster, J. C., Xu, L., Karnell, F. G., et al. (2000). Essential roles for ankyrin repeat and transactivation domains in induction of T-cell leukemia by Notch1. *Molecular and Cellular Biology, 20*, 7505–7515.
75. Aster, J. C., Bodnar, N., Xu, L., et al. (2011). Notch ankyrin repeat domain variation influences leukemogenesis and Myc transactivation. *PLoS One, 6*, e25645.
76. Weng, A. P., Nam, Y., Wolfe, M. S., et al. (2003). Growth suppression of pre-T acute lymphoblastic leukemia cells by inhibition of notch signaling. *Molecular and Cellular Biology, 23*, 655–664.
77. Wu, Y., Cain-Hom, C., Choy, L., et al. (2010a). Therapeutic antibody targeting of individual Notch receptors. *Nature, 464*, 1052–1057.
78. Weng, A. P., Ferrando, A. A., Lee, W., et al. (2004a). Activating mutations of NOTCH1 in human T cell acute lymphoblastic leukemia. *Science, 306*, 269–271.
79. Mansour, M. R., Sulis, M. L., Duke, V., et al. (2009a). Prognostic implications of NOTCH1 and FBXW7 mutations in adults with T-cell acute lymphoblastic leukemia treated on the MRC UKALLXII/ECOG E2993 protocol. *Journal of Clinical Oncology, 27*, 4352–4356.
80. Asnafi, V., Buzyn, A., Le Noir, S., et al. (2009). NOTCH1/FBXW7 mutation identifies a large subgroup with favorable outcome in adult T-cell acute lymphoblastic leukemia (T-ALL): A Group for Research on Adult Acute Lymphoblastic Leukemia (GRAALL) study. *Blood, 113*, 3918–3924.

81. Zhu, Y. M., Zhao, W. L., Fu, J. F., et al. (2006). NOTCH1 mutations in T-cell acute lymphoblastic leukemia: Prognostic significance and implication in multifactorial leukemogenesis. *Clinical Cancer Research, 12*, 3043–3049.
82. Park, M. J., Taki, T., Oda, M., et al. (2009). FBXW7 and NOTCH1 mutations in childhood T cell acute lymphoblastic leukaemia and T cell non-Hodgkin lymphoma. *British Journal of Haematology, 145*, 198–206.
83. van Grotel, M., Meijerink, J. P., Beverloo, H. B., et al. (2006). The outcome of molecular-cytogenetic subgroups in pediatric T-cell acute lymphoblastic leukemia: A retrospective study of patients treated according to DCOG or COALL protocols. *Haematologica, 91*, 1212–1221.
84. Breit, S., Stanulla, M., Flohr, T., et al. (2006). Activating NOTCH1 mutations predict favorable early treatment response and long-term outcome in childhood precursor T-cell lymphoblastic leukemia. *Blood, 108*, 1151–1157.
85. Larson Gedman, A., Chen, Q., Kugel Desmoulin, S., et al. (2009). The impact of NOTCH1, FBW7 and PTEN mutations on prognosis and downstream signaling in pediatric T-cell acute lymphoblastic leukemia: A report from the Children's Oncology Group. *Leukemia, 23*, 1417–1425.
86. Zhang, J., Ding, L., Holmfeldt, L., et al. (2012). The genetic basis of early T-cell precursor acute lymphoblastic leukaemia. *Nature, 481*, 157–163.
87. Neumann, M., Vosberg, S., Schlee, C., et al. (2015). Mutational spectrum of adult T-ALL. *Oncotarget, 6*, 2754–2766.
88. Homminga, I., Pieters, R., Langerak, A. W., et al. (2011). Integrated transcript and genome analyses reveal NKX2-1 and MEF2C as potential oncogenes in T cell acute lymphoblastic leukemia. *Cancer Cell, 19*, 484–497.
89. Fabbri, G., Rasi, S., Rossi, D., et al. (2011). Analysis of the chronic lymphocytic leukemia coding genome: Role of NOTCH1 mutational activation. *The Journal of Experimental Medicine, 208*, 1389–1401.
90. Fabbri, G., Khiabanian, H., Holmes, A. B., et al. (2013). Genetic lesions associated with chronic lymphocytic leukemia transformation to Richter syndrome. *The Journal of Experimental Medicine, 210*, 2273–2288.
91. Puente, X. S., Pinyol, M., Quesada, V., et al. (2011). Whole-genome sequencing identifies recurrent mutations in chronic lymphocytic leukaemia. *Nature, 475*, 101–105.
92. Andersson, E. R., Sandberg, R., & Lendahl, U. (2011). Notch signaling: Simplicity in design, versatility in function. *Development, 138*, 3593–3612.
93. Sportoletti, P., Baldoni, S., Del Papa, B., et al. (2014). A revised NOTCH1 mutation frequency still impacts survival while the allele burden predicts early progression in chronic lymphocytic leukemia. *Leukemia, 28*, 436–439.
94. Kridel, R., Meissner, B., Rogic, S., et al. (2012). Whole transcriptome sequencing reveals recurrent NOTCH1 mutations in mantle cell lymphoma. *Blood, 119*, 1963–1971.
95. Beà, S., Valdés-Mas, R., Navarro, A., et al. (2013). Landscape of somatic mutations and clonal evolution in mantle cell lymphoma. *Proceedings of the National Academy of Sciences, 110*, 18250–18255.
96. Rossi, D., Trifonov, V., Fangazio, M., et al. (2012). The coding genome of splenic marginal zone lymphoma: Activation of NOTCH2 and other pathways regulating marginal zone development. *The Journal of Experimental Medicine, 209*, 1537–1551.
97. Kiel, M. J., Velusamy, T., Betz, B. L., et al. (2012). Whole-genome sequencing identifies recurrent somatic NOTCH2 mutations in splenic marginal zone lymphoma. *The Journal of Experimental Medicine, 209*, 1553–1565.
98. Lee, S. Y., Kumano, K., Nakazaki, K., et al. (2009). Gain-of-function mutations and copy number increases of Notch2 in diffuse large B-cell lymphoma. *Cancer Science, 100*, 920–926.
99. Malecki, M. J., Sanchez-Irizarry, C., Mitchell, J. L., et al. (2006). Leukemia-associated mutations within the NOTCH1 heterodimerization domain fall into at least two distinct mechanistic classes. *Molecular and Cellular Biology, 26*, 4642–4651.

100. Sulis, M. L., Williams, O., Palomero, T., et al. (2008). NOTCH1 extracellular juxtamembrane expansion mutations in T-ALL. *Blood, 112*, 733–740.
101. O'Neil, J., Grim, J., Strack, P., et al. (2007a). FBW7 mutations in leukemic cells mediate NOTCH pathway activation and resistance to {gamma}-secretase inhibitors. *The Journal of Experimental Medicine, 204*, 1813–1824.
102. Thompson, B. J., Buonamici, S., Sulis, M. L., et al. (2007a). The SCFFBW7 ubiquitin ligase complex as a tumor suppressor in T cell leukemia. *The Journal of Experimental Medicine, 204*, 1825–1835.
103. Chiang, M. Y., Xu, M. L., Histen, G., et al. (2006). Identification of a conserved negative regulatory sequence that influences the leukemogenic activity of NOTCH1. *Molecular and Cellular Biology, 26*, 6261–6271.
104. Welcker, M., Orian, A., Jin, J., et al. (2004a). The Fbw7 tumor suppressor regulates glycogen synthase kinase 3 phosphorylation-dependent c-Myc protein degradation. *Proceedings of the National Academy of Sciences of the United States of America, 101*, 9085–9090.
105. Onoyama, I., Tsunematsu, R., Matsumoto, A., et al. (2007). Conditional inactivation of Fbxw7 impairs cell-cycle exit during T cell differentiation and results in lymphomatogenesis. *The Journal of Experimental Medicine, 204*, 2875–2888.
106. Malyukova, A., Dohda, T., von der Lehr, N., et al. (2007). The tumor suppressor gene hCDC4 is frequently mutated in human T-cell acute lymphoblastic leukemia with functional consequences for Notch signaling. *Cancer Research, 67*, 5611–5616.
107. King, B., Trimarchi, T., Reavie, L., et al. (2013a). The ubiquitin ligase FBXW7 modulates leukemia-initiating cell activity by regulating MYC stability. *Cell, 153*, 1552–1566.
108. Welcker, M., Orian, A., Grim, J. E., et al. (2004b). A nucleolar isoform of the Fbw7 ubiquitin ligase regulates c-Myc and cell size. *Current Biology, 14*, 1852–1857.
109. Mantha, S., Ward, M., McCafferty, J., et al. (2007). Activating Notch1 mutations are an early event in T-cell malignancy of Ikaros point mutant plastic/+ mice. *Leukemia Research, 31*, 321–327.
110. Reschly, E. J., Spaulding, C., Vilimas, T., et al. (2006). Notch1 promotes survival of E2A-deficient T cell lymphomas through pre-T cell receptor-dependent and -independent mechanisms. *Blood, 107*, 4115–4121.
111. Maser, R. S., Choudhury, B., Campbell, P. J., et al. (2007). Chromosomally unstable mouse tumours have genomic alterations similar to diverse human cancers. *Nature, 447*, 966–971.
112. O'Neil, J., Calvo, J., McKenna, K., et al. (2006). Activating Notch1 mutations in mouse models of T-ALL. *Blood, 107*, 781–785.
113. Lin, Y. W., Nichols, R. A., Letterio, J. J., et al. (2006). Notch1 mutations are important for leukemic transformation in murine models of precursor-T leukemia/lymphoma. *Blood, 107*, 2540–2543.
114. Dumortier, A., Jeannet, R., Kirstetter, P., et al. (2006). Notch activation is an early and critical event during T-Cell leukemogenesis in Ikaros-deficient mice. *Molecular and Cellular Biology, 26*, 209–220.
115. Tsuji, H., Ishii-Ohba, H., Ukai, H., et al. (2003). Radiation-induced deletions in the 5' end region of Notch1 lead to the formation of truncated proteins and are involved in the development of mouse thymic lymphomas. *Carcinogenesis, 24*, 1257–1268.
116. Ashworth, T. D., Pear, W. S., Chiang, M. Y., et al. (2010). Deletion-based mechanisms of Notch1 activation in T-ALL: Key roles for RAG recombinase and a conserved internal translational start site in Notch1. *Blood, 116*, 5455–5464.
117. Kox, C., Zimmermann, M., Stanulla, M., et al. (2010). The favorable effect of activating NOTCH1 receptor mutations on long-term outcome in T-ALL patients treated on the ALL-BFM 2000 protocol can be separated from FBXW7 loss of function. *Leukemia, 24*, 2005–2013.
118. Clappier, E., Collette, S., Grardel, N., et al. (2010). NOTCH1 and FBXW7 mutations have a favorable impact on early response to treatment, but not on outcome, in children with T-cell

acute lymphoblastic leukemia (T-ALL) treated on EORTC trials 58881 and 58951. *Leukemia, 24*, 2023–2031.
119. Zuurbier, L., Homminga, I., Calvert, V., et al. (2010). NOTCH1 and/or FBXW7 mutations predict for initial good prednisone response but not for improved outcome in pediatric T-cell acute lymphoblastic leukemia patients treated on DCOG or COALL protocols. *Leukemia, 24*, 2014–2022.
120. Real, P. J., Tosello, V., Palomero, T., et al. (2009a). [gamma]-secretase inhibitors reverse glucocorticoid resistance in T cell acute lymphoblastic leukemia. *Nature Medicine, 15*, 50–58.
121. Bellavia, D., Campese, A. F., Checquolo, S., et al. (2002). Combined expression of pTalpha and Notch3 in T cell leukemia identifies the requirement of preTCR for leukemogenesis. *Proceedings of the National Academy of Sciences of the United States of America, 99*, 3788–3793.
122. Felli, M. P., Vacca, A., Calce, A., et al. (2005). PKC theta mediates pre-TCR signaling and contributes to Notch3-induced T-cell leukemia. *Oncogene, 24*, 992–1000.
123. Jeannet, R., Mastio, J., Macias-Garcia, A., et al. (2010). Oncogenic activation of the Notch1 gene by deletion of its promoter in Ikaros-deficient T-ALL. *Blood, 116*, 5443–5454.
124. Palomero, T., Sulis, M. L., Cortina, M., et al. (2007). Mutational loss of PTEN induces resistance to NOTCH1 inhibition in T-cell leukemia. *Nature Medicine, 13*, 1203–1210.
125. Gonzalez-Garcia, S., Garcia-Peydro, M., Martin-Gayo, E., et al. (2009). CSL-MAML-dependent Notch1 signaling controls T lineage-specific IL-7R{alpha} gene expression in early human thymopoiesis and leukemia. *The Journal of Experimental Medicine, 206*, 779–791.
126. Barata, J. T., Silva, A., Brandao, J. G., et al. (2004). Activation of PI3K is indispensable for interleukin 7-mediated viability, proliferation, glucose use, and growth of T cell acute lymphoblastic leukemia cells. *The Journal of Experimental Medicine, 200*, 659–669.
127. Medyouf, H., Gusscott, S., Wang, H., et al. (2011a). High-level IGF1R expression is required for leukemia-initiating cell activity in T-ALL and is supported by Notch signaling. *The Journal of Experimental Medicine, 208*, 1809–1822.
128. Correia, N. C., Gírio, A., Antunes, I., et al. (2014). The multiple layers of non-genetic regulation of PTEN tumour suppressor activity. *European Journal of Cancer, 50*, 216–225.
129. Silva, A., Yunes, J. A., Cardoso, B. A., et al. (2008). PTEN posttranslational inactivation and hyperactivation of the PI3K/Akt pathway sustain primary T cell leukemia viability. *The Journal of Clinical Investigation, 118*, 3762–3774.
130. Herranz, D., Ambesi-Impiombato, A., Sudderth, J., et al. (2015). Metabolic reprogramming induces resistance to anti-NOTCH1 therapies in T cell acute lymphoblastic leukemia. *Nature Medicine, 21*, 1182–1189.
131. Medyouf, H., Gao, X., Armstrong, F., et al. (2010). Acute T-cell leukemias remain dependent on Notch signaling despite PTEN and INK4A/ARF loss. *Blood, 115*, 1175–1184.
132. Vilimas, T., Mascarenhas, J., Palomero, T., et al. (2007a). Targeting the NF-kappaB signaling pathway in Notch1-induced T-cell leukemia. *Nature Medicine, 13*, 70–77.
133. Oswald, F., Liptay, S., Adler, G., et al. (1998). NF-kappaB2 is a putative target gene of activated Notch-1 via RBP- Jkappa. *Molecular and Cellular Biology, 18*, 2077–2088.
134. Vilimas, T., Mascarenhas, J., Palomero, T., et al. (2007b). Targeting the NF-[kappa]B signaling pathway in Notch1-induced T-cell leukemia. *Nature Medicine, 13*, 70–77.
135. Shin, H. M., Minter, L. M., Cho, O. H., et al. (2006). Notch1 augments NF-κB activity by facilitating its nuclear retention. *The EMBO Journal, 25*, 129–138.
136. Espinosa, L., Cathelin, S., D'Altri, T., et al. (2010). The Notch/Hes1 pathway sustains NF-κB activation through CYLD repression in T cell leukemia. *Cancer Cell, 18*, 268–281.
137. Clarke, M. F., Dick, J. E., Dirks, P. B., et al. (2006). Cancer stem cells--perspectives on current status and future directions: AACR workshop on cancer stem cells. *Cancer Research, 66*, 9339–9344.
138. Bonnet, D., & Dick, J. E. (1997). Human acute myeloid leukemia is organized as a hierarchy that originates from a primitive hematopoietic cell. *Nature Medicine, 3*, 730–737.

139. Cox, C. V., Martin, H. M., Kearns, P. R., et al. (2007). Characterization of a progenitor cell population in childhood T-cell acute lymphoblastic leukemia. *Blood, 109*, 674–682.
140. Chiu, P. P., Jiang, H., & Dick, J. E. (2010). Leukemia-initiating cells in human T-lymphoblastic leukemia exhibit glucocorticoid resistance. *Blood, 116*, 5268–5279.
141. Gerby, B., Clappier, E., Armstrong, F., et al. (2011). Expression of CD34 and CD7 on human T-cell acute lymphoblastic leukemia discriminates functionally heterogeneous cell populations. *Leukemia, 25*, 1249–1258.
142. Guo, W., Lasky, J. L., Chang, C. J., et al. (2008). Multi-genetic events collaboratively contribute to Pten-null leukaemia stem-cell formation. *Nature, 453*, 529–533.
143. Tremblay, M., Tremblay, C. S., Herblot, S., et al. (2010). Modeling T-cell acute lymphoblastic leukemia induced by the SCL and LMO1 oncogenes. *Genes & Development, 24*, 1093–1105.
144. Giambra, V., Jenkins, C. R., Wang, H., et al. (2012a). NOTCH1 promotes T cell leukemia-initiating activity by RUNX-mediated regulation of PKC-theta and reactive oxygen species. *Nature Medicine, 18*, 1693–1698.
145. Tatarek, J., Cullion, K., Ashworth, T., et al. (2011). Notch1 inhibition targets the leukemia-initiating cells in a Tal1/Lmo2 mouse model of T-ALL. *Blood, 118*, 1579–1590.
146. Giambra, V., Jenkins, C. E., Lam, S. H., et al. (2015). Leukemia stem cells in T-ALL require active Hif1α and Wnt signaling. *Blood, 125*, 3917–3927.
147. Chiang, M. Y., Shestova, O., Xu, L., et al. (2013). Divergent effects of supraphysiologic Notch signals on leukemia stem cells and hematopoietic stem cells. *Blood, 121*, 905–917.
148. Armstrong, F., Brunet de la Grange, P., Gerby, B., et al. (2009). NOTCH is a key regulator of human T-cell acute leukemia initiating cell activity. *Blood, 113*, 1730–1740.
149. Giambra, V., Jenkins, C. R., Wang, H., et al. (2012b). NOTCH1 promotes T cell leukemia-initiating activity by RUNX-mediated regulation of PKC-θ and reactive oxygen species. *Nature Medicine, 18*, 1693–1698.
150. Ma, W., Gutierrez, A., Goff, D. J., et al. (2012). NOTCH1 signaling promotes human T-cell acute lymphoblastic leukemia initiating cell regeneration in supportive niches. *PLoS One, 7*, e39725.
151. Giambra, V., Gusscott, S., Gracias, D., et al. (2018). Epigenetic restoration of fetal-like IGF1 signaling inhibits leukemia stem cell activity. *Cell Stem Cell, 23*, 714–726. https://doi.org/10.1016/j.stem.2018.08.018.
152. Roderick, J. E., Tesell, J., Shultz, L. D., et al. (2014). c-Myc inhibition prevents leukemia initiation in mice and impairs the growth of relapsed and induction failure pediatric T-ALL cells. *Blood, 123*, 1040–1050.
153. Tanigaki, K., Han, H., Yamamoto, N., et al. (2002). Notch-RBP-J signaling is involved in cell fate determination of marginal zone B cells. *Nature Immunology, 3*, 443–450.
154. Saito, T., Chiba, S., Ichikawa, M., et al. (2003). Notch2 is preferentially expressed in mature B cells and indispensable for marginal zone B lineage development. *Immunity, 18*, 675–685.
155. Wu, L., Maillard, I., Nakamura, M., et al. (2007). The transcriptional coactivator Maml1 is required for Notch2-mediated marginal zone B-cell development. *Blood, 110*, 3618–3623.
156. Oyama, T., Harigaya, K., Muradil, A., et al. (2007). Mastermind-1 is required for Notch signal-dependent steps in lymphocyte development in vivo. *Proceedings of the National Academy of Sciences of the United States of America, 104*, 9764–9769.
157. Song, R., Kim, Y. W., Koo, B. K., et al. (2008). Mind bomb 1 in the lymphopoietic niches is essential for T and marginal zone B cell development. *The Journal of Experimental Medicine, 205*, 2525–2536.
158. Gibb, D. R., El Shikh, M., Kang, D. J., et al. (2010). ADAM10 is essential for Notch2-dependent marginal zone B cell development and CD23 cleavage in vivo. *The Journal of Experimental Medicine, 207*, 623–635.
159. Wendorff, A. A., Koch, U., Wunderlich, F. T., et al. (2010). Hes1 is a critical but context-dependent mediator of canonical Notch signaling in lymphocyte development and transformation. *Immunity, 33*, 671–684.

160. Zweidler-McKay, P. A., He, Y., Xu, L., et al. (2005). Notch signaling is a potent inducer of growth arrest and apoptosis in a wide range of B-cell malignancies. *Blood, 106*, 3898–3906.
161. Kuang, S. Q., Fang, Z., Zweidler-McKay, P. A., et al. (2013). Epigenetic inactivation of Notch-Hes pathway in human B-cell acute lymphoblastic leukemia. *PLoS One, 8*, e61807.
162. Hamblin, T. J., Davis, Z., Gardiner, A., et al. (1999). Unmutated Ig VH genes are associated with a more aggressive form of chronic lymphocytic leukemia. *Blood, 94*, 1848–1854.
163. Hubmann, R., Schwarzmeier, J. D., Shehata, M., et al. (2002). Notch2 is involved in the overexpression of CD23 in B-cell chronic lymphocytic leukemia. *Blood, 99*, 3742–3747.
164. Rosati, E., Sabatini, R., Rampino, G., et al. (2009). Constitutively activated Notch signaling is involved in survival and apoptosis resistance of B-CLL cells. *Blood, 113*, 856–865.
165. Balatti, V., Bottoni, A., Palamarchuk, A., et al. (2012). NOTCH1 mutations in CLL associated with trisomy 12. *Blood, 119*, 329–331.
166. Del Giudice, I., Rossi, D., Chiaretti, S., et al. (2012). NOTCH1 mutations in +12 chronic lymphocytic leukemia (CLL) confer an unfavorable prognosis, induce a distinctive transcriptional profiling and refine the intermediate prognosis of +12 CLL. *Haematologica, 97*, 437–441.
167. Nadeu, F., Delgado, J., Royo, C., et al. (2016). Clinical impact of clonal and subclonal TP53, SF3B1, BIRC3, NOTCH1, and ATM mutations in chronic lymphocytic leukemia. *Blood, 127*, 2122–2130.
168. Rossi, D., Rasi, S., Fabbri, G., et al. (2012). Mutations of NOTCH1 are an independent predictor of survival in chronic lymphocytic leukemia. *Blood, 119*(2), 521–529.
169. Puente, X. S., Bea, S., Valdes-Mas, R., et al. (2015). Non-coding recurrent mutations in chronic lymphocytic leukaemia. *Nature, 526*, 519–524.
170. Kluk, M. J., Ashworth, T., Wang, H., et al. (2013). Gauging NOTCH1 activation in cancer using immunohistochemistry. *PLoS One, 8*, e67306.
171. Onaindia, A., Gomez, S., Piris-Villaespesa, M., et al. (2014). Chronic lymphocytic leukemia cells in lymph nodes show frequent NOTCH1 activation. *Haematologica, 100*, e200–e203.
172. Arruga, F., Gizdic, B., Serra, S., et al. (2014). Functional impact of NOTCH1 mutations in chronic lymphocytic leukemia. *Leukemia, 28*, 1060–1070.
173. Jares, P., Colomer, D., & Campo, E. (2007). Genetic and molecular pathogenesis of mantle cell lymphoma: Perspectives for new targeted therapeutics. *Nature Reviews. Cancer, 7*, 750–762.
174. Salido, M., Baró, C., Oscier, D., et al. (2010). Cytogenetic aberrations and their prognostic value in a series of 330 splenic marginal zone B-cell lymphomas: A multicenter study of the Splenic B-Cell Lymphoma Group. *Blood, 116*, 1479–1488.
175. Rossi, D., Deaglio, S., Dominguez-Sola, D., et al. (2011). Alteration of BIRC3 and multiple other NF-κB pathway genes in splenic marginal zone lymphoma. *Blood, 118*, 4930–4934.
176. Arcaini, L., Paulli, M., Boveri, E., et al. (2004). Splenic and nodal marginal zone lymphomas are indolent disorders at high hepatitis C virus seroprevalence with distinct presenting features but similar morphologic and phenotypic profiles. *Cancer, 100*, 107–115.
177. Hermine, O., Lefrère, F., Bronowicki, J.-P., et al. (2002). Regression of splenic lymphoma with villous lymphocytes after treatment of hepatitis C virus infection. *New England Journal of Medicine, 347*, 89–94.
178. Link, B. K., Maurer, M. J., Nowakowski, G. S., et al. (2013). Rates and outcomes of follicular lymphoma transformation in the immunochemotherapy era: A report from the University of Iowa/Mayo Clinic Specialized Program of Research Excellence Molecular Epidemiology Resource. *Journal of Clinical Oncology, 31*, 3272–3278.
179. Martinez, D., Royo, C., Castillo, P., et al. (2013). Recurrent mutations Of NOTCH genes in follicular lymphoma. *Blood, 122*, 4253–4253.
180. Arcaini, L., Rossi, D., Lucioni, M., et al. (2015). The NOTCH pathway is recurrently mutated in diffuse large B-cell lymphoma associated with hepatitis C virus infection. *Haematologica, 100*, 246–252.

181. Jundt, F., Probsting, K. S., Anagnostopoulos, I:, et al. (2004). Jagged1-induced Notch signaling drives proliferation of multiple myeloma cells. *Blood, 103*, 3511–3515.
182. Houde, C., Li, Y., Song, L., et al. (2004). Overexpression of the NOTCH ligand JAG2 in malignant plasma cells from multiple myeloma patients and cell lines. *Blood, 104*, 3697–3704.
183. Mirandola, L., Apicella, L., Colombo, M., et al. (2013). Anti-Notch treatment prevents multiple myeloma cells localization to the bone marrow via the chemokine system CXCR4/SDF-1. *Leukemia, 27*, 1558+.
184. Nefedova, Y., Sullivan, D. M., Bolick, S. C., et al. (2008a). Inhibition of Notch signaling induces apoptosis of myeloma cells and enhances sensitivity to chemotherapy. *Blood, 111*, 2220–2229.
185. Kanzler, H., Küppers, R., Hansmann, M. L., et al. (1996). Hodgkin and Reed-Sternberg cells in Hodgkin's disease represent the outgrowth of a dominant tumor clone derived from (crippled) germinal center B cells. *The Journal of Experimental Medicine, 184*, 1495–1505.
186. Jundt, F., Anagnostopoulos, I., Forster, R., et al. (2002). Activated Notch1 signaling promotes tumor cell proliferation and survival in Hodgkin and anaplastic large cell lymphoma. *Blood, 99*, 3398–3403.
187. Skrtic, A., Korac, P., Kristo, D. R., et al. (2010). Immunohistochemical analysis of NOTCH1 and JAGGED1 expression in multiple myeloma and monoclonal gammopathy of undetermined significance. *Human Pathology, 41*, 1702–1710.
188. Schwarzer, R., Dorken, B., & Jundt, F. (2012). Notch is an essential upstream regulator of NF-kappaB and is relevant for survival of Hodgkin and Reed-Sternberg cells. *Leukemia, 26*, 806–813.
189. Bigas, A., Martin, D. I., & Milner, L. A. (1998). Notch1 and Notch2 inhibit myeloid differentiation in response to different cytokines. *Molecular and Cellular Biology, 18*, 2324–2333.
190. Milner, L. A., Bigas, A., Kopan, R., et al. (1996). Inhibition of granulocytic differentiation by mNotch1. *Proceedings of the National Academy of Sciences of the United States of America, 93*, 13014–13019.
191. Ohishi, K., Varnum-Finney, B., Serda, R. E., et al. (2001). The Notch ligand, Delta-1, inhibits the differentiation of monocytes into macrophages but permits their differentiation into dendritic cells. *Blood, 98*, 1402–1407.
192. Schroeder, T., Kohlhof, H., Rieber, N., et al. (2003). Notch signaling induces multilineage myeloid differentiation and up-regulates PU.1 expression. *Journal of Immunology, 170*, 5538–5548.
193. Mercher, T., Cornejo, M. G., Sears, C., et al. (2008). Notch signaling specifies megakaryocyte development from hematopoietic stem cells. *Cell Stem Cell, 3*, 314–326.
194. Poirault-Chassac, S., Six, E., Catelain, C., et al. (2010). Notch/Delta4 signaling inhibits human megakaryocytic terminal differentiation. *Blood, 116*, 5670–5678.
195. Chiaramonte, R., Basile, A., Tassi, E., et al. (2005). A wide role for NOTCH1 signaling in acute leukemia. *Cancer Letters, 219*, 113–120.
196. Tohda, S., & Nara, N. (2001). Expression of Notch1 and Jagged1 proteins in acute myeloid leukemia cells. *Leukemia & Lymphoma, 42*, 467–472.
197. Tohda, S., Kogoshi, H., Murakami, N., et al. (2005). Diverse effects of the Notch ligands Jagged1 and Delta1 on the growth and differentiation of primary acute myeloblastic leukemia cells. *Experimental Hematology, 33*, 558–563.
198. Tohda, S., Sakano, S., Ohsawa, M., et al. (2002). A novel cell line derived from de novo acute myeloblastic leukaemia with trilineage myelodysplasia which proliferates in response to a Notch ligand, Delta-1 protein. *British Journal of Haematology, 117*, 373–378.
199. Tohda, S., Murata-Ohsawa, M., Sakano, S., et al. (2003). Notch ligands, Delta-1 and Delta-4 suppress the self-renewal capacity and long-term growth of two myeloblastic leukemia cell lines. *International Journal of Oncology, 22*, 1073–1079.
200. Kannan, S., Sutphin, R. M., Hall, M. G., et al. (2013). Notch activation inhibits AML growth and survival: A potential therapeutic approach. *The Journal of Experimental Medicine, 210*, 321–337.

201. Lobry, C., Ntziachristos, P., Ndiaye-Lobry, D., et al. (2013). Notch pathway activation targets AML-initiating cell homeostasis and differentiation. *The Journal of Experimental Medicine, 210*, 301–319.
202. Tian, C., Yu, Y., Jia, Y., et al. (2015). HES1 activation suppresses proliferation of leukemia cells in acute myeloid leukemia. *Annals of Hematology, 94*, 1477–1483.
203. Kato, T., Sakata-Yanagimoto, M., Nishikii, H., et al. (2015). Hes1 suppresses acute myeloid leukemia development through FLT3 repression. *Leukemia, 29*, 576–585.
204. Klinakis, A., Lobry, C., Abdel-Wahab, O., et al. (2011). A novel tumour-suppressor function for the Notch pathway in myeloid leukaemia. *Nature, 473*, 230–233.
205. Evin, G., Sernee, M. F., & Masters, C. L. (2006). Inhibition of gamma-secretase as a therapeutic intervention for Alzheimer's disease: Prospects, limitations and strategies. *CNS Drugs, 20*, 351–372.
206. Luistro, L., He, W., Smith, M., et al. (2009). Preclinical profile of a potent gamma-secretase inhibitor targeting notch signaling with in vivo efficacy and pharmacodynamic properties. *Cancer Research, 69*, 7672–7680.
207. Kolb, E. A., Gorlick, R., Keir, S. T., et al. (2012). Initial testing (stage 1) by the pediatric preclinical testing program of RO4929097, a gamma-secretase inhibitor targeting notch signaling. *Pediatric Blood & Cancer, 58*, 815–818.
208. Tammam, J., Ware, C., Efferson, C., et al. (2009). Down-regulation of the Notch pathway mediated by a gamma-secretase inhibitor induces anti-tumour effects in mouse models of T-cell leukaemia. *British Journal of Pharmacology, 158*, 1183–1195.
209. DeAngelo, D., Stone, R., Silverman, L., et al. (2006). A phase I clinical trial of the notch inhibitor MK-0752 in patients with T-cell acute lymphoblastic leukemia/lymphoma (T-ALL) and other leukemias. *Journal of Clinical Oncology, ASCO Annual Meeting Proceedings Part I, 24*, 6585.
210. Riccio, O., van Gijn, M. E., Bezdek, A. C., et al. (2008). Loss of intestinal crypt progenitor cells owing to inactivation of both Notch1 and Notch2 is accompanied by derepression of CDK inhibitors p27Kip1 and p57Kip2. *EMBO Reports, 9*, 377–383.
211. van Es, J. H., van Gijn, M. E., Riccio, O., et al. (2005). Notch/[gamma]-secretase inhibition turns proliferative cells in intestinal crypts and adenomas into goblet cells. *Nature, 435*, 959–963.
212. Moellering, R. E., Cornejo, M., Davis, T. N., et al. (2009). Direct inhibition of the NOTCH transcription factor complex. *Nature, 462*, 182–188.
213. Maillard, I., Weng, A. P., Carpenter, A. C., et al. (2004). Mastermind critically regulates Notch-mediated lymphoid cell fate decisions. *Blood, 104*, 1696–1702.
214. Aste-Amezaga, M., Zhang, N., Lineberger, J. E., et al. (2010). Characterization of Notch1 antibodies that inhibit signaling of both normal and mutated Notch1 receptors. *PLoS One, 5*, e9094.
215. Li, K., Li, Y., Wu, W., et al. (2008b). Modulation of Notch signaling by antibodies specific for the extracellular negative regulatory region of NOTCH3. *The Journal of Biological Chemistry, 283*, 8046–8054.
216. Agnusdei, V., Minuzzo, S., Frasson, C., et al. (2014). Therapeutic antibody targeting of Notch1 in T-acute lymphoblastic leukemia xenografts. *Leukemia, 28*, 278–288.
217. Yen, W. C., Fischer, M. M., Axelrod, F., et al. (2015). Targeting Notch signaling with a Notch2/Notch3 antagonist (tarextumab) inhibits tumor growth and decreases tumor-initiating cell frequency. *Clinical Cancer Research, 21*, 2084–2095.
218. Ridgway, J., Zhang, G., Wu, Y., et al. (2006). Inhibition of Dll4 signalling inhibits tumour growth by deregulating angiogenesis. *Nature, 444*, 1083–1087.
219. Noguera-Troise, I., Daly, C., Papadopoulos, N. J., et al. (2006). Blockade of Dll4 inhibits tumour growth by promoting non-productive angiogenesis. *Nature, 444*, 1032–1037.

Chapter 9
The Role of Notch in Breast Cancer

Jeffrey C. Bloodworth and Clodia Osipo

Abstract Women have a one in eight lifetime risk of being diagnosed with breast cancer. Breast cancer is the second leading cause of cancer-related mortality in women worldwide. Notch signaling is critical for proper mammary development and homeostasis. Notch is emerging as an important targetable oncogene in breast cancer. Notch signaling promotes a number of cancer phenotypes including stem cell survival, self-renewal, and differentiation. This chapter will describe research advancements and clinical implications of Notch signaling in the context of the normal mammary gland and in breast cancer. Notch is involved in cross talk with several other signaling pathways. Estrogen receptor alpha and ErbB2 are commonly overexpressed breast oncogenes. Therapies designed to target these receptors are indicated for the majority of invasive breast cancer cases. However, breast tumors are often able to overcome these therapies, and upregulation of Notch is implicated in the development of drug resistance.

Keywords Breast cancer · Notch · Gamma secretase · Mammary · Breast cancer stem cell

9.1 Notch Signaling in the Normal Breast

Owing to its role in tissue patterning and development, Notch signaling is critical for proper breast development and function [1]. The epithelial cells within the mammary epithelial ducts and glands form a highly branched arboreal structure. The epithelium within the mammary tree system can be subdivided into ducts and terminal end buds which are comprised of a wide variety of cells that are specialized for the production and secretion of milk [2].

Proper mammary development and maturation are highly dependent upon four endocrine hormones: estrogen, progesterone, insulin-like growth factor, and growth

J. C. Bloodworth · C. Osipo (✉)
Loyola University Chicago, Department of Microbiology and Immunology, Oncology Research Institute, Biochemistry and Molecular Biology Program, Maywood, IL, USA
e-mail: cosipo@luc.edu

L. Miele, S. Artavanis-Tsakonas (eds.), *Targeting Notch in Cancer*,
https://doi.org/10.1007/978-1-4939-8859-4_9

hormone [3]. During puberty, these hormones drive proper morphology by signaling cells of the epithelia and stroma. Throughout life, the mammary epithelia remain highly responsive to fluctuations in hormone levels. Monthly estrogen/progesterone cycles maintain the mammary epithelium in a poised state. During pregnancy, the mammary epithelia become highly proliferative and thoroughly invade the breast stroma to form fully functional mammary glands. After weening, the epithelium undergoes massive apoptosis causing the mammary ductal system to regress to a prepregnancy state [4].

The Notch signaling pathway is employed in a wide variety of physiological processes. From a single-cell point of view, Notch signaling influences cellular survival and proliferation [5], migration, polarity, and cell fate decisions [6]. From a more holistic point of view, it can be seen that this signaling system orchestrates the elegant processes of embryogenesis [7], tissue patterning [8], organogenesis [9], angiogenesis [10], and wound healing [11]. The ability of cells to regulate the fate of neighboring cells is a concept that is central to developmental biology. Notch serves as a signaling prototype for two cooperating phenomena known as lateral inhibition and lateral induction [12, 13]. Lateral inhibition and lateral induction constitute negative and positive feedback loops (respectively) between cells that are in direct contact [12]. The Notch pathway operates on this same design [13]. Intracellular Notch signaling can be classified by considering cells as either "signal-sending" or "signal-receiving." This mechanism makes Notch ideal for propagating lateral inhibition and lateral induction [12]. Thus, Notch signaling coordinates the development of structures whose morphology and/or function depend upon cell-cell contacts [13].

Notch signaling can be briefly summarized beginning with posttranslational Golgi processing. Notch is glycosylated and cleaved in the Golgi apparatus and exists on the cell membrane as a heterodimer of the two cleavage products [14, 15]. Notch is recognized by one of its ligands, which is expressed on an opposing cell [16]. Ligand binding triggers cleavage by an ADAM/TACE family proteinase [17]. This newly truncated Notch is recognized and cleaved further by the γ-secretase complex [18]. Cleavage by γ-secretase releases the Notch intracellular domain allowing it to translocate to the nucleus where it acts as a transcriptional activator of numerous target genes [18]. Several strategies for targeting Notch have been proposed. The two classes of drugs to reach clinical trials are the γ-secretase inhibitors and Notch-specific monoclonal antibodies.

Notch signaling is required for proper organization of mammary tissue [19]. Notch3 facilitates differentiation of mammary progenitor cells into the luminal lineage [20]. Notch activity is required for the maintenance of the luminal cell layer in the mammary gland [21]. Others have shown that cJun N-terminal kinase2 inhibits Notch1 activity, which in turn facilitates development of the myoepithelial mammary cell layer [22]. Moreover, aberrant activation of Notch1 yields hyperplasia of cells in the luminal layer [21]. Indeed, Notch signaling is essential for normal breast development. However, in the context of breast cancer, Notch signaling can become dysregulated giving rise to tumor advancement and confounding therapeutic approaches (Fig. 9.1).

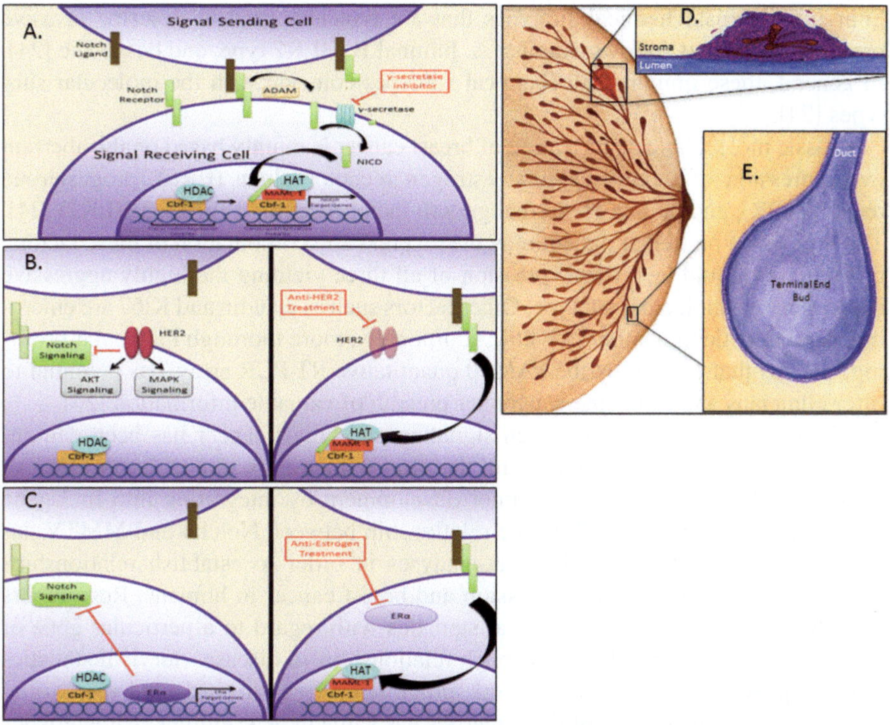

Fig. 9.1 Notch Signaling controls a number of characteristics that are central to normal mammary development and tumorigenesis. (**a**) Canonical Notch signaling requires a series of proteolytic cleavage steps. The resulting Notch intracellular domain translocates to the nucleus and directs the transcription of its target genes. (**b**) Aberrant HER2 overexpression suppresses Notch signaling. However, when anti-HER2 treatment is administered, Notch often becomes hyperactived which can sustain tumor survival and confer stem-like characteristics. (**c**) Similar to HER2 positive breast cancer, aberrant ERα overexpression suppresses Notch signaling, which is reversed upon anti-estrogen treatment. (**d**) Notch signaling controls several features of invasive breast cancer including proliferation, invasion, metastasis, aberrant angiogenesis, etc. (**e**) Notch signaling controls cell fate decisions in the normal mammary gland

9.2 An Overview of Breast Cancer

Breast tumors can often be noticed as a palpable mass embedded in the breast tissue, and mammography is typically employed to confirm differences in tissue density [23]. Breast cancer is a highly heterogeneous disease making biopsy of the tumor mass necessary for characterization. Breast cancer is subtyped on the basis of gross histology of the tumor and the presence/absence of well-described molecular markers. Histological classification assesses a number of factors such as invasiveness and whether the tumor arises from the mammary duct or lobule. Diagnosis of breast cancer subtype based on the molecular profile allows physicians to assess risk and choose appropriate treatment options with a higher degree of accuracy.

Four immunohistochemical subtypes that are typically used to describe invasive breast cancer are as follows: luminal A, luminal B, HER2 type, and basal-like [24]. In general, these immunohistochemical subtypes coincide with the molecular subtypes [24].

Classic molecular categorization of breast cancer is mainly based on the aberrant overexpression of three receptors: estrogen receptor alpha (ERα), progesterone receptor (PR), and human epidermal growth factor receptor 2 (ErbB-2/HER2) [24]. The tumor of a particular patient may overexpress any combination of these factors, or the tumor could lack overexpression of all three yielding the highly aggressive triple-negative molecular subtype. Other factors such as claudin and Ki67 are emerging as prognostic indicators [25, 26]. Additionally, more thorough molecular profiling, such as that offered by the PAM50 quantitative RT-PCR array, has potential to offer clinicians and researchers a greater breadth of valuable information [27].

The relationship between Notch signaling and breast cancer has been demonstrated by investigators working with the mouse mammary tumor virus (MMTV) [28]. MMTV can induce breast tumor development by integrating into Int3 gene locus (mouse Notch4) [28, 29]. The relationship between Notch4 and MMTV has been followed up by multiple meta-analyses in order to establish relationships between Notch family gene expression and breast cancer in humans. Researchers and clinicians often refer to survival statistics with regard to a particular gene or treatment modality in order to establish relationships in disease. Survival statistics may be presented as overall survival, progression-free survival, and regression/disease-free survival. Each of these metrics has value in determining characteristics of the disease, gene, and treatments being investigated. The Notch pathway is frequently dysregulated in breast cancer as revealed by these statistical techniques. Meta-analyses demonstrate a positive correlation between high Notch1 expression and poor overall and regression-free survival in all breast cancer subtypes [30, 31]. Co-overexpression of Notch1 and its ligand, Jagged1 (Jag1), is a strong indicator of poor overall survival in advanced breast cancer [30]. A follow-up of these studies underpins a correlation between Jag1 and progression of early-stage breast tumors [32]. Conversely, Notch2 tends to correlate with survival [33].

Notchl is suggested to be sufficient in driving breast oncogenesis [21]. Moreover, mounting evidence suggests that Notch can contribute to secondary tumor characteristics, which make the disease more aggressive and difficult to overcome. Notch has been shown to cross talk with the oncogenic Akt [5], NF-κB [34], and MAP kinase [35] pathways. The breast oncogene, c-Myc, is a direct target of Notch1 transcriptional activation, and Notch1-mediated c-Myc activation is sufficient to drive breast oncogenesis [36]. Furthermore, in vitro studies show that Notch1 and Notch3 augment cell proliferation by binding to the promoter region and activating CyclinD1 [37].

The DNA damage response (DDR) is critical for genomic fidelity, and mutations in DDR genes are frequently occurring facilitators of breast oncogenesis. Notch is known to promote oncogenesis by interacting with DDR genes and proteins. Subsequent to γ-secretase cleavage, the Notch1 intracellular domain has been shown to interact with ATM, a DDR element that arrests mitosis by stabilizing p53 [38]. This interaction confers a Notch1-dependent negative regulatory effect to the

ATM kinase domain rendering it unable to phosphorylate and stabilize p53 [38]. The tumor suppressor p53 is often subject to inactivating mutations, which facilitates tumorigenesis. Notch1 inhibits apoptosis by interfering with p53-mediated induction of the proapoptotic effectors Puma and Noxa [39]. In addition, p53 feeds back into Notch signaling by directly binding to MAML1 thus impeding the formation of the Notch activation complex [40].

9.3 Notch Signaling in Cancer Stem Cells

The therapeutic strategies currently at our disposal yield a high rate of initial tumor regression in some breast cancer patients. However, drug resistance and tumor relapse have emerged as major therapeutic hurdles [41]. Recent attention in breast cancer research has turned to preventing tumor relapse by targeting the breast cancer stem cell (BCSC). The BCSC hypothesis posits the existence of a small population of multipotent cells that are capable of giving rise to a heterogeneous tumor mass. Cancer stem cells possess a number of phenotypes that make them prone to therapeutic resistance.

A number of lines of evidence exist in support of the BCSC hypothesis. Transplant studies that date back to the late 1950s demonstrate the ability of certain cells to repopulate the mammary fat pad [42]. The technique involves surgically removing the mammary epithelium from the fat pad of young mice and subsequently repopulating the fat pad with cells or tissue of choice. These transplant studies were developed in order to demonstrate the ability of precancerous mammary nodules to give rise to tumors [42]. The researchers included a comparison between normal mammary tissue and precancerous nodules. Interestingly, the normal mammary tissue is able to repopulate the fat pad with a structurally normal mammary epithelial complex [42].

A subpopulation of tumor cells identified as $CD44^{+}/CD24^{-/low}/ALDH1^{high}$ has been shown to bear stem cell characteristics [43]. $CD44^{+}/CD24^{-/low}/ALDH1^{high}$ cells are highly efficient at forming mammospheres and tumor xenografts [44]. Notch4 is strongly implicated in BCSC activity [45]. Anti-Notch targeted therapies currently undergoing clinical trials are mainly focused on inhibiting the survival and differentiation potential of the BCSCs [46].

9.4 Notch Signaling in Metastasis

Metastasis presents one of the most challenging features of breast cancer with regard to treatment. The presence and number of metastatic lesions are used clinically to stage breast cancer [47]. The lymph nodes that occupy the chest walls are frequently the first organs to experience metastatic invasion. Metastasis to distant organs such as the bone, lung, and brain is characteristic of the most advanced stage, and these patients exhibit the poorest prognosis. The metastatic process involves a number of steps wherein cancer cells depart from the primary tumor, enter the blood or lymphatic systems, and colonize a distant site. JAG1 has been shown to facilitate bone metastasis in mice, a process that can be inhibited by γ-secretase inhibition [48]. In addition, γ-secretase inhibition hinders the ability of the metastatic breast cancer cell line MDA-MB-231-Br to colonize the brain [49].

Epithelial-mesenchymal transition (EMT) is a key cellular phenomenon that a cancer cell must undergo in order for metastasis to occur. Epithelial cells are characteristically polar and dependent on attachment to a basal membrane. Mesenchymal cells are devoid of polarity and are resistant to anoikis, a type of cell death associated with detachment from a basement membrane. A number of salient genes have emerged as promoters of EMT. The transcription factors Snail, Slug, and Twist are known to promote the EMT process by suppressing epithelial factors such as E-cadherin and augmenting expression of mesenchymal factors such as N-cadherin [50]. The transforming growth factor-β (TGF-β) signaling pathway is a prominent facilitator of EMT. However, other signaling pathways, including Notch, are emerging as regulators of this process. The JAG1-Notch1 signaling axis has been shown to directly promote EMT and anoikis resistance by promoting Slug expression [6, 51]. Slug in turn suppresses E-cadherin expression while upregulating N-cadherin and vimentin expression: hallmarks of EMT [6, 51]. The vacuolar ATPase DMXL2, a novel regulator of Notch signaling, has been shown to facilitate EMT via Notch activation which further implicates Notch in the EMT process [52].

9.5 Notch Signaling in Different Breast Cancer Subtypes

Histological and immunohistochemical subtyping is an immensely valuable method of classifying breast cancer in a clinical setting. However, the research literature often refers to breast cancers based on molecular subtype. Molecular characterization relies upon the identification of "driver oncogenes." As such, it is more logical to consider interacting molecular pathways with respect to the driver oncogene than to structural characteristics. We will proceed by examining Notch signaling in the context of different molecular subtypes of breast cancer. One exception will be for ductal carcinoma in situ for which molecular subtyping is not usually indicated.

9.6 Ductal Carcinoma In Situ

Ductal carcinoma in situ (DCIS) is a type of mammary lesion that is frequently encountered in the clinic. Though DCIS is considered a preinvasive neoplastic lesion, the disease can progress to an invasive tumor if left untreated. The standard of care typically involves surgical resection followed by radiation or antihormonal therapy if the tumor expresses ER/PR. Histological classification is generally sufficient to diagnose and successfully treat DCIS patients, and molecular subtyping is rarely indicated. DCIS usually presents a favorable prognosis with current therapeutic modalities.

Breast cancer development is a poorly understood process, and our lack of understanding presents a major drawback to diagnosis and treatment of the disease. Active research surrounding DCIS provides an avenue for improved understanding of breast oncogenesis. Notch signaling has emerged as a potential suspect for the progression of DCIS to invasive carcinoma [31]. Stem cell activity is implicated in the advancement of DCIS to invasive disease, and inhibition of Notch signaling reduces DCIS mammosphere formation [53]. Further studies underpin Notch as a promoter of stem cell activity in DCIS [54].

9.7 Estrogen/Progesterone Positive Breast Cancer

ERα and PR are ovarian hormone receptors that play a critical role in breast development and function [3]. Aberrant overexpression of ERα is sufficient to drive oncogenic transformation [55]. The role of PR is debated because many studies show protective effects of progesterone and PR in breast cancer. In addition, compared to ER+/PR- patients, ER+/PR+ patients have a more favorable response to antihormone therapy [41]. Unlike ERα, no studies exist that single out PR with regard to interaction with Notch signaling.

ERα is a nuclear hormone receptor which is overexpressed in about 60% of all breast cancers. ERα-targeted therapies are commonly prescribed and are successful at inducing tumor regression [41]. Strategies that interfere with estrogen signaling involve either targeting ERα directly or inhibiting the aromatase enzyme responsible for synthesizing estrogen. ERα inhibitors fall under two classes, selective estrogen receptor modulators (SERMs) and selective estrogen receptor downregulators (SERDs). SERMs, including tamoxifen and raloxifene, act on estrogen signaling by binding to ER and inhibiting its ability to recruit transcriptional co-activators to its target genes [56]. SERDs, such as fulvestrant, inhibit estrogen signaling by promoting proteasomal degradation of ERα [57]. Aromatase inhibitors, such as letrozole, anastrozole, and exemestane, are effective but are generally indicated in postmenopausal women due to gynecological complications that they cause in pre-menopausal patients [58].

Recent evidence suggests a close interdependence between Notch and estrogen signaling in ERα+ breast cancer [59]. Estrogen has been shown to upregulate Notch1 expression but decrease cleavage of Notch1 in ERα+ breast cancer cell lines [59]. Conversely, Notch1 signaling can act cooperatively with other factors such as IKK-alpha to activate ERα providing yet another avenue for aberrant cell proliferation [60].

In contrast with its role on Notch1, ERα activity suppresses the expression of Notch4, a phenotype that is reversed by estrogen deprivation or treatment with tamoxifen or fulvestrant [61, 62]. Recently, it has been shown that in ERα+ cell line populations and in patient-derived xenografts, ERα expression is significantly lower in a subpopulation of cells that express high levels of Notch4 [61]. Tamoxifen and fulvestrant are ineffective at killing these cells, an expected outcome due to the lack of a molecular target. Thus, the $ER\alpha^{lo}$/$Notch4^{hi}$ population is suggested to give rise to tumors that are inherently hormone therapy-resistant. The estrogen-dependent control of Notch4 has come under scrutiny due to its hypothesized role in BCSC activity [45]. Studies identifying an $ER\alpha^{lo}$/$Notch4^{hi}$ population of cells demonstrate putative signs of breast cancer stemness such as high ALDH activity and high mammosphere-forming efficiency.

Currently, the major goal in improving treatment of ERα+ breast cancer is to prevent tumor relapse. Notch is strongly implicated as a BCSC maintenance factor. In turn, Notch signaling is hypothesized to promote inherent and acquired drug resistance especially through Notch4 activity. Thus, clinical trials combining γ-secretase inhibitors (targeting Notch activation) with antihormone therapy are being conducted.

9.8 HER2-Positive Breast Cancer

HER2, also known as ErbB2, is a receptor tyrosine kinase that is overexpressed in about 20% of all breast cancers. HER2 has no known ligand. Instead, the receptor is constitutively active and exerts its effects by dimerizing with other EGF receptor family members. As with other receptor tyrosine kinases, HER2 acts as a potent mitogenic and pro-survival factor by activating MAP kinase and PI3K/AKT signaling cascades. Two therapies exist which target the HER2 protein directly: Monoclonal antibodies such as trastuzumab, pertuzumab, TDM-1, and/or small molecules such as lapatinib. Trastuzumab is a humanized, monoclonal antibody that targets the extracellular domain of HER2. Trastuzumab and other antibody-based biologics trigger a number of cytotoxic events that lead to growth arrest and apoptosis. Lapatinib is a small molecule tyrosine kinase inhibitor, which exhibits efficacy against both HER2 and HER1. Both drugs are administered as adjuvants to chemotherapeutic regimens including doxorubicin, paclitaxel, and 5-fluorouracil.

HER2+ tumors are prone to drug resistance and relapse, and multiple mechanisms of resistance have been proposed and investigated [63]. Notch signaling components are upregulated upon anti-HER2 therapy [64, 65]. Studies in mice show that when a γ-secretase inhibitor is given in combination with trastuzumab, tumors are less prone to acquiring trastuzumab resistance [65, 66]. The trastuzumab-dependent increase in Notch1 activity is sufficient to make HER2+ cell lines susceptible to the anti-Notch effects of γ-secretase inhibition [65]. Others have taken a genetic approach to demonstrating the relationship between Notch and HER2 wherein doxycycline-induced ablation of HER2 causes an increase in Notch1 expression and activity [66]. Sustainment of Notch1 in the absence of HER2 allows dormant breast cancer cells to relapse, and relapse can be inhibited by the administration of a γ-secretase inhibitor [66]. One mode of HER2-mediated

Notch1 suppression involves cross talk with PKCα [67]. HER2 activates PKCα, and PKCα in turn attenuates Jagged-mediated activation of Notch1 [67]. This series of interactions is associated with sensitivity to anti-HER2 therapy, which is underscored by clinical observations wherein PKCα is a predictor for positive response to HER2 therapy [68].

9.9 Triple-Negative Breast Cancer

The triple-negative breast cancer (TNBC) subtype is associated with poor prognosis and receives a considerable amount of research attention. TNBC accounts for about 15% of all breast cancers. Unlike other subtypes, no universal driver oncogene is attributed to TNBC, but some typical genetic alterations exist such as BRCA1 [69], ATM [70], and PTEN [71]. Mutations in the PEST-negative regulatory region of Notch have been identified in a few isolated cases, which are sufficient to drive oncogenesis [72]. However, mutations in Notch genes are rare in breast cancer. Instead, abnormalities in Notch signaling are usually due to alterations in the overall expression or posttranslational regulation of Notch pathway components.

In general, a TNBC diagnosis limits therapeutic options to chemotherapy. It is possible to identify certain mutations and to adjust treatment regimens accordingly. The feasibility of screening for BRCA1/2 mutations in all TNBC patients has been considered, especially with the advent of PARP inhibitors [73]. Nonetheless, TNBC remains an extremely heterogeneous disease, and in lieu of large-scale genetic screening of each patient, researchers are tasked with searching for a central targetable node.

Notch is a commonly upregulated factor in TNBC [74]. Immunohistochemistry and microarray database analyses reveal a significant proportion of patients with high Notch1 expression profiles [75]. Furthermore, patients with high Notch1 expression demonstrate poorer overall survival than those with low Notch1 expression [75]. A more recent study validated the elevated expression of Notch1 and also indicated upregulation of Notch4 in a cohort of 29 TNBC cases [74]. One possible mechanism for this upregulation of Notch is expression of an Ets transcription factor, PEA3. PEA3 has been shown to activate Notch1 and Notch4 gene expression in MDA-MB-231 cells, a common TNBC cell line [76].

One hallmark of TNBC tumors is the high degree of cellular heterogeneity, which makes the disease prone to rapid advancement and evasion of therapeutic intervention. One explanation for this heterogeneity is the particularly active stem cell population present in these tumors. Some hypothesize that by targeting BCSCs in this breast cancer subtype, the more threatening phenotypes attributed to this disease can be halted or reversed. Notch signaling facilitates stemness in TNBC by interacting with a number of pathways. NFκB has been shown to promote Jagged1 expression, which in turn facilitates stem cell expansion by activating Notch [34, 77]. Inhibition of TORC1/2 causes an increase in stemness in TNBC cell lines, but this effect is attenuated by simultaneously treating with γ-secretase inhibitors [78]. Similar results are seen when the VEGF receptor inhibitor sunitinib is administered to the triple-negative MDA-MB-468 cells [79]. Sunitinib administration increases the $CD44^{hi}/CD24^{low}$ population, and this effect is reversed upon γ-secretase inhibition [79].

9.10 Conclusion

The emergence of resistance to targeted therapies as well as to chemotherapy is a major obstacle to achieving a cure for breast cancer. Notch is a druggable signaling pathway that is frequently dysregulated in breast cancer. Though Notch can facilitate proliferation and pro-survival programs in certain contexts, the main goal of anti-Notch therapy is to inhibit stem cell activity. Several clinical trials aim to determine the efficacy of γ-secretase inhibitors or selective antibodies against Notch and its ligands in breast cancer. Additionally, novel classes of Notch inhibitors, particularly in combination with targeted agents, are being developed and may find applications in breast cancer, most likely in combinations with other targeted agents or chemotherapy.

References

1. Buono, K. D., et al. (2006). The canonical Notch/RBP-J signaling pathway controls the balance of cell lineages in mammary epithelium during pregnancy. *Developmental Biology, 293*(2), 565–580.
2. Van Keymeulen, A., et al. (2011). Distinct stem cells contribute to mammary gland development and maintenance. *Nature, 479*(7372), 189–193.
3. Kleinberg, D. L., & Ruan, W. (2008). IGF-I, GH, and sex steroid effects in normal mammary gland development. *Journal of Mammary Gland Biology and Neoplasia, 13*(4), 353–360.
4. Quarrie, L. H., Addey, C. V., & Wilde, C. J. (1996). Programmed cell death during mammary tissue involution induced by weaning, litter removal, and milk stasis. *Journal of Cellular Physiology, 168*(3), 559–569.
5. Meurette, O., et al. (2009). Notch activation induces Akt signaling via an autocrine loop to prevent apoptosis in breast epithelial cells. *Cancer Research, 69*(12), 5015–5022.
6. Shao, S., et al. (2015). Notch1 signaling regulates the epithelial-mesenchymal transition and invasion of breast cancer in a Slug-dependent manner. *Molecular Cancer, 14*, 28.
7. Angerer, L. M., & Angerer, R. C. (1999). Regulative development of the sea urchin embryo: Signalling cascades and morphogen gradients. *Seminars in Cell & Developmental Biology, 10*(3), 327–334.
8. Kurata, S., et al. (2000). Notch signaling and the determination of appendage identity. *Proceedings of the National Academy of Sciences of the United States of America, 97*(5), 2117–2122.
9. Zhu, X., et al. (2006). Sustained Notch signaling in progenitors is required for sequential emergence of distinct cell lineages during organogenesis. *Genes & Development, 20*(19), 2739–2753.
10. Dufraine, J., Funahashi, Y., & Kitajewski, J. (2008). Notch signaling regulates tumor angiogenesis by diverse mechanisms. *Oncogene, 27*(38), 5132–5137.

11. Chigurupati, S., et al. (2007). Involvement of notch signaling in wound healing. *PLoS One, 2*(11), e1167.
12. Petrovic, J., et al. (2014). Ligand-dependent Notch signaling strength orchestrates lateral induction and lateral inhibition in the developing inner ear. *Development, 141*(11), 2313–2324.
13. Barad, O., Hornstein, E., & Barkai, N. (2011). Robust selection of sensory organ precursors by the Notch-Delta pathway. *Current Opinion in Cell Biology, 23*(6), 663–667.
14. Logeat, F., et al. (1998). The Notch1 receptor is cleaved constitutively by a furin-like convertase. *Proceedings of the National Academy of Sciences of the United States of America, 95*(14), 8108–8112.
15. Rand, M. D., et al. (2000). Calcium depletion dissociates and activates heterodimeric notch receptors. *Molecular and Cellular Biology, 20*(5), 1825–1835.
16. D'Souza, B., Meloty-Kapella, L., & Weinmaster, G. (2010). Canonical and non-canonical Notch ligands. *Current Topics in Developmental Biology, 92*, 73–129.
17. Hartmann, D., et al. (2002). The disintegrin/metalloprotease ADAM 10 is essential for Notch signalling but not for alpha-secretase activity in fibroblasts. *Human Molecular Genetics, 11*(21), 2615–2624.
18. Sastre, M., et al. (2001). Presenilin-dependent gamma-secretase processing of beta-amyloid precursor protein at a site corresponding to the S3 cleavage of Notch. *EMBO Reports, 2*(9), 835–841.
19. Dontu, G., et al. (2004). Role of Notch signaling in cell-fate determination of human mammary stem/progenitor cells. *Breast Cancer Research, 6*(6), R605–R615.
20. Lafkas, D., et al. (2013). Notch3 marks clonogenic mammary luminal progenitor cells in vivo. *The Journal of Cell Biology, 203*(1), 47–56.
21. Bouras, T., et al. (2008). Notch signaling regulates mammary stem cell function and luminal cell-fate commitment. *Cell Stem Cell, 3*(4), 429–441.
22. Cantrell, M. A., et al. (2015). C-Jun N-terminal kinase 2 prevents luminal cell commitment in normal mammary glands and tumors by inhibiting p53/Notch1 and breast cancer gene 1 expression. *Oncotarget, 6*(14), 11863–11881.
23. Domingo, L., et al. (2014). Tumor phenotype and breast density in distinct categories of interval cancer: Results of population-based mammography screening in Spain. *Breast Cancer Research, 16*(1), R3.
24. Schnitt, S. J. (2010). Classification and prognosis of invasive breast cancer: From morphology to molecular taxonomy. *Modern Pathology, 23*(Suppl 2), S60–S64.
25. Prat, A., et al. (2010). Phenotypic and molecular characterization of the claudin-low intrinsic subtype of breast cancer. *Breast Cancer Research, 12*(5), R68.
26. Yerushalmi, R., et al. (2010). Ki67 in breast cancer: Prognostic and predictive potential. *The Lancet Oncology, 11*(2), 174–183.
27. Bastien, R. R., et al. (2012). PAM50 breast cancer subtyping by RT-qPCR and concordance with standard clinical molecular markers. *BMC Medical Genomics, 5*, 44.
28. Gallahan, D., & Callahan, R. (1997). The mouse mammary tumor associated gene INT3 is a unique member of the NOTCH gene family (NOTCH4). *Oncogene, 14*(16), 1883–1890.
29. Gallahan, D., Kozak, C., & Callahan, R. (1987). A new common integration region (int-3) for mouse mammary tumor virus on mouse chromosome 17. *Journal of Virology, 61*(1), 218–220.
30. Reedijk, M., et al. (2005). High-level coexpression of JAG1 and NOTCH1 is observed in human breast cancer and is associated with poor overall survival. *Cancer Research, 65*(18), 8530–8537.
31. Yuan, X., et al. (2015). Expression of Notch1 correlates with breast cancer progression and prognosis. *PLoS One, 10*(6), e0131689.
32. Reedijk, M., et al. (2008). JAG1 expression is associated with a basal phenotype and recurrence in lymph node-negative breast cancer. *Breast Cancer Research and Treatment, 111*(3), 439–448.
33. Chu, D., et al. (2011). Notch1 and Notch2 have opposite prognostic effects on patients with colorectal cancer. *Annals of Oncology, 22*(11), 2440–2447.

34. Li, L., et al. (2014). Notch-1 signaling promotes the malignant features of human breast cancer through NF-kappaB activation. *PLoS One, 9*(4), e95912.
35. Tremblay, I., et al. (2013). The MEK/ERK pathway promotes NOTCH signalling in pancreatic cancer cells. *PLoS One, 8*(12), e85502.
36. Klinakis, A., et al. (2006). Myc is a Notch1 transcriptional target and a requisite for Notch1-induced mammary tumorigenesis in mice. *Proceedings of the National Academy of Sciences of the United States of America, 103*(24), 9262–9267.
37. Cohen, B., et al. (2010). Cyclin D1 is a direct target of JAG1-mediated Notch signaling in breast cancer. *Breast Cancer Research and Treatment, 123*(1), 113–124.
38. Vermezovic, J., et al. (2015). Notch is a direct negative regulator of the DNA-damage response. *Nature Structural & Molecular Biology, 22*(5), 417–424.
39. Stylianou, S., Clarke, R. B., & Brennan, K. (2006). Aberrant activation of notch signaling in human breast cancer. *Cancer Research, 66*(3), 1517–1525.
40. Yun, J., et al. (2015). p53 modulates Notch signaling in MCF-7 breast cancer cells by associating with the Notch transcriptional complex via MAML1. *Journal of Cellular Physiology, 230*(12), 3115–3127.
41. Early Breast Cancer Trialists' Collaborative, G, et al. (2011). Relevance of breast cancer hormone receptors and other factors to the efficacy of adjuvant tamoxifen: patient-level meta-analysis of randomised trials. *Lancet, 378*(9793), 771–784.
42. Deome, K. B., et al. (1959). Development of mammary tumors from hyperplastic alveolar nodules transplanted into gland-free mammary fat pads of female C3H mice. *Cancer Research, 19*(5), 515–520.
43. Ricardo, S., et al. (2011). Breast cancer stem cell markers CD44, CD24 and ALDH1: Expression distribution within intrinsic molecular subtype. *Journal of Clinical Pathology, 64*(11), 937–946.
44. Neumeister, V., et al. (2010). In situ identification of putative cancer stem cells by multiplexing ALDH1, CD44, and cytokeratin identifies breast cancer patients with poor prognosis. *The American Journal of Pathology, 176*(5), 2131–2138.
45. Harrison, H., et al. (2010). Regulation of breast cancer stem cell activity by signaling through the Notch4 receptor. *Cancer Research, 70*(2), 709–718.
46. Grudzien, P., et al. (2010). Inhibition of Notch signaling reduces the stem-like population of breast cancer cells and prevents mammosphere formation. *Anticancer Research, 30*(10), 3853–3867.
47. Park, Y. H., et al. (2011). Clinical relevance of TNM staging system according to breast cancer subtypes. *Annals of Oncology, 22*(7), 1554–1560.
48. Sethi, N., et al. (2011). Tumor-derived JAGGED1 promotes osteolytic bone metastasis of breast cancer by engaging notch signaling in bone cells. *Cancer Cell, 19*(2), 192–205.
49. McGowan, P. M., et al. (2011). Notch1 inhibition alters the CD44hi/CD24lo population and reduces the formation of brain metastases from breast cancer. *Molecular Cancer Research, 9*(7), 834–844.
50. Martin, T. A., et al. (2005). Expression of the transcription factors snail, slug, and twist and their clinical significance in human breast cancer. *Annals of Surgical Oncology, 12*(6), 488–496.
51. Leong, K. G., et al. (2007). Jagged1-mediated Notch activation induces epithelial-to-mesenchymal transition through slug-induced repression of E-cadherin. *The Journal of Experimental Medicine, 204*(12), 2935–2948.
52. Faronato, M., et al. (2015). DMXL2 drives epithelial to mesenchymal transition in hormonal therapy resistant breast cancer through Notch hyper-activation. *Oncotarget, 6*(26), 22467–22479.
53. Farnie, G., et al. (2007). Novel cell culture technique for primary ductal carcinoma in situ: Role of Notch and epidermal growth factor receptor signaling pathways. *Journal of the National Cancer Institute, 99*(8), 616–627.

54. Farnie, G., et al. (2013). Combined inhibition of ErbB1/2 and Notch receptors effectively targets breast ductal carcinoma in situ (DCIS) stem/progenitor cell activity regardless of ErbB2 status. *PLoS One, 8*(2), e56840.
55. Tanos, T., et al. (2012). ER and PR signaling nodes during mammary gland development. *Breast Cancer Research, 14*(4), 210.
56. Katzenellenbogen, B. S., & Katzenellenbogen, J. A. (2000). Estrogen receptor transcription and transactivation: Estrogen receptor alpha and estrogen receptor beta: Regulation by selective estrogen receptor modulators and importance in breast cancer. *Breast Cancer Research, 2*(5), 335–344.
57. Wardell, S. E., Marks, J. R., & McDonnell, D. P. (2011). The turnover of estrogen receptor alpha by the selective estrogen receptor degrader (SERD) fulvestrant is a saturable process that is not required for antagonist efficacy. *Biochemical Pharmacology, 82*(2), 122–130.
58. Goss, P. E., & Strasser, K. (2001). Aromatase inhibitors in the treatment and prevention of breast cancer. *Journal of Clinical Oncology, 19*(3), 881–894.
59. Rizzo, P., et al. (2008). Cross-talk between notch and the estrogen receptor in breast cancer suggests novel therapeutic approaches. *Cancer Research, 68*(13), 5226–5235.
60. Hao, L., et al. (2010). Notch-1 activates estrogen receptor-alpha-dependent transcription via IKKalpha in breast cancer cells. *Oncogene, 29*(2), 201–213.
61. Simoes, B. M., et al. (2015). Anti-estrogen resistance in human breast tumors is driven by JAG1-NOTCH4-dependent cancer stem cell activity. *Cell Reports, 12*(12), 1968–1977.
62. Lombardo, Y., et al. (2014). Nicastrin and Notch4 drive endocrine therapy resistance and epithelial to mesenchymal transition in MCF7 breast cancer cells. *Breast Cancer Research, 16*(3), R62.
63. Arteaga, C. L., et al. (2012). Treatment of HER2-positive breast cancer: Current status and future perspectives. *Nature Reviews. Clinical Oncology, 9*(1), 16–32.
64. Han, M., Deng, H. Y., & Jiang, R. (2012). Effect of trastuzumab on Notch-1 signaling pathway in breast cancer SK-BR3 cells. *Chinese Journal of Cancer Research, 24*(3), 213–219.
65. Osipo, C., et al. (2008). ErbB-2 inhibition activates Notch-1 and sensitizes breast cancer cells to a gamma-secretase inhibitor. *Oncogene, 27*(37), 5019–5032.
66. Abravanel, D. L., et al. (2015). Notch promotes recurrence of dormant tumor cells following HER2/neu-targeted therapy. *Journal of Clinical Investigation, 125*(6), 2484–2496.
67. Pandya, K., et al. (2016). PKCalpha attenuates Jagged-1-mediated Notch signaling in ErbB-2-positive breast cancer to reverse trastuzumab resistance. *Clinical Cancer Research, 22*(1), 175–186.
68. Manni, A., et al. (1996). Induction of a less aggressive breast cancer phenotype by protein kinase C-alpha and -beta overexpression. *Cell Growth & Differentiation, 7*(9), 1187–1198.
69. Severson, T. M., et al. (2015). BRCA1-like signature in triple negative breast cancer: Molecular and clinical characterization reveals subgroups with therapeutic potential. *Molecular Oncology, 9*(8), 1528–1538.
70. Tommiska, J., et al. (2008). The DNA damage signalling kinase ATM is aberrantly reduced or lost in BRCA1/BRCA2-deficient and ER/PR/ERBB2-triple-negative breast cancer. *Oncogene, 27*(17), 2501–2506.
71. Ross, J. S., et al. (2015). Comprehensive genomic profiling of inflammatory breast cancer cases reveals a high frequency of clinically relevant genomic alterations. *Breast Cancer Research and Treatment, 154*(1), 155–162.
72. Wang, K., et al. (2015). PEST domain mutations in Notch receptors comprise an oncogenic driver segment in triple-negative breast cancer sensitive to a gamma-secretase inhibitor. *Clinical Cancer Research, 21*(6), 1487–1496.
73. Phuah, S. Y., et al. (2012). Triple-negative breast cancer and PTEN (phosphatase and tensin homologue) loss are predictors of BRCA1 germline mutations in women with early-onset and familial breast cancer, but not in women with isolated late-onset breast cancer. *Breast Cancer Research, 14*(6), R142.

74. Speiser, J., et al. (2012). Notch-1 and Notch-4 biomarker expression in triple-negative breast cancer. *International Journal of Surgical Pathology, 20*(2), 139–145.
75. Lee, C. W., et al. (2008). A functional Notch-survivin gene signature in basal breast cancer. *Breast Cancer Research, 10*(6), R97.
76. Clementz, A. G., et al. (2011). NOTCH-1 and NOTCH-4 are novel gene targets of PEA3 in breast cancer: Novel therapeutic implications. *Breast Cancer Research, 13*(3), R63.
77. Yamamoto, M., et al. (2013). NF-kappaB non-cell-autonomously regulates cancer stem cell populations in the basal-like breast cancer subtype. *Nature Communications, 4*, 2299.
78. Bhola, N. E., et al. (2016). Treatment of triple negative breast cancer with TORC1/2 inhibitors sustains a drug-resistant and Notch-dependent cancer stem cell population. *Cancer Research, 76*(2), 440–452.
79. Chinchar, E., et al. (2014). Sunitinib significantly suppresses the proliferation, migration, apoptosis resistance, tumor angiogenesis and growth of triple-negative breast cancers but increases breast cancer stem cells. *Vascular Cell, 6*, 12.

Chapter 10
Notch in Lung Cancer

Sara L. Sinicropi-Yao, Michael J. Koenig, and David P. Carbone

Abstract Lung cancer is the deadliest malignancy in the world. The Notch signaling pathway plays an important role in both normal lung development and the pathobiology of lung cancer. By understanding the function of the Notch pathway in normal development, we can begin to appreciate the intricate role that it plays in lung cancer. The complexity of Notch signaling includes multiple Notch receptors and ligands, posttranslational modifications affecting Notch receptor function, and significant cross talk with other signaling pathways. Dysregulation of the Notch signaling pathway occurs in every type of lung cancer, but the specific role of the Notch pathway in the different subtypes of lung cancer is still unclear. There is evidence that Notch can act in a pro-tumorigenic manner under some circumstances and in an anti-tumorigenic manner under others. Notch can facilitate tumor growth and proliferation, apoptosis, cell differentiation, survival, immune response, angiogenesis, cancer stem cell biology, and chemoresistance. Understanding how Notch naturally usurps these mechanisms to promote or suppress tumors can provide new insights regarding therapeutic intervention while minimizing toxicity.

Keywords Lung cancer · Notch signaling · Cancer stem cell · Tumor microenvironment · Immune response · Therapy

S. L. Sinicropi-Yao · M. J. Koenig
The Ohio State University Comprehensive Cancer Center, Columbus, OH, USA
e-mail: Sara.Sinicropi-Yao@osumc.edu; Michael.Koenig@osumc.edu

D. P. Carbone (✉)
The Ohio State University Comprehensive Cancer Center, Columbus, OH, USA

Division of Medical Oncology, Department of Internal Medicine, Columbus, OH, USA

The James Thoracic Oncology Center, Columbus, OH, USA
e-mail: David.Carbone@osumc.edu

L. Miele, S. Artavanis-Tsakonas (eds.), *Targeting Notch in Cancer*,
https://doi.org/10.1007/978-1-4939-8859-4_10

10.1 Introduction to the Notch Signaling Pathway in Lung Cancer

Notch signaling plays a prominent role in early lung development promoting cell fate determination, cell differentiation and the coordination of alveolar development. In humans, there are four Notch receptors (NOTCH1, NOTCH2, NOTCH3, and NOTCH4) and five ligands (DLL1, DLL3, DLL4, JAGGED1, and JAGGED2). Notch receptors and ligands are membrane bound and act in both a juxtacrine and autocrine manner. Notch receptors are first synthesized as precursor polypeptides that are cleaved in the Golgi apparatus by a furin-like convertase (S1 cleavage). The resulting extracellular domain (ECD) and intracellular domain (ICD) are maintained by a non-covalent bond between the N- and C- terminal halves and present at the cell surface. The second proteolytic cleavage site, S2, is buried within the negative regulatory region (NRR). Notch ligands DLL1, DLL4, JAGGED1, and JAGGED2 transactivate the Notch receptor and induce a conformational change that exposes the NRR and triggers the second cleavage (S2) by ADAM10(Kuz)/17(TACE) protease. Cleavage by the γ-secretase complex at a third site (S3) releases the ICD, which translocates to the nucleus and regulates gene expression by cooperating with the DNA binding protein CSL (CBF-1/SU(H)/Lag-1) and co-activator MamL1-3 (Fig. 10.1).

The Notch signaling cascade does not rely on an enzymatic amplification step. Instead precise stoichiometry of receptor-ligand complexes is required for Notch

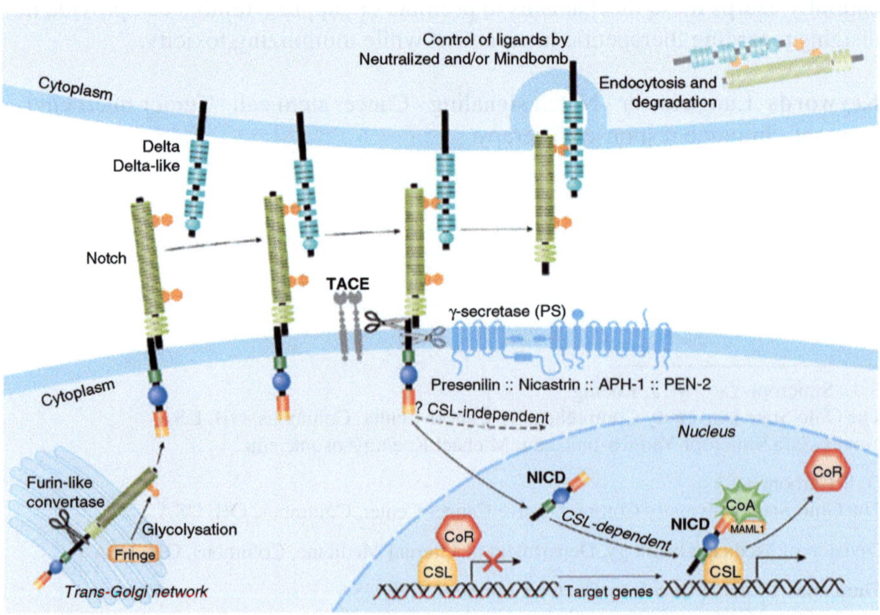

Fig. 10.1 Overview of the Notch signaling pathway. (Modified from [1] by [2])

activation [3]. This likely allows for the precise regulation of Notch signaling and partially explains the sensitivity of Notch signals to small perturbations.

Aberrant Notch signaling has been reported in 20% of all cancers [4]. Likewise, 25% of small cell lung cancer (SCLC) [5] tumors and 33% of non-small cell lung cancer (NSCLC) [6] tumors have altered Notch signaling, and is correlated with poor overall survival [7, 8]. It has become increasingly clear that the outcomes of Notch signaling alterations are context dependent and can have opposing roles in different subtypes of lung cancer. The divergent impact of Notch receptor or ligand expression at the RNA or protein level may be related to its context-dependent role as oncogene or tumor suppressor [9–15]. Given the complexity of Notch signaling, modulated by the expression of multiple combinations of Notch receptors and ligands and their state of posttranslational modification, numerous target genes and crosstalk with other signaling cascades, it is crucial to understand Notch biology to predict the outcome of Notch therapies [12]. Pan-inhibition of Notch receptors or their ligands may not be optimal, and therapies that target individual receptors or ligands may be necessary. Successful development of targeted and combination therapies will require a better understanding of the role of each Notch receptor and ligand in each tumor and how targeting them affects different aspects of cell behavior.

10.2 Modulation of Notch Signaling by Posttranslational Modification

Regulation of the Notch receptor and Notch-ICD occurs throughout maturation with signaling and turnover affected by a number of posttranslational modifications that include glycosylation, ubiquitination, and phosphorylation events [3, 6, 16–30]. How these modifications affect Notch activity, signaling, and turnover is not yet fully understood.

With the exception of the loss of NUMB, a negative regulator of Notch that promotes ubiquitylation and degradation of NOTCH1, posttranslational modifications of Notch have not been extensively studied in the context of lung cancer [6]. One study identified manic fringe as a tumor suppressor in lung cancer [30]. Because JAGGED1 is often upregulated in lung cancer and manic fringe was found to be downregulated, the authors hypothesized that manic fringe expression in lung cancer would suppress Notch-Jagged activation. They found that re-expressing manic fringe downregulated NOTCH3 signaling through increased protein turnover. More studies are needed to better understand the role of modifications in the context of lung cancer. Mechanisms such as posttranslational modifications can alter Notch signaling activity without affecting Notch expression itself and thus represent potential targets for therapeutic modulation.

10.3 Notch Signaling in Normal Lung Development and Homeostasis

Notch plays an integral role in the development of the lung, a stratified structure composed of a number of specialized cells each with specific functions (Fig. 10.2).

Notch pathway genes are expressed during tracheobronchial bud formation and regulate proximal and distal cell fates. Within the budding epithelium, NOTCH1, JAGGED1, and JAGGED2 expressions are localized to distal areas of the bud, whereas DLL1 expression occurs proximally [31, 32]. This pattern suggests that Notch signaling mediates cell fate determination along the proximodistal axis. In mouse embryos, pan-Notch inhibition using a γ-secretase inhibitor has been shown to disrupt the proximodistal axis of the budding lung epithelium by causing an expansion of distal progenitors and loss of proximal structure formation [31].

Notch signaling regulates the development of undifferentiated precursor populations into specialized cell types. In basal cells, NOTCH1-mediated lateral inhibition appears to regulate the adoption of a club (secretory), ciliated, or pulmonary neuroendocrine cell (PNEC) fate [33]. Morimoto et al. found that deletion of the Notch effector protein RBPJ (CSL) redirects cells from a club fate to a ciliated fate. They also found that NOTCH2 determines club cell fate independently of NOTCH1 and NOTCH3 [33, 34]. Moreover, using an injury model, the authors found that CC10-positive club cells arise from a population of CC10-negative cells that activate the Notch signaling pathway and develop into club cells [33].

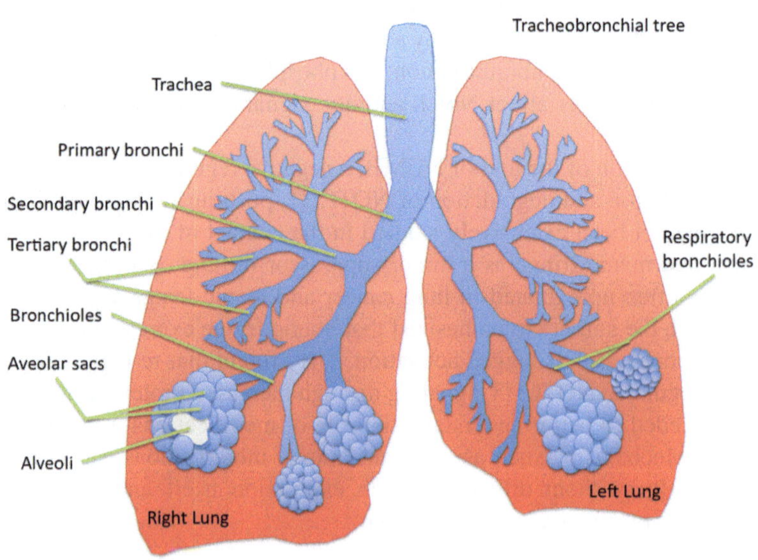

Fig. 10.2 The tracheobronchial tree

Similarly, Notch signaling controls the binary cell fate decision of neuroendocrine versus non-neuroendocrine cells [34, 35]. Morimoto et al. found that NOTCH1, NOTCH2, and NOTCH3 contribute to development of PNECs and observed a mutually exclusive relationship between expression of HES1, which is expressed in non-neuroendocrine cells, and ASH1, which is expressed in neuroendocrine cells. PNECs express DLL1, which activates Notch receptors on adjacent cells to produce HES1. HES1 functions as a transcriptional repressor of ASH1, which is required for neuroendocrine cell differentiation. Thus pulmonary neuroendocrine cells that express the Notch ligand DLL1 suppress adjacent cells from developing into pulmonary neuroendocrine cells themselves [35, 36]. Morimoto et al. propose that this traditional model may be incomplete and suggest that DLL1 expression by pulmonary neuroendocrine cells does not merely inhibit adjacent cells from developing a neuroendocrine cell phenotype but rather drives the development of a specialized group of cells surrounding the neuroendocrine cells. They call these specialized cells stage-specific embryonic antigen-1 (SSEA-1)-positive, peri-neuroepithelial body, Notch-active, CC10-negative cells (SPNCs) [34]. Deletion of JAGGED1 in non-neuroendocrine cells has also been reported to increase the number of neuroendocrine cells [36]. Zhang et al. hypothesize that JAGGED1 may be able to activate Notch receptors in neighboring SPNCs and prevent their adoption of a neuroendocrine cell fate [36]. Recent studies by Lafkas et al. demonstrate that under normal conditions, JAGGED1 prevents differentiated secretory cells from adopting a ciliated fate; on the other hand, inhibition of JAGGED1 promotes the conversion of secretory cells to a ciliated fate [37]. It appears that DLL3 may act as a negative regulator of Notch and DLL1 by redirecting them to internal degradation pathways [38, 39]. DLL3 is a direct downstream target of ASCL1, a basic helix-loop-helix (bHLH) transcription factor involved in neuronal cell differentiation [40, 41]. Saunders et al. suggest that DLL3 is associated with a neuroendocrine cell phenotype and contributes to neuroendocrine tumorigenesis [42]. They found that targeting DLL3 with an antibody-drug conjugate (ADC) known as SC16LD6.5 (Rova-T) suppressed tumor growth in SCLC patient-derived xenograft (PDX)'s [42].

Pulmonary goblet cell fate is also regulated by Notch. In murine airway tracheal explant studies, addition of the Notch agonist Dll4 increased the percentage of Muc5ac-positive expressing goblet cells [43]. Presumably overexpression of Notch1-ICD increased goblet cell numbers in the proximal airways driving a goblet cell fate over a ciliated one [43]. Conversely when a diazepine inhibitor of γ-secretase (DBZ) was added to mouse tracheal explants, the fraction of ciliated cells increased, and the number of mucus-secreting cells decreased [43].

In the distal lung, Notch signaling regulates alveolar development that is necessary for alveoli formation [44]. Constitutive activation of Notch1 in the distal lung epithelium stops alveolar development [43]. Distal cysts form and cells within these structures stop expressing alveolar markers [43]. Similarly, constitutive expression of Notch3-ICD in the distal lung epithelium arrests alveolar epithelium differentiation, stalls maturation of Type II pneumocytes, and prevents the formation of Type I pneumocytes in the lungs of transgenic mice [45]. This study suggests that constitutive expression of the Notch3 receptor is essential for proper microvasculature development in the alveoli of the embryonic lung.

While Notch signaling plays a critical role in cell fate determination, maintenance of adult airways, and tissue architecture, it has also been investigated for its role in stem cell maintenance [46–48]. Throughout the lung, specific stem/progenitor cells have been identified that are capable of self-renewal and regeneration into specialized cell types [46]. The role of Notch in lung stem cells was recently reviewed by Carraro et al. [46]. In cancer, the lung epithelium undergoes pathological remodeling with large changes to the proportion of cell types [49–51], recapitulating what happens during development. Notch contributes to the dedifferentiated state of tumor cells [52]. A deeper understanding of the mechanisms regulating lung maintenance and repair by stem cells is needed for the development of new therapies.

10.4 Notch Signaling in Lung Tumorigenesis: Preclinical and Clinical Relevance

The contribution of Notch signaling to lung tumorigenesis is poorly understood. Notch's oncogenic role in lung cancer was supported by the discovery of a chromosome 15:19 translocation in a case of poorly differentiated lung cancer in 2000 [53]. The position of this translocation upstream of the NOTCH3 locus on chromosome 19 was associated with massive overexpression of NOTCH3 [53]. While translocation-mediated oncogene activation is common in leukemia and increasingly recognized in other solid tumor types, this was the first reported case of a translocation in a cancer of epithelial origin and the first to implicate NOTCH3 as an oncogene in lung cancer.

Notch has been implicated as both an oncogene and a suppressor in lung cancer. These contrasting roles may be a result of the complexity of the pathway, interactions with other signaling pathways, lack of specific inhibitors, and the fact that Notch signaling is context-dependent. For example, NOTCH1 can play opposing roles in different subtypes of lung cancer (Table 10.1). A review of Notch mutation rates and copy number alterations is provided in Table 10.2. The tumor microenvironment can also influence Notch's role in cancer, as Notch exerts opposing effects in the same tissue type under hypoxic versus normoxic conditions [67].

Table 10.1 Hypothesized role of Notch receptors in specific cancer subtypes

Notch receptor	Small cell lung cancer	Adenocarcinoma	Squamous cell carcinoma
NOTCH1	Tumor suppressor [5, 54, 55]	Oncogene [9–11, 56]	Tumor suppressor [57, 58]
NOTCH2	Tumor suppressor [5, 57]	Tumor suppressor [9]	Unknown
NOTCH3	Tumor suppressor [59]	Oncogene [60, 61]	Unknown
NOTCH4	Unknown	Oncogene [62]	Unknown

Table 10.2 Frequency of Notch pathway mutations and copy number alterations in lung cancer[a]

Notch receptor	Small cell lung cancer ($N = 110$)[b]	Adenocarcinoma ($N = 230$)	Squamous cell carcinoma ($N = 178$)
NOTCH1	14.55%	5.22%	8.99%
NOTCH2	4.55%	18.7%	12.92%
NOTCH3	9.09%	1.74%	6.74%
NOTCH4	2.73%	13.48%	2.81%
JAGGED1	1.82%	3.04%	3.93%
JAGGED2	2.73%	2.17%	5.62%
DLL1	1.82%	2.61%	2.25%
DLL3	2.73%	3.48%	7.87%
DLL4	1.82%	2.91%	0.56%

[a]Percentages represent the prevalence of mutation and copy number alterations obtained from the cBioPortal for Cancer Genomics (www.cbioportal.org) [63, 64] using the TCGA provisional datasets [65, 66] and from the small cell lung cancer dataset from U Cologne [5]
[b]Percentages from the small cell lung cancer dataset represent the prevalence of mutations but not copy number alterations

10.4.1 Role of Notch in Small Cell Lung Cancer (SCLC)

SCLC comprises 15% of all lung cancers and typically arises in heavy smokers [68]. SCLC is an aggressive neuroendocrine carcinoma that is homogeneously poorly differentiated, has a very high mitotic rate, arises in the central airways, and infiltrates the bronchial airways. SCLC is distinguished by a rapid growth rate and early spread to regional lymph nodes and distant sites. While chemotherapy is often temporarily effective, recurrence is nearly universal, with death occurring within weeks or months [69].

Notch signaling has a tumor-suppressive role in PNECs [70] including the neuroendocrine cells in SCLC and other neuroendocrine tumors [5, 54]. For example, overexpression of active NOTCH1 or NOTCH2 caused growth arrest of SCLC cells [54]. There are two known mechanisms of Notch-mediated tumor suppression in SCLC [71]. The first mechanism occurs through the transcriptional regulatory cascade whereby Notch signaling causes transactivation of HES1, a transcriptional repressor of hASH1, which leads to repression of neural determination and differentiation genes. The second mechanism involves a novel pathway of NOTCH1 signaling that enhances hASH1 ubiquitination and targets it for degradation through a proteasome-dependent pathway.

Since SCLC is rarely treated surgically, it has been difficult to acquire a large number of high-quality surgical resections that are needed for large genomic studies. In 2012 two independent studies performed comprehensive genomic characterization of SCLC tumors [72, 73]. In an analysis of 36 primary human SCLC samples, Rudin et al. found mutations clustering in the Notch (NOTCH1, NOTCH2, and NOTCH3) family genes [72]. Scientists at the University of Cologne in Germany sequenced the genome of 110 resected SCLCs [5]. Using unsupervised hierarchical clustering of tumor transcriptomes, they observed that the majority (53/69) of tumors had high expression of neuroendocrine markers and low Notch pathway activity as indicated by high levels of DLK1, a noncanonical inhibitor of Notch signaling, and ASCL1 whose expression is inhibited by active Notch signaling [5]. Damaging mutations were enriched in the extracellular domains of Notch receptors suggesting a tumor-suppressive role of Notch in SCLC. In concordance with the earlier study by Rudin et al., the University of Cologne's study determined that Notch family genes were affected by predicted functional genomic alterations in 25% of tumors [5]. A review of mutation rates in SCLC from the University of Cologne study is provided in Table 10.2 [5]. It is possible that alterations in other pathway genes could make the frequency of functional Notch inactivation even higher. Notch receptor/ligand mutations were mutually exclusive of mutations in other frequently altered pro-tumorigenic genes such as CREBBP, EP300, TP73, RBL1, and RBL2. In the University of Cologne dataset, NOTCH1 and JAGGED1 ($p = 0.02$) as well as DLL1 and DLL4 ($p = 0.04$) had a significant association toward co-occurrence [63]. Mutations in Notch were not significantly associated with the total number of mutations, overall survival, or other clinical parameters.

Lim et al. identified that activation of Notch in SCLC models leads some cells to undergo a neuroendocrine to non-neuroendocrine shift [55]. These non-neuroendocrine cells are slow growing, chemoresistant and stimulate neuroendocrine tumor cell growth [55]. This lineage switch requires the expression of the Notch-targeted transcription factor Rest (NRSF), an inhibitor of neuroendocrine fate [55].

Activation of Notch1 or Notch2 signaling in murine SCLC models is associated with increases in Hes1 expression, suppression of neuroendocrine differentiation, and significantly reduced tumor formation [5]. Consistent with earlier studies, expression of NOTCH1-ICD inhibited tumor growth, and expression of NOTCH2-ICD prolonged overall survival. In a SCLC cell line, inhibition of NOTCH3 promoted tumor growth supporting a tumor-suppressive role [59]. Taken together this data supports a tumor-suppressive role for Notch in SCLC that parallels its role as a regulator of lineage specification in PNECs during lung development. The finding of frequent DLL3 overexpression in SCLC (a suppressive Notch ligand) supports this hypothesis [42].

10.4.2 Role of Notch in Non-small Cell Lung Cancer (NSCLC)

10.4.2.1 Altered Expression, Mutations, and SNPs

Many studies have characterized mutations in Notch genes that are involved with the pathogenesis of NSCLC [6, 74–76]. A 2015 article by Guo et al. reviewed the role of Notch in lung cancer [77]. In a cohort of 49 NSCLC cancers, Westhoff et al. found a subset of patients had NOTCH1 gain-of-function mutations [6]. The authors reported that 30% of NSCLC tumors lose expression of NUMB, a negative regulator of Notch, whose loss leads to increased NOTCH1 expression and activity [6]. A review of mutation rates in NSCLC from The Cancer Genome Atlas (TCGA) is provided in Table 10.2 [65, 66].

Multiple studies have examined the value of Notch signaling as a prognostic indicator in patients with NSCLC [8, 78–80]. Studies show that NSCLCs have higher NOTCH1 expression compared to normal lung tissue and that the expression of NOTCH1 is positively correlated with disease progression, metastasis, and poorer overall survival [78]. Mariscal et al. showed that high NOTCH1 expression in circulating tumor cells is a negative prognostic factor for progression-free survival, suggesting its potential utility in liquid biopsy [81]. Another recent study found that patients with lung adenocarcinoma have higher NOTCH2 expression, which is positively correlated with recurrence. This study identified high NOTCH1 and NOTCH3 expression as negative prognostic indicators in adenocarcinoma [82].

A meta-analysis by Yuan et al. examining 3663 patients across 19 studies found that high expression of NOTCH1 was associated with higher tumor, lymph node, and metastasis (TNM) stage and higher risk of lymph node metastasis [78]. NOTCH1 and NOTCH3 overexpression was linked to poor overall survival (NOTCH1, HR, 1.29; 95% CI, 1.06–1.57, $p = 0.468$, and I2 = 0.0%; NOTCH3, HR, 1.57; 95%CI, 1.04–2.36, $p = 0.445$, and I2 = 0.0%). The study also identified that DLL4 expression and HES1 expression were associated with poor overall survival in NSCLC. There was no association found between DLL1 and DLL3 expression and overall survival.

The studies reviewed by Yuan [78], Westhoff [6], and Andersen [80] stand out for their size and significance. Westhoff et al. identified NOTCH1 expression as a poor prognostic marker, and the Andersen et al. study identified NOTCH1 and HIF1α co-expression as a poor prognostic marker. Similarly, a 2007 study by Jiang et al. showed that JAGGED1 expression was correlated with lymph node metastasis [79]. Jiang et al. also found that high NOTCH1 expression in adenocarcinoma samples was associated with poorer overall survival and that high co-expression of NOTCH1 and VEGF-A was associated with poorer overall survival in all types of NSCLC. In squamous cell carcinoma, low DLL4 expression was an indicator of poor prognosis [7, 8].

According to dbSNP, the single-nucleotide polymorphism (SNP) rs2229968(V1671I) occurs in African American ancestry populations with a frequency of approximately 3.4% but not in populations of European ancestry [83]. A study by Bollig-Fischer et al. observed that in 472 patients (137 African American ancestry, 335 European ancestry) with NSCLC, the frequency of NOTCH1 V1671I was increased in the African American (9%) versus European ancestry (0%) population ($p < 0.0001$) [84]. These results from Bollig-Fisher associate this SNP with a higher risk of cancer. Another study by Lee and colleagues suggest that the DTX1 rs1732786A>G promoter region polymorphism may affect DTX1 expression and is associated with better overall survival and disease-free survival [85]. Results from Quan et al. suggest that the NOTCH1 SNP rs3124599 may be associated with a predisposition to SCLC in northeast Chinese non-smoking women but had no prognostic effect [86].

10.4.2.2 Notch Signaling in Adenocarcinoma

Several studies have shown that NOTCH1 directly contributes to lung adenocarcinoma carcinogenesis and is critical for invasion, metastasis, and malignant transformation [9–11, 56]. Allen et al. demonstrated that continuous expression of activated Notch1-ICD in the alveolar epithelium of transgenic mice induced lung adenoma formation [56]. After seven days of induction of Notch1-ICD expression, mice began to develop alveolar hyperplasia, which progressed to adenoma after eight months. When crossed with mice overexpressing Myc in the alveolar epithelium, adenocarcinoma developed. Further studies by Baumgart et al. demonstrated that the loss of Notch1 substantially reduced tumor formation in mouse lung adenocarcinoma models driven by *Kras*^{G12D} mutations [9]. In agreement with these studies, Licciulli et al. demonstrated Notch1 function is required for tumor initiation through suppression of p53-mediated apoptosis [10]. Following knockdown of the individual NOTCH1-3 receptors *in vitro*, Licciulli et al. found a dramatic decrease in cell numbers *only* after NOTCH1 knockdown [10]. In *Kras*^{G12D} *Notch1*$^{flox/flox}$ mice, six weeks after tumor initiation, *Kras*^{G12D} mice with the conditional Notch1 knocked out had two lung lesions versus 13 lesions in the *Kras*^{G12D} control animals. Additionally, substantially lower tumor-to-lung ratios were observed in mice without Notch1 function. These combined findings demonstrate the role of NOTCH1 in tumor initiation and promotion of lung adenocarcinoma.

In contrast NOTCH2 has been demonstrated to mediate differentiation and function as a tumor suppressor in lung adenocarcinoma. Conditional ablation of Notch2 in vivo led to upregulation of β-catenin and development of a higher number of tumors in a shorter period of time [9]. Furthermore, Notch2 has been shown to regulate E-cadherin levels, cell migration, and invasiveness.

Evidence for an oncogenic role of NOTCH3 is provided by experiments that demonstrated *in vitro* and *in vivo* suppression of NOTCH3 results in loss of the malignant phenotype [60]. NOTCH3 is elevated in 30–40% of primary lung tumors and frequently co-expressed with EGFR [61, 87]. In cells co-expressing NOTCH3 and EGFR, NOTCH3 suppression sensitizes cells to EGFR inhibitors. Studies by Haruki et al. showed that expression of dominant-negative (DN) NOTCH3 receptor, with a nonfunctional intracellular domain, antagonized NOTCH3 signaling, slowed growth, and induced apoptosis [61]. While all four Notch receptors are present in tumor propagating cells, studies by Zheng et al. showed that only NOTCH3 played a functionally non-redundant role in tumor cell propagation in *Kras*-driven NSCLC [88]. A study by Arasada et al. showed that NOTCH3 is tyrosine phosphorylated in an EGFR-dependent manner, the functional consequences of which still need to be determined [89]. The authors also demonstrated that erlotinib-mediated EGFR inhibition increased the cancer stemlike cell population and was dependent on activation of NOTCH3 [89]. Knocking down NOTCH3, but not NOTCH1, was shown to eliminate the erlotinib-induced ALDH^{+} stemlike population, which also suggests a non-redundant role for NOTCH3 in this process [89].

Likewise, NOTCH4 expression has been linked to cancer stem cells in adenocarcinoma models [90]. The frequency of NOTCH4 alterations in white non-Hispanics in adenocarcinoma is approximately 5.5% but approximately 20% in the Hispanic/Latino cohort. Moreover, 7/12 (58.4%) of amino acid substitutions occurred in the NRR of Notch [62]. Expression of one of these NRR domain mutations (P1663Q) by Gordian et al. in the lung adenocarcinoma, A549 cell line model, suggests NOTCH4 may have an oncogenic role in lung adenocarcinoma [62].

10.4.2.3 Notch Signaling in Squamous Cell Carcinoma

To date, the role for Notch receptors in lung squamous cell carcinoma has focused on NOTCH1 signaling but very little on other Notch receptors. Downregulation of NOTCH1 is often associated with dysfunctional (or aberrant) squamous cell differentiation and the development of squamous cell carcinoma [91]. However, early studies demonstrated that Notch signaling drove cell cycle arrest and differentiation in keratinocytes and that loss of NOTCH1 in epidermal keratinocytes promoted tumorigenesis [92, 93]. Subsequent studies by Nicolas et al. demonstrated that conditional ablation of Notch1 in the mouse epidermis resulted in epidermal hyperplasia, skin carcinoma, and basal and squamous carcinomas, thus implying a tumor-suppressive role for NOTCH1 [14]. While the tumor-suppressive role for NOTCH1 has been primarily studied in skin cancer, Li et al. reported that an increase in NOTCH1 signaling in lung squamous cell carcinoma was associated with squamous lung cell differentiation and corresponded with a lengthened survival, low grade, and low stage [94]. Interestingly, studies have shown inhibition of Notch1 in a *Kras*-driven mouse model of lung cancer strongly decreased adenocarcinoma formation but promoted squamous hyperplasia in the alveoli [11].

The TCGA dataset for lung squamous cell carcinoma identified alterations in Notch receptors in 39% (69/178) of cases [74–76]. Additionally a comparative genomic analysis by Kim et al. of 104 squamous cell carcinoma tumors from East Asia with 178 tumors from mostly white patients from the United States suggests that the frequency of Notch mutations in squamous cell carcinoma may vary by ethnic group [57]. Although the frequency of mutations in NOTCH1 (7% and 9%) was similar between the two cohorts, NOTCH2 mutations occurred in 4% of East Asian versus 13% of tumors from the Unites States and found that 10% East Asian tumors versus 7% of tumors from the United States had mutations in NOTCH3 [57, 66]. Although these results were not statistically significant, a larger study in lung squamous cell carcinoma may be able to identify the frequency of Notch alterations among ethnic groups. Furthermore Kim et al. found that eight of the 17 samples with NOTCH1 mutations had truncating mutations suggesting loss of function [57]. Moreover, NOTCH1 mutations have been reported in cutaneous squamous cell carcinoma and head and neck squamous cell carcinoma [74–76]. Experiments by Brooks et al. show that ER-ß is a direct positive regulator of NOTCH1 expression in lung keratinocyte-derived squamous cell carcinoma cells [58]. The authors demonstrate that *in vitro* and *in vivo* overexpression of ER-ß induces NOTCH1 expression and suppresses proliferation in lung squamous cell carcinoma [58]. This finding is consistent with clinical epidemiological studies that have shown in postmenopausal women that estrogen exposure is associated with reduced risk of NSCLC and that nuclear ER-ß expression is a positive prognostic marker for male NSCLC patients [95–97].

10.4.3 Conflicting Roles of Notch in Cancer Subtypes

Despite ample experimental evidence for an oncogenic role for NOTCH1 in NSCLC, conflicting data exist [58, 77, 98, 99]. A study by Zheng et al. demonstrated Notch signaling inhibited growth of A549 lung adenocarcinoma cells suggesting a tumor suppressive rather than oncogenic role for Notch in lung adenocarcinoma [100]. Other studies support an oncogenic role of NOTCH1 in squamous lung cancer [101]. Wael et al. used siRNAs to knockdown NOTCH1 in the adenocarcinoma (A549) and lung squamous cell carcinoma (H2170) cell line and reported that knockdown of NOTCH1 had a tumor-suppressive function in the lung adenocarcinoma (A549) cells and no effect on biological functions in the H2170 squamous cell carcinoma line [99]. One possible explanation for these apparently conflicting data is that the Notch output is highly context and cell of origin dependent. The precise underlying mechanisms of this difference remain to be unraveled.

Hallmarks of cancer such as the tumor microenvironment and interaction with the immune system may be involved in mechanisms that favor an oncogenic versus tumor-suppressive role for Notch in different cellular contexts.

10.4.4 Notch and the Tumor Microenvironment

The tumor microenvironment, including oxygen levels, angiogenesis, paracrine signaling, and immune cells, may contribute to the apparent discrepancies in experimental findings associated with the role of Notch in NSCLC. Maintenance of normal oxygen concentrations is important for normal lung physiology, and tissue hypoxia is common in many tumors including NSCLC [102–104].

Regulation of mitochondrial metabolism may also depend on the interaction between tumor cells and the microenvironment. Hypoxia has an important role in lung cancer progression and been shown to decrease therapeutic efficacy of some forms of radiotherapy and chemotherapy [102, 105–107]. Notch signaling in lung tumor cell lines is dramatically elevated under hypoxic conditions [108], and Notch signaling is necessary to maintain tumor cells in an undifferentiated state and allow them to survive in these hypoxic microenvironments [109]. Under normoxic conditions, NOTCH1 expression promotes apoptosis, but in hypoxic conditions, NOTCH1 signaling stimulates cell survival by inhibiting PTEN and activating the IGF-1R pathway [110]. Lung adenocarcinoma studies have shown that inhibition of the mitochondrial electron transport chain induced cell cycle arrest and triggered apoptosis [111]. In contrast, a recent comparison of the metabolic phenotype of lung adenocarcinoma and squamous cell carcinoma identified elevated expression of the GLUT1 glucose transporter selectively in lung squamous cell carcinoma [112]. While squamous cells were sensitive to glucose deprivation, adenocarcinoma cells exhibited glucose intolerance [112]. Different phenotypes such as hypoxic versus normoxic have different metabolic requirements. Researchers speculate that differences in signaling pathways mediated in part by Notch may drive divergent metabolic phenotypes [113]. Studies such as these underscore the complexity of the pathway and the importance of the controlling the tumor microenvironment for studies focused on Notch signaling therapeutics.

Studies in mammary epithelial cells indicate that the phenotypic response to Notch is determined by the degree of pathway activation [114]. It is likely that the amount of Notch signaling in lung cancer similarly affects the balance between growth-stimulating and growth-suppressing effects [114]. In squamous cell carcinoma keratinocytes, high levels of Notch1 cause growth arrest but at low levels cause transformation [115]. It is likely that mechanisms have evolved for cells with excessive Notch expression to undergo programmed cell death [108]. A study by Chen et al. suggested that under hypoxic conditions, which potentiate the strength of Notch signaling, total Notch1 protein levels increase, but active Notch1 levels remain relatively unchanged. The low levels of active Notch1-ICD may be a reflection of rapid activation-degradation to prevent pathway hyperactivation and maintain Notch signaling homeostasis [108]. These studies suggest that this pathway, like most other crucial pathways, is self-regulating/negatively regulating and underscores the fragile nature and context dependency of Notch signaling.

10.5 Notch and the Immune Response to Lung Cancer

The immune system plays a critical role in the suppression of tumors, and immune evasion is a hallmark of malignancy [116–118]. Notch signaling has been found to play a critical role in normal immune system activation and T cell differentiation (Fig. 10.3). Proliferating helper T cells develop into two major subtypes known as TH1 and TH2 cells. TH1 helpers are host immunity effectors against bacterial and protozoa, while TH2 helpers are host immunity effectors against extracellular parasites. A new lineage of T cells has been designated as TH18 cells that produce proinflammatory cytokines and are thought to play an essential role in host defense against extracellular bacteria and fungi and be involved in autoimmune disease.

Notch has been implicated as a general coactivator of T cells [119] and a pathway that favors polarization of activated macrophages toward the M1 state [120, 121], both of which could augment the host immune response against cancer in the local microenvironment. This signaling is often ligand-specific, as specific ligands can elicit the development of different immune cells. DLL4 expressed by antigen-presenting cells specifically directs the differentiation and activation of $CD8^{+}$ T cells [122, 123]. On the other hand, expression of JAGGED1 by antigen-presenting cells

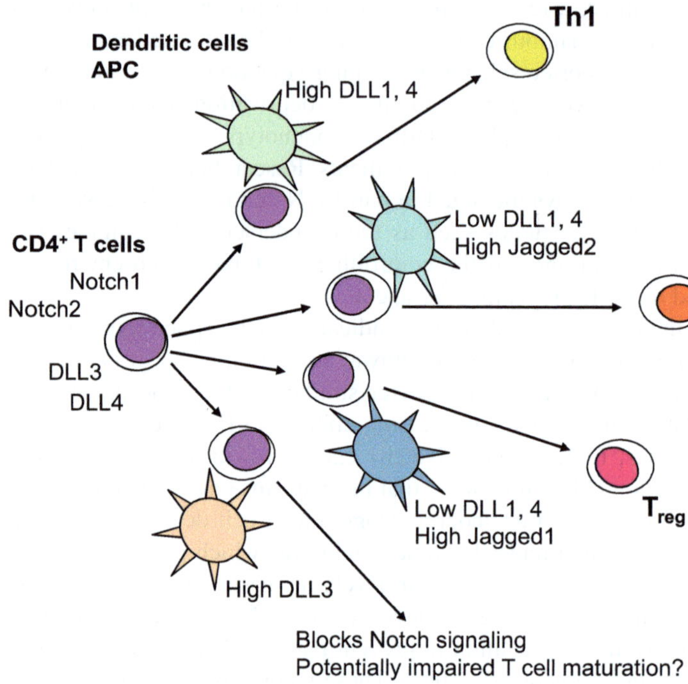

Fig. 10.3 Schema of Notch's role directing T cell fate. (Figure illustrated by Mikhail Dikov, Translational Therapeutics, The Ohio State University)

induces a T regulatory phenotype and subsequent immune suppression [124]. Expression of DLL1 or DLL4 leads to induction of T cell development and suppression of B cell development [125, 126]. Moreover, DLL4 is the essential and non-redundant ligand for NOTCH1 in T cell development [127]. Reduction in DLL1 and DLL4 in the hematopoietic microenvironment allows tumors to escape T cell immunity by elevating circulating VEGF [128]. This tumor-mediated suppression of T cell activity can be reversed by activation of Notch signaling using multivalent Dll1 in mouse xenograft models [129]. This activation is specific to the DLL1 ligand. For example, since DLL3 does not activate Notch signaling, it is not presumed to have an effect on T cell maturation [130]. JAGGED1 and JAGGED2 expression is thought to induce a Th2 fate [131]. NOTCH1 activation also directs T cells to a Th17 fate, although the specific ligand interaction mediating this fate is not known [132].

Notch1 and Notch2 are the receptors that mediate this signaling axis. It has been shown that Notch1 and Notch2 are necessary for the proliferation of activated $CD8^+$ T cells and tumor-infiltrating T cells [133]. T cell differentiation is primarily mediated through Notch1. Eliminating Notch1 signaling results in impaired T cell development and increased B cell development [134]. Conversely, inducing constitutive Notch1 signaling promotes T cell development and reduces B cell development

[135]. Furthermore, myeloid-derived suppressor cells, another immune-suppressing cell, block Notch1 and Notch2 expression in T cells, and this suppression can be circumvented by exogenously expressing Notch1-ICD in transgenic mouse models [133].

DLL1 plays a critical role in immunotherapy. DLL1 stimulation increases the number of infiltrating T cells and decreases the number of immune-suppressing regulatory T cells [129]. Combination of multivalent DLL1 and bortezomib, which sensitizes tumors to death signals, has been shown to restore the ability of the immune system to attack lung cancer cells [129]. Treatment with DLL1 has also been shown to improve progression-free survival in mice when combined with erlotinib by inducing T cell immunity [129, 136]. Importantly, DLL1 therapy does not have a proliferative or clonogenic effect on lung cancer cells, which suggests that Notch pathways can be targeted in the immune compartment without promoting tumor growth or aggressiveness.

In contrast to these studies, it has been shown that continued activation of the Notch signaling pathway in $CD8^+$ T cells results in an increase in PD-1 expression and suppression of T cell activation [137]. Notch1-ICD specifically occupies the Pdcd1 promoter and can thus downregulate T cell activation [137]. Moreover, combination dosing of PD-1 and anti-DLL4 in a syngeneic CT26 model resulted in enhanced long-term memory, reduced suppressive functions of MDSC and Tregs, increased CD8 T cells, IL2 and IFN-γ levels [138].

Because of the complexity of these roles and the difficulty of measuring Notch activation and downstream effects in tumors, there remains uncertainty about the contribution of Notch signaling in stromal cells to cancer biology. Nonetheless, some intriguing preclinical data have emerged that suggest that modulation of host responses with selective Notch pathway inhibitors holds therapeutic promise. For example, short-term treatment with Dll4- or Notch1-blocking antibodies in the immediate posttransplant setting abrogates graft-versus-host disease without any measurable deleterious effect on graft-versus-leukemia activity [139], possibly because of a role for Dll4 expressed on lymph node stromal cells in the priming of Notch-expressing T cells [140]. Further investigation of Notch effects on host immunity in various disease settings clearly appears to be merited.

10.6 Notch as a Therapeutic Target

Many features unique to the Notch pathway must be considered when developing cancer therapies targeting Notch. The *first key feature* is that the Notch signaling cascade does not rely on an enzymatic amplification step by a phospholipase, nucleotide cyclase, or protein kinase [115, 141]. Instead, the Notch signaling cascade is triggered by receptor-ligand interaction and regulated by a series of proteolytic cleavages, protein stability, and cellular compartment changes. The “strength” of the Notch signal is proportional to the nuclear accumulation of cleaved intracellular “active” Notch [115]. As a consequence, Notch signaling is dose-dependent and can be regulated by factors that control the expression of ligands, expression of receptors, export of ligands and receptors to the membrane, receptor-ligand interaction, proteolytic cleavage, and endocytosis. Thus, complete shutdown of the pathway may be neither necessary nor ideal to achieve therapeutic effect [115]. *A second key feature* is that the intracellular half-life of cleaved intracellular "active" Notch is very short, resulting in a pulse of gene regulation and implying that intermittent inhibition may be sufficient to disrupt Notch signaling [52, 141]. The *third key feature* is that Notch signaling in the lung is context-dependent. While Notch signaling has an oncogenic role in adenocarcinoma, it is a tumor suppressor in SCLC and squamous cell carcinoma.

Additionally, the outcome of aberrant Notch activity is dependent on the spatial and temporal context of Notch activation. During the initial stages of tumor initiation, Notch signaling can prevent tumor formation, while in later stages of tumor development, Notch activation is required for maintenance of the tumor [142]. Furthermore, Notch activity can exert opposing effects in the same tissue under different microenvironmental conditions such as hypoxia.

The most established method of therapeutically targeting Notch signaling has been through inhibition of γ-secretase in tumors with Notch gain-of-function mutations. However, this approach needs to be carefully considered for use in cancers such as SCLC and squamous cell carcinoma, where NOTCH1 has been identified as a tumor suppressor. When designing therapies for the Notch pathway, it is important to consider the broad implications and multiple effects that Notch may have in different cell types. Clearly, having well-defined patient-stratification biomarkers is required for the development of effective Notch inhibitors.

A multitude of therapeutic approaches have been explored that include γ-secretase inhibitors (GSIs), antibodies against Notch ligands, therapies targeting the Notch receptor negative regulatory region (NRR), and antibodies against Notch receptors. Table 10.3 summarizes drugs in development, and Table 10.4 summarizes clinical trials targeting the Notch signaling pathway.

10.6.1 γ-Secretase Inhibitors (GSIs)

To date, the most widely studied inhibitors of the Notch pathway are γ-secretase inhibitors. γ-secretase inhibitors were originally developed to treat Alzheimer's disease. γ-secretase inhibitors target all four Notch receptors, ligands including DLL1 and JAGGED2, as well as many other proteins involved in Notch signal transduction, transcriptional regulation, and differentiation [149–152]. A number of small molecules that inhibit the γ-secretase complex with variable specificity and selectivity have been developed. These γ-secretase inhibitors inhibit Notch signaling by preventing presenilin-1 substrate binding and S3 proteolytic cleavage of Notch receptors. Early studies with γ-secretase inhibitors suggested that these agents might be useful as Notch-targeted therapies.

Table 10.3 Preclinical lung cancer studies targeting the Notch signaling pathway

Compound	Target	Drug type	Tumor model	Conclusion	Authors
MRK-003	Notch (γ-secretase)	Small molecule	Human cell lines	Inhibition of γ-secretase activity caused apoptosis in lung adenocarcinomas Reintroduction of NOTCH1-ICD reduced cell death	Chen et al. [108]
MRK-003	Notch (γ-secretase)	Small molecule	Human cell lines	Inhibition of γ-secretase activity prevents NOTCH3 activation, causes apoptosis, and decreases proliferation	Konishi et al. [60]
DAPT/ MRK-003	Notch (γ-secretase)	Small molecule	Human cell lines	Inhibition of γ-secretase activity caused apoptosis in cell lines with NOTCH1 gain-of-function mutations	Westoff et al. [6]
DAPT	Notch (γ-secretase)	Small molecule	Xenograft mouse models	γ-Secretase inhibitors caused dose-dependent inhibition of proliferation and differentiation in human lung adenocarcinoma tumors xenotransplanted into nude mice	Paris et al. [143]
LSN-4111575	Notch (γ-secretase)	Small molecule	GEMM models	In vivo therapeutic potential of γ-secretase in NSCLC. Treatment with γ-secretase decreased HES1 which directly represses DUSP1	Maraver et al. [144]
A5226A	Nicastrin; Notch (γ-secretase)	Antibody	Human cell lines	A5226A inhibits γ-secretase activity and reduced cell viability	Hayashi et al. [145]
YW152F	DLL4/ Notch1	Antibody	Human cell lines/in vivo	Blocking DLL4/Notch alters neovascularization and results in inhibited tumor growth in a lung adenocarcinoma xenograft. However chronic inhibition of DLL4 poses the risk of inducing vascular neoplasms	Ridgway et al. [146] and Yan et al. [147]
TBD-Genentech	NRR1/NRR2	Antibody	Human cell lines	Antitumor efficacy and decreased tumor angiogenesis in Calu-6 xenografts	Wu et al. [148]
JAG1.b70 and JAG2.b33	Jagged1/ Jagged2	Antibody	Normal mouse and human models	Anti-Jag1.b70 alone or in combination with anti-Jag2.b33 reversed goblet cell metaplasia in vivo	Lafkas et al. [37]

Table 10.4 Ongoing and completed clinical trials targeting the Notch signaling pathway

Molecular target	Therapy	Study identifier	Phase	Status
Pan-Notch (γ-secretase)	RO-4929097 plus erlotinib hydrochloride in metastatic or recurrent NSCLC	NCT01193881	Phase 1	Terminated
	RO-4929097 in recurrent or refractory NSCLC	NCT01070927	Phase 2	Completed
	BMS-906024 plus weekly paclitaxel, 5FU + irinotecan, or carboplatin+paclitaxel in metastatic/advanced solid tumors	NCT01653470	Phase 1	Completed
	PF-03084014 in desmoid/aggressive fibromatosis	NCT01981551	Phase 2	Active, not recruiting
NOTCH1	OMP-52M51 in solid tumors	NCT01778439	Phase 1	Completed
	OMP-52M51 in lymphoid malignancies	NCT01703572	Phase 1	Completed
	OMP-52M51 plus chemotherapy in previously treated metastatic colorectal cancer	NCT03031691	Phase 1	Completed
NOTCH2/NOTCH3	OMP-59R5 in solid tumors	NCT01277146	Phase 1	Completed
	OMP-59R5 plus etoposide and platinum therapy in untreated stage IV SCLC	NCT01859741	Phase 1/2	Completed
	OMP-59R5 plus nab-paclitaxel and gemcitabine in untreated stage IV pancreatic cancer	NCT01647828	Phase 1/2	Completed
DLL3	SC15LD6.5 (Rova-T) in recurrent SCLC	NCT01901653	Phase 1/2	Completed
	SC15LD6.5 (Rova-T) in combination with nivolumab with or without ipilimumab in extensive stage SCLC	NCT03026166	Phase 1/2	Active, not recruiting
	SC16LD6.5 (Rova-T) in the frontline treatment of patients with DLL3-expressing extensive stage SCLC	NCT02819999	Phase 1	Recruiting
	Rova-T as maintenance therapy following first-line platinum-based chemotherapy in participants with extensive stage SCLC	NCT03033511	Phase 3	Recruiting
DLL4	REGN421 in advanced solid malignancies	NCT00871559	Phase 1	Completed
	OMP-21M18 plus pembrolizumab in locally advanced or metastatic solid tumors	NCT02722954	Phase 1	Completed
	OMP-21M18 plus paclitaxel in platinum-resistant ovarian	NCT01952249	Phase 1/2	Completed
	OMP-21M18 plus carboplatin and pemetrexed in non-squamous NSCLC	NCT01189968	Phase 1	Completed

In vitro, γ-secretase inhibitors induce apoptosis in human lung cancer lines. For example, under hypoxia, which potentiates the strength of Notch signaling in adenocarcinoma, Chen et al. demonstrated that treatment with the γ-secretase inhibitor MRK-003 caused a potent apoptotic response as early as 48 h after treatment [108]. Reintroduction of active NOTCH1 led to a twofold reduction in cell death despite MRK-003 treatment [108], supporting an essential role for NOTCH1 in survival of adenocarcinoma cells. Similarly, Westhoff et al. demonstrated that primary cell cultures with NOTCH1 gain-of-function mutations were selectively killed by treatment with γ-secretase inhibitor's DAPT and MRK-003 [6]. Additionally, Konoshi et al. investigated the *in vitro* and *in vivo* properties of MRK-003 in NSCLC and showed that MRK-003 inhibited NOTCH3 signaling, reduced tumor cell proliferation, and induced apoptosis [60]. Loss of NOTCH3 rendered the γ-secretase inhibitor ineffective, suggesting that the antitumor effect was NOTCH3 dependent [60]. Downregulation of pMAPK following MRK-003 treatment suggested that NOTCH3 may regulate apoptosis by modulating pERK and the pro-survival BCL-2 proteins [153]. A study by Kaur and colleagues demonstrated that SCLC cell lines are not responsive to γ-secretase inhibitors alone or in combination with etoposide or carboplatin [154].

In vivo studies have demonstrated that γ-secretase inhibitors slow the growth of subcutaneous lung cancer xenografts. In an adenocarcinoma xenograft model, Paris and colleagues demonstrated that treatment with the γ-secretase inhibitor DAPT resulted in dose-dependent inhibition of proliferation and differentiation [143]. Using a transgenic lung GEMM, Maraver et al. also demonstrated the efficacy of γ-secretase inhibitors [144]. Likewise, the γ-secretase inhibitor, LSN-4111575, exhibited antitumor efficacy in a *KRAS*^{G12V}-driven NSCLC mouse model [144]. Treatment with the γ-secretase inhibitor correlated with decreased expression of HES1, a Notch target gene and a negative regulator of DUSP1, a phosphatase that acts on the MAPKs [144]. The researchers demonstrated that increased expression of DUSP1 led to a decrease in pERK without changes in phosphorylated MEK [144]. In human lung tumor samples, high HES1 and low DUSP1 are associated with a poor outcome. Ambrogio et al. found that in *KRAS*-driven lung adenocarcinoma, inhibition of DDR1 in combination with Notch (using either LY-411575 or demcizumab) showed a survival benefit in patient-derived xenografts [155]. The authors hypothesized that this synergy was due to Notch and DDR1s combined role maintaining MAPK activity in *KRAS*-driven lung adenocarcinoma. Interestingly, the γ-secretase inhibitor JLK-6, a mechanism-based inhibitor of serine proteases, does not affect the Notch pathway and was shown to have a dose-dependent antitumor effect in lung adenocarcinoma xenografts [143]. Additionally JLK-6 inhibited the growth and vascularization of the human lung adenocarcinoma xenografts [143].

γ-secretase inhibitors have been evaluated in Phase I clinical trials in lung cancer. A Phase I clinical trial (NCT01193881) involving 16 patients with Stage IV or recurrent NSCLC was carried out to evaluate Roche's γ-secretase inhibitor R04929097 [156, 157] in combination with erlotinib. The study showed improved median progression-free survival (PFS) for patients with a prior history of progression on erlotinib alone (64 versus 42 days) and four patients had stable disease at six weeks. While the combination was considered safe and feasible [156], adverse events included hypophosphatemia, rash, neuropathic pain and nausea. The manufacturer discontinued the development of R04929097 following completion of the Phase I cohort. The Bristol-Myers Squibb pan-Notch/γ-secretase inhibitor, BMS-906024, is currently in Phase I clinical trial (NCT01653470) alone and in combination with paclitaxel, FOLFIRI, or carboplatin plus paclitaxel to determine safe and tolerable dose in patients with solid tumors including lung cancer.

γ-secretase inhibitors have many advantages including ease of administration, oral bioavailability and low cost. Two main challenges facing the development of γ-secretase inhibitors include (a) substrate specificity since γ-secretase cleaves more than 60 substrates in addition to Notch [158] and (b) toxicity since pan-Notch inhibition has been linked with severe GI toxicity. These problems could be circumvented by developing substrate-specific γ-secretase inhibitors. Recent efforts have targeted Nicastrin, one of the subunits of γ-secretase that appears to be a main discriminator in γ-secretase substrate selectivity. Nicastrin is the target of the novel monoclonal antibody A5226A, developed by Hayashi et al. at the University of Tokyo. Hayashi et al. have demonstrated A5226A reduced cell viability of A549 cells [145]. Intriguingly, A5226A treatment further reduced the viability of DAPT-treated A549 cells [145].

10.6.2 Notch Antibodies

A number of biologics have been approved for the treatment of lung cancer. Moreover, a number of antibodies targeting Notch ligands, Notch receptors, and the NRR of Notch receptors are in clinical development. Some of these drugs have shown promising results in early clinical trials.

10.6.2.1 Ligand-Targeted Antibodies

Inhibitory antibodies directed against Notch ligands DLL3, DLL4, JAGGED1, and JAGGED2 have been developed. Preclinical studies by Genentech using an anti-DLL4 antibody, YW152F, demonstrated targeting DLL4/NOTCH1 signaling could have a profound impact by suppressing tumor angiogenesis and growth [146, 159]. Unfortunately, these studies also identified a number of significant safety concerns associated with this approach. *In vitro* studies with the anti-DLL4 antibody showed dysregulation of endothelium-specific genes as well as genes critical for proliferation and cell cycle regulation, while *in vivo* mice developed histopathological changes in the liver, sinusoidal dilation, and centrilobular hepatocyte atrophy. These preclinical findings suggest an essential role of DLL4 for maintaining the structural and functional integrity of the liver sinusoidal epithelium and hepatocyte homeostasis [159]. Genentech has also generated synthetic therapeutic antibodies targeting JAGGED1 and JAGGED2 [37]. JAGGED1 is overexpressed in many cancer types and has been implicated as a target for antitumor therapy [160]. Future studies will need to assess the clinical implications of using these antibodies in the context of lung cancer.

More recently, clinical trials of Regeneron's anti-DLL4 antibody enoticumab (REGN421) and OncoMed Pharmaceutical's antibody demcizumab (OMP-21M18) have shown dose-limiting adverse toxicity (nausea, abdominal pain, hypertension, fatigue and headache) [161] in clinical trials despite promising antitumor activity in the preclinical setting. No clinical benefit was seen in the Phase I clinical trial of enoticumab (NCT00871559). However, partial response was observed in a NSCLC bronchioloalveolar carcinoma patient with a β-catenin mutation [162]. Because tumor angiogenesis involves both VEGF and Notch, future studies may want to target both the VEGF and Notch pathway to increase efficacy or specifically investigate use of the DLL4 inhibitor in specific subtypes of cancers such as lung cancer patients with dysregulated Notch/β-catenin signaling. Anti-DLL4 treatment (OMP-21M18 targeting human and 21R30 targeting mouse) combination with chemotherapy inhibited tumor growth and appeared to decrease the frequency of tumor-initiating cells in a series of NSCLC PDX models [163]. Phase Ib clinical trials (NCT01189968) of demcizumab in combination with carboplatin and pemetrexed (Alimta) in patients with non-squamous NSCLC demonstrated promising results (RECIST response rate of 50%) and benefit for patient survival (overall clinical benefit rate of 88%). These results are being confirmed in an ongoing Phase II trial known as DENALI (NCT02259582) of demcizumab with carboplatin and pemetrexed in first-line non-squamous NSCLC patients [164].

Antibody-drug conjugates (ADCs) are therapies that combine the precision of an antibody linked with the cytotoxic power of a payload. DLL3 is a promising target for the treatment of SCLC, since DLL3 is expressed by both SCLC and large cell neuroendocrine carcinoma (LCNEC) tumors and tumor-initiating cells but is not expressed by normal cells [42]. AbbVie Stemcentrx is evaluating SC15LD6.5 that consists of an anti-DLL3 monoclonal antibody conjugated to a potent DNA-damaging pyrrolobenzodiazepine (PBD) dimer toxin. SC15LD6.5 dosed at one mg/kg, intravenous (iv), once a week for a total of four weeks (qwX4) demonstrated durable complete regression for up to 144 days of observation in preclinical mouse xenograft models [42]. Mechanism-of-action studies suggest that the rapid tumor debulking is a result of DLL3 expression on most tumor cells and suggest that the durability in response to SC16LD6.5 is due to eradication of DLL3-expressing tumor-initiating cells (TICs). Moreover, SC16LD6.5 is efficacious in relapsed and refractory SCLC PDX models and is thus a potentially promising option for patients in the setting of second and third-line treatment. The safety and efficacy of SC16LD6.5 have been evaluated in an ongoing Phase 1 clinical trial (NCT01901653) in recurrent or refractory high-grade pulmonary and/or neuroendocrine cancer patients [165]. Rova-T demonstrated an acceptable safety profile in this trial and showed a confirmed objective response in 10/26 patients with elevated tumor DLL3 expression. Phase 1/2/3 trials with Rova-T are active (NCT03026166, NCT02819999, NCT03033511).

10.6.2.2 Targeted Antibodies Against the Negative Regulatory Region (NRR) of the Notch Receptor

The NRR domain plays a critical role in preventing activation of the receptors in the absence of ligand. The three cysteine-rich Lin12 Notch repeats (LNR) and heterodimerization (HD) domain of the NRR interact to keep the S2 cleavage site buried and prevent cleavage. During canonical Notch signaling, ligand binding to the receptor at the extracellular domain triggers a conformational change in the NRR exposing the S2 site for cleavage by ADAM proteases [166]. Li et al. demonstrated the potential of antibodies to target and stabilize the NRR domain in an "inactive" conformation where the S2 cleavage site remains buried within the NRR [167]. The inhibitory antibodies they identified by functional screening reverted the phenotypes of 293T cells induced by NOTCH3 signaling [167]. Scientists at Genentech have also developed antibodies to the NRR domain of NOTCH1 (NRR1) and NOTCH2 (NRR2). Antibodies targeted to the NRR1 demonstrated antitumor efficacy and decreased tumor angiogenesis in a Calu-6 lung adenocarcinoma mouse xenograft model [148]. Using ligand-competitive assays, researchers at Merck demonstrated that NRR-specific antibodies blocked JAGGED2-stimulated NOTCH1 activity, presumably by stabilizing the NRR domain in an auto-inhibited conformation [168]. While the NRR antibodies maximally inhibited NOTCH1 signaling, they did not significantly inhibit ligand-stimulated NOTCH2 or NOTCH3 [168]. Moreover, the NRR antibodies developed by Merck had variable efficacy in colorectal carcinoma and T-ALL cell lines, suggesting binding of the NRR is complex and that epitope masking by glycosylation or other posttranslational modifications of NOTCH1 may be cell type specific [168].

10.6.2.3 Receptor-Targeted Antibodies

The extracellular domains (ECD) of the four Notch receptors are composed of EGF-like repeats, which are of variable length. For example, NOTCH1 and NOTCH2 each contain 36 EGF-like repeats, whereas NOTCH3 contains 34, and NOTCH4 contains 29 EGF-like repeats in the extracellular domain. Antibodies that target the ligand-binding domain and compete with the endogenous ligand represent a promising novel therapeutic approach.

Tarextumab (OMP-59R5) which targets the ligand-binding domain of NOTCH2 and NOTCH3 has recently completed Phase IIb trials (NCT01859741) in SCLC [169]. It demonstrated dose-dependent antitumor efficacy and corresponding biomarker-driven activity in a Phase I trial. However the randomized 145 Phase 2 PINNACLE clinical trial in combination with chemotherapy (etoposide plus cisplatin or carboplatin) in previously untreated SCLC patients with extensive disease showed *no* benefit over placebo [170]. The median progression-free survival for tarextumab plus chemotherapy was 5.6 months versus 5.5 months for the placebo plus chemotherapy group. Median overall survival was 9.4 months in the treated versus 10.3 months (HR = 1.01) in the placebo group. The overall response rates were 68.5% in the treated and 70.8% in the placebo group. The Notch biomarkers that were evaluated in the study (HES1, HES6, HEY1, HEY2, and NOTCH3) failed to identify a subset of patients with treatment effect on progression-free or overall survival [170]. Furthermore, increased diarrhea and thrombocytopenia were observed in the placebo arm.

There is some early evidence that Notch overexpression may predict response to tarextumab, a NOTCH2/3 inhibitor, in SCLC. This comes from a Phase Ib dose escalation trial of tarextumab in SCLC [171]. In this study, patients were treated with etoposide, platinum, and tarextumab. NOTCH3 expression was determined by RT-PCR. Extensive disease patients with high NOTCH3 expression fared better with tarextumab than patients with low NOTCH3 expression. Although this trend was striking, it was not significant due to small patient numbers. Further analysis of NOTCH3 as a predictive marker of tarextumab response will take place when the Phase II trial of the drug is completed.

Another human monoclonal antibody brontictuzumab (OMP-52M51) targets the ligand-binding domain of NOTCH1 and demonstrated antitumor efficacy in early studies [172]. One potential concern was that chronic reduction of Notch1 signaling in mice promoted widespread vascular tumor formation in preclinical studies [173]. Additionally enrollment for Phase 1B clinical trials in combination with trifluridine/tipiracil in third-line colorectal patients was abruptly ended and was not tolerated in that patient population [170]. A clinical trial for brontictuzumab in relapsed or refractory solid tumors (including SCLC) with activated NOTCH1 has been completed (OncoMed Pharmaceuticals, NCT01778439). Preliminary findings demonstrated general tolerability at 1.5 mg/kg Q3W. The main toxicity was off-target diarrhea, but patients also exhibited fatigue, nausea and vomiting. In patients with high NOTCH1, there were a few patients with stable disease 42.9% (6/14), and one (7.1%; 1/14) patient had partial response [174]. Patients with low NOTCH1 did not respond and had stable 9.1% (1/11) or progressive disease 90.9% (10/11) [174]. Oncomed has halted clinical trials with brontictuzumab.

The Notch receptor is also an ideal target for antibody-drug conjugates. Pfizer is currently evaluating the safety and efficacy of their non-inhibitory anti-NOTCH3 antibody-drug conjugate PF-06650808 in a Phase I clinical trial (NCT02129205) for patients with solid tumors that have a history of metastatic triple-negative breast cancer [175].

Monoclonal antibodies provide a number of advantages including improved half-life, immune-mediated efficacy through antibody-dependent cell-mediated cytotoxicity and complement-dependent cytotoxicity, as well as specificity allowing members of the Notch signaling pathway to be targeted with high affinity. While antibodies are generally well tolerated, it is critical to identify the right combination of tumor and drug to derive maximal therapeutic benefit. Additional challenges with antibody-targeted therapies are their complex dose-response curves in vivo and long half-lives. While small molecules are typically excreted in hours, most antibodies remain in circulation for days. This may pose a problem, as the consequences of sustained inhibition of the Notch signaling pathway are not fully understood. For example, studies with anti-Dll4 antibodies in rat models have shown that prolonged blockade of the ligand resulted in severe disruption of normal tissue homeostasis, activation of endothelial cells and led to development of vascular/endothelial-based tumors resembling hemangioblastoma in the heart and lung [147]. These studies raise significant concern that chronic blockade of Notch signaling pathways may disrupt normal organ homeostasis and potentially produce disease in multiple organs. In that case, single-chain antibodies with short half-lives may be preferable.

10.6.3 Radiotherapy

Although radiation has been reported to induce Notch activation, very little is known about the relationship between radiation and the Notch pathway. Studies have proposed a synergistic effect of Notch-targeted therapy following radiation therapy of lung cancer *in vitro* and *in vivo*. Mizugaki et al. combined γ-secretase inhibitor and radiation in escalating doses in three Notch-expressing NSCLC cell lines (H460, A549, and H1395) [176]. γ-secretase inhibitor treatment following radiation suppressed growth most effectively *in vitro* and *in vivo*. The combination induced apoptosis via MAPK and Bcl2 family proteins. They found that blocking activation of Notch by using γ-secretase inhibitors after radiation treatment prevents Notch-induced radiation resistance. Ikezawa et al. determined that the induction of NOTCH3 following radiotherapy is caused by HIF-1α and found that co-treatment with HIF inhibitor YC-1 improved radiosensitivity of tumors in conjunction with a γ-secretase inhibitor [177].

10.6.4 Summary of Therapeutic Approaches

Each of the therapeutic approaches described above has potential advantages and disadvantages. While γ-secretase inhibitors have demonstrated preclinical activity, their clinical utility for lung cancer remains to be demonstrated. Targeted and selective biologics including antibody-drug conjugates (ADCs) are likely to be the treatment of choice with fewer side effects. Alternatively, bispecific antibodies may offer a useful strategy for Notch-targeted drug development in the future, for example, combining a Notch antibody with a T cell antibody to direct the immune response to Notch-expressing tumor cells. It will be critical to have a strong companion biomarker package in place to select patients and optimize clinical benefit. A better understanding of the transcriptional, translational, and posttranslational regulation of the Notch signaling pathway is needed to understand the implications that these specific therapies may have for lung cancer patients. The cellular context of the cancer will be very important, as roles of Notch in adenocarcinoma will be very different than in squamous cell carcinoma. The ability to identify subgroups of cancer patients that will benefit from Notch-targeted therapies will be essential if they are to be of clinical utility.

10.7 Targeting Notch in Cancer Stem Cells and Rational Combinations of Therapies with Notch Inhibitors

As discussed in Section 10.3, the Notch signaling pathway has been shown to have a role in the survival and maintenance of stem cell populations in the lung [46–48, 185]. Cancer stemlike cells are undifferentiated cancer cells that share properties of normal stem cells such as self-renewal, asymmetric cell division, clonogenicity, and resistance to chemotherapies. Cancer stemlike cells are thought to exist in small numbers as a distinct population of cells within tumors. Their quiescent nature allows them to escape standard therapies and even after periods of apparent complete remission cause recurrence or metastasis. Targeted therapeutics to eradicate cancer stemlike cells should theoretically result in more durable responses and improve survival outcomes.

Cancer stemlike cells can be isolated on the basis of the expression of cancer stemlike cell markers, but the accuracy and relevance of these markers remains controversial [186, 187]. Research has identified CD44 [188], CD133 [189–191] and aldehyde dehydrogenase (ALDH) [192–194] as potential markers of lung cancer stemlike cells [195]. Sullivan et al. compared the expression of three putative lung cancer stemlike cell markers (ALDH1A1, ALDH3A1 and CD133) and found that the markers identified distinct tumor subpopulations [194]. Elevated expression of NOTCH1, NOTCH2, NOTCH3, HES1, and HEY1 in $ALDH^+$ cells versus $ALDH^-$ cells, indicated Notch pathway activation in the $ALDH^+$ subpopulation [194]. NOTCH3 had the strongest correlation with $ALDH^+$ expression in NSCLC and suppression of NOTCH3 expression reduced the ALDH positive population and reduced tumor cell proliferation [194]. Other studies have supported a role of ALDH as a marker for stemlike lung cancer cells. Studies by Li et al. isolated $ALDH^+$ lung cancer cells and demonstrated the population was capable of colony formation, proliferation, growth, migration and resulted in tumors in mice that represented characteristics of the parental lung cancer cells [193]. Futhermore, γ-secretase inhibitor therapy reduced the ADLH+ population, supporting a role of Notch signaling in maintenance of the cancer stemlike cell population [194]. In addition to NSCLC, Notch drives stemlike properties in esophageal adenocarcinoma [196]. Another research group has identified that MAP17-mediated sequestration of Numb promotes Notch signaling and cancer stemlike cell phenotypes [197].

Experimental studies have found that pretreatment of H460 and H661 lung cancer cell lines with low-dose cisplatin resulted in enrichment of $CD133^+$cells and appeared to be mediated through Notch signaling [198]. Pretreatment with the γ-secretase inhibitor, DAPT, or a NOTCH1-targeted shRNA reduced enrichment of $CD133^+$cells and increased sensitivity to doxorubicin and paclitaxel. Additionally, re-expression of NOTCH1-ICD was shown to reverse the action of DAPT on drug sensitivity. Immunohistochemistry of relapsed NSCLC lung tumors that had been treated with cisplatin showed a significant increase in $CD133^+$ expression in three out of six patients. In vivo studies demonstrated cisplatin treatment increased NOTCH1 cleavage and suggested that cisplatin-induced enrichment of $CD133^+$ cells was mediated through activation of Notch signaling.

It has also been shown that treating lung cancer cells with erlotinib enriches $ALDH^+$ stemlike cells through activation of Notch3 [89]. Similarly, a study by Rosell et al. identified that gefitinib treatment in EGFR-mutant cell lines induced YAP1-Notch signaling in a compensatory manner [199]. These studies may shed light on the perplexing observation that the addition of EGFR TKIs to curative-intent therapies (chemoradiation [200] or surgery [201]) actually results in an increased risk of death. Clinical benefit in these situations may depend on the elimination of cancer stemlike cells as well as the primary tumor. Together, these studies-suggest that dual targeting of the stem cells using Notch therapies together with targeted TKI's or standard chemotherapies may result in more durable responses in lung cancer patients.

10.8 Conclusion

Notch plays essential role in early lung development, maintenance of adult airways, and cancer. Genome sequencing studies have identified Notch mutations in a small percentage of lung cancers. Recent literature has highlighted the significant role that Notch signaling plays in lung tumorigenesis even in the absence of mutational evidence. Despite the low number of mutations, dysregulation of the Notch signaling pathway is associated with 25% of SCLC and 33% of NSCLCs. This makes Notch an attractive target for therapy since it plays critical roles in the regulation of tumor growth and proliferation, apoptosis, cell differentiation, survival, immune response, angiogenesis, cancer stem cell biology, and chemoresistance. Unfortunately, efforts to target Notch therapeutically still face a number of hurdles. Successful development of targeted therapies that can be used in combination with other approaches will require a deeper understanding of the mechanisms that enable different cell-type specific responses of Notch in lung cancer.

Acknowledgments We would like to thank Joseph Amann, Yung-Mae Yao, Susan Cole, and Rajeswara Arasada for the critical review of this manuscript. We would like to thank Mikhail Dikov for providing a schematic of Notch's role in T cell maturation.

References

1. Radtke, F., Schweisguth, F., & Pear, W. (2005). The Notch 'gospel'. *EMBO Reports, 6*(12), 1120–1125.
2. Gazave, E., et al. (2009). Origin and evolution of the Notch signalling pathway: An overview from eukaryotic genomes. *BMC Evolutionary Biology, 9*(1), 249.
3. Aster, J. C., Pear, W. S., & Blacklow, S. C. (2017). The varied roles of notch in cancer. *Annual Review of Pathology: Mechanisms of Disease, 12*, 245–275.
4. Leiserson, M. D., et al. (2015). Pan-cancer network analysis identifies combinations of rare somatic mutations across pathways and protein complexes. *Nature Genetics, 47*(2), 106–114.

5. George, J., et al. (2015). Comprehensive genomic profiles of small cell lung cancer. *Nature, 524*(7563), 47–53.
6. Westhoff, B., et al. (2009). Alterations of the Notch pathway in lung cancer. *Proceedings of the National Academy of Sciences, 106*(52), 22293–22298.
7. Capaccione, K. M., & Pine, S. R. (2013). The Notch signaling pathway as a mediator of tumor survival. *Carcinogenesis, 34*(7), 1420–1430. p. bgt127.
8. Donnem, T., et al. (2010). Prognostic impact of Notch ligands and receptors in nonsmall cell lung cancer. *Cancer, 116*(24), 5676–5685.
9. Baumgart, A., et al. (2015). Opposing role of Notch1 and Notch2 in a Kras G12D-driven murine non-small cell lung cancer model. *Oncogene, 34*(5), 578.
10. Licciulli, S., et al. (2013). Notch1 is required for Kras-induced lung adenocarcinoma and controls tumor cell survival via p53. *Cancer Research, 73*(19), 5974–5984.
11. Xu, X., et al. (2014). The cell of origin and subtype of K-Ras-induced lung tumors are modified by Notch and Sox2. *Genes & Development, 28*(17), 1929–1939.
12. Duan, L., et al. (2006). Growth suppression induced by Notch1 activation involves Wnt—β-catenin down-regulation in human tongue carcinoma cells. *Biology of the Cell, 98*(8), 479–490.
13. Radtke, F., Fasnacht, N., & MacDonald, H. R. (2010). Notch signaling in the immune system. *Immunity, 32*(1), 14–27.
14. Nicolas, M., et al. (2003). Notch1 functions as a tumor suppressor in mouse skin. *Nature Genetics, 33*(3), 416–421.
15. Leong, K. G., & Karsan, A. (2006). Recent insights into the role of Notch signaling in tumorigenesis. *Blood, 107*(6), 2223–2233.
16. Espinoza, I., & Miele, L. (2013). Notch inhibitors for cancer treatment. *Pharmacology & Therapeutics, 139*(2), 95–110.
17. Stanley, P., & Okajima, T. (2010). Chapter four-roles of glycosylation in Notch signaling. *Current Topics in Developmental Biology, 92*, 131–164.
18. Shi, S., & Stanley, P. (2003). Protein O-fucosyltransferase 1 is an essential component of Notch signaling pathways. *Proceedings of the National Academy of Sciences of the United States of America, 100*(9), 5234–5239.
19. Fernandez-Valdivia, R., et al. (2011). Regulation of mammalian Notch signaling and embryonic development by the protein O-glucosyltransferase Rumi. *Development, 138*(10), 1925–1934.
20. Takeuchi, H., & Haltiwanger, R. S. (2014). Significance of glycosylation in Notch signaling. *Biochemical and Biophysical Research Communications, 453*(2), 235–242.
21. Andersson, E. R., & Lendahl, U. (2014). Therapeutic modulation of Notch signalling [mdash] are we there yet? *Nature Reviews. Drug Discovery, 13*(5), 357–378.
22. Le Bras, S., Loyer, N., & Le Borgne, R. (2011). The multiple facets of ubiquitination in the regulation of notch signaling pathway. *Traffic, 12*(2), 149–161.
23. O'Neil, J., et al. (2007). FBW7 mutations in leukemic cells mediate NOTCH pathway activation and resistance to γ-secretase inhibitors. *The Journal of Experimental Medicine, 204*(8), 1813–1824.
24. Matsuno, K., et al. (2002). Involvement of a proline-rich motif and RING-H2 finger of Deltex in the regulation of Notch signaling. *Development, 129*(4), 1049–1059.
25. Matsuno, K., et al. (1995). Deltex acts as a positive regulator of Notch signaling through interactions with the Notch ankyrin repeats. *Development, 121*(8), 2633–2644.
26. Espinosa, L., et al. (2003). Phosphorylation by glycogen synthase kinase-3β down-regulates Notch activity, a link for Notch and Wnt pathways. *Journal of Biological Chemistry, 278*(34), 32227–32235.
27. McGill, M. A., & McGlade, C. J. (2003). Mammalian numb proteins promote Notch1 receptor ubiquitination and degradation of the Notch1 intracellular domain. *Journal of Biological Chemistry, 278*(25), 23196–23203.

28. Housden, B. E., et al. (2013). Transcriptional dynamics elicited by a short pulse of notch activation involves feed-forward regulation by E (spl)/Hes genes. *PLoS Genetics, 9*(1), e1003162.
29. Lamar, E., et al. (2001). Nrarp is a novel intracellular component of the Notch signaling pathway. *Genes & Development, 15*(15), 1885–1899.
30. Yi, F., Amarasinghe, B., & Dang, T. P. (2013). Manic fringe inhibits tumor growth by suppressing Notch3 degradation in lung cancer. *American Journal of Cancer Research, 3*(5), 490–499.
31. Tsao, P.-N., et al. (2008). γ-secretase activation of Notch signaling regulates the balance of proximal and distal fates in progenitor cells of the developing lung. *Journal of Biological Chemistry, 283*(43), 29532–29544.
32. Kong, Y., et al. (2004). Functional diversity of notch family genes in fetal lung development. *American Journal of Physiology-Lung Cellular and Molecular Physiology, 286*(5), L1075–L1083.
33. Morimoto, M., et al. (2010). Canonical Notch signaling in the developing lung is required for determination of arterial smooth muscle cells and selection of Clara versus ciliated cell fate. *Journal of Cell Science, 123*(2), 213–224.
34. Morimoto, M., et al. (2012). Different assemblies of Notch receptors coordinate the distribution of the major bronchial Clara, ciliated and neuroendocrine cells. *Development (Cambridge, England), 139*(23), 4365–4373.
35. Ito, T., et al. (2000). Basic helix-loop-helix transcription factors regulate the neuroendocrine differentiation of fetal mouse pulmonary epithelium. *Development, 127*(18), 3913–3921.
36. Zhang, S., et al. (2013). Jagged1 is the major regulator of notch-dependent cell fate in proximal airways. *Developmental Dynamics, 242*(6), 678–686.
37. Lafkas, D., et al. (2015). Therapeutic antibodies reveal Notch control of transdifferentiation in the adult lung. *Nature, 528*(7580), 127–131.
38. Chapman, G., et al. (2011). Notch inhibition by the ligand DELTA-LIKE 3 defines the mechanism of abnormal vertebral segmentation in spondylocostal dysostosis. *Human Molecular Genetics, 20*(5), 905–916.
39. Serth, K., et al. (2015). O-fucosylation of DLL3 is required for its function during somitogenesis. *PLoS One, 10*(4), e0123776.
40. Henke, R. M., et al. (2009). Ascl1 and Neurog2 form novel complexes and regulate Delta-like3 (Dll3) expression in the neural tube. *Developmental Biology, 328*(2), 529–540.
41. Augustyn, A., et al. (2014). ASCL1 is a lineage oncogene providing therapeutic targets for high-grade neuroendocrine lung cancers. *Proceedings of the National Academy of Sciences, 111*(41), 14788–14793.
42. Saunders, L. R., et al. (2015). A DLL3-targeted antibody-drug conjugate eradicates high-grade pulmonary neuroendocrine tumor-initiating cells in vivo. *Science Translational Medicine, 7*(302), 302ra136.
43. Guseh, J. S., et al. (2009). Notch signaling promotes airway mucous metaplasia and inhibits alveolar development. *Development, 136*(10), 1751–1759.
44. Xu, K., et al. (2010). Lunatic Fringe-mediated Notch signaling is required for lung alveogenesis. *American Journal of Physiology-Lung Cellular and Molecular Physiology, 298*(1), L45–L56.
45. Dang, T. P., et al. (2003). Constitutive activation of Notch3 inhibits terminal epithelial differentiation in lungs of transgenic mice. *Oncogene, 22*(13), 1988–1997.
46. Carraro, G., & Stripp, B. R. (2015). A new Notch for lung stem cells. *Cell Stem Cell, 16*(2), 107–109.
47. Pardo-Saganta, A., et al. (2015). Injury induces direct lineage segregation of functionally distinct airway basal stem/progenitor cell subpopulations. *Cell Stem Cell, 16*(2), 184–197.
48. Vaughan, A. E., et al. (2015). Lineage-negative progenitors mobilize to regenerate lung epithelium after major injury. *Nature, 517*(7536), 621–625.

49. Randell, S. H. (2006). Airway epithelial stem cells and the pathophysiology of chronic obstructive pulmonary disease. *Proceedings of the American Thoracic Society, 3*(8), 718–725.
50. Rock, J. R., Randell, S. H., & Hogan, B. L. (2010). Airway basal stem cells: A perspective on their roles in epithelial homeostasis and remodeling. *Disease Models & Mechanisms, 3*(9–10), 545–556.
51. Shi, W., Chen, F., & Cardoso, W. V. (2009). Mechanisms of lung development: Contribution to adult lung disease and relevance to chronic obstructive pulmonary disease. *Proceedings of the American Thoracic Society, 6*(7), 558–563.
52. Custodio, A., & Barriuso, J. (2014). What is the meaning of notch pathway and how can we selectively do the targeting? In *Stem cells in Cancer: Should we believe or not?* (pp. 23–65). Dordrecht: Springer.
53. Dang, T. P., et al. (2000). Chromosome 19 translocation, overexpression of Notch3, and human lung cancer. *Journal of the National Cancer Institute, 92*(16), 1355–1357.
54. Sriuranpong, V., et al. (2001). Notch signaling induces cell cycle arrest in small cell lung cancer cells. *Cancer Research, 61*(7), 3200–3205.
55. Lim, J. S., et al. (2017). Intratumoural heterogeneity generated by Notch signalling promotes small-cell lung cancer. *Nature, 545*(7654), 360.
56. Allen, T. D., et al. (2011). Activated Notch1 induces lung adenomas in mice and cooperates with Myc in the generation of lung adenocarcinoma. *Cancer Research, 71*(18), 6010–6018.
57. Kim, Y., et al. (2014). Integrative and comparative genomic analysis of lung squamous cell carcinomas in East Asian patients. *Journal of Clinical Oncology, 32*(2), 121–128.
58. Brooks, Y. S., et al. (2014). Multifactorial ERβ and NOTCH1 control of squamous differentiation and cancer. *The Journal of Clinical Investigation, 124*(5), 2260.
59. Hassan, W. A., et al. (2016). Evaluation of role of Notch3 signaling pathway in human lung cancer cells. *Journal of Cancer Research and Clinical Oncology, 142*(5), 981–993.
60. Konishi, J., et al. (2007). γ-Secretase inhibitor prevents Notch3 activation and reduces proliferation in human lung cancers. *Cancer Research, 67*(17), 8051–8057.
61. Haruki, N., et al. (2005). Dominant-negative Notch3 receptor inhibits mitogen-activated protein kinase pathway and the growth of human lung cancers. *Cancer Research, 65*(9), 3555–3561.
62. Gordian, E., et al. (2017). Novel oncogenic function of Notch4 in Hispanic lung cancer. In *AACR. Proceedings: AACR annual meeting 2017*. Washington, DC.: http://cancerres.aacrjournals.org/content/77/13_Supplement/4456.short.
63. Cerami, E., et al. (2012). The cBio cancer genomics portal: An open platform for exploring multidimensional cancer genomics data. *Cancer Discovery, 2*, 401–404. https://doi.org/10.1158/2159-8290.CD-12-0095. PubMed: 22588877.
64. Gao, J., et al. (2013). Integrative analysis of complex cancer genomics and clinical profiles using the cBioPortal. *Science Signaling, 6*(269), pl1.
65. Ding, L., et al. (2008). Somatic mutations affect key pathways in lung adenocarcinoma. *Nature, 455*(7216), 1069–1075.
66. Network, C. G. A. R. (2012). Comprehensive genomic characterization of squamous cell lung cancers. *Nature, 489*(7417), 519–525.
67. Barse, L., & Bocchetta, M. (2015). Non-small-cell lung carcinoma: Role of the Notch signaling pathway. *Lung Cancer (Auckl), 6*, 43–53.
68. Society,A.C.*Lungcancer(Non-SmallCell):Whatisnon-smallcelllungcancer*.201603/04/2015 12 January 2016]. Available from: http://www.cancer.org/cancer/lungcancer-non-smallcell/detailedguide/non-small-cell-lung-cancer-what-is-non-small-cell-lung-cancer.
69. van Meerbeeck, J. P., Fennell, D. A., & De Ruysscher, D. K. (2011). Small-cell lung cancer. *The Lancet, 378*(9804), 1741–1755.
70. Kunnimalaiyaan, M., & Chen, H. (2007). Tumor suppressor role of Notch-1 signaling in neuroendocrine tumors. *The Oncologist, 12*(5), 535–542.
71. Sriuranpong, V., et al. (2002). Notch signaling induces rapid degradation of achaete-scute homolog 1. *Molecular and Cellular Biology, 22*(9), 3129–3139.

72. Rudin, C. M., et al. (2012). Comprehensive genomic analysis identifies SOX2 as a frequently amplified gene in small-cell lung cancer. *Nature Genetics, 44*(10), 1111–1116.
73. Peifer, M., et al. (2012). Integrative genome analyses identify key somatic driver mutations of small-cell lung cancer. *Nature Genetics, 44*(10), 1104–1110.
74. Wang, N. J., et al. (2011). Loss-of-function mutations in Notch receptors in cutaneous and lung squamous cell carcinoma. *Proceedings of the National Academy of Sciences, 108*(43), 17761–17766.
75. Agrawal, N., et al. (2011). Exome sequencing of head and neck squamous cell carcinoma reveals inactivating mutations in NOTCH1. *Science, 333*(6046), 1154–1157.
76. Stransky, N., et al. (2011). The mutational landscape of head and neck squamous cell carcinoma. *Science, 333*(6046), 1157–1160.
77. Guo, L., et al. (2015). Roles of NOTCH1 as a therapeutic target and a biomarker for lung cancer: Controversies and perspectives. *Disease Markers, 2015*, 520590.
78. Yuan, X., et al. (2015). Meta-analysis reveals the correlation of Notch signaling with non-small cell lung cancer progression and prognosis. *Scientific Reports, 5*, 10338.
79. Jiang, X., et al. (2007). Expression and significance of Notch1, Jagged1 and VEGF in human non-small cell lung cancer. *Zhong nan da xue xue bao. Yi xue ban= Journal of Central South University. Medical Sciences, 32*(6), 1031–1036.
80. Andersen, S., et al. (2011). Correlation and coexpression of HIFs and NOTCH markers in NSCLC. *Anticancer Research, 31*(5), 1603–1606.
81. Mariscal, J., et al. (2016). Molecular profiling of circulating tumour cells identifies notch1 as a principal regulator in advanced non-small cell lung cancer. *Scientific Reports, 6*, 37820.
82. Chen, C.-Y., et al. (2017). Expression of notch gene and its impact on survival of patients with resectable non-small cell lung cancer. *Journal of Cancer, 8*(7), 1292.
83. Sherry, S. T., et al. (2001). dbSNP: The NCBI database of genetic variation. *Nucleic Acids Research, 29*(1), 308–311.
84. Bollig-Fischer, A., et al. (2015). Racial diversity of actionable mutations in non–small cell lung cancer. *Journal of Thoracic Oncology, 10*(2), 250–255.
85. Lee, S. Y., et al. (2017). A functional polymorphism in DTX1 gene of notch pathway predicts the prognosis of surgically resected non-small cell lung cancer. AACR Proceedings: AACR annual meeting 2017; Washington, DC http://cancerres.aacrjournals.org/content/77/13_Supplement/5727.short.
86. Quan, X., et al. (2017). Single nucleotide polymorphism rs3124599 in Notch1 is associated with the risk of lung cancer in northeast Chinese non-smoking females. *Oncotarget, 8*(19), 31180.
87. Xu, K., Moghal, N., & Egan, S. E. (2012). Notch signaling in lung development and disease. In *Notch signaling in embryology and Cancer* (pp. 89–98). Springer, New York, NY.
88. Zheng, Y., et al. (2013). A rare population of CD24+ ITGB4+ Notch hi cells drives tumor propagation in NSCLC and requires Notch3 for self-renewal. *Cancer Cell, 24*(1), 59–74.
89. Arasada, R. R., et al. (2014). EGFR blockade enriches for lung cancer stem–like cells through Notch3-dependent signaling. *Cancer Research, 74*(19), 5572–5584.
90. Justilien, V., et al. (2012). Matrix metalloproteinase-10 is required for lung cancer stem cell maintenance, tumor initiation and metastatic potential. *PLoS One, 7*(4), e35040.
91. Lefort, K., & Dotto, G. P. (2004). Notch signaling in the integrated control of keratinocyte growth/differentiation and tumor suppression. *Seminars in Cancer Biology, 14* (5), 374–386. Academic Press.
92. Lowell, S., et al. (2000). Stimulation of human epidermal differentiation by Delta–Notch signalling at the boundaries of stem-cell clusters. *Current Biology, 10*(9), 491–500.
93. Rangarajan, A., et al. (2001). Notch signaling is a direct determinant of keratinocyte growth arrest and entry into differentiation. *The EMBO Journal, 20*(13), 3427–3436.
94. Li, L., Sheehan, C., & Ross, J. (2009). Notch signaling in non small cell lung cancers (NSCLC) is associated with squamous differentiation and favorable clinical outcome.

Laboratory Investigation. Nature Publishing Group 75 varick st, 9TH FLR, New York, NY 10013-1917 USA.

95. Schwartz, A. G., et al. (2007). Reproductive factors, hormone use, estrogen receptor expression and risk of non–small-cell lung cancer in women. *Journal of Clinical Oncology, 25*(36), 5785–5792.
96. Schwartz, A. G., et al. (2005). Nuclear estrogen receptor β in lung cancer: Expression and survival differences by sex. *Clinical Cancer Research, 11*(20), 7280–7287.
97. Skov, B. G., Fischer, B. M., & Pappot, H. (2008). Oestrogen receptor β over expression in males with non-small cell lung cancer is associated with better survival. *Lung Cancer, 59*(1), 88–94.
98. Zhang, M., et al. (2016). Does Notch play a tumor suppressor role across diverse squamous cell carcinomas? *Cancer Medicine, 5*(8), 2048–2060.
99. Wael, H., et al. (2014). Notch1 signaling controls cell proliferation, apoptosis and differentiation in lung carcinoma. *Lung Cancer, 85*(2), 131–140.
100. Zheng, Q., et al. (2007). Notch signaling inhibits growth of the human lung adenocarcinoma cell line A549. *Oncology Reports, 17*(4), 847–852.
101. Baumgart, A., et al. (2010). ADAM17 regulates epidermal growth factor receptor expression through the activation of Notch1 in non–small cell lung cancer. *Cancer Research, 70*(13), 5368–5378.
102. Meng, X., & Yu, J. (2012). Implementation of hypoxia measurement into lung cancer therapy. *Lung Cancer, 75*(2), 146–150.
103. Graves, E. E., et al. (2010). Hypoxia in models of lung cancer: Implications for targeted therapeutics. *Clinical Cancer Research, 16*(19), 4843–4852.
104. Le, Q.-T., et al. (2006). An evaluation of tumor oxygenation and gene expression in patients with early stage non–small cell lung cancers. *Clinical Cancer Research, 12*(5), 1507–1514.
105. Graves, E. E., Maity, A., & Le, Q.-T. (2010). The tumor microenvironment in non–small-cell lung cancer. *Seminars in Radiation Oncology*, *20*(3), 156–163. WB Saunders.
106. Mees, G., et al. (2009). Molecular imaging of hypoxia with radiolabelled agents. *European Journal of Nuclear Medicine and Molecular Imaging, 36*(10), 1674–1686.
107. Vikram, D. S., Zweier, J. L., & Kuppusamy, P. (2007). Methods for noninvasive imaging of tissue hypoxia. *Antioxidants & Redox Signaling, 9*(10), 1745–1756.
108. Chen, Y., et al. (2007). Oxygen concentration determines the biological effects of NOTCH-1 signaling in adenocarcinoma of the lung. *Cancer Research, 67*(17), 7954–7959.
109. Gustafsson, M. V., et al. (2005). Hypoxia requires notch signaling to maintain the undifferentiated cell state. *Developmental Cell, 9*(5), 617–628.
110. Eliasz, S., et al. (2010). Notch-1 stimulates survival of lung adenocarcinoma cells during hypoxia by activating the IGF-1R pathway. *Oncogene, 29*(17), 2488–2498.
111. Han, Y. H., et al. (2008). Antimycin A as a mitochondrial electron transport inhibitor prevents the growth of human lung cancer A549 cells. *Oncology Reports, 20*(3), 689–693.
112. Goodwin, J., et al. (2017). The distinct metabolic phenotype of lung squamous cell carcinoma defines selective vulnerability to glycolytic inhibition. *Nature Communications, 8*, 15503.
113. Peiris-Pagès, M., et al. (2016). Cancer stem cell metabolism. *Breast Cancer Research, 18*(1), 55.
114. Mazzone, M., et al. (2010). Dose-dependent induction of distinct phenotypic responses to Notch pathway activation in mammary epithelial cells. *Proceedings of the National Academy of Sciences, 107*(11), 5012–5017.
115. Miele, L., Golde, T., & Osborne, B. (2006). Notch signaling in cancer. *Current Molecular Medicine, 6*(8), 905–918.
116. Bachireddy, P., Rakhra, K., & Felsher, D. (2012). Immunology in the clinic review series; focus on cancer: Multiple roles for the immune system in oncogene addiction. *Clinical & Experimental Immunology, 167*(2), 188–194.

117. Rakhra, K., et al. (2010). CD4+ T cells contribute to the remodeling of the microenvironment required for sustained tumor regression upon oncogene inactivation. *Cancer Cell, 18*(5), 485–498.
118. Odunsi, K., & Old, L. J. (2007). Tumor infiltrating lymphocytes: Indicators of tumor-related immune responses. *Cancer Immunity., 7*(3). http://cancerimmunolres.aacrjournals.org/content/canimmarch/7/1/3.full-text.pdf.
119. Bailis, W., et al. (2013). Notch simultaneously orchestrates multiple helper T cell programs independently of cytokine signals. *Immunity, 39*(1), 148–159.
120. Xu, H., et al. (2012). Notch-RBP-J signaling regulates the transcription factor IRF8 to promote inflammatory macrophage polarization. *Nature Immunology, 13*(7), 642–650.
121. Xu, J., et al. (2015). NOTCH reprograms mitochondrial metabolism for proinflammatory macrophage activation. *The Journal of Clinical Investigation, 125*(4), 1579.
122. Sauma, D., et al. (2012). Notch signalling regulates cytokine production by CD8+ and CD4+ T cells. *Scandinavian Journal of Immunology, 75*(4), 389–400.
123. Kassner, N., et al. (2010). Cutting edge: Plasmacytoid dendritic cells induce IL-10 production in T cells via the Delta-like-4/Notch axis. *The Journal of Immunology, 184*(2), 550–554.
124. Yvon, E. S., et al. (2003). Overexpression of the Notch ligand, Jagged-1, induces alloantigen-specific human regulatory T cells. *Blood, 102*(10), 3815–3821.
125. Delaney, C., et al. (2005). Dose-dependent effects of the Notch ligand Delta1 on ex vivo differentiation and in vivo marrow repopulating ability of cord blood cells. *Blood, 106*(8), 2693–2699.
126. Dorsch, M., et al. (2002). Ectopic expression of Delta4 impairs hematopoietic development and leads to lymphoproliferative disease. *Blood, 100*(6), 2046–2055.
127. Koch, U., et al. (2008). Delta-like 4 is the essential, nonredundant ligand for Notch1 during thymic T cell lineage commitment. *The Journal of Experimental Medicine, 205*(11), 2515–2523.
128. Huang, Y., et al. (2011). Resuscitating cancer immunosurveillance: Selective stimulation of DLL1-Notch signaling in T cells rescues T cell function and inhibits tumor growth. *Cancer Research, 71*(19), 6122–6131.
129. Shanker, A., et al. (2014). Cancer therapy by resuscitating Notch immune surveillance. *Journal for Immunotherapy of Cancer, 2*(Suppl 1), O1.
130. Ladi, E., et al. (2005). The divergent DSL ligand Dll3 does not activate Notch signaling but cell autonomously attenuates signaling induced by other DSL ligands. *The Journal of Cell Biology, 170*(6), 983–992.
131. Amsen, D., Antov, A., & Flavell, R. A. (2009). The different faces of Notch in T-helper-cell differentiation. *Nature Reviews. Immunology, 9*(2), 116–124.
132. Keerthivasan, S., Suleiman, R., Lawlor, R., Roderick, J., Bates, T., Minter, L., ... & Miele, L. (2011). Notch signaling regulates mouse and human Th17 differentiation. *The Journal of Immunology*, 1003658.
133. Sierra, R. A., et al. (2014). Rescue of Notch 1 signaling in antigen-specific CD8+ T cells overcomes tumor-induced T cell suppression and enhances immunotherapy in cancer. *Cancer Immunology Research, 2*(8), 800–811.
134. Radtke, F., et al. (1999). Deficient T cell fate specification in mice with an induced inactivation of Notch1. *Immunity, 10*(5), 547–558.
135. Pear, W. S., et al. (1996). Exclusive development of T cell neoplasms in mice transplanted with bone marrow expressing activated Notch alleles. *The Journal of Experimental Medicine, 183*(5), 2283–2291.
136. Biktasova, A. K., et al. (2015). Multivalent forms of the Notch ligand DLL-1 enhance antitumor T cell immunity in lung cancer and improve efficacy of EGFR targeted therapy. *Cancer Research*: p. canres. 1154.2014.
137. Mathieu, M., et al. (2013). Notch signaling regulates PD-1 expression during CD8+ T-cell activation. *Immunology and Cell Biology, 91*(1), 82–88.

138. Srivastava, M., et al. (2015). Dual targeting of delta-like ligand 4 (DLL4) and programmed death 1 (PD1) inhibits tumor growth and generates enhanced long-term immunological memory. *Cancer Research, 75*(15 Suppl), 255–255.
139. Tran, I. T., et al. (2013). Blockade of individual Notch ligands and receptors controls graft-versus-host disease. *The Journal of Clinical Investigation, 123*(4), 1590–1604.
140. Fasnacht, N., et al. (2014). Specific fibroblastic niches in secondary lymphoid organs orchestrate distinct Notch-regulated immune responses. *Journal of Experimental Medicine, 211*(11), 2265–2279.
141. Rizzo, P., et al. (2008). Rational targeting of Notch signaling in cancer. *Oncogene, 27*(38), 5124–5131.
142. Ranganathan, P., Weaver, K. L., & Capobianco, A. J. (2011). Notch signalling in solid tumours: A little bit of everything but not all the time. *Nature Reviews Cancer, 11*(5), 338–351.
143. Paris, D., et al. (2005). Inhibition of angiogenesis and tumor growth by β and γ-secretase inhibitors. *European Journal of Pharmacology, 514*(1), 1–15.
144. Maraver, A., et al. (2012). Therapeutic effect of γ-secretase inhibition in Kras G12V-driven non-small cell lung carcinoma by derepression of DUSP1 and inhibition of ERK. *Cancer Cell, 22*(2), 222–234.
145. Hayashi, I., et al. (2012). Neutralization of the γ-secretase activity by monoclonal antibody against extracellular domain of nicastrin. *Oncogene, 31*(6), 787–798.
146. Ridgway, J., et al. (2006). Inhibition of Dll4 signalling inhibits tumour growth by deregulating angiogenesis. *Nature, 444*(7122), 1083–1087.
147. Yan, M., et al. (2010). Chronic DLL4 blockade induces vascular neoplasms. *Nature, 463*(7282), E6–E7.
148. Wu, Y., et al. (2010). Therapeutic antibody targeting of individual Notch receptors. *Nature, 464*(7291), 1052–1057.
149. Nickoloff, B. J., Osborne, B. A., & Miele, L. (2003). Notch signaling as a therapeutic target in cancer: A new approach to the development of cell fate modifying agents. *Oncogene, 22*(42), 6598–6608.
150. Kopan, R., & Ilagan, M. X. G. (2004). γ-secretase: Proteasome of the membrane? *Nature Reviews Molecular Cell Biology, 5*(6), 499–504.
151. Maetzel, D., et al. (2009). Nuclear signalling by tumour-associated antigen EpCAM. *Nature Cell Biology, 11*(2), 162–171.
152. Takebe, N., Nguyen, D., & Yang, S. X. (2014). Targeting notch signaling pathway in cancer: Clinical development advances and challenges. *Pharmacology & Therapeutics, 141*(2), 140–149.
153. Konishi, J., et al. (2010). Notch3 cooperates with the EGFR pathway to modulate apoptosis through the induction of bim. *Oncogene, 29*(4), 589–596.
154. Kaur, G., et al. (2016). Bromodomain and hedgehog pathway targets in small cell lung cancer. *Cancer Letters, 371*(2), 225–239.
155. Ambrogio, C., et al. (2016). Combined inhibition of DDR1 and Notch signaling is a therapeutic strategy for KRAS-driven lung adenocarcinoma. *Nature Medicine, 22*(3), 270.
156. Gold, K. A., et al. (2013). A phase I/II trial combining erlotinib with gamma secretase inhibitor RO4929097 in advanced non-small cell lung cancer (NSCLC). *Journal of Clinical Oncology*. American Society of Clinical Oncology 2318 MILL ROAD, STE 800, ALEXANDRIA, VA 22314 USA.
157. Luistro, L., et al. (2009). Preclinical profile of a potent γ-secretase inhibitor targeting notch signaling with in vivo efficacy and pharmacodynamic properties. *Cancer Research, 69*(19), 7672–7680.
158. De Strooper, B., Iwatsubo, T., & Wolfe, M. S. (2012). Presenilins and γ-secretase: Structure, function, and role in Alzheimer disease. *Cold Spring Harbor Perspectives in Medicine, 2*(1), a006304.
159. Yan, M. (2011). Therapeutic promise and challenges of targeting DLL4/NOTCH1. *Vascular Cell, 3*, 17.

160. Li, D., et al. (2014). The notch ligand JAGGED1 as a target for anti-tumor therapy. *Frontiers in Oncology, 4*, 254.
161. Alketbi, A., & Attoub, S. (2015). Notch signaling in cancer: Rationale and strategies for targeting. *Current Cancer Drug Targets, 15*(5), 364–374.
162. Chiorean, E. G., et al. (2015). A phase I first-in-human study of enoticumab (REGN421), a fully human Delta-like ligand 4 (Dll4) monoclonal antibody in patients with advanced solid tumors. *Clinical Cancer Research, 21*(12), 2695–2703.
163. Brunner, A., et al. (2016). Effects of anti-DLL4 treatment on non-small cell lung cancer (NSCLC) human xenograft tumors. AACR. (http://cancerres.aacrjournals.org/content/76/14_Supplement/4652.short) Proceedings: AACR 107th Annual Meeting 2016; April 16–20, 2016; New Orleans, LA.
164. Globenewswire.com. (2015). Oncomed presents demcizumab data from phase 1B clinical trial in non-small cell lung cancer patients at the European lucg cancer conference. Available from: http://globenewswire.com/news-release/2015/04/16/725132/10129223/en/OncoMed-Presents-Demcizumab-Data-From-Phase-1b-Clinical-Trial-in-Non-Small-Cell-Lung-Cancer-Patients-at-the-European-Lung-Cancer-Conference.html?print=1.
165. Rudin, C. M., et al. (2017). Rovalpituzumab tesirine, a DLL3-targeted antibody-drug conjugate, in recurrent small-cell lung cancer: A first-in-human, first-in-class, open-label, phase 1 study. *The Lancet Oncology, 18*(1), 42–51.
166. Gordon, W. R., et al. (2007). Structural basis for autoinhibition of Notch. *Nature Structural & Molecular Biology, 14*(4), 295–300.
167. Li, K., et al. (2008). Modulation of Notch signaling by antibodies specific for the extracellular negative regulatory region of NOTCH3. *Journal of Biological Chemistry, 283*(12), 8046–8054.
168. Aste-Amézaga, M., et al. (2010). Characterization of Notch1 antibodies that inhibit signaling of both normal and mutated Notch1 receptors. *PLoS One, 5*(2), e9094.
169. Daniel, D. B., Rudin, C. M., Hart, L., Spigel, D. R., Edelman, M. J., Goldschmidt, J., Bordoni, R., et al. (2017). 1530PDResults of a randomized, placebo-controlled, phase 2 study of tarextumab (TRXT, anti-Notch2/3) in combination with etoposide and platinum (EP) in patients (pts) with untreated extensive-stage small-cell lung cancer (ED-SCLC). *Annals of Oncology, 28*(suppl_5).
170. OncoMed Pharmaceuticals, I. (2017). OncoMed's phase 2 trial of tarextumab in small cell lung cancer does not meet endpoints. In *Company also announces discontinuation of brontictuzumab phase 1b study*. OncoMed Pharmaceuticals, Inc: Online.
171. Chiang, A., Mclaughlin, J., Pietanza, M. C., Spira, A., Jotte, R., Gadgeel, S., Mita, A. et al. (2015). NOTCH3 protein expression and outcome in small cell lung Cancer (SCLC) and therapeutic targeting with Tarextumab (anti-NOTCH 2/3). *Journal of Thoracic Oncology, 10*(9), S361. New York, NY: Elsevier Science Inc.
172. Davis, S. L., et al. (2013). A first-in-human phase I study of the novel cancer stem cell (CSC) targeting antibody OMP-52M51 (anti-Notch1) administered intravenously to patients with certain advanced solid tumors. In *Proceedings of the AACR-NCI-EORTC International Conference: Molecular Targets and Cancer Therapeutics*.
173. Liu, Z., et al. (2011). Notch1 loss of heterozygosity causes vascular tumors and lethal hemorrhage in mice. *The Journal of Clinical Investigation, 121*(2), 800.
174. Pamela Munster, S. G. E., Patnaik, A., Shields, A., Tolcher, A. W., Davis, S. L., Heymach, J. V., Xu, L., Kapoun, A. M., Faoro, L., Dupont, J., & Ferrarotto, R. (2015). Safety and preliminary efficacy results of a first-in-human phase I study of the novel cancer stem cell (CSC) targeting antibody brontictuzumab (OMP-52M51, anti-Notch1) administered intravenously to patients with certain advanced solid tumors. [Poster] [cited 2018 January 24 2018]. Available from: http://posters.omed.s3.amazonaws.com/2015_N1_solid_tumor_triple_meeting.pdf.
175. Geles, K. G., et al. (2015). Therapeutic targeting the NOTCH3 receptor with antibody drug conjugates. *Cancer Research, 75*(15 Suppl), 1697–1697.

176. Mizugaki, H., et al. (2012). γ-Secretase inhibitor enhances antitumour effect of radiation in Notch-expressing lung cancer. *British Journal of Cancer, 106*(12), 1953–1959.
177. Ikezawa, Y., et al. (2017). Inhibition of Notch and HIF enhances the antitumor effect of radiation in Notch expressing lung cancer. *International Journal of Clinical Oncology, 22*(1), 59–69.
178. Purow, B. W., et al. (2008). Notch-1 regulates transcription of the epidermal growth factor receptor through p53. *Carcinogenesis, 29*(5), 918–925.
179. Jin, S., et al. (2008). Notch signaling regulates platelet-derived growth factor receptor-β expression in vascular smooth muscle cells. *Circulation Research, 102*(12), 1483–1491.
180. Yuan, X., et al. (2014). Notch signaling and EMT in non-small cell lung cancer: Biological significance and therapeutic application. *Journal of Hematology & Oncology, 7*(1), 87.
181. Tammela, T., et al. (2008). Blocking VEGFR-3 suppresses angiogenic sprouting and vascular network formation. *Nature, 454*(7204), 656–660.
182. Funahashi, Y., et al. (2010). Notch regulates the angiogenic response via induction of VEGFR-1. *Journal of Angiogenesis Research, 2*(3), 2.
183. Espinosa, L., et al. (2002). p65-NFκB synergizes with Notch to activate transcription by triggering cytoplasmic translocation of the nuclear receptor corepressor N-CoR. *Journal of Cell Science, 115*(6), 1295–1303.
184. Wang, Z., et al. (2010). Targeting Notch signaling pathway to overcome drug resistance for cancer therapy. *Biochimica et Biophysica Acta (BBA)-Reviews on Cancer, 1806*(2), 258–267.
185. Mori, M., et al. (2015). Notch3-Jagged signaling controls the pool of undifferentiated airway progenitors. *Development, 142*(2), 258–267.
186. Ranganathan, P., et al. (2011). Hierarchical phosphorylation within the ankyrin repeat domain defines a phosphoregulatory loop that regulates Notch transcriptional activity. *Journal of Biological Chemistry, 286*(33), 28844–28857.
187. Alamgeer, M., et al. (2013). Cancer stem cells in lung cancer: Evidence and controversies. *Respirology, 18*(5), 757–764.
188. Leung, E. L.-H., et al. (2010). Non-small cell lung cancer cells expressing CD44 are enriched for stem cell-like properties. *PLoS One, 5*(11), e14062.
189. Eramo, A., et al. (2008). Identification and expansion of the tumorigenic lung cancer stem cell population. *Cell Death & Differentiation, 15*(3), 504–514.
190. Bertolini, G., et al. (2009). Highly tumorigenic lung cancer CD133+ cells display stem-like features and are spared by cisplatin treatment. *Proceedings of the National Academy of Sciences, 106*(38), 16281–16286.
191. Chen, Y.-C., et al. (2008). Oct-4 expression maintained cancer stem-like properties in lung cancer-derived CD133-positive cells. *PLoS One, 3*(7), e2637.
192. Jiang, F., et al. (2009). Aldehyde dehydrogenase 1 is a tumor stem cell-associated marker in lung cancer. *Molecular Cancer Research, 7*(3), 330–338.
193. Shi, Y., et al. (2012). The side population in human lung cancer cell line NCI-H460 is enriched in stem-like cancer cells. *PLoS One, 7*(3), e33358.
194. Sullivan, J. P., et al. (2010). Aldehyde dehydrogenase activity selects for lung adenocarcinoma stem cells dependent on notch signaling. *Cancer Research, 70*(23), 9937–9948.
195. Okudela, K., et al. (2012). Expression of the potential cancer stem cell markers, CD133, CD44, ALDH1, and β-catenin, in primary lung adenocarcinoma—their prognostic significance. *Pathology International, 62*(12), 792–801.
196. Wang, Z., et al. (2014). Notch signaling drives stemness and tumorigenicity of esophageal adenocarcinoma. *Cancer Research, 74*(21), 6364–6374.
197. Garcia-Heredia, J. M., et al. (2017). The cargo protein MAP17 (PDZK1IP1) regulates the cancer stem cell pool activating the Notch pathway by abducting NUMB. *Clinical Cancer Research, 23*(14), 3871–3883.
198. Liu, Y.-P., et al. (2013). Cisplatin selects for multidrug-resistant CD133+ cells in lung adenocarcinoma by activating Notch signaling. *Cancer Research, 73*(1), 406–416.

199. Rosell, R., et al. (2017). OA10.03 YAP-NOTCH and STAT3 signaling rebound as a compensatory response to gefitinib or osimertinib treatment in EGFR mutant lung cancer. *Journal of Thoracic Oncology, 12*(1), S281–S282.
200. Kelly, K., et al. (2008). Phase III trial of maintenance gefitinib or placebo after concurrent chemoradiotherapy and docetaxel consolidation in inoperable stage III non-small-cell lung cancer: SWOG S0023. *Journal of Clinical Oncology, 26*(15), 2450–2456.
201. Goss, G. D., et al. (2010). A phase III randomized, double-blind, placebo-controlled trial of the epidermal growth factor receptor inhibitor gefitinb in completely resected stage IB-IIIA non-small cell lung cancer (NSCLC): NCIC CTG BR.19. *Journal of Clinical Oncology, 28*(18s), abstr LBA7005.

Chapter 11
Notch Signaling in Pediatric Soft Tissue Sarcoma

Cristina Cossetti, Alberto Gualtieri, Silvia Pomella, Elena Carcarino, and Rossella Rota

Abstract Etiology, biology, response to treatment, and outcome greatly differ between adult and childhood cancers. Soft tissue sarcoma encompasses a heterogeneous group of pediatric sarcomas characterized by a high capacity to invade neighboring tissues. Although in the last years the overall survival in childhood cancers has improved to over 70% for the nonmetastatic forms, subgroups of young patients with metastatic and aggressive disease still show a poor outcome. Moreover, survivors often suffer from long-term morbidity due to the effects of therapy. It is widely accepted that soft tissue sarcomas of childhood develop from mesenchymal progenitor cells affected by chromosomal aberrations and mutations in genetic and epigenetic pathways during development. Therefore, pathways driving tissue differentiation are particularly relevant. Among these, the Notch signaling pathway plays one of the major roles. Notch signaling is evolutionarily conserved among species, working as a cell-to-cell communication system strictly defining cell fate, stem cell renewal, and tissue homeostasis during embryo development and in postnatal life. In the present chapter, we describe recent insights on Notch deregulation in the most prominent pediatric soft tissue sarcomas: rhabdomyosarcomas, Ewing sarcomas, and synovial sarcomas. We also summarize the challenges and opportunities in inhibiting Notch signaling for the treatment of this group of tumors.

Keywords Notch signaling · Notch receptors · Gamma-secretase · Soft tissue sarcoma · Rhabdomyosarcoma · Ewing sarcoma · Synovial sarcoma

---

C. Cossetti · A. Gualtieri · S. Pomella · E. Carcarino · R. Rota (✉)
Laboratory of Angiogenesis, Department of Oncohematology, Ospedale Pediatrico Bambino Gesù, Rome, Italy
e-mail: cristina.cossetti@opbg.net; alberto.gualtieri@opbg.net; silvia.pomella@opbg.net; elena.carcarino@opbg.net; rossella.rota@opbg.net

L. Miele, S. Artavanis-Tsakonas (eds.), *Targeting Notch in Cancer*,
https://doi.org/10.1007/978-1-4939-8859-4_11

Abbreviations

DLL1, 3, 4	Delta-like 1, 3, 4
ES	Ewing sarcoma
GEMM	Genetically engineered mice models
GSI	Gamma secretase inhibitors
MAML1	Mastermind-like 1
NEC	Notch extracellular domain
NEXT	Notch extracellular truncation
NICD	Notch intracellular domain
NTM	Notch transmembrane domain
RMS	Rhabdomyosarcoma
SS	Synovial sarcoma

11.1 Introduction

11.1.1 Childhood Versus Adult Cancers

Conversely to adult tumors, whose pathogenesis is related to environment-/age-dependent genetic and epigenetic alterations, pediatric cancers originate from progenitor cells in which developmental pathways governing embryonic life are deregulated. In line with this, tumors of childhood often contain a clonal population of presumably tumor-initiating cells expressing fusion products of genes that guide tissue development.

Increasing knowledge of the landscape of molecular networks involving genetic and epigenetic mechanisms acting in childhood cancers have opened the way to the discovery of novel potential approaches to treat the disease.

Crucial developmental pathways involved in pediatric tumor biology are Sonic Hedgehog (SHH), Wingless (WNT), and Notch signaling. These pathways are fundamental for proper cell differentiation and tissue lineage commitment of progenitor cells and, more importantly, cooperate and cross talk each other (reviewed in [1–6]). Considering the crucial role of Notch signaling in developmental processes, it is not surprising that it has been found affected in several diseases ([7–15] and reviewed in [16]).

An oncogenic role of Notch signaling has been highlighted for the first time in pediatric acute T-cell leukemia (T-ALL). Indeed, two groups demonstrated that (i) mutations of the Notch1 receptor resulted in the constitutive production of an activated form of Notch1, i.e., the Notch1 intracellular domain, in patients with T-ALL [17], and that (ii) this Notch1 constitutive activation is sufficient for tumorigenesis [18]: an observation confirmed later also in adult cancers [19]. In the last few years, the deregulation of Notch signaling has been shown to be involved in several types of pediatric solid tumors. Recently, we and others have shown Notch signaling abnormalities are pathogenetic events in pediatric soft tissue sarcomas, a heterogeneous group of solid tumors affecting mainly soft tissue and bone of young patients.

As for adult cancers, where several clinical trials with Notch signaling inhibitors are being evaluated, the modulation of the Notch signaling is under preclinical study as an anticancer strategy in this type of pediatric tumors.

11.1.2 Pediatric Soft Tissue Sarcomas

Pediatric soft tissue sarcomas include a group of tumors derived from the mesenchymal compartment that are highly heterogeneous in terms of clinical behavior and genomic alterations [20].

Collectively, they represent about 8–10% of all childhood tumors and about 15% of tumors outside the central nervous system [21]. Multimodal approach with chemotherapy and surgery is the usual treatment of pediatric soft tissue sarcoma, while radiation is rarely used in young children due to its side effects on a growing organism [22]. Advances in treatments have improved the overall survival in all childhood cancers to over 70% today. However, although the prognosis of soft tissue sarcoma has improved considerably, a group of patients still shows a dismal prognosis. Indeed, metastatic forms and subsets of tumors harboring specific oncogenic mutations/chromosomal translocations are often incurable. Additionally, young survivors often suffer from long-term side effects linked to therapy. An additional clinical challenge to eradicate soft tissue sarcomas is due to the high ability of tumor cells to invade the neighboring tissues [22].

Therefore, the scientific community is focusing on finding a therapy that is more specific and less toxic for these young patients. This can be achieved only through the knowledge of the molecular pathogenetic mechanisms responsible for the development and maintenance of these tumors.

The three major groups of pediatric soft tissue sarcomas include rhabdomyosarcoma (RMS), Ewing sarcoma (ES), and synovial sarcoma (SS). Although they have different and peculiar characteristics, experimental evidences clearly indicate that all can develop from mesenchymal progenitor cells affected by chromosomal aberrations and/or gene mutations. It is widely accepted that the dysregulation of the major embryonic developmental molecular pathways plays a fundamental role in the pathogenesis of pediatric soft tissue sarcomas. In agreement, small populations of cells that remain undifferentiated and maintain self-renewal capacity seem to represent the tumor ancestor cells unresponsive to therapy [23, 24].

Therefore, the modulation of developmental pathways regulating stem cell properties, such as the Notch pathway, might be a potential strategy to improve the clinical response of this type of tumors affecting young patients.

In the last several years, we and others have reported preclinical experimental proofs of principle indicating Notch signaling modulation as a potential approach to reduce the tumorigenesis of pediatric soft tissue sarcomas.

11.1.3 Structure of Notch Receptors and Ligands

The Notch pathway is one of the fundamental signaling pathways strictly defining developmental processes regulating cell fate and tissue differentiation and homeostasis in embryo and in the postnatal life. The pathway signals through cell-to-cell interaction between a signal-sending cell (expressing Notch ligands) and a signal-receiving cell (expressing Notch receptors) (Fig. 11.1) [25, 26]. This type of cell communication relies on the particular structure of ligands and receptors.

Notch receptors While in the fruit fly *Drosophila melanogaster* only a single Notch gene exists (reviewed in [27]), in mammals four Notch receptors have been identified, i.e., Notch 1–4 [28]. They are encoded by four different gene loci on chro-

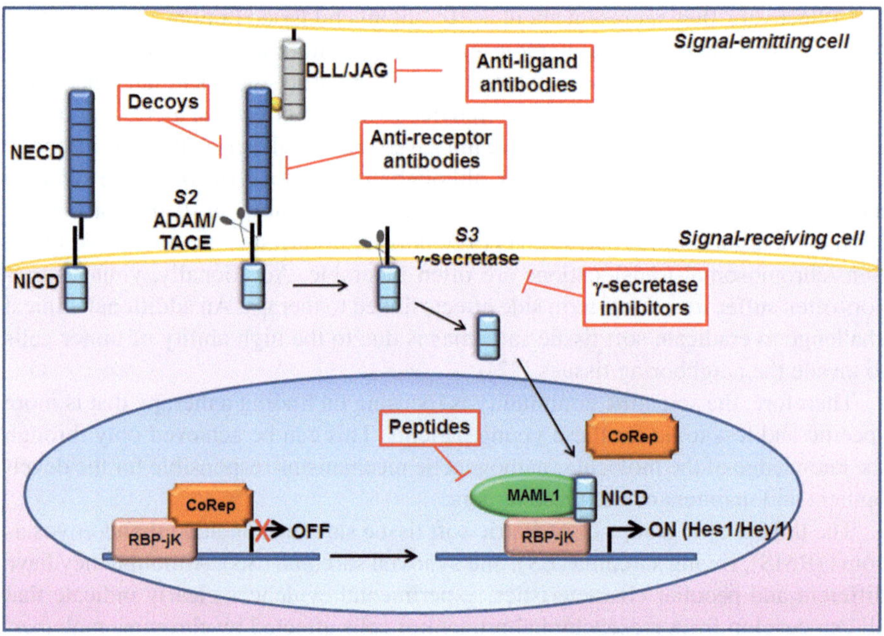

Fig. 11.1 After proteolytic processing maturation, Notch receptors are expressed on the cell membrane as an extracellular domain (NECD) non-covalently associated with a transmembrane portion and an intracellular domain (NICD). Notch signaling is initiated by a Notch receptor-Delta/Jagged-type (DLL/JAG) ligand interaction between two neighboring cells *in trans*, which induces two successive proteolytic cleavages. The first one is operated on the S2 site by "a disintegrin and metalloprotease" 10 (ADAM10) or ADAM17, which is followed by an S3 cleavage by a presenilin complex (γ-secretase). The S3 cleavage gives rise to the NICD fragment that translocates into the nucleus, where it binds to a protein complex containing recombination signal-binding protein Jk (RBP-Jk) relieving the repressor complex (CoRep). This event modulates chromatin activity recruiting activators such as MAML1 and converts RBP-Jk from a transcriptional repressor to an activator, leading to the transcription of hairy/enhancer of split (Hes) and Hey family genes, which work as transcriptional repressors. Several stages of the Notch signaling pathway are prone to pharmacological intervention. Decoys, anti-ligand antibodies, anti-receptor-antibodies, γ-secretase inhibitors, and peptide inhibitors are labeled in the red boxes

mosome (Chr) 9, Chr 1, Chr 19, and Chr 6, respectively, and are about 60% homologous to each other. Each Notch paralog is translated as a single-pass transmembrane protein that is subjected to posttranslational modifications before being expressed on the surface of the cells: a single-chain precursor is cleaved by furin-like proteases in the Golgi compartment (S1 cleavage), resulting in an N-terminal extracellular domain (NECD) and a C-terminal portion encompassing both a Notch transmembrane (NTM) and intracellular domain (NICD). The two fragments are non-covalently reassembled on the Golgi membranes and, then, expressed on the surface of the plasma membrane ([29] and reviewed in [30]).

The NECD is formed by a number of epidermal growth factor (EGF)-like repeats responsible for the binding of ligands [31]. Important under a functional point of view, a specific number of EGF repeats characterize each Notch receptor, Notch1 containing 36 EGF repeats [32], whereas Notch2 presenting 35 EGF repeats [33], Notch3 34 EGF repeats [34], and Notch4, the shorter Notch receptor, only 29 EGF repeats [35]. A negative regulatory region (NRR), composed of three cysteine-rich Lin12/Notch repeats (LNR) [36, 37], followed by a juxtamembrane hydrophobic region, is responsible for the heterodimerization of the NECD and the NTM-NICD portions of the receptor. The LNR regulates the auto-inhibition of the Notch receptor preventing the receptor for being cleaved without binding to the ligand [37, 38].

The intracellular region NICD contains a module, named RAM, which recognizes the recombination signal-binding protein Jk (RBP-Jk) supporting the transcriptional role for the NICD that can interact with the transcriptional coactivator RBP-jK in the CSL complex (RBP-jK/CBF-1/KBF2 in mammals) [39]. The RAM region is followed by seven ankyrin (ANK) repeats important for the interaction with CSL and other transcriptional regulators [40, 41], two nuclear localization signals (NLS) [42], a transactivation domain (TAD) [43], and a C-terminal PEST sequence (rich in proline, glutamic acid, serine, and threonine) [44]. The PEST sequence is highly important since it can be phosphorylated, thus regulating the ubiquitination of the NICD and, consequently, its stability and signaling ability [44]. Notably, the strength of the TAD sequence in transactivating gene transcription is different among the paralogs being strong for Notch1, weak for Notch2, and strong but highly specific for Notch3, while Notch4 does not have a TAD [43, 45]. These differences in the structure and activity explain the diverse and somewhat divergent functions of the Notch receptor family.

Notch ligands Only two canonical ligands of the Delta-Serrate family are expressed in *Drosophila*, while mammalian cells express three ligands of the Delta family, Delta-like 1 (DLL1), DLL3, and DLL4 [46–48], and two of the Serrate family, JAG1 and JAG2 [49, 50]. All the five mammalian ligands are type I transmembrane proteins containing an N-terminal region and a cysteine-rich domain (DSL for Delta, Serrate, and LAG-2), followed by a number of EGF-like repeats. In particular, the N-terminal region with DSL and the first two EGF-repeats are responsible for the interaction with the EGF-like repeats of Notch receptors ([51, 52] and reviewed in [25]). The structure of the intracellular region of the canonical ligands is not conserved among species and regulates ligand interactions with the cellular cytoskeleton.

Additional noncanonical ligands can interact with and activate Notch receptors, either transmembrane or soluble proteins, such as DLK1, DLK2, DNER, the EGF-like protein7 (EGFL7), or the F3/contactin ([53, 54] and reviewed in [25, 55, 56]). They do not contain a DSL domain but are all characterized by the presence of EGF-like repeats.

Another level of complexity is added by the posttranslational modifications of Notch receptors, operated in the cytoplasmic compartment, which strictly regulate their half-life, selectivity, and activity [25, 57]. Among those are the glycosylation, ubiquitylation, phosphorylation, and acetylation.

Fringe glycosyltransferases, firstly identified in Drosophila, glycosylate specific EGF-like repeats of the Notch heterodimer in the Golgi compartment [58–60]: a modification that affects the affinity of the receptor for the ligands, specifically preventing Jagged-dependent activation [61, 62]. Three mammalian fringe enzymes are known, i.e., lunatic fringe (LFNG), manic fringe (MFNG), and radical fringe (RFNG) [63]. It is arguable that dysregulation of these enzymes can lead to imbalance in the expression/activity of Notch components since it can induce the Notch receptors to be cleaved with higher rate than in normal tissue (reviewed in [64]), as demonstrated for breast cancer cells [65].

The lysosomal degradation or, conversely, the recycling to the plasma membrane of the cleaved Notch is regulated by polyubiquitylation, a process governed by several E3 ubiquitin ligases such as Deltex, β-arrestin/Kurtz, Itch, NEDD4 (neural precursor cell expressed developmentally downregulated 4), Cbl (casitas B-lineage lymphoma), and Fbw7/Sel-10 ([66–69] and reviewed in [70]). The inclusion of Notch in the early endosomes can be regulated by Numb, a cytoplasmic negative regulator of the pathway [71], and it is followed by proteasome-mediated degradation [72]. The phosphorylation of NICD to the ANK and/or PEST domain along with acetylation modulates the stability and the activity of the cleaved receptor [73–77]. Further, NICD can interact in the cytoplasm with several molecules among which Nemo-like kinase NLK, which suppresses Notch signaling [78], or Pin1, which conversely amplifies Notch activation [79–82].

11.1.4 Notch Signaling Pathway

The Notch signaling is critical in embryos during the differentiation of stem cells when a ligand-expressing cell interacts with a Notch-expressing cell and, then, the former undergoes differentiation while the latter remains in an undifferentiated state [30]. However, the results of this cell-to-cell communication highly depend on the molecular, cellular, and environmental contexts, making a simple mechanism extremely versatile [83–85].

When a canonical ligand on a cell binds to the specific EGF-like repeats of a Notch receptor on a neighboring cell (in *trans*), the resulting mechanical stretch favors the cleavage (at site S2) of the heterodimeric portion just outside the plasma membrane by the a disintegrin and metalloprotease 10 (ADAM10) or 17 (ADAM17) [86].

A requirement for this process is the ubiquitination and subsequent endocytosis of the ligand (reviewed by [87]). Then, the remaining membrane-tethered intermediate, named NEXT (Notch extracellular truncation), is subsequently cleaved in an intracellular region (at sites S3 and S4) by a γ-secretase complex formed by four subunits [88–93]. This last cleavage results in an intracellular activated form, NICD, which translocates to the nucleus, binds the CSL complex (RBP-Jk/CBF-1/KBF2 in mammals) and activates the transcription of canonical Notch target genes [94]. To do so, the CSL/Notch complex recruits several transcriptional coactivators such as Mastermind-like 1 (MAML1) and the acetyltransferases CBP/p300 or PCAF/GCN5 ([41, 95–97] and reviewed in [98]). The canonical target genes belong to the basic helix-loop-helix (bHLH) families of hairy/enhancer of split (Hes) and Hey (subfamily of Hes, related with YRPW motif) repressors [25]. The result is the transcriptional repression of multiple differentiation genes. Interestingly, conversely to the classical view based on the recruitment of NICD by RBP-jK already bound to the DNA in a repressor state [83, 99], more recently the group of Tajbakhsh demonstrates that in mammalian myoblasts (i) NICD recruits free RBP-jK to the chromatin on specific enhancers, while (ii) the amount of RBP-jK constitutively bound to the DNA is unaffected by Notch activation [100]. This finding further highlights the importance of the cellular and molecular context for the regulation and effects of Notch signaling pathway. In addition to the Hes and Hey genes, Notch signaling can activate in a context-/tissue-dependent manner the transcription of, among others, Deltex or members of NF-kB family, the cyclin-dependent kinase inhibitor $p21^{Cip1}$, cyclin D1 or MYC [101–106]. Notch signaling can be also activated in a noncanonical way that can be (i) independent from CSL, (ii) independent from the S3 cleavage, or (iii) in the absence of Notch cleavage and NICD formation (reviewed in [55, 107, 108]). Finally, ligand-receptor interactions on the same cell can be also in *cis* and results in inhibition of the signaling [109–112]. Importantly, the structural molecular features of Notch components that allow several types of modifications concurring to the diverse mechanisms of signalization represent a platform for therapeutical interventions with modulators of the pathway (Fig. 11.1). Notably, being Notch signaling tissue- and context-specific and paralogs similar but not identical, the signal triggered by different Notch receptors in different tissues is somewhat specific and can be even opposite (reviewed in [25]).

11.2 Notch Signaling Deregulation in Pediatric Soft Tissue Sarcomas

11.2.1 Notch Signaling in Rhabdomyosarcoma

Rhabdomyosarcoma (RMS) is the most common soft tissue tumor of childhood of myogenic origins accounting for about 8% of all pediatric tumors [113]. Despite the expression of the master regulators of skeletal muscle differentiation such as MYOD and myogenin, also used for diagnostic purposes to exclude other small round blue cell tumors, RMS cells do not differentiate in multifiber structures and proliferate indefinitely ([114, 115] reviewed in [116]). To date, we and others have shown that the modulation of differentiation represents a potential approach to restore the cell cycle checkpoints inhibiting tumor cell proliferation [117, 118]. However, as shown in genetically modified mice models (GEMM) of spontaneous RMS, this sarcoma could originate from a heterogeneous group of mesenchymal-derived cells, even if mesenchymal precursors with different degrees of skeletal muscle commitment have been implicated as the major tumor-prone subset [119–124]. Two major histological subtypes are included in pediatric RMS: the embryonal (ERMS) and the alveolar (ARMS) variants. ERMS represents about 70–75% of all cases of pediatric RMS and primarily affects young children arising in the head and neck and retroperitoneum and showing, when nonmetastatic, a good prognosis with an overall survival of about 80% [125, 126]. ERMS is characterized by somatic gene mutations in the *RAS* gene family, *TP53*, *FGFR4*, *PIK3CA*, *CTNNB1*, *FBXW7*, and *BCOR,* associated with genomic instability including loss of imprinting and loss of heterozygosity of specific chromosomal regions, among which the Chr. 11p.15 region, and gain of regions of chromosomes 2, 7, 8, 11, 12, 13, and 20 [127–129]. Moreover, ERMS pathogenesis has been related to mutation/dysfunction of components of one of the major developmental pathways, i.e., Hedgehog [130–133]. Interestingly, the *MYOD* gene has been shown to be mutated in a group of older adolescent with an aggressive form of ERMS [134]. The p.Leu122Arg substitution leads to a MYOD protein capable to activate gene transcription in a "MYC-like" manner, once more highlighting the strong involvement of malfunction of myogenic factors in RMS. Collectively, these findings emphasize the heterogeneous molecular features of the ERMS variant. An about 20% of ARMS behave clinically and show molecular alterations similar to the ERMS subtype [127, 135], whereas the majority of ARMS is characterized by clonal cell populations with specific chromosomal translocations, defining a subset of RMS clinically and molecularly different from fusion-negative RMS [127, 135].

The most frequent chromosomal translocations in ARMS are t(2;13) (q35;q14) or t(1;13) (q36;q14), which result in the expression of the two oncogenic proteins PAX3-FOXO1 and PAX7-FOXO1, respectively [136, 137]. Both are transcription factors formed by the DNA-binding domain of PAX3/7 and the transactivation domain of FOXO1. The result is a constitutive activation of a PAX3/7 transcriptional gene profile. In addition, PAX3-FOXO1 acquires transcriptional ability that is absent in PAX3 alone (reviewed in [138]). Fusion-positive ARMS affects mainly older children and adolescents arising in legs and trunk. The expression of the fusion proteins is a negative prognostic factor per se independent from histology, identifying a subset of patients at high risk frequently with metastatic disease at diagnosis. Fusion-positive ARMS but also metastatic fusion-negative RMS represent a challenge for clinicians since they are often unresponsive to treatments with a high chance to recur. The demonstration of the expression of the fusion products is entering the clinical practice to help in the risk stratification of patients, and, more recently, the Shipley group demonstrated that those patients characterized by a PAX3-FOXO1 protein expression are at ultrahigh risk showing a 5-year overall survival (OS) less than 15% [139]. Taken together, these clinical data indicate that to halt the disease, it is imperative to hamper PAX3-FOXO1 activity. Despite improvements in the therapeutic strategies, the outcome of high-risk patients remains poor. Therefore, the need of a deeper knowledge of the mechanisms underlying the development and progression/recurrence of RMS is urgent. However, transcription factors such as PAX3-FOXO1 are difficult to target. Therefore, targeting PAX3-FOXO1 downstream molecules could be an acceptable approach to block its signaling. The developmental networks appear to be good targets due to their involvement in the differentiation of mesenchymal cells in addition to the PAX3 program. In particular, Notch signaling plays one of the major roles among the crucial regulators of skeletal muscle differentiation, maintenance, and homeostasis, both in embryo and in the postnatal life [140].

To date, several recent experimental findings by our group and other laboratories demonstrate that Notch signaling pathway is deregulated in RMS (Table 11.1). The first evidence of an implication of a Notch component in RMS stems from the work of Sang et al. [151] showing that the Notch target gene *HES1*, encoding for a transcriptional repressor, was able to halt the muscle-like differentiation when expressed in fibroblasts engineered with a plasmid encoding MYOD. This effect was reversed by treatment with a γ-secretase inhibitor (GSI), which blocks the cleavage of Notch receptors, or by silencing a corepressor working with HES1, i.e., TLE1/groucho. *HES1* transcripts were then shown to be overexpressed in RMS tumors and cell lines compared to normal skeletal muscle tissue. Then, the authors elegantly demonstrated that inhibition of the HES1 function using either a mutant HES1, defective

Table 11.1 Notch signaling in STS

Tumor	Notch deregulated component	Functions	Ref.
Synovial sarcoma	Notch1, JAG1, and TLEs	Oncogenic	[141]
	TLE1	Oncogenic	[142, 143]
	TLE1	Oncogenic	[144]
Ewing sarcoma	MFNG		[145]
	MNFG and Notch1	Regulator of differentiation	[146]
	JAG1 and HEY1	Onco-suppressor	[147]
	Notch1 and Notch3	Onco-suppressor	[148]
	HEY1 and Notch1	Onco-suppressor	[149]
	DLL1, Notch1, and Notch3	Oncogenic	[150]
Rhabdomyosarcoma	HES1	Oncogenic	[151]
	Notch2 and HEY1	Oncogenic	[152]
	Notch1 and HEY1	Oncogenic	[153]
	Notch3 and HES1	Oncogenic	[154]
	RBP-jK	Oncogenic	[155]
	DLL1, JAG1, Notch3	Oncogenic	[156]
	JAG1	Oncogenic	[157]
	Dll1	Oncogenic	[123]

in the DNA binding, or a dominant-negative HES1 form, lacking the domain that mediates the interaction between HES1 and its corepressors, halted cell proliferation and facilitated muscle-like differentiation of fusion-positive ARMS cell lines [151]. Similar results, associated to a diminution of the levels of HES1, were obtained inhibiting Notch signaling with a GSI, establishing that the effects seen were, at least in part, dependent from the Notch signaling activation.

Subsequently, the group of Gallego published a report showing a general deregulation in transcripts of the Notch pathway in 37 primary RMS samples, irrespective of the fusion status [152]. The authors showed significant upregulation of *Notch2* and *HEY1* compared to normal muscles. No overt difference in the levels of *Notch4* and *Notch1* transcripts in RMS compared to control tissues was seen, while *HES1* transcripts resulted modestly overexpressed in ERMS. However, the expression of the HES1 protein by immunohistochemistry was more elevated in RMS either fusion-negative or fusion-positive compared to muscle tissues. Interestingly, HES1 expression levels well correlated with the invasive capabilities of RMS cells with the lowest expression in low-invasive ERMS cell lines, and highest expression in PAX3-FOXO1 cells, which are the most invasive subtype [152]. The importance of Notch signaling in the invasive features of RMS cells was then confirmed either (i) inhibiting the γ-secretase-dependent cleavage of Notch receptors with several GSIs or (ii) transfecting RMS cells with a dominant-negative form of MAML1 (dnMAML1), which forms inactive RBP-jK/NICD/MAML1 complexes on DNA [158]. In both cases, HES1 transcript and protein levels were negatively affected by each of the two approaches, supporting the view of a Notch-dependent direct or indirect mechanism for HES1 overexpression. In a more recent work, Belyea et al. [153], interrogating previously published gene expression datasets [135], showed a marked upregulation of *HEY1* transcripts in ERMS compared not only to muscle tissues but also to ARMS samples. The results were confirmed in ERMS cell lines with respect to fusion-positive ARMS cells. The authors investigated the protein levels of HEY1 along with those of nuclear Notch1 in primary samples by immunohistochemistry and found that both were remarkably higher in ERMS compared to ARMS or to normal muscle tissue. HEY1 or Notch1 genetic depletion through shRNAs led to impaired ERMS cell proliferation in vitro and enhanced expression of the differentiation gene myogenin, particularly when cells were cultured in differentiation medium (low serum). However, despite the upregulation of myogenin and the phenotypic changes from round- to spindle-shaped cells, only a few myofiber-like structures were formed in these experimental conditions. Since Notch1 down-regulation induced HEY1 decrease, suggesting that HEY1 was directly or indirectly targeted by Notch1 signaling in ERMS cells, the Notch1-HEY1 axis seems to be a regulator of cell cycle rather than of terminal differentiation in the ERMS context [153]. These effects were phenocopied by two GSIs and, more importantly, rescued in GSI-treated cells by vector-induced N1ICD forced expression, supporting the hypothesis of a Notch1-specific effect. Moreover, these approaches worked also in in vivo models of ERMS xenografts, which showed reduced tumor growth for those formed by cells depleted of Notch1 or in animals treated with a GSI [153]. This last treatment resulted in the reduction of Notch1 levels in tumor samples, confirming the involvement of the Notch paralog signaling in the development of tumor masses [153]. Recently, the RBP-jK transcription factor has been shown to indicate a trend for a bad prognosis in RMS patients [135], and its modulation in ERMS cells clarified that Notch signaling aberrant functions in ERMS relies partly on a canonical signaling [155]. In fact, RBP-jK knockdown in ERMS cells downregulated HES1 expression and reduced colony formation in soft agar, while its overexpression behaved in the opposite manner [155]. ERMS cells depleted of RBP-jK formed smaller tumors in vivo and showed downregulation of pro-proliferative markers associated with upregulation of the cyclin-dependent inhibitor $p21^{Cip1}$ [155].

The metastatic behavior is recognized as extremely important for the response to therapy and outcome of RMS patients, and metastasis formation has been related to Notch activation in cancer [159–161]. Therefore, starting from the findings of a correlation of HES1 or HEY1 levels with cell invasion in vitro in RMS cell lines, the Rome group further clarified the role of Notch1 and HES1 in the invasiveness of RMS cells [162]. Pharmacological treatment with a GSI of one fusion-negative- and one PAX7-FOXO1- and one PAX3-FOXO1-positive cell line led to a marked decrease of cell adhesion on two different substrates and negatively modulated N-cadherin and α9-integrin transcriptional expression, together with those of the Notch target gene HES1, resulting in the lowering of protein levels [162]. These findings were in agreement with the observation that Notch1 and Notch3 upregulate N-cadherin in melanoma cells [163, 164]. In patients with RMS, a positive correlation between N-cadherin and α9-integrin with HES1 was seen. In line with the hypothesis of an involvement of Notch signaling in this phenomenon, RMS cells transfected with a plasmid expressing a dominant-negative form of MAML1 [152] showed a response similar to that of cells treated with a GSI. Conversely, RMS cells in which an exogenous DLL1 was forcedly overexpressed, thus leading to Notch signaling over-activation, enhanced the expression of all the three genes. These effects appeared quite specific since the level of the usual partner of α9-integrin, i.e., β1-integrin, was unaffected. Interestingly from a translational point of view, the authors showed that cell adhesion on fibronectin and the invasive capabilities of the cells in vitro were markedly reduced using an anti-N-cadherin-blocking antibody, whereas anti-α9-integrin-blocking antibody was able to impair only the tumor cell adhesive properties. Chromatin-immunoprecipitation assays demonstrated a possible direct regulation of Notch1 on the two gene promoters. However, HES1 seemed also to bind those promoters, but its role in regulating these genes should be clarified in future studies. This pro-invasive role of Notch signaling in RMS seems to be counteracted by the restoration of the expression of miR-203, a microRNA often downregulated epigenetically by promoter hypermethylation in RMS primary samples and cell lines and re-expressed after treatment with the DNA methyltransferase 1 inhibitor 5-AZA [157]. When miR-203 was re-expressed in vitro in one ERMS and one PAX3-FOXO1 ARMS cell line, it inhibited cell proliferation inducing the myogenic conversion of the tumor cells, decreasing the levels of the transcription factor p63, an inducer of JAG1 and of HES1. Similar results were obtained silencing p63. These findings suggest that the promyogenic role of miR-203 relies, at least in part, on its ability to down-modulate p63. Moreover, miR-203 forced expression blocked both cell migration and invasion. Tumor growth in vivo was also hampered in RMS cells overexpressing miR-203 or in ERMS-xenografted mice treated with 5-AZA. It could be interesting to evaluate whether the re-expression of miR-203 could have similar effects in vivo also in PAX3-FOXO1 ARMS cells, which are less prone to differentiate.

Previously, our findings unveiled a role for Notch3 in RMS [154]. Genetic down-regulation of Notch3 by silencing in fusion-negative and fusion-positive RMS cell lines overexpressing nuclear Notch1–3-activated forms compared to myoblasts resulted in a blockade of cell cycle in the G1 phase and formation of myofiber-like structures even when the cells were cultured in medium containing serum. In agreement with this phenotype, p21 was upregulated together with members of the differentiation machinery such as myogenin, MHC, and troponin. Moreover, p38MAPK, AKT, and mTOR were activated as during myogenesis. In parallel, HES1 levels were decreased suggesting that Notch3 can have a direct or indirect effect on its expression. Concordantly, HES1 depletion mimicked, as already reported by Sang et al. [151], as well as reinforced the effects of Notch3 silencing, while, conversely, its forced overexpression partially overcame them. Moreover, silencing Notch3 even in a fraction of cells inhibited tumor growth in vivo. Interestingly, (i) the depletion of Notch1, which was also hyperactivated in RMS cell lines, reduced the proliferation of the cells and, only in fusion-negative cells, favored the formation of some myotube-like structures, but was ineffective in fusion-positive cells; and (ii) the knockdown of Notch2, whose levels were higher in myoblasts, reduced the expression of myogenin and led to HES1 levels upregulation.

Consistent with a role of Notch3 in RMS, tumor cells forcedly expressing an exogenous N3ICD form proliferated faster in vitro and formed more colonies in soft agar irrespective of their fusion status [156]. Notably, the antiproliferative effects of a GSI were counteracted by N3ICD overexpression. We also confirmed that N3ICD influences tumor growth in vivo showing that PAX3-FOXO1/N3ICD xenografted cells produced bigger masses with a higher expression of Ki67 and HES1 [156]. Of note, we also showed that HES1 and Notch3 protein levels correlated with those of Ki67 in samples from RMS patients [156].

Since a very low number of mutations of Notch paralogs have been found in RMS primary samples [128, 129, 165], it is arguable that the hyperactivation of Notch receptors in tumor cells could be due to other reasons such as to the binding to the Notch ligands. As a matter of fact, downregulating DLL1 and JAG1, whose transcripts were found expressed in RMS cell lines [153] and primary specimens [135, 155], led to the inhibition of cell proliferation of ERMS and PAX3-FOXO1 ARMS cells associated with the lowering of N3ICD and HES1 levels [154, 156]. Summarizing all these results, it appears clear that a general dysregulation of the Notch signaling characterizes the RMS setting opening the way to potential targeted therapy for this sarcoma.

One of the characteristics of Notch signaling is the capacity to cross talk with several key pathways that regulate stem cell fate and are involved in cancer pathogenesis and maintenance. The Hedgehog pathway is one of the major regulators of the myogenesis in vertebrates, by maintaining the expression of the myogenic regulatory factors (MRFs) such as MYF5 and modulating survival and proliferation of developing myoblasts [166]. In particular, it supports the proliferation of myogenic precursors repressing terminal differentiation and apoptosis [167–169]. A dysregulation of Hedgehog seems to be one of the drivers of ERMS development, as highlighted by studies in humans and GEMM [170–173]. Recently, alterations of Hedgehog signaling have been recently shown to be interconnected to that of Notch in the pathogenesis of ERMS [132]. In this work the authors demonstrated that in mice heterozygous for the negative regulator of Hedgehog signaling *ptch1*, which spontaneously develop ERMS, the cells of origin of the tumor are derived from those expressing the Notch ligand *Dll1* and concomitantly negative for *Myf5*, *myogenin*, and *Pax3* expression [132]. This type of cells is prone to undergo myogenic differentiation but is not yet stably committed. These results, on one hand, imply that Hedgehog and Notch cross talk to define the fate of some cells during myogenesis, and on another hand highlight the importance of the molecular degree of differentiation and commitment for subsets of cells to behave as tumor-initiating RMS cells, as already demonstrated by the group of Keller [122, 174]. Importantly under a translational point of view, Hedgehog signaling activation is able to induce HES1 expression in both mesodermal and neural cells independently from Notch, suggesting combinatorial inhibition of the two pathways [175].

Several points on the impact of Notch signaling deregulation in RMS remain to be investigated among which the expression of protein levels of Notch ligands in RMS patients, its role in the invasiveness and metastasis in in vivo models, and its effects in GEMM of RMS. However, it appears evident that this signaling pathway could be activated in both ARMS and ERMS thus representing a potential target for therapy in both RMS variants.

11.2.2 Notch Signaling in Ewing Sarcoma

Ewing sarcoma (ES) is the second most common bone and soft tissue sarcoma of childhood. It arises most commonly in adolescents showing a median age of 15 years, even if cases of ES in neonates and infants have been reported [176, 177]. The most frequently affected sites are the lower extremities and pelvis for bone and the trunk and extremities for soft tissue disease. It is an aggressive malignancy, metastatic at diagnosis in about 25% of young patients [176]. Improvements in therapy have enhanced the survival rates for localized forms, but the outcome and disease-free survival of patients with metastatic disease remain poor [178–180]. ES often shows gains of chromosomes 8, 12, 20, and 1q, losses of 1p36 and 16q, and homozygous deletion of *CDKN2A*, but the mutation rate is low and mostly involves *STAG2* or *TP53* (5–20% of cases), making finding actionable therapeutic targets difficult ([181–183] and reviewed in [180]). In about 90% of cases, ES is characterized by typical chromosomal translocations t(11;22)(q24;q12) resulting in the fusion of the amino-terminal-encoding portion of EWSR1 to the carboxyl-terminal DNA-binding domain of the FLI1 gene of the ETS family genes, generating the EWS-FLI1 fusion product with transcriptional regulatory functions ([184, 185] and reviewed in [186]). The translocation can involve several different portions of the genes, due to different breakpoints in each of the sequences, but without effects on the prognosis [187, 188]. Variants of fusion products involving or not EWS have also been observed in a number of cases (reviewed in [186]). When expressed in a "permissive" cell of origin context, i.e., mesenchymal- and neural crest-derived progenitors, EWS-FLI1 shows transforming capacity [185, 189–192]. EWS-FLI1 is a transcription factor with higher potency compared to FLI1 that binds to ETS consensus sequences across the genome [185, 193] and whose mechanism of action has been recently unraveled. It binds several types of chromatin regions, from promoters to intra- and intergenic regions, repressing but also inducing a high number of genes [194–197] with a function that can be context-dependent [198]. When exogenously expressed in murine fibroblasts, EWS-FLI1 induced the transcription of the Notch signaling enzymatic component Mfng [145], a result in agreement with transcript *MNFG* upregulation found in ES patients (Table 11.1) [146], even if in human ES cells, the transcriptional effect on *MNFG* is weaker [199]. Recently, the group of Kovar unveiled the mechanism through which EWS-FLI1 was able to overcome cell cycle arrest in a context of wild-type *TP53* [147]. The authors demonstrated that, by repressing the expression of the Notch ligand *JAG1*, EWS-FLI1 reduced the activation of Notch3 necessary for the induction of the Notch target gene *HEY1* that, in turn, stabilized and activated p53 [147]. Indeed, in *TP53* wild-type ES cell lines, (i) *EWS-FLI1* silencing promoted p53 and $p21^{Cip1}$ expression followed by cell cycle arrest; (ii) this effect was associated with the induction of *JAG1* and *HEY1*, often barely expressed in ES primary samples; (iii) Notch2 and Notch3 were expressed in both ES cell lines and primary samples, and Notch3 resulted activated only in *TP53* wild-type cells by JAG1; and (iv) in EWS-FLI1-depleted cells, *JAG1* or *HEY1* silencing, treatment with a GSI, or expression of the negative regulator of Notch, NUMB, prevented p53 and $p21^{Cip1}$ induction, while forced expression of either exogenous JAG1, HEY1, or N3ICD reversed the effects. Therefore, in ES cells with wild-type *TP53*, Notch signaling seems to act as an onco-suppressor stabilizing p53 with an unknown mechanism involving HEY1. Interestingly, when Notch signaling was inhibited in the presence of EWS-FLI1, no HEY1 expression was observed, suggesting that the pathway could be inactive under these cell conditions [147]. This was consistent with the observation of a lack of nuclear expression of NICD and HES1 in ES tumors, despite the mRNA upregulation of the latter [148]. Moreover, the transcriptional overexpression of *HES1* was independent from Notch activation and also from EWS-FLI1 expression.

ES pathogenesis implies an aberrant chromatin remodeling due to the influence of the fusion proteins on epigenetic machinery (reviewed in [186]). Accordingly, pharmacological inhibition of the lysine demethylase LSD1 (or KDM1A), upregulated in a large cohort of sarcomas including ES, led to p53 expression in ES cell lines through the methylation of Lys 4 on histone H3 (H3K4) followed by cell cycle arrest [200]. In other cell systems, LSD1 is able, as a component of a corepressor complex with the deacetylase SIRT1, to inhibit Notch signaling by recruiting the RBP-jK complexes and repressing the expression of Notch target genes, including *HEY1* [201–203]. Starting from this observation, the same group sheds light on the mechanism of p53 induction after EWS-FLI1 depletion showing that ectopically expressed HEY1 prevented the expression of the deacetylase SIRT1, which in turn was responsible for the posttranslational modification that leads to p53 destabilization and deactivation [149]. This effect was obtained also by ectopic expression of NICD, demonstrating that it is Notch-dependent, and also demonstrated in other cell contexts in which Notch signaling can act similarly, such as B-cell tumors and primary human keratinocytes lacking *HEY1* expression. Consistently, genetic and pharmacologic inhibition of SIRT1 was sufficient to increase p53 acetylation and target genes activation, in ES cells in the presence of EWS-FLI1, resulting in tumor cell death, while its overexpression reverted the phenotype [149]. An antitumorigenic effect was also seen in vivo after pharmacological treatment of xenografted zebrafish models. Finally, the screening of about 400 ES human tumor samples by immunohistochemistry showed that SIRT1 expression could be correlated to disseminated disease due to the highest levels of staining in metastatic patients. Thus, on one hand, this work unveils a novel epigenetic Notch-dependent mechanism to regulate cell cycle and on the other hand points to SIRT1 as a pharmacologically targetable factor in ES. Although EWS-FLI1 is necessary for tumorigenesis, it requires a "permissive" cellular background for transformation. Among the involved adjuvant molecules is CD99 [204], a cell surface protein involved in cell migration, proliferation, and differentiation [205, 206]. As a matter of fact, EWS-FLI1 is able to upregulate CD99 that, in turn, facilitates the oncogenic function of the fusion protein [204, 207, 208]. However, although CD99 contributes to the oncogenic phenotype defined by the fusion gene, EWS-FLI1 is able to induce a neuroblastic phenotype while CD99 counteracts this effect [204]. Since ES cells are unable to completely differentiate, a recent work demonstrates that a network CD99-miR-34a-Notch-NF-kB underpins the mechanism underlying the anti-differentiative phenotype and suggests novel avenues for intervention [150].

The work showed that CD99, by inducing the expression of the Notch ligand DLL1, resulted in Notch1 and Notch3 activation paralleled by a concomitant activation of NF-kB, all effects prevented by CD99 depletion or GSI treatment. In turn, the CD99-dependent activity of NF-kB, or NF-kBp65 forced overexpression in a CD99 knockdown context, affected the neural phenotype due to the presence of EWS-FLI1, whereas, conversely, its silencing enhanced the proneural differentiation [150]. Elegantly, the authors then demonstrate that all the molecular and phenotypic effects of CD99 depletion, including Notch components regulation, can be phenocopied by a microRNA previously involved in ES and able to regulate Notch signaling, i.e., miR-34a [209–212], which was induced by CD99 knockdown. Thus, the presence of CD99 prevented miR-34a expression thus allowing Notch and NF-kB activation [150]. Interestingly, Notch and NF-kB pathways cross talk in several systems mainly in a noncanonical way (reviewed in [213]), which is in agreement with the inactivation of canonical Notch signaling found in ES, despite the expression of Notch receptors [147]. Strikingly, the effects of CD99 expression spread to neighboring cells through exosomes bearing CD99 from ES cells, and, consequently, when CD99 was depleted, exosomes lacking CD99 and containing high levels of the induced miR-34a carried a proneural signal to the target cells. These important results are in agreement with a previous report showing that Notch signaling inhibition induced neuroectodermal differentiation of tumor xenografts in ES with low impact on tumor cell proliferation [146]. Taken together, the reported findings further complicate the scenario of an role of Notch signaling in ES, showing an antiproliferative but also anti-differentiative role for this pathway. The predominance of a canonical versus noncanonical Notch signaling activation depends on the molecular context of the cells and deserves further investigations.

11.2.3 Notch Signaling in Synovial Sarcoma

Synovial sarcoma (SS) is a soft tissue sarcoma developing most commonly in the lower limbs of adolescents and young adults and showing a high metastatic potential ([214]; and reviewed in [215, 216]). It accounts for about 10–20% of all soft tissue sarcomas in young patients [217]. SS includes three histological subtypes: monophasic (only spindle cells), biphasic (both spindle and epithelial cells), and poorly differentiated. In addition to the soft tissue adjacent to the joints (i.e., synovial), it can develop in extra-synovial tissues. Localized disease can be treated by surgical intervention followed by adjuvant radiotherapy, but it often shows early and even late recurrences with 50% 10-year disease-free survival [218]. Molecularly, SS is characterized by the chromosomal translocation t(X,18; p11,q11) involving *SS18* (previously *SYT*) on chromosome 18q11 and either *SSX1*, *SSX2*, or very rarely *SSX4* on chromosome Xp11. The results are fusion proteins formed by almost all the SS18 sequence with the C-terminal portion of the SSX paralogs. That SS18-SSX proteins are the oncogenic drivers of the malignancy was demonstrated by the observations that their expression in vitro is sufficient to transform the cells, while their silencing reverts the malignant phenotype [219, 220]. SS is considered to be derived from mesenchymal stem cells in which the fusion proteins behave as oncogenes [221, 222]. In agreement with the importance of a specific cell of origin for tumorigenesis, the SS1-SSX oncoproduct induces spontaneous SS in transgenic mice in vivo with 100% penetrance when expressed in mesenchymal-derived progenitors expressing Myf5 [223]. However, conversely to myogenic sarcomas, no expression of myogenic markers has been unveiled in SS murine models or in SS patients. The evidence of the presence of the fusion both in primary and metastatic lesions and the apoptotic effects linked to its depletion concur to suggest a master role for SS18-SSX in the development of SS [220, 224]. Although SS18 is a transcriptional activator and SSX functions as a repressor and both bind several partners, SS18-SSX does not contain a DNA-binding domain making difficult the identification of direct target genes [219]. However, it acts as a transcriptional regulator controlling gene expression by chromatin remodeling (reviewed in [225]). Indeed, both SS18 and SS18-SSX associate with the SWI/SNF chromatin remodeling complex, which in normal cells/tissues facilitates gene transcriptional programs creating nucleosome-depleted regions at core promoters and regulatory regions [226–229]. The inclusion of SS18-SSX fusion products in the SWI/SNF complex dysregulates the function of the complex [229]. This is due to the repressor intrinsic properties of the SSX portion that can interact with gene repressor complexes, thus behaving in an opposite manner compared to SS18 itself [230]. SS shows no additional chromosomal imbalance in young patients; however it is characterized by a high expression of components of molecular pathways strictly involved in early embryogenesis. Among these are WNT, Hedgehog, BMP, and Notch pathways. Studies aimed at unveiling binding partners for the SS18-SSX factor demonstrated an interaction of the SSX portion with the corepressor TLE1 (Table 11.1) [144]. *TLE* genes encode for TLE1–4 proteins that are corepressors and, in particular TLE1, components of the Notch signaling the regulate stemness of embryonic progenitors during development. As a matter of fact, TLE1 is recruited by the Notch target HES1 on promoters to prevent gene expression [231]. SS18-SSX/TLE1 complex was found linked to ATF2, a transcriptional activator and DNA-binding protein, and was able to turn the ATF2 activator program in a repressor program [144]. The ultimate result is the repression of apoptotic/cell cycle blocker genes *EGR1*, *p21Cip1*, and *ATF3* and the promotion of tumor cell survival, which was impaired by SS18-SSX silencing. The intrinsic mechanism of this effect on ATF2 was related to the interaction of SS18-SSX with the polycomb repressor complexes PRC2 and PRC1 [232], whose repressor activity was further enhanced by the presence of TLE1 in the complex. A deregulated transcript expression of TLE1 has been found by expression profiling experiments in primary SS [141] and the nuclear expression of the protein confirmed by immunohistochemistry [142, 233]. To date, the evidence of an overexpression of TLE1 has currently entered the clinical use to discriminate among other soft tissue sarcomas [143]. In addition to TLE1, also other Notch-related factors have been shown to be upregulated in SS, such as Notch1 and JAG1 [141], although no evidence for functional roles for these proteins in SS pathogenesis has been described so far. However, results from a randomized Phase I/II clinical trial using the GSI RO4229097 in association with the Hedgehog inhibitor vismodegib for adult and adolescent patients with advanced and metastatic sarcomas, among which SS (Table 11.2), will give some information about the potentiality of Notch signaling inhibition in SS.

11.3 Approaches to Inhibit Notch Signaling

Considering the structure, regulation, and function of Notch components, several steps of the signaling pathway can be targeted for inhibition.

11.3.1 γ-Secretase Inhibitors (GSI)

The most widely used approach to hamper Notch signaling is based on the inhibition of γ-secretase activity resulting in Notch cleavage blockade. GSI showed antitumorigenic activities in various cancer cells in preclinical models, and some of them are currently in clinical trials for oncologic diseases, mostly for adult patients. However, over the last years, several Phase I/II studies have been started involving also pediatric and adolescent oncologic patients (Table 11.2).

MK-0752 is a clinical GSI that was evaluated in several Phase I clinical trials for treatment in pediatric and adult malignancies (Table 11.2) [234–236]. Another GSI, RO4929097 [237], was evaluated in several NCI-sponsored Phase I/II clinical trials for treatment of solid tumors and T-ALL (Table 11.2). RO4929097 has been used in combinatorial adjuvant regimens with other anticancer drugs, and it is recently in Phase I/II associated with vismodegib, an inhibitor of Hedgehog signaling, for treatment of advanced and metastatic sarcomas for adults and pediatric patients (Table 11.2).

The Phase II clinical trial with the GSI PF-03084014 for pediatric patients is ongoing for desmoid tumors and aggressive fibromatosis and is progressing to a Phase II for T-ALL and solid tumors (Table 11.2) [238]. In preclinical models, GSIs have shown also anti-angiogenic effects that could contribute to their efficacy in vivo. However, (i) GSI are unable to discriminate among Notch receptors and (ii) γ-secretase have a plethora of targets, and, thus, these chemicals can have off-target effects in vivo [239]. Among these, the most evident is the goblet cell metaplasia of the small intestine due to Notch2 inhibition in the intestinal epithelial stem cells compartment. Even if this effect can be partly prevented by coadministration of glucocorticoids, often the treatment with GSI) requires a lowering in the doses and intermittent administration. Moreover, the evidence of Notch target inhibition in tumor tissue, to decide the dose escalation, is often difficult since the modulated clinical targets not always are the Notch targets found in preclinical studies but can depend on the tissue-context of the patient.

11.3.2 Antibodies Against Notch Signaling Components

Although all Notch paralogs have similar mechanisms of signalization, paralog-specific and even opposite downstream effects have been reported [154, 240–246]. Therefore, specific monoclonal antibodies against individual receptors or ligands have been developed so far. Although no Notch monoclonal antibody has been evaluated in pediatric tumors, some of them are being evaluated in clinical trials for adult tumors. The binding of the Notch component by the antibody results in the blockade of interaction between the receptor and the ligand and hampers the activation of the signaling. Among the antibodies against DLL4, the ligands responsible for the sprouting of endothelial cells and formation of new vessels that have been evaluated in

Table 11.2 Completed and ongoing clinical trials with γ-secretase inhibitors in pediatric/young adult oncologic patients

Compound	Combined	Clinical trials. Gov Identifier	Clinical studies	Cancer type	Patients age
MK0752		NCT00106145	Phase I	Breast and advanced solid tumors	18 years and older
MK0752		NCT00100152	Phase I	T-ALL	12 months[a] and older
PF-03084014		NCT01981551	Phase II	Desmoid tumors/ aggressive fibromatosis	18 years[a] and older
PF-03084014		NCT00878189	Phase I	Advanced solid tumors T-ALL	16 years and older
RO4929097		NCT01269411	Phase I	Gliomas	18 years and older
RO4929097	WBRT SRS	NCT01217411	Phase I/ II	Breast cancer, lung cancer, melanoma	18 years and older
RO4929097	Dexamethasone	NCT01088763	Phase I	Leukemia, solid tumors, lymphoma	1 year to[a] 21 years
RO4929097	Vismodegib	NCT01154452	Phase I/ II	Advanced or metastatic sarcoma	18 years and older
RO4929097	Carboplatin/paclitaxel	NCT01238133	Phase I	Breast cancer	18 years and older
RO4929097	Cisplatin, vinblastine, and temozolomide	NCT01196416	Phase I/ II	Recurrent or metastatic melanoma	18 years and older
RO4929097	Cediranib maleate	NCT01131234	Phase I	Advanced solid tumors	18 years and older
RO4929097		NCT01232829	Phase II	Metastatic pancreas cancer	18 years and older
RO4929097	Gemcitabine hydrochloride	NCT01145456	Phase I	Advanced solid tumors	18 years and older
RO4929097	Temozolomide and radiation therapy	NCT01119599	Phase 1	Malignant glioma	19 years and older
RO4929097	Ketoconazole, rifampin midazolam, hydrochloride, omeprazole, tolbutamide, dextromethorphan, hydrobromide	NCT01218620	Phase I	Adult solid neoplasm	18 years and older
RO4929097	Bicalutamide	NCT01200810	Phase II	Prostate cancer	18 years and older

(continued)

Table 11.2 (continued)

Compound	Combined	Clinical trials. Gov Identifier	Clinical studies	Cancer type	Patients age
RO4929097		NCT01141569	Phase II	Renal cell carcinoma	18 years and older
RO4929097		NCT01192763	Phase I	Pancreatic cancer	18 years and older
RO4929097	Letrozole	NCT01208441	Phase I	Breast cancer	18 years and older
RO4929097	Exemestane, goserelin acetate	NCT01149356	Phase I	Metastatic breast cancer	18 years and older
RO4929097		NCT01175343	Phase II	Metastatic epithelial ovarian cancer, fallopian tube cancer, and primary peritoneal cancer	18 years and older
RO4929097	Capecitabine	NCT01158274	Phase I	Solid tumors	18 years and older
RO4929097		NCT01116687	Phase II	Colon cancer, rectal cancer	18 years and older
RO4929097	Cetuximab	NCT01198535	Phase I	Metastatic colorectal cancer	18 years and older
RO4929097		NCT01070927	Phase II	Non-squamous non-small cell lung cancer	18 years and older
RO4929097	Bevacizumab	NCT01189240	Phase I/II	Glioma	18 years and older
RO4929097	Erlotinib hydrochloride	NCT01193881	Phase I	Lung cancer	18 years and older
RO4929097	Vismodegib	NCT01071564	Phase I	Breast cancer	18 years and older
RO4929097		NCT01193868	Phase II	Advanced non-small cell lung cancer	18 years and older
RO4929097	Temsirolimus	NCT01198184	Phase I	Advanced solid tumors	18 years and older
RO4929097		NCT01096355	Phase I	Solid malignancies	18 years and older

http://clinicaltrials.gov
T-ALL T-cell acute lymphoblastic leukemia/lymphoma
[a]Enrollment of children

clinical trials for adult malignancies are MEDI0639 (NCT01577745, recruiting Phase I), OMP-21M18 (NCT01189929; NCT01952249; NCT01189942; NCT01189968 Phase I and Ib), and REGN421 (Phase I completed, showing good tolerability and two partial responses [247]). The specific antibody OMP-52M51 against Notch1 is in clinical trial Phase I, NCT01778439; NCT01703572) and the antibody OMP-59R5 against Notch2/3 in Phase I/II trials (NCT01647828; NCT01859741).

11.3.3 Blocking Peptides

Preclinical studies demonstrated that it is possible to interfere with the transcriptional machinery of Notch signaling with inhibitory peptides. This is the case of a dnMAML1 used to block the RBP-jK-dependent transcription due to Notch activation. Stapled peptides competing with MAML are able to prevent gene transcription in murine models of T-ALL [248, 249]. One characteristic of this stapled peptide is the ability to bind also to preassembled Notch1–CSL complexes to inhibit the binding of the endogenous MAML1 [249]. These peptides have relatively small size and are highly cell-permeable. However, if they target only the transcriptional activity of Notch signaling, they can be ineffective in cancers in which the Notch pathway works in a noncanonical way. Nonetheless, dnMAML peptides could act also sequestering NICD in the cytoplasm, thus hampering also noncanonical roles of the cleaved protein.

11.3.4 Decoys

Soluble forms of the extracellular domains of Notch receptors and their ligands have been studied as decoys to inhibit the signaling. Decoys function by binding to endogenous ligands or receptors preventing the endogenous counterpart to be bound, and, since it lacks intracellular domains, the signaling of the pathway is completely abrogated [250–252]. Interestingly, endogenous soluble Notch ligands can be produced by metalloproteases, but their physiologic role still needs to be clarified [253, 254].

11.4 Conclusions

In conclusion, we summarized the role of Notch signaling in pediatric soft tissue sarcomas, giving an overview of the potentiality in targeting the pathway. Notch signaling plays a major role in the determination and homeostasis of tissues of mesenchymal origin in the embryo and postnatal life. Here we highlighted a role of Notch signaling deregulation in pediatric soft tissue sarcomas in the preclinical setting, reporting evidence that Notch modulation regulates cell proliferation, differentiation, and motility/invasion of tumor cells. To date, the majority of approaches against Notch signaling activation rely on the use of GSI even if promising monoclonal antibodies and cell-permeable small molecules are being developed for adult cancers. It is arguable that the pharmacokinetics properties and the biodistribution of decoys and antibodies are the limiting factors for their therapeutic application. Interestingly, for those patients with tumors in which Notch pathway works as a tumor suppressor, such as in EWS, agents stimulating its activity or downstream effects should be considered. In summary, potentially a Notch-based therapy might represent one of the future personalized strategies for young patients with soft tissue sarcomas.

Acknowledgments This work was financially supported by the Italian Association for Cancer Research (AIRC IG 15312).

Conflict of Interest/Disclosures No conflict of interest

References

1. Visweswaran, M., Pohl, S., Arfuso, F., Newsholme, P., Dilley, R., Pervaiz, S., et al. (2015). Multi-lineage differentiation of mesenchymal stem cells – To Wnt, or not Wnt. *The International Journal of Biochemistry & Cell Biology, 68*, 139–147.
2. Happe, C. L., & Engler, A. J. (2016). Mechanical forces reshape differentiation cues that guide cardiomyogenesis. *Circulation Research, 118*(2), 296–310.
3. Briscoe, J., & Small, S. (2015). Morphogen rules: Design principles of gradient-mediated embryo patterning. *Development, 142*(23), 3996–4009.
4. Luo, S. X., & Huang, E. J. (2015). Dopaminergic neurons and brain reward pathways: From neurogenesis to circuit assembly. *The American Journal of Pathology, 186*(3), 478–488.
5. Li, X. Y., Zhai, W. J., & Teng, C. B. (2015). Notch signaling in pancreatic development. *International Journal of Molecular Sciences, 17*(1), 48.
6. Luxan, G., D'Amato, G., MacGrogan, D., & de la Pompa, J. L. (2016). Endocardial Notch signaling in cardiac development and disease. *Circulation Research, 118*(1), e1–e18.
7. Krantz, I. D., Colliton, R. P., Genin, A., Rand, E. B., Li, L., Piccoli, D. A., et al. (1998). Spectrum and frequency of jagged1 (JAG1) mutations in Alagille syndrome patients and their families. *American Journal of Human Genetics, 62*(6), 1361–1369.
8. McDaniell, R., Warthen, D. M., Sanchez-Lara, P. A., Pai, A., Krantz, I. D., Piccoli, D. A., et al. (2006). NOTCH2 mutations cause Alagille syndrome, a heterogeneous disorder of the notch signaling pathway. *American Journal of Human Genetics, 79*(1), 169–173.
9. Federico, A., Bianchi, S., & Dotti, M. T. (2005). The spectrum of mutations for CADASIL diagnosis. *Neurological Sciences, 26*(2), 117–124.
10. Sparrow, D. B., Chapman, G., Wouters, M. A., Whittock, N. V., Ellard, S., Fatkin, D., et al. (2006). Mutation of the LUNATIC FRINGE gene in humans causes spondylocostal dysostosis with a severe vertebral phenotype. *American Journal of Human Genetics, 78*(1), 28–37.
11. Lee, S. J., Kim, K. H., Pak, S. C., Kang, Y. N., Yoon, G. S., & Park, K. K. (2015). Notch signaling affects biliary fibrosis via transcriptional regulation of RBP-jkappa in an animal model of chronic liver disease. *International Journal of Clinical and Experimental Pathology, 8*(10), 12688–12697.
12. Bansal, R., van Baarlen, J., Storm, G., & Prakash, J. (2015). The interplay of the Notch signaling in hepatic stellate cells and macrophages determines the fate of liver fibrogenesis. *Scientific Reports, 5*, 18272.
13. Vieira, N. M., Elvers, I., Alexander, M. S., Moreira, Y. B., Eran, A., Gomes, J. P., et al. (2015). Jagged 1 rescues the duchenne muscular dystrophy phenotype. *Cell, 163*(5), 1204–1213.
14. Lafkas, D., Shelton, A., Chiu, C., de Leon Boenig, G., Chen, Y., Stawicki, S. S., et al. (2015). Therapeutic antibodies reveal Notch control of transdifferentiation in the adult lung. *Nature, 528*(7580), 127–131.
15. Hu, B., Wu, Z., Bai, D., Liu, T., Ullenbruch, M. R., & Phan, S. H. (2015). Mesenchymal deficiency of Notch1 attenuates bleomycin-induced pulmonary fibrosis. *The American Journal of Pathology, 185*(11), 3066–3075.

16. Louvi, A., & Artavanis-Tsakonas, S. (2012). Notch and disease: A growing field. *Seminars in Cell & Developmental Biology, 23*(4), 473–480.
17. Ellisen, L. W., Bird, J., West, D. C., Soreng, A. L., Reynolds, T. C., Smith, S. D., et al. (1991). TAN-1, the human homolog of the Drosophila notch gene, is broken by chromosomal translocations in T lymphoblastic neoplasms. *Cell, 66*(4), 649–661.
18. Pear, W. S., Aster, J. C., Scott, M. L., Hasserjian, R. P., Soffer, B., Sklar, J., et al. (1996). Exclusive development of T cell neoplasms in mice transplanted with bone marrow expressing activated Notch alleles. *The Journal of Experimental Medicine, 183*(5), 2283–2291.
19. Weng, A. P., Ferrando, A. A., Lee, W., JPt, M., Silverman, L. B., Sanchez-Irizarry, C., et al. (2004). Activating mutations of NOTCH1 in human T cell acute lymphoblastic leukemia. *Science, 306*(5694), 269–271.
20. Bovee, J. V., & Hogendoorn, P. C. (2010). Molecular pathology of sarcomas: Concepts and clinical implications. *Virchows Archiv, 456*(2), 193–199.
21. Grunewald, T. G., & Fulda, S. (2016). Editorial: Biology-driven targeted therapy of pediatric soft-tissue and bone tumors: Current opportunities and future challenges. *Frontiers in Oncology, 6*, 39.
22. Thacker, M. M. (2013). Malignant soft tissue tumors in children. *The Orthopedic Clinics of North America, 44*(4), 657–667.
23. Walter, D., Satheesha, S., Albrecht, P., Bornhauser, B. C., D'Alessandro, V., Oesch, S. M., et al. (2011). CD133 positive embryonal rhabdomyosarcoma stem-like cell population is enriched in rhabdospheres. *PLoS One, 6*(5), e19506.
24. De Vito, C., Riggi, N., Cornaz, S., Suva, M. L., Baumer, K., Provero, P., et al. (2012). A TARBP2-dependent miRNA expression profile underlies cancer stem cell properties and provides candidate therapeutic reagents in Ewing sarcoma. *Cancer Cell, 21*(6), 807–821.
25. Espinoza, I., & Miele, L. (2013). Notch inhibitors for cancer treatment. *Pharmacology & Therapeutics, 139*(2), 95–110.
26. Teodorczyk, M., & Schmidt, M. H. (2015). Notching on cancer's door: Notch signaling in brain tumors. *Frontiers in Oncology, 4*, 341.
27. Dominguez, M. (2014). Oncogenic programmes and Notch activity: An 'organized crime'? *Seminars in Cell & Developmental Biology, 28*, 78–85.
28. Lardelli, M., Williams, R., & Lendahl, U. (1995). Notch-related genes in animal development. *The International Journal of Developmental Biology, 39*(5), 769–780.
29. Blaumueller, C. M., Qi, H., Zagouras, P., & Artavanis-Tsakonas, S. (1997). Intracellular cleavage of Notch leads to a heterodimeric receptor on the plasma membrane. *Cell, 90*(2), 281–291.
30. Hori, K., Sen, A., & Artavanis-Tsakonas, S. (2013). Notch signaling at a glance. *Journal of Cell Science, 126*(Pt 10), 2135–2140.
31. Rebay, I., Fleming, R. J., Fehon, R. G., Cherbas, L., Cherbas, P., & Artavanis-Tsakonas, S. (1991). Specific EGF repeats of Notch mediate interactions with Delta and Serrate: Implications for Notch as a multifunctional receptor. *Cell, 67*(4), 687–699.
32. del Amo, F. F., Gendron-Maguire, M., Swiatek, P. J., Jenkins, N. A., NG, C., & Gridley, T. (1993). Cloning, analysis, and chromosomal localization of Notch-1, a mouse homolog of Drosophila Notch. *Genomics, 15*(2), 259–264.
33. Weinmaster, G., Roberts, V. J., & Lemke, G. (1992). Notch2: A second mammalian Notch gene. *Development, 116*(4), 931–941.
34. Lardelli, M., Dahlstrand, J., & Lendahl, U. (1994). The novel Notch homologue mouse Notch 3 lacks specific epidermal growth factor-repeats and is expressed in proliferating neuroepithelium. *Mechanisms of Development, 46*(2), 123–136.
35. Uyttendaele, H., Marazzi, G., Wu, G., Yan, Q., Sassoon, D., & Kitajewski, J. (1996). Notch4/int-3, a mammary proto-oncogene, is an endothelial cell-specific mammalian Notch gene. *Development, 122*(7), 2251–2259.

36. Aster, J. C., Simms, W. B., Zavala-Ruiz, Z., Patriub, V., North, C. L., & Blacklow, S. C. (1999). The folding and structural integrity of the first LIN-12 module of human Notch1 are calcium-dependent. *Biochemistry, 38*(15), 4736–4742.
37. Gordon, W. R., Vardar-Ulu, D., Histen, G., Sanchez-Irizarry, C., Aster, J. C., & Blacklow, S. C. (2007). Structural basis for autoinhibition of Notch. *Nature Structural & Molecular Biology, 14*(4), 295–300.
38. Sanchez-Irizarry, C., Carpenter, A. C., Weng, A. P., Pear, W. S., Aster, J. C., & Blacklow, S. C. (2004). Notch subunit heterodimerization and prevention of ligand-independent proteolytic activation depend, respectively, on a novel domain and the LNR repeats. *Molecular and Cellular Biology, 24*(21), 9265–9273.
39. Tamura, K., Taniguchi, Y., Minoguchi, S., Sakai, T., Tun, T., Furukawa, T., et al. (1995). Physical interaction between a novel domain of the receptor Notch and the transcription factor RBP-J kappa/Su(H). *Current Biology, 5*(12), 1416–1423.
40. Lubman, O. Y., Korolev, S. V., & Kopan, R. (2004). Anchoring notch genetics and biochemistry; structural analysis of the ankyrin domain sheds light on existing data. *Molecular Cell, 13*(5), 619–626.
41. Nam, Y., Sliz, P., Song, L., Aster, J. C., & Blacklow, S. C. (2006). Structural basis for cooperativity in recruitment of MAML coactivators to Notch transcription complexes. *Cell, 124*(5), 973–983.
42. Lieber, T., Kidd, S., Alcamo, E., Corbin, V., & Young, M. W. (1993). Antineurogenic phenotypes induced by truncated Notch proteins indicate a role in signal transduction and may point to a novel function for Notch in nuclei. *Genes & Development, 7*(10), 1949–1965.
43. Kurooka, H., Kuroda, K., & Honjo, T. (1998). Roles of the ankyrin repeats and C-terminal region of the mouse notch1 intracellular region. *Nucleic Acids Research, 26*(23), 5448–5455.
44. Rechsteiner, M. (1988). Regulation of enzyme levels by proteolysis: The role of pest regions. *Advances in Enzyme Regulation, 27*, 135–151.
45. Ong, C. T., Cheng, H. T., Chang, L. W., Ohtsuka, T., Kageyama, R., Stormo, G. D., et al. (2006). Target selectivity of vertebrate notch proteins. Collaboration between discrete domains and CSL-binding site architecture determines activation probability. *The Journal of Biological Chemistry, 281*(8), 5106–5119.
46. Bettenhausen, B., Hrabe de Angelis, M., Simon, D., Guenet, J. L., & Gossler, A. (1995). Transient and restricted expression during mouse embryogenesis of Dll1, a murine gene closely related to Drosophila Delta. *Development, 121*(8), 2407–2418.
47. Dunwoodie, S. L., Henrique, D., Harrison, S. M., & Beddington, R. S. (1997). Mouse Dll3: A novel divergent Delta gene which may complement the function of other Delta homologues during early pattern formation in the mouse embryo. *Development, 124*(16), 3065–3076.
48. Shutter, J. R., Scully, S., Fan, W., Richards, W. G., Kitajewski, J., Deblandre, G. A., et al. (2000). Dll4, a novel Notch ligand expressed in arterial endothelium. *Genes & Development, 14*(11), 1313–1318.
49. Lindsell, C. E., Shawber, C. J., Boulter, J., & Weinmaster, G. (1995). Jagged: A mammalian ligand that activates Notch1. *Cell, 80*(6), 909–917.
50. Shawber, C., Boulter, J., Lindsell, C. E., & Weinmaster, G. (1996). Jagged2: A serrate-like gene expressed during rat embryogenesis. *Developmental Biology, 180*(1), 370–376.
51. Parks, A. L., Stout, J. R., Shepard, S. B., Klueg, K. M., Dos Santos, A. A., Parody, T. R., et al. (2006). Structure-function analysis of delta trafficking, receptor binding and signaling in Drosophila. *Genetics, 174*(4), 1947–1961.
52. Shimizu, K., Chiba, S., Kumano, K., Hosoya, N., Takahashi, T., Kanda, Y., et al. (1999). Mouse jagged1 physically interacts with notch2 and other notch receptors. Assessment by quantitative methods. *The Journal of Biological Chemistry, 274*(46), 32961–32969.
53. Schmidt, M. H., Bicker, F., Nikolic, I., Meister, J., Babuke, T., Picuric, S., et al. (2009). Epidermal growth factor-like domain 7 (EGFL7) modulates Notch signalling and affects neural stem cell renewal. *Nature Cell Biology, 11*(7), 873–880.

54. Hu, Q. D., Ang, B. T., Karsak, M., Hu, W. P., Cui, X. Y., Duka, T., et al. (2003). F3/contactin acts as a functional ligand for Notch during oligodendrocyte maturation. *Cell, 115*(2), 163–175.
55. Ayaz, F., & Osborne, B. A. (2014). Non-canonical notch signaling in cancer and immunity. *Frontiers in Oncology, 4*, 345.
56. D'Souza, B., Meloty-Kapella, L., & Weinmaster, G. (2010). Canonical and non-canonical Notch ligands. *Current Topics in Developmental Biology, 92*, 73–129.
57. Guruharsha, K. G., Kankel, M. W., & Artavanis-Tsakonas, S. (2012). The Notch signalling system: Recent insights into the complexity of a conserved pathway. *Nature Reviews. Genetics, 13*(9), 654–666.
58. Bruckner, K., Perez, L., Clausen, H., & Cohen, S. (2000). Glycosyltransferase activity of Fringe modulates Notch-Delta interactions. *Nature, 406*(6794), 411–415.
59. Moloney, D. J., Panin, V. M., Johnston, S. H., Chen, J., Shao, L., Wilson, R., et al. (2000). Fringe is a glycosyltransferase that modifies Notch. *Nature, 406*(6794), 369–375.
60. Moloney, D. J., Shair, L. H., Lu, F. M., Xia, J., Locke, R., Matta, K. L., et al. (2000). Mammalian Notch1 is modified with two unusual forms of O-linked glycosylation found on epidermal growth factor-like modules. *The Journal of Biological Chemistry, 275*(13), 9604–9611.
61. Okajima, T., Xu, A., & Irvine, K. D. (2003). Modulation of notch-ligand binding by protein O-fucosyltransferase 1 and fringe. *The Journal of Biological Chemistry, 278*(43), 42340–42345.
62. Panin, V. M., Papayannopoulos, V., Wilson, R., & Irvine, K. D. (1997). Fringe modulates Notch-ligand interactions. *Nature, 387*(6636), 908–912.
63. Cohen, B., Bashirullah, A., Dagnino, L., Campbell, C., Fisher, W. W., Leow, C. C., et al. (1997). Fringe boundaries coincide with Notch-dependent patterning centres in mammals and alter Notch-dependent development in Drosophila. *Nature Genetics, 16*(3), 283–288.
64. Pakkiriswami, S., Couto, A., Nagarajan, U., & Georgiou, M. (2016). Glycosylated Notch and cancer. *Frontiers in Oncology, 6*, 37.
65. Xu, K., Usary, J., Kousis, P. C., Prat, A., Wang, D. Y., Adams, J. R., et al. (2012). Lunatic fringe deficiency cooperates with the Met/Caveolin gene amplicon to induce basal-like breast cancer. *Cancer Cell, 21*(5), 626–641.
66. Mukherjee, A., Veraksa, A., Bauer, A., Rosse, C., Camonis, J., & Artavanis-Tsakonas, S. (2005). Regulation of Notch signalling by non-visual beta-arrestin. *Nature Cell Biology, 7*(12), 1191–1201.
67. Qiu, L., Joazeiro, C., Fang, N., Wang, H. Y., Elly, C., Altman, Y., et al. (2000). Recognition and ubiquitination of Notch by Itch, a hect-type E3 ubiquitin ligase. *The Journal of Biological Chemistry, 275*(46), 35734–35737.
68. Sakata, T., Sakaguchi, H., Tsuda, L., Higashitani, A., Aigaki, T., Matsuno, K., et al. (2004). Drosophila Nedd4 regulates endocytosis of notch and suppresses its ligand-independent activation. *Current Biology, 14*(24), 2228–2236.
69. Jehn, B. M., Dittert, I., Beyer, S., von der Mark, K., & Bielke, W. (2002). c-Cbl binding and ubiquitin-dependent lysosomal degradation of membrane-associated Notch1. *The Journal of Biological Chemistry, 277*(10), 8033–8040.
70. Conner, S. D. (2016). Regulation of Notch signaling through intracellular transport. *International Review of Cell and Molecular Biology, 323*, 107–127.
71. Santolini, E., Puri, C., Salcini, A. E., Gagliani, M. C., Pelicci, P. G., Tacchetti, C., et al. (2000). Numb is an endocytic protein. *The Journal of Cell Biology, 151*(6), 1345–1352.
72. McGill, M. A., & McGlade, C. J. (2003). Mammalian numb proteins promote Notch1 receptor ubiquitination and degradation of the Notch1 intracellular domain. *The Journal of Biological Chemistry, 278*(25), 23196–23203.
73. Foltz, D. R., Santiago, M. C., Berechid, B. E., & Nye, J. S. (2002). Glycogen synthase kinase-3beta modulates notch signaling and stability. *Current Biology, 12*(12), 1006–1011.

74. Ingles-Esteve, J., Espinosa, L., Milner, L. A., Caelles, C., & Bigas, A. (2001). Phosphorylation of Ser2078 modulates the Notch2 function in 32D cell differentiation. *The Journal of Biological Chemistry, 276*(48), 44873–44880.
75. Fryer, C. J., White, J. B., & Jones, K. A. (2004). Mastermind recruits CycC:CDK8 to phosphorylate the Notch ICD and coordinate activation with turnover. *Molecular Cell, 16*(4), 509–520.
76. Popko-Scibor, A. E., Lindberg, M. J., Hansson, M. L., Holmlund, T., & Wallberg, A. E. (2011). Ubiquitination of Notch1 is regulated by MAML1-mediated p300 acetylation of Notch1. *Biochemical and Biophysical Research Communications, 416*(3–4), 300–306.
77. Palermo, R., Checquolo, S., Giovenco, A., Grazioli, P., Kumar, V., Campese, A. F., et al. (2012). Acetylation controls Notch3 stability and function in T-cell leukemia. *Oncogene, 31*(33), 3807–3817.
78. Ishitani, T., Hirao, T., Suzuki, M., Isoda, M., Ishitani, S., Harigaya, K., et al. (2010). Nemo-like kinase suppresses Notch signalling by interfering with formation of the Notch active transcriptional complex. *Nature Cell Biology, 12*(3), 278–285.
79. Rustighi, A., Tiberi, L., Soldano, A., Napoli, M., Nuciforo, P., Rosato, A., et al. (2009). The prolyl-isomerase Pin1 is a Notch1 target that enhances Notch1 activation in cancer. *Nature Cell Biology, 11*(2), 133–142.
80. Rustighi, A., Zannini, A., Tiberi, L., Sommaggio, R., Piazza, S., Sorrentino, G., et al. (2014). Prolyl-isomerase Pin1 controls normal and cancer stem cells of the breast. *EMBO Molecular Medicine, 6*(1), 99–119.
81. Baik, S. H., Fane, M., Park, J. H., Cheng, Y. L., Yang-Wei Fann, D., Yun, U. J., et al. (2015). Pin1 promotes neuronal death in stroke by stabilizing Notch intracellular domain. *Annals of Neurology, 77*(3), 504–516.
82. Franciosa, G., Diluvio, G., Del Gaudio, F., Giuli, M. V., Palermo, R., Grazioli, P., et al. (2016). Prolyl-isomerase Pin1 controls Notch3 protein expression and regulates T-ALL progression. *Oncogene, 35*(36), 4741–4751.
83. Cho, S., Lu, M., He, X., Ee, P. L., Bhat, U., Schneider, E., et al. (2011). Notch1 regulates the expression of the multidrug resistance gene ABCC1/MRP1 in cultured cancer cells. *Proceedings of the National Academy of Sciences of the United States of America, 108*(51), 20778–20783.
84. Wang, Z., Li, Y., Ahmad, A., Banerjee, S., Azmi, A. S., Kong, D., et al. (2011). Down-regulation of Notch-1 is associated with Akt and FoxM1 in inducing cell growth inhibition and apoptosis in prostate cancer cells. *Journal of Cellular Biochemistry, 112*(1), 78–88.
85. Zhao, B., Zou, J., Wang, H., Johannsen, E., Peng, C. W., Quackenbush, J., et al. (2011). Epstein-Barr virus exploits intrinsic B-lymphocyte transcription programs to achieve immortal cell growth. *Proceedings of the National Academy of Sciences of the United States of America, 108*(36), 14902–14907.
86. Brou, C., Logeat, F., Gupta, N., Bessia, C., LeBail, O., Doedens, J. R., et al. (2000). A novel proteolytic cleavage involved in Notch signaling: The role of the disintegrin-metalloprotease TACE. *Molecular Cell, 5*(2), 207–216.
87. Musse, A. A., Meloty-Kapella, L., & Weinmaster, G. (2012). Notch ligand endocytosis: Mechanistic basis of signaling activity. *Seminars in Cell & Developmental Biology, 23*(4), 429–436.
88. Saxena, M. T., Schroeter, E. H., Mumm, J. S., & Kopan, R. (2001). Murine notch homologs (N1-4) undergo presenilin-dependent proteolysis. *The Journal of Biological Chemistry, 276*(43), 40268–40273.
89. Schroeter, E. H., Kisslinger, J. A., & Kopan, R. (1998). Notch-1 signalling requires ligand-induced proteolytic release of intracellular domain. *Nature, 393*(6683), 382–386.
90. Chen, F., Hasegawa, H., Schmitt-Ulms, G., Kawarai, T., Bohm, C., Katayama, T., et al. (2006). TMP21 is a presenilin complex component that modulates gamma-secretase but not epsilon-secretase activity. *Nature, 440*(7088), 1208–1212.

91. Zhang, Y. W., Luo, W. J., Wang, H., Lin, P., Vetrivel, K. S., Liao, F., et al. (2005). Nicastrin is critical for stability and trafficking but not association of other presenilin/gamma-secretase components. *The Journal of Biological Chemistry, 280*(17), 17020–17026.
92. Lee, S. F., Shah, S., Yu, C., Wigley, W. C., Li, H., Lim, M., et al. (2004). A conserved GXXXG motif in APH-1 is critical for assembly and activity of the gamma-secretase complex. *The Journal of Biological Chemistry, 279*(6), 4144–4152.
93. Prokop, S., Shirotani, K., Edbauer, D., Haass, C., & Steiner, H. (2004). Requirement of PEN-2 for stabilization of the presenilin N-/C-terminal fragment heterodimer within the gamma-secretase complex. *The Journal of Biological Chemistry, 279*(22), 23255–23261.
94. Fortini, M. E., & Artavanis-Tsakonas, S. (1994). The suppressor of hairless protein participates in notch receptor signaling. *Cell, 79*(2), 273–282.
95. Wu, L., Aster, J. C., Blacklow, S. C., Lake, R., Artavanis-Tsakonas, S., & Griffin, J. D. (2000). MAML1, a human homologue of Drosophila mastermind, is a transcriptional co-activator for NOTCH receptors. *Nature Genetics, 26*(4), 484–489.
96. Wallberg, A. E., Pedersen, K., Lendahl, U., & Roeder, R. G. (2002). p300 and PCAF act cooperatively to mediate transcriptional activation from chromatin templates by notch intracellular domains in vitro. *Molecular and Cellular Biology, 22*(22), 7812–7819.
97. Kurooka, H., & Honjo, T. (2000). Functional interaction between the mouse notch1 intracellular region and histone acetyltransferases PCAF and GCN5. *The Journal of Biological Chemistry, 275*(22), 17211–17220.
98. Kitagawa, M. (2016). Notch signalling in the nucleus: Roles of Mastermind-like (MAML) transcriptional coactivators. *Journal of Biochemistry, 159*(3), 287–294.
99. Wang, Z., Ahmad, A., Li, Y., Azmi, A. S., Miele, L., & Sarkar, F. H. (2011). Targeting notch to eradicate pancreatic cancer stem cells for cancer therapy. *Anticancer Research, 31*(4), 1105–1113.
100. Castel, D., Mourikis, P., Bartels, S. J., Brinkman, A. B., Tajbakhsh, S., & Stunnenberg, H. G. (2013). Dynamic binding of RBPJ is determined by Notch signaling status. *Genes & Development, 27*(9), 1059–1071.
101. Choi, J. W., Pampeno, C., Vukmanovic, S., & Meruelo, D. (2002). Characterization of the transcriptional expression of Notch-1 signaling pathway members, Deltex and HES-1, in developing mouse thymocytes. *Developmental and Comparative Immunology, 26*(6), 575–588.
102. Oswald, F., Liptay, S., Adler, G., & Schmid, R. M. (1998). NF-kappaB2 is a putative target gene of activated Notch-1 via RBP-Jkappa. *Molecular and Cellular Biology, 18*(4), 2077–2088.
103. Cheng, P., Zlobin, A., Volgina, V., Gottipati, S., Osborne, B., Simel, E. J., et al. (2001). Notch-1 regulates NF-kappaB activity in hemopoietic progenitor cells. *Journal of Immunology, 167*(8), 4458–4467.
104. Rangarajan, A., Talora, C., Okuyama, R., Nicolas, M., Mammucari, C., Oh, H., et al. (2001). Notch signaling is a direct determinant of keratinocyte growth arrest and entry into differentiation. *The EMBO Journal, 20*(13), 3427–3436.
105. Ronchini, C., & Capobianco, A. J. (2001). Induction of cyclin D1 transcription and CDK2 activity by Notch(ic): Implication for cell cycle disruption in transformation by Notch(ic). *Molecular and Cellular Biology, 21*(17), 5925–5934.
106. Weng, A. P., Millholland, J. M., Yashiro-Ohtani, Y., Arcangeli, M. L., Lau, A., Wai, C., et al. (2006). c-Myc is an important direct target of Notch1 in T-cell acute lymphoblastic leukemia/lymphoma. *Genes & Development, 20*(15), 2096–2109.
107. Andersen, P., Uosaki, H., Shenje, L. T., & Kwon, C. (2012). Non-canonical Notch signaling: Emerging role and mechanism. *Trends in Cell Biology, 22*(5), 257–265.
108. Sanalkumar, R., Dhanesh, S. B., & James, J. (2010). Non-canonical activation of Notch signaling/target genes in vertebrates. *Cellular and Molecular Life Sciences, 67*(17), 2957–2968.
109. de Celis, J. F., & Bray, S. (1997). Feed-back mechanisms affecting Notch activation at the dorsoventral boundary in the Drosophila wing. *Development, 124*(17), 3241–3251.

110. Li, Y., & Baker, N. E. (2004). The roles of cis-inactivation by Notch ligands and of neuralized during eye and bristle patterning in Drosophila. *BMC Developmental Biology, 4*, 5.
111. Miller, A. C., Lyons, E. L., & Herman, T. G. (2009). cis-Inhibition of Notch by endogenous Delta biases the outcome of lateral inhibition. *Current Biology, 19*(16), 1378–1383.
112. Becam, I., Fiuza, U. M., Arias, A. M., & Milan, M. (2010). A role of receptor Notch in ligand cis-inhibition in Drosophila. *Current Biology, 20*(6), 554–560.
113. Loeb, D. M., Thornton, K., & Shokek, O. (2008). Pediatric soft tissue sarcomas. *The Surgical Clinics of North America, 88*(3), 615–627. vii.
114. Tapscott, S. J., Thayer, M. J., & Weintraub, H. (1993). Deficiency in rhabdomyosarcomas of a factor required for MyoD activity and myogenesis. *Science, 259*(5100), 1450–1453.
115. De Giovanni, C., Landuzzi, L., Nicoletti, G., Lollini, P. L., & Nanni, P. (2009). Molecular and cellular biology of rhabdomyosarcoma. *Future Oncology, 5*(9), 1449–1475.
116. Parham, D. M., & Barr, F. G. (2013). Classification of rhabdomyosarcoma and its molecular basis. *Advances in Anatomic Pathology, 20*(6), 387–397.
117. Taulli, R., Bersani, F., Foglizzo, V., Linari, A., Vigna, E., Ladanyi, M., et al. (2009). The muscle-specific microRNA miR-206 blocks human rhabdomyosarcoma growth in xenotransplanted mice by promoting myogenic differentiation. *The Journal of Clinical Investigation, 119*(8), 2366–2378.
118. Ciarapica, R., Carcarino, E., Adesso, L., De Salvo, M., Bracaglia, G., Leoncini, P. P., et al. (2014). Pharmacological inhibition of EZH2 as a promising differentiation therapy in embryonal RMS. *BMC Cancer, 14*, 139.
119. Kikuchi, K., Taniguchi, E., Chen, H. I., Svalina, M. N., Abraham, J., Huang, E. T., et al. (2013). Rb1 loss modifies but does not initiate alveolar rhabdomyosarcoma. *Skeletal Muscle, 3*(1), 27.
120. Chen, E. Y., Dobrinski, K. P., Brown, K. H., Clagg, R., Edelman, E., Ignatius, M. S., et al. (2013). Cross-species array comparative genomic hybridization identifies novel oncogenic events in zebrafish and human embryonal rhabdomyosarcoma. *PLoS Genetics, 9*(8), e1003727.
121. Hettmer, S., Liu, J., Miller, C. M., Lindsay, M. C., Sparks, C. A., Guertin, D. A., et al. (2011). Sarcomas induced in discrete subsets of prospectively isolated skeletal muscle cells. *Proceedings of the National Academy of Sciences of the United States of America, 108*(50), 20002–20007.
122. Abraham, J., Nunez-Alvarez, Y., Hettmer, S., Carrio, E., Chen, H. I., Nishijo, K., et al. (2014). Lineage of origin in rhabdomyosarcoma informs pharmacological response. *Genes & Development, 28*(14), 1578–1591.
123. Nitzki, F., Zibat, A., Frommhold, A., Schneider, A., Schulz-Schaeffer, W., Braun, T., et al. (2011). Uncommitted precursor cells might contribute to increased incidence of embryonal rhabdomyosarcoma in heterozygous Patched1-mutant mice. *Oncogene, 30*(43), 4428–4436.
124. Hatley, M. E., Tang, W., Garcia, M. R., Finkelstein, D., Millay, D. P., Liu, N., et al. (2012). A mouse model of rhabdomyosarcoma originating from the adipocyte lineage. *Cancer Cell, 22*(4), 536–546.
125. Meza, J. L., Anderson, J., Pappo, A. S., Meyer, W. H., & Children's Oncology G. (2006). Analysis of prognostic factors in patients with nonmetastatic rhabdomyosarcoma treated on intergroup rhabdomyosarcoma studies III and IV: The Children's Oncology Group. *Journal of Clinical Oncology, 24*(24), 3844–3851.
126. Arndt, C. A., Stoner, J. A., Hawkins, D. S., Rodeberg, D. A., Hayes-Jordan, A. A., Paidas, C. N., et al. (2009). Vincristine, actinomycin, and cyclophosphamide compared with vincristine, actinomycin, and cyclophosphamide alternating with vincristine, topotecan, and cyclophosphamide for intermediate-risk rhabdomyosarcoma: Children's oncology group study D9803. *Journal of Clinical Oncology, 27*(31), 5182–5188.
127. Williamson, D., Missiaglia, E., de Reynies, A., Pierron, G., Thuille, B., Palenzuela, G., et al. (2010). Fusion gene-negative alveolar rhabdomyosarcoma is clinically and molecularly indistinguishable from embryonal rhabdomyosarcoma. *Journal of Clinical Oncology, 28*(13), 2151–2158.

128. Chen, X., Stewart, E., Shelat, A. A., Qu, C., Bahrami, A., Hatley, M., et al. (2013). Targeting oxidative stress in embryonal rhabdomyosarcoma. *Cancer Cell, 24*(6), 710–724.
129. Shern, J. F., Chen, L., Chmielecki, J., Wei, J. S., Patidar, R., Rosenberg, M., et al. (2014). Comprehensive genomic analysis of rhabdomyosarcoma reveals a landscape of alterations affecting a common genetic axis in fusion-positive and fusion-negative tumors. *Cancer Discovery, 4*(2), 216–231.
130. Hahn, H., Wojnowski, L., Zimmer, A. M., Hall, J., Miller, G., & Zimmer, A. (1998). Rhabdomyosarcomas and radiation hypersensitivity in a mouse model of Gorlin syndrome. *Nature Medicine, 4*(5), 619–622.
131. Zibat, A., Missiaglia, E., Rosenberger, A., Pritchard-Jones, K., Shipley, J., Hahn, H., et al. (2010). Activation of the hedgehog pathway confers a poor prognosis in embryonal and fusion gene-negative alveolar rhabdomyosarcoma. *Oncogene, 29*(48), 6323–6330.
132. Nitzki, F., Cuvelier, N., Drager, J., Schneider, A., Braun, T., & Hahn, H. (2016). Hedgehog/Patched-associated rhabdomyosarcoma formation from delta1-expressing mesodermal cells. *Oncogene, 35*(22), 2923–2931.
133. Pressey, J. G., Anderson, J. R., Crossman, D. K., Lynch, J. C., & Barr, F. G. (2011). Hedgehog pathway activity in pediatric embryonal rhabdomyosarcoma and undifferentiated sarcoma: A report from the Children's Oncology Group. *Pediatric Blood & Cancer, 57*(6), 930–938.
134. Kohsaka, S., Shukla, N., Ameur, N., Ito, T., Ng, C. K., Wang, L., et al. (2014). A recurrent neomorphic mutation in MYOD1 defines a clinically aggressive subset of embryonal rhabdomyosarcoma associated with PI3K-AKT pathway mutations. *Nature Genetics, 46*(6), 595–600.
135. Davicioni, E., Anderson, J. R., Buckley, J. D., Meyer, W. H., & Triche, T. J. (2010). Gene expression profiling for survival prediction in pediatric rhabdomyosarcomas: A report from the children's oncology group. *Journal of Clinical Oncology, 28*(7), 1240–1246.
136. Galili, N., Davis, R. J., Fredericks, W. J., Mukhopadhyay, S., Rauscher, F. J., 3rd, Emanuel, B. S., et al. (1993). Fusion of a fork head domain gene to PAX3 in the solid tumour alveolar rhabdomyosarcoma. *Nature Genetics, 5*(3), 230–235.
137. Davis, R. J., D'Cruz, C. M., Lovell, M. A., Biegel, J. A., & Barr, F. G. (1994). Fusion of PAX7 to FKHR by the variant t(1;13)(p36;q14) translocation in alveolar rhabdomyosarcoma. *Cancer Research, 54*(11), 2869–2872.
138. Marshall, A. D., Picchione, F., Geltink, R. I., & Grosveld, G. C. (2013). PAX3-FOXO1 induces up-regulation of Noxa sensitizing alveolar rhabdomyosarcoma cells to apoptosis. *Neoplasia, 15*(7), 738–748.
139. Missiaglia, E., Williamson, D., Chisholm, J., Wirapati, P., Pierron, G., Petel, F., et al. (2012). PAX3/FOXO1 fusion gene status is the key prognostic molecular marker in rhabdomyosarcoma and significantly improves current risk stratification. *Journal of Clinical Oncology, 30*(14), 1670–1677.
140. Mourikis, P., & Tajbakhsh, S. (2014). Distinct contextual roles for Notch signalling in skeletal muscle stem cells. *BMC Developmental Biology, 14*, 2.
141. Francis, P., Namlos, H. M., Muller, C., Eden, P., Fernebro, J., Berner, J. M., et al. (2007). Diagnostic and prognostic gene expression signatures in 177 soft tissue sarcomas: Hypoxia-induced transcription profile signifies metastatic potential. *BMC Genomics, 8*, 73.
142. Terry, J., Saito, T., Subramanian, S., Ruttan, C., Antonescu, C. R., Goldblum, J. R., et al. (2007). TLE1 as a diagnostic immunohistochemical marker for synovial sarcoma emerging from gene expression profiling studies. *The American Journal of Surgical Pathology, 31*(2), 240–246.
143. Jagdis, A., Rubin, B. P., Tubbs, R. R., Pacheco, M., & Nielsen, T. O. (2009). Prospective evaluation of TLE1 as a diagnostic immunohistochemical marker in synovial sarcoma. *The American Journal of Surgical Pathology, 33*(12), 1743–1751.
144. Su, L., Sampaio, A. V., Jones, K. B., Pacheco, M., Goytain, A., Lin, S., et al. (2012). Deconstruction of the SS18-SSX fusion oncoprotein complex: Insights into disease etiology and therapeutics. *Cancer Cell, 21*(3), 333–347.

145. May, W. A., Arvand, A., Thompson, A. D., Braun, B. S., Wright, M., & Denny, C. T. (1997). EWS/FLI1-induced manic fringe renders NIH 3T3 cells tumorigenic. *Nature Genetics, 17*(4), 495–497.
146. Baliko, F., Bright, T., Poon, R., Cohen, B., Egan, S. E., & BA, A. (2007). Inhibition of notch signaling induces neural differentiation in Ewing sarcoma. *The American Journal of Pathology, 170*(5), 1686–1694.
147. Ban, J., Bennani-Baiti, I. M., Kauer, M., Schaefer, K. L., Poremba, C., Jug, G., et al. (2008). EWS-FLI1 suppresses NOTCH-activated p53 in Ewing's sarcoma. *Cancer Research, 68*(17), 7100–7109.
148. Bennani-Baiti, I. M., Aryee, D. N., Ban, J., Machado, I., Kauer, M., Muhlbacher, K., et al. (2011). Notch signalling is off and is uncoupled from HES1 expression in Ewing's sarcoma. *The Journal of Pathology, 225*(3), 353–363.
149. Ban, J., Aryee, D. N., Fourtouna, A., van der Ent, W., Kauer, M., Niedan, S., et al. (2014). Suppression of deacetylase SIRT1 mediates tumor-suppressive NOTCH response and offers a novel treatment option in metastatic Ewing sarcoma. *Cancer Research, 74*(22), 6578–6588.
150. Ventura, S., Aryee, D. N., Felicetti, F., De Feo, A., Mancarella, C., Manara, M. C., et al. (2016). CD99 regulates neural differentiation of Ewing sarcoma cells through miR-34a-Notch-mediated control of NF-kappaB signaling. *Oncogene, 35*(30), 3944–3954.
151. Sang, L., Coller, H. A., & Roberts, J. M. (2008). Control of the reversibility of cellular quiescence by the transcriptional repressor HES1. *Science, 321*(5892), 1095–1100.
152. Roma, J., Masia, A., Reventos, J., Sanchez de Toledo, J., & Gallego, S. (2011). Notch pathway inhibition significantly reduces rhabdomyosarcoma invasiveness and mobility in vitro. *Clinical Cancer Research, 17*(3), 505–513.
153. Belyea, B. C., Naini, S., Bentley, R. C., & Linardic, C. M. (2011). Inhibition of the Notch-Hey1 axis blocks embryonal rhabdomyosarcoma tumorigenesis. *Clinical Cancer Research, 17*(23), 7324–7336.
154. Raimondi, L., Ciarapica, R., De Salvo, M., Verginelli, F., Gueguen, M., Martini, C., et al. (2012). Inhibition of Notch3 signalling induces rhabdomyosarcoma cell differentiation promoting p38 phosphorylation and p21(Cip1) expression and hampers tumour cell growth in vitro and in vivo. *Cell Death and Differentiation, 19*(5), 871–881.
155. Nagao, H., Setoguchi, T., Kitamoto, S., Ishidou, Y., Nagano, S., Yokouchi, M., et al. (2012). RBPJ is a novel target for rhabdomyosarcoma therapy. *PLoS One, 7*(7), e39268.
156. De Salvo, M., Raimondi, L., Vella, S., Adesso, L., Ciarapica, R., Verginelli, F., et al. (2014). Hyper-activation of Notch3 amplifies the proliferative potential of rhabdomyosarcoma cells. *PLoS One, 9*(5), e96238.
157. Diao, Y., Guo, X., Jiang, L., Wang, G., Zhang, C., Wan, J., et al. (2014). miR-203, a tumor suppressor frequently down-regulated by promoter hypermethylation in rhabdomyosarcoma. *The Journal of Biological Chemistry, 289*(1), 529–539.
158. Kitagawa, M., Oyama, T., Kawashima, T., Yedvobnick, B., Kumar, A., Matsuno, K., et al. (2001). A human protein with sequence similarity to Drosophila mastermind coordinates the nuclear form of notch and a CSL protein to build a transcriptional activator complex on target promoters. *Molecular and Cellular Biology, 21*(13), 4337–4346.
159. Hu, Y. Y., Zheng, M. H., Zhang, R., Liang, Y. M., & Han, H. (2012). Notch signaling pathway and cancer metastasis. *Advances in Experimental Medicine and Biology, 727*, 186–198.
160. Liu, Z. H., Dai, X. M., & Du, B. (2015). Hes1: A key role in stemness, metastasis and multidrug resistance. *Cancer Biology & Therapy, 16*(3), 353–359.
161. Weidle, U. H., Birzele, F., & Kruger, A. (2015). Molecular targets and pathways involved in liver metastasis of colorectal cancer. *Clinical & Experimental Metastasis, 32*(6), 623–635.
162. Masia, A., Almazan-Moga, A., Velasco, P., Reventos, J., Toran, N., Sanchez de Toledo, J., et al. (2012). Notch-mediated induction of N-cadherin and alpha9-integrin confers higher invasive phenotype on rhabdomyosarcoma cells. *British Journal of Cancer, 107*(8), 1374–1383.
163. Liu, Z. J., Xiao, M., Balint, K., Smalley, K. S., Brafford, P., Qiu, R., et al. (2006). Notch1 signaling promotes primary melanoma progression by activating mitogen-activated protein

kinase/phosphatidylinositol 3-kinase-Akt pathways and up-regulating N-cadherin expression. *Cancer Research, 66*(8), 4182–4190.
164. Wang, T., Holt, C. M., Xu, C., Ridley, C., POJ, R., Baron, M., et al. (2007). Notch3 activation modulates cell growth behaviour and cross-talk to Wnt/TCF signalling pathway. *Cellular Signalling, 19*(12), 2458–2467.
165. Shukla, N., Ameur, N., Yilmaz, I., Nafa, K., Lau, C. Y., Marchetti, A., et al. (2012). Oncogene mutation profiling of pediatric solid tumors reveals significant subsets of embryonal rhabdomyosarcoma and neuroblastoma with mutated genes in growth signaling pathways. *Clinical Cancer Research, 18*(3), 748–757.
166. Gustafsson, M. K., Pan, H., Pinney, D. F., Liu, Y., Lewandowski, A., Epstein, D. J., et al. (2002). Myf5 is a direct target of long-range Shh signaling and Gli regulation for muscle specification. *Genes & Development, 16*(1), 114–126.
167. Straface, G., Aprahamian, T., Flex, A., Gaetani, E., Biscetti, F., Smith, R. C., et al. (2009). Sonic hedgehog regulates angiogenesis and myogenesis during post-natal skeletal muscle regeneration. *Journal of Cellular and Molecular Medicine, 13*(8B), 2424–2435.
168. Koleva, M., Kappler, R., Vogler, M., Herwig, A., Fulda, S., & Hahn, H. (2005). Pleiotropic effects of sonic hedgehog on muscle satellite cells. *Cellular and Molecular Life Sciences, 62*(16), 1863–1870.
169. Bren-Mattison, Y., & Olwin, B. B. (2002). Sonic hedgehog inhibits the terminal differentiation of limb myoblasts committed to the slow muscle lineage. *Developmental Biology, 242*(2), 130–148.
170. Hahn, H., Nitzki, F., Schorban, T., Hemmerlein, B., Threadgill, D., & Rosemann, M. (2004). Genetic mapping of a Ptch1-associated rhabdomyosarcoma susceptibility locus on mouse chromosome 2. *Genomics, 84*(5), 853–858.
171. Calzada-Wack, J., Schnitzbauer, U., Walch, A., Wurster, K. H., Kappler, R., Nathrath, M., et al. (2002). Analysis of the PTCH coding region in human rhabdomyosarcoma. *Human Mutation, 20*(3), 233–234.
172. Bridge, J. A., Liu, J., Weibolt, V., Baker, K. S., Perry, D., Kruger, R., et al. (2000). Novel genomic imbalances in embryonal rhabdomyosarcoma revealed by comparative genomic hybridization and fluorescence in situ hybridization: An intergroup rhabdomyosarcoma study. *Genes, Chromosomes & Cancer, 27*(4), 337–344.
173. Tostar, U., Malm, C. J., Meis-Kindblom, J. M., Kindblom, L. G., Toftgard, R., & Unden, A. B. (2006). Deregulation of the hedgehog signalling pathway: A possible role for the PTCH and SUFU genes in human rhabdomyoma and rhabdomyosarcoma development. *The Journal of Pathology, 208*(1), 17–25.
174. Rubin, B. P., Nishijo, K., Chen, H. I., Yi, X., Schuetze, D. P., Pal, R., et al. (2011). Evidence for an unanticipated relationship between undifferentiated pleomorphic sarcoma and embryonal rhabdomyosarcoma. *Cancer Cell, 19*(2), 177–191.
175. Ingram, W. J., McCue, K. I., Tran, T. H., Hallahan, A. R., & Wainwright, B. J. (2008). Sonic Hedgehog regulates Hes1 through a novel mechanism that is independent of canonical Notch pathway signalling. *Oncogene, 27*(10), 1489–1500.
176. Esiashvili, N., Goodman, M., & Marcus, R. B., Jr. (2008). Changes in incidence and survival of Ewing sarcoma patients over the past 3 decades: Surveillance Epidemiology and End Results data. *Journal of Pediatric Hematology/Oncology, 30*(6), 425–430.
177. van den Berg, H., Dirksen, U., Ranft, A., & Jurgens, H. (2008). Ewing tumors in infants. *Pediatric Blood & Cancer, 50*(4), 761–764.
178. Grier, H. E., Krailo, M. D., Tarbell, N. J., Link, M. P., Fryer, C. J., Pritchard, D. J., et al. (2003). Addition of ifosfamide and etoposide to standard chemotherapy for Ewing's sarcoma and primitive neuroectodermal tumor of bone. *The New England Journal of Medicine, 348*(8), 694–701.
179. Womer, R. B., West, D. C., Krailo, M. D., Dickman, P. S., Pawel, B. R., Grier, H. E., et al. (2012). Randomized controlled trial of interval-compressed chemotherapy for the treat-

ment of localized Ewing sarcoma: A report from the Children's Oncology Group. *Journal of Clinical Oncology, 30*(33), 4148–4154.
180. Gaspar, N., Hawkins, D. S., Dirksen, U., Lewis, I. J., Ferrari, S., Le Deley, M. C., et al. (2015). Ewing sarcoma: Current management and future approaches through collaboration. *Journal of Clinical Oncology, 33*(27), 3036–3046.
181. Roberts, P., Burchill, S. A., Brownhill, S., Cullinane, C. J., Johnston, C., Griffiths, M. J., et al. (2008). Ploidy and karyotype complexity are powerful prognostic indicators in the Ewing's sarcoma family of tumors: A study by the United Kingdom Cancer Cytogenetics and the Children's Cancer and Leukaemia Group. *Genes, Chromosomes & Cancer, 47*(3), 207–220.
182. Postel-Vinay, S., Veron, A. S., Tirode, F., Pierron, G., Reynaud, S., Kovar, H., et al. (2012). Common variants near TARDBP and EGR2 are associated with susceptibility to Ewing sarcoma. *Nature Genetics, 44*(3), 323–327.
183. Tuna, M., Ju, Z., CI, A., & Mills, G. B. (2012). Soft tissue sarcoma subtypes exhibit distinct patterns of acquired uniparental disomy. *BMC Medical Genomics, 5*, 60.
184. Delattre, O., Zucman, J., Plougastel, B., Desmaze, C., Melot, T., Peter, M., et al. (1992). Gene fusion with an ETS DNA-binding domain caused by chromosome translocation in human tumours. *Nature, 359*(6391), 162–165.
185. May, W. A., Gishizky, M. L., Lessnick, S. L., Lunsford, L. B., Lewis, B. C., Delattre, O., et al. (1993). Ewing sarcoma 11;22 translocation produces a chimeric transcription factor that requires the DNA-binding domain encoded by FLI1 for transformation. *Proceedings of the National Academy of Sciences of the United States of America, 90*(12), 5752–5756.
186. Lawlor, E. R., & Sorensen, P. H. (2015). Twenty years on: What do we really know about Ewing sarcoma and what is the path forward? *Critical Reviews in Oncogenesis, 20*(3–4), 155–171.
187. van Doorninck, J. A., Ji, L., Schaub, B., Shimada, H., Wing, M. R., Krailo, M. D., et al. (2010). Current treatment protocols have eliminated the prognostic advantage of type 1 fusions in Ewing sarcoma: A report from the Children's Oncology Group. *Journal of Clinical Oncology, 28*(12), 1989–1994.
188. Le Deley, M. C., Delattre, O., Schaefer, K. L., Burchill, S. A., Koehler, G., Hogendoorn, P. C., et al. (2010). Impact of EWS-ETS fusion type on disease progression in Ewing's sarcoma/peripheral primitive neuroectodermal tumor: Prospective results from the cooperative Euro-E.W.I.N.G. 99 trial. *Journal of Clinical Oncology, 28*(12), 1982–1988.
189. Riggi, N., Cironi, L., Provero, P., Suva, M. L., Kaloulis, K., Garcia-Echeverria, C., et al. (2005). Development of Ewing's sarcoma from primary bone marrow-derived mesenchymal progenitor cells. *Cancer Research, 65*(24), 11459–11468.
190. Riggi, N., Suva, M. L., & Stamenkovic, I. (2009). Ewing's sarcoma origin: From duel to duality. *Expert Review of Anticancer Therapy, 9*(8), 1025–1030.
191. Riggi, N., Suva, M. L., De Vito, C., Provero, P., Stehle, J. C., Baumer, K., et al. (2010). EWS-FLI-1 modulates miRNA145 and SOX2 expression to initiate mesenchymal stem cell reprogramming toward Ewing sarcoma cancer stem cells. *Genes & Development, 24*(9), 916–932.
192. von Levetzow, C., Jiang, X., Gwye, Y., von Levetzow, G., Hung, L., Cooper, A., et al. (2011). Modeling initiation of Ewing sarcoma in human neural crest cells. *PLoS One, 6*(4), e19305.
193. May, W. A., Lessnick, S. L., Braun, B. S., Klemsz, M., Lewis, B. C., Lunsford, L. B., et al. (1993). The Ewing's sarcoma EWS/FLI-1 fusion gene encodes a more potent transcriptional activator and is a more powerful transforming gene than FLI-1. *Molecular and Cellular Biology, 13*(12), 7393–7398.
194. Bilke, S., Schwentner, R., Yang, F., Kauer, M., Jug, G., Walker, R. L., et al. (2013). Oncogenic ETS fusions deregulate E2F3 target genes in Ewing sarcoma and prostate cancer. *Genome Research, 23*(11), 1797–1809.
195. Patel, M., Simon, J. M., Iglesia, M. D., Wu, S. B., McFadden, A. W., Lieb, J. D., et al. (2012). Tumor-specific retargeting of an oncogenic transcription factor chimera results in dysregulation of chromatin and transcription. *Genome Research, 22*(2), 259–270.
196. Owen, L. A., Kowalewski, A. A., & Lessnick, S. L. (2008). EWS/FLI mediates transcriptional repression via NKX2.2 during oncogenic transformation in Ewing's sarcoma. *PLoS One, 3*(4), e1965.

197. Stoll, G., Surdez, D., Tirode, F., Laud, K., Barillot, E., Zinovyev, A., et al. (2013). Systems biology of Ewing sarcoma: A network model of EWS-FLI1 effect on proliferation and apoptosis. *Nucleic Acids Research, 41*(19), 8853–8871.
198. Zwerner, J. P., Guimbellot, J., & May, W. A. (2003). EWS/FLI function varies in different cellular backgrounds. *Experimental Cell Research, 290*(2), 414–419.
199. Smith, R., Owen, L. A., Trem, D. J., Wong, J. S., Whangbo, J. S., Golub, T. R., et al. (2006). Expression profiling of EWS/FLI identifies NKX2.2 as a critical target gene in Ewing's sarcoma. *Cancer Cell, 9*(5), 405–416.
200. Bennani-Baiti, I. M., Machado, I., Llombart-Bosch, A., & Kovar, H. (2012). Lysine-specific demethylase 1 (LSD1/KDM1A/AOF2/BHC110) is expressed and is an epigenetic drug target in chondrosarcoma, Ewing's sarcoma, osteosarcoma, and rhabdomyosarcoma. *Human Pathology, 43*(8), 1300–1307.
201. Mulligan, P., Yang, F., Di Stefano, L., Ji, J. Y., Ouyang, J., Nishikawa, J. L., et al. (2011). A SIRT1-LSD1 corepressor complex regulates Notch target gene expression and development. *Molecular Cell, 42*(5), 689–699.
202. Wang, J., Scully, K., Zhu, X., Cai, L., Zhang, J., Prefontaine, G. G., et al. (2007). Opposing LSD1 complexes function in developmental gene activation and repression programmes. *Nature, 446*(7138), 882–887.
203. Di Stefano, L., Walker, J. A., Burgio, G., Corona, D. F., Mulligan, P., Naar, A. M., et al. (2011). Functional antagonism between histone H3K4 demethylases in vivo. *Genes & Development, 25*(1), 17–28.
204. Rocchi, A., Manara, M. C., Sciandra, M., Zambelli, D., Nardi, F., Nicoletti, G., et al. (2010). CD99 inhibits neural differentiation of human Ewing sarcoma cells and thereby contributes to oncogenesis. *The Journal of Clinical Investigation, 120*(3), 668–680.
205. Schenkel, A. R., Mamdouh, Z., Chen, X., Liebman, R. M., & Muller, W. A. (2002). CD99 plays a major role in the migration of monocytes through endothelial junctions. *Nature Immunology, 3*(2), 143–150.
206. Alberti, I., Bernard, G., Rouquette-Jazdanian, A. K., Pelassy, C., Pourtein, M., Aussel, C., et al. (2002). CD99 isoforms expression dictates T cell functional outcomes. *The FASEB Journal, 16*(14), 1946–1948.
207. Miyagawa, Y., Okita, H., Nakaijima, H., Horiuchi, Y., Sato, B., Taguchi, T., et al. (2008). Inducible expression of chimeric EWS/ETS proteins confers Ewing's family tumor-like phenotypes to human mesenchymal progenitor cells. *Molecular and Cellular Biology, 28*(7), 2125–2137.
208. Hu-Lieskovan, S., Zhang, J., Wu, L., Shimada, H., Schofield, D. E., & Triche, T. J. (2005). EWS-FLI1 fusion protein up-regulates critical genes in neural crest development and is responsible for the observed phenotype of Ewing's family of tumors. *Cancer Research, 65*(11), 4633–4644.
209. Nakatani, F., Ferracin, M., Manara, M. C., Ventura, S., Del Monaco, V., Ferrari, S., et al. (2012). miR-34a predicts survival of Ewing's sarcoma patients and directly influences cell chemo-sensitivity and malignancy. *The Journal of Pathology, 226*(5), 796–805.
210. Marino, M. T., Grilli, A., Baricordi, C., Manara, M. C., Ventura, S., Pinca, R. S., et al. (2014). Prognostic significance of miR-34a in Ewing sarcoma is associated with cyclin D1 and ki-67 expression. *Annals of Oncology, 25*(10), 2080–2086.
211. Li, Y., Guessous, F., Zhang, Y., Dipierro, C., Kefas, B., Johnson, E., et al. (2009). MicroRNA-34a inhibits glioblastoma growth by targeting multiple oncogenes. *Cancer Research, 69*(19), 7569–7576.
212. Bu, P., Chen, K. Y., Chen, J. H., Wang, L., Walters, J., Shin, Y. J., et al. (2013). A microRNA miR-34a-regulated bimodal switch targets Notch in colon cancer stem cells. *Cell Stem Cell, 12*(5), 602–615.
213. Osipo, C., Golde, T. E., Osborne, B. A., & Miele, L. A. (2008). Off the beaten pathway: The complex cross talk between Notch and NF-kappaB. *Laboratory Investigation, 88*(1), 11–17.
214. Ducimetiere, F., Lurkin, A., Ranchere-Vince, D., Decouvelaere, A. V., Péoc'h, M., Istier, L., et al. (2011). Incidence of sarcoma histotypes and molecular subtypes in a prospective epi-

demiological study with central pathology review and molecular testing. *PLoS One, 6*(8), e20294.

215. Palmerini, E., Paioli, A., & Ferrari, S. (2014). Emerging therapeutic targets for synovial sarcoma. *Expert Review of Anticancer Therapy, 14*(7), 791–806.
216. Nielsen, T. O., Poulin, N. M., & Ladanyi, M. (2015). Synovial sarcoma: Recent discoveries as a roadmap to new avenues for therapy. *Cancer Discovery, 5*(2), 124–134.
217. Herzog, C. E. (2005). Overview of sarcomas in the adolescent and young adult population. *Journal of Pediatric Hematology/Oncology, 27*(4), 215–218.
218. Sultan, I., Rodriguez-Galindo, C., Saab, R., Yasir, S., Casanova, M., & Ferrari, A. (2009). Comparing children and adults with synovial sarcoma in the Surveillance, Epidemiology, and End Results program, 1983 to 2005: An analysis of 1268 patients. *Cancer, 115*(15), 3537–3547.
219. Nagai, M., Tanaka, S., Tsuda, M., Endo, S., Kato, H., Sonobe, H., et al. (2001). Analysis of transforming activity of human synovial sarcoma-associated chimeric protein SYT-SSX1 bound to chromatin remodeling factor hBRM/hSNF2 alpha. *Proceedings of the National Academy of Sciences of the United States of America, 98*(7), 3843–3848.
220. Carmody Soni, E. E., Schlottman, S., Erkizan, H. V., Uren, A., & Toretsky, J. A. (2014). Loss of SS18-SSX1 inhibits viability and induces apoptosis in synovial sarcoma. *Clinical Orthopaedics and Related Research, 472*(3), 874–882.
221. Naka, N., Takenaka, S., Araki, N., Miwa, T., Hashimoto, N., Yoshioka, K., et al. (2010). Synovial sarcoma is a stem cell malignancy. *Stem Cells, 28*(7), 1119–1131.
222. Cironi, L., Provero, P., Riggi, N., Janiszewska, M., Suva, D., Suva, M. L., et al. (2009). Epigenetic features of human mesenchymal stem cells determine their permissiveness for induction of relevant transcriptional changes by SYT-SSX1. *PLoS One, 4*(11), e7904.
223. Haldar, M., Randall, R. L., & Capecchi, M. R. (2008). Synovial sarcoma: From genetics to genetic-based animal modeling. *Clinical Orthopaedics and Related Research, 466*(9), 2156–2167.
224. Panagopoulos, I., Mertens, F., Isaksson, M., Limon, J., Gustafson, P., Skytting, B., et al. (2001). Clinical impact of molecular and cytogenetic findings in synovial sarcoma. *Genes, Chromosomes & Cancer, 31*(4), 362–372.
225. Zollner, S. K., Rossig, C., & Toretsky, J. A. (2015). Synovial sarcoma is a gateway to the role of chromatin remodeling in cancer. *Cancer Metastasis Reviews, 34*(3), 417–428.
226. Thaete, C., Brett, D., Monaghan, P., Whitehouse, S., Rennie, G., Rayner, E., et al. (1999). Functional domains of the SYT and SYT-SSX synovial sarcoma translocation proteins and co-localization with the SNF protein BRM in the nucleus. *Human Molecular Genetics, 8*(4), 585–591.
227. Kato, H., Tjernberg, A., Zhang, W., Krutchinsky, A. N., An, W., Takeuchi, T., et al. (2002). SYT associates with human SNF/SWI complexes and the C-terminal region of its fusion partner SSX1 targets histones. *The Journal of Biological Chemistry, 277*(7), 5498–5505.
228. Middeljans, E., Wan, X., Jansen, P. W., Sharma, V., Stunnenberg, H. G., & Logie, C. (2012). SS18 together with animal-specific factors defines human BAF-type SWI/SNF complexes. *PLoS One, 7*(3), e33834.
229. Kadoch, C., & Crabtree, G. R. (2013). Reversible disruption of mSWI/SNF (BAF) complexes by the SS18-SSX oncogenic fusion in synovial sarcoma. *Cell, 153*(1), 71–85.
230. Soulez, M., Saurin, A. J., Freemont, P. S., & Knight, J. C. (1999). SSX and the synovial-sarcoma-specific chimaeric protein SYT-SSX co-localize with the human Polycomb group complex. *Oncogene, 18*(17), 2739–2746.
231. Grbavec, D., & Stifani, S. (1996). Molecular interaction between TLE1 and the carboxyl-terminal domain of HES-1 containing the WRPW motif. *Biochemical and Biophysical Research Communications, 223*(3), 701–705.
232. Su, L., Cheng, H., Sampaio, A. V., Nielsen, T. O., & Underhill, T. M. (2010). EGR1 reactivation by histone deacetylase inhibitors promotes synovial sarcoma cell death through the PTEN tumor suppressor. *Oncogene, 29*(30), 4352–4361.

233. Valente, A. L., Tull, J., & Zhang, S. (2013). Specificity of TLE1 expression in unclassified high-grade sarcomas for the diagnosis of synovial sarcoma. *Applied Immunohistochemistry & Molecular Morphology, 21*(5), 408–413.
234. Macy, M. E., Sawczyn, K. K., Garrington, T. P., Graham, D. K., & Gore, L. (2008). Pediatric developmental therapies: Interesting new drugs now in early-stage clinical trials. *Current Oncology Reports, 10*(6), 477–490.
235. Zweidler-McKay, P. A. (2008). Notch signaling in pediatric malignancies. *Current Oncology Reports, 10*(6), 459–468.
236. Fouladi, M., Stewart, C. F., Olson, J., Wagner, L. M., Onar-Thomas, A., Kocak, M., et al. (2011). Phase I trial of MK-0752 in children with refractory CNS malignancies: A pediatric brain tumor consortium study. *Journal of Clinical Oncology, 29*(26), 3529–3534.
237. Luistro, L., He, W., Smith, M., Packman, K., Vilenchik, M., Carvajal, D., et al. (2009). Preclinical profile of a potent gamma-secretase inhibitor targeting notch signaling with in vivo efficacy and pharmacodynamic properties. *Cancer Research, 69*(19), 7672–7680.
238. Messersmith, W. A., Shapiro, G. I., Cleary, J. M., Jimeno, A., Dasari, A., Huang, B., et al. (2015). A Phase I, dose-finding study in patients with advanced solid malignancies of the oral gamma-secretase inhibitor PF-03084014. *Clinical Cancer Research, 21*(1), 60–67.
239. De Strooper, B., Iwatsubo, T., & Wolfe, M. S. (2012). Presenilins and gamma-secretase: Structure, function, and role in Alzheimer disease. *Cold Spring Harbor Perspectives in Medicine, 2*(1), a006304.
240. Bigas, A., Martin, D. I., & Milner, L. A. (1998). Notch1 and Notch2 inhibit myeloid differentiation in response to different cytokines. *Molecular and Cellular Biology, 18*(4), 2324–2333.
241. Fan, X., Mikolaenko, I., Elhassan, I., Ni, X., Wang, Y., Ball, D., et al. (2004). Notch1 and notch2 have opposite effects on embryonal brain tumor growth. *Cancer Research, 64*(21), 7787–7793.
242. Shimizu, K., Chiba, S., Saito, T., Kumano, K., Hamada, Y., & Hirai, H. (2002). Functional diversity among Notch1, Notch2, and Notch3 receptors. *Biochemical and Biophysical Research Communications, 291*(4), 775–779.
243. Nefedova, Y., Cheng, P., Alsina, M., Dalton, W. S., & Gabrilovich, D. I. (2004). Involvement of Notch-1 signaling in bone marrow stroma-mediated de novo drug resistance of myeloma and other malignant lymphoid cell lines. *Blood, 103*(9), 3503–3510.
244. Graziani, I., Eliasz, S., De Marco, M. A., Chen, Y., Pass, H. I., De May, R. M., et al. (2008). Opposite effects of Notch-1 and Notch-2 on mesothelioma cell survival under hypoxia are exerted through the Akt pathway. *Cancer Research, 68*(23), 9678–9685.
245. Sun, Y., Lowther, W., Kato, K., Bianco, C., Kenney, N., Strizzi, L., et al. (2005). Notch4 intracellular domain binding to Smad3 and inhibition of the TGF-beta signaling. *Oncogene, 24*(34), 5365–5374.
246. Verginelli, F., Adesso, L., Limon, I., Alisi, A., Gueguen, M., Panera, N., et al. (2015). Activation of an endothelial Notch1-Jagged1 circuit induces VCAM1 expression, an effect amplified by interleukin-1beta. *Oncotarget, 6*(41), 43216–43229.
247. Chiorean, E. G., LoRusso, P., Strother, R. M., Diamond, J. R., Younger, A., Messersmith, W. A., et al. (2015). A phase I first-in-human study of enoticumab (REGN421), a fully human Delta-like ligand 4 (Dll4) monoclonal antibody in patients with advanced solid tumors. *Clinical Cancer Research, 21*(12), 2695–2703.
248. Weng, A. P., Nam, Y., Wolfe, M. S., Pear, W. S., Griffin, J. D., Blacklow, S. C., et al. (2003). Growth suppression of pre-T acute lymphoblastic leukemia cells by inhibition of notch signaling. *Molecular and Cellular Biology, 23*(2), 655–664.
249. Moellering, R. E., Cornejo, M., Davis, T. N., Del Bianco, C., Aster, J. C., Blacklow, S. C., et al. (2009). Direct inhibition of the NOTCH transcription factor complex. *Nature, 462*(7270), 182–188.
250. Funahashi, Y., Hernandez, S. L., Das, I., Ahn, A., Huang, J., Vorontchikhina, M., et al. (2008). A notch1 ectodomain construct inhibits endothelial notch signaling, tumor growth, and angiogenesis. *Cancer Research, 68*(12), 4727–4735.

251. Varnum-Finney, B., Wu, L., Yu, M., Brashem-Stein, C., Staats, S., Flowers, D., et al. (2000). Immobilization of Notch ligand, Delta-1, is required for induction of notch signaling. *Journal of Cell Science, 113*(Pt 23), 4313–4318.
252. Small, D., Kovalenko, D., Kacer, D., Liaw, L., Landriscina, M., Di Serio, C., et al. (2001). Soluble Jagged 1 represses the function of its transmembrane form to induce the formation of the Src-dependent chord-like phenotype. *The Journal of Biological Chemistry, 276*(34), 32022–32030.
253. Six, E., Ndiaye, D., Laabi, Y., Brou, C., Gupta-Rossi, N., Israel, A., et al. (2003). The Notch ligand Delta1 is sequentially cleaved by an ADAM protease and gamma-secretase. *Proceedings of the National Academy of Sciences of the United States of America, 100*(13), 7638–7643.
254. LaVoie, M. J., Fraering, P. C., Ostaszewski, B. L., Ye, W., Kimberly, W. T., Wolfe, M. S., et al. (2003). Assembly of the gamma-secretase complex involves early formation of an intermediate subcomplex of Aph-1 and nicastrin. *The Journal of Biological Chemistry, 278*(39), 37213–37222.

Chapter 12
Notch Ligands in Hematopoietic Stem Cell Production

Anna Bigas, Cristina Ruiz-Herguido, Rosa Aligué, and Lluís Espinosa

Abstract Hematopoietic transplantation has been a therapeutic option for leukemia patients for more than 50 years. Its possible applications have expanded in recent years with the success of gene therapy and gene-editing approaches that can now offer promising treatments for monogenic incurable diseases. Nowadays, the main limitation to apply this therapy is the availability of compatible donor stem cells and the complications of hematopoietic recovery, which could be attenuated by the recent breakthrough discoveries on the field of reprogramming. However, our knowledge how to produce hematopoietic stem cells is still limited to safely use this technology. In this review, we covered the key elements that should be considered for a better understanding of hematopoietic cell production in the embryo proper or from in vitro protocols and how Notch participates in this process.

Keywords Embryonic hematopoiesis · HSC · AGM · Fetal liver · Bone marrow · ES cells

12.1 Hematopoietic Stem Cells

12.1.1 Overview of Hematopoietic Stem Cell Production

Hematopoiesis is the process that generates the different types of blood cells and takes place during the whole life of an organism. Blood cells derive from a common ancestor or hematopoietic stem cell (HSC). HSCs are somatic, tissue-specific stem cells with multipotency and self-renewal capacity [4]. A single HSC is able to reconstitute the whole hematopoietic system of an immunodeficient receptor, and

A. Bigas (✉) · C. Ruiz-Herguido · L. Espinosa
Program in Cancer Research, CIBERONC, Institut Hospital del Mar d'Investigacions Mèdiques (IMIM), Barcelona, Spain
e-mail: abigas@imim.es

R. Aligué
Department of Cell Biology, CIBERONC, Facultat de Medicina. Universitat de Barcelona, Barcelona, Spain

L. Miele, S. Artavanis-Tsakonas (eds.), *Targeting Notch in Cancer*,
https://doi.org/10.1007/978-1-4939-8859-4_12

this unique trait is used to define a bona fide functional stem cell [27]. Thus, HSCs are the most robust source of blood cells, being the base of the hematopoietic transplantation therapies, which are common practice for leukemia treatments and other blood-related diseases. The main limitation for these treatments is the source of HLA-matched immune cells, which usually relies on family members or rare unrelated altruistic donors. Obtaining an unlimited source of compatible blood cells in vitro that could be used for transplantation would provide an alternative option for many patients. The understanding of the process that regulates HSC maintenance and differentiation is crucial for this purpose.

In the recent years, the stem cell scientific community has turned the focus of the investigations onto reprogramming and generation of newly formed HSC from embryonic cells. This is a promising and exciting field not only for hematopoietic production but also for other somatic stem cell types that could provide different sources of cell replacement. The demonstration that a combination of transcription factors can reprogram differentiated cells into pluripotent stem (PS) cells [82] led to a change of the paradigm and laid high expectations about the possibility of generating HSCs from autologous induced PS (iPS) or to directly reprogram cells into HSCs (iHSC). Investigations on this area have revealed striking parallelisms between the molecular mechanisms for HSC generation in vitro and the developmental processes that lead to HSC specification in the embryo. Thus, there is a clear need for a better understanding of this embryonic process.

Studies focused on the regulation of de novo formation or the expansion of HSCs in the embryo have identified candidate signals that will be relevant for this process.

For example, and after many years of discussion, Notch signaling is slowly settling in the field as a promising tool to amplify or generate HSC in vitro. However, many questions still remain related to the physiological Notch function in the hematopoietic system, likely associated with its complex and context-dependent effects. In this review, we will discuss the physiological involvement of Notch in the formation and maintenance of the hematopoietic system and how this signal can be manipulated to our benefit.

12.1.1.1 Overview of Embryonic and Adult Hematopoietic Development

Hematopoietic development in the vertebrate embryo occurs in waves (reviewed in [22]), adapted to fulfill the embryo necessities likely as a result of an evolutionary process. In the mammalian embryo, the first wave of hematopoietic cells takes place in the yolk sac, and it is known as primitive hematopoiesis. In the yolk sac, endothelial-like cells organize in vessel structures called blood islands where the first erythrocytes and macrophages are found. Next, the yolk sac will produce progenitors with definitive characteristics and erythroid/myeloid potential (EMPs) but without or with limited capacity to self-renew [17]. After the organization of the embryonic vascular tubes and alongside with artery specification, the next wave of hematopoiesis takes place closely associated with the endothelium of the aorta, the

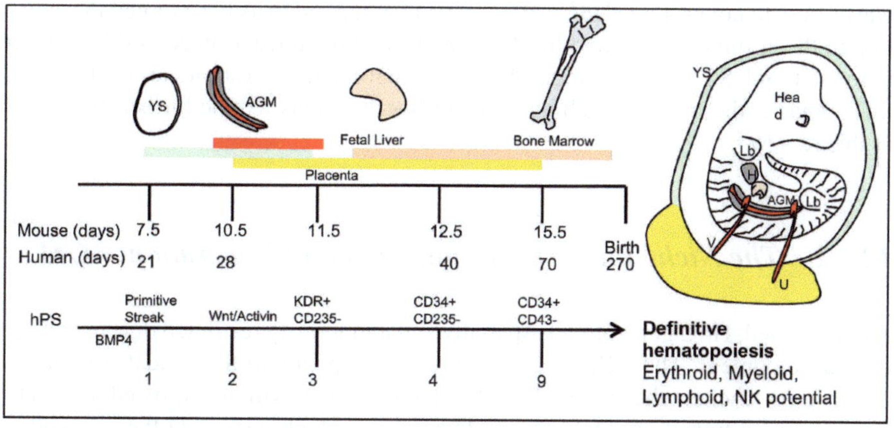

Fig. 12.1 Timing of hematopoietic development waves in the mouse and human embryo (upper) and in vitro human pluripotent (hPS) differentiation protocol for definitive hematopoiesis (lower) adapted from [80] (YS, yolk sac; Lb, limb buds; NK, natural killer; V, vitellin; U, umbilical)

umbilical and vitelline arteries, and the placenta [22] restricted to a very limited temporal window (E10–E12 in the mouse and week 4–5 in human). The aorta surrounded by the gonad and mesonephros (AGM) structures is the best characterized hemogenic tissue, both in mouse and human, with the capacity for HSC production [39, 57]. Cells with endothelial characteristics transit into a hematopoietic (EHT) phenotype and form cell clusters that emerge into the lumen of the aorta. It is within these clusters that a few cells are specified as definitive HSCs. Hematopoietic cells formed in the different embryonic sites (including the HSCs) and migrate then to the fetal liver, which becomes the main hematopoietic organ after E12 and until birth. Close to birth, hematopoiesis moves to the bone marrow of the long and flat bones, where it will reside through life (see scheme in Fig. 12.1).

12.1.1.2 Development of the Hematopoietic System In Vitro

Following the establishment of murine and human embryonic stem cell (ESC) lines [25, 83], important progress has been made to induce the differentiation into hematopoietic products and, ideally, use them as a source of HSCs [60]. Unfortunately, engraftment of ESC-derived hematopoietic cells has reproducibly failed. More recently, the implementation of induced pluripotent stem (iPS) cell techniques and the generation of personalized HSCs for clinical applications are viewed as realistic goals. Since in vitro HSC production is still a big limitation, a diversity of cytokine cocktails and differentiation protocols have been developed to mimic the normal differentiation of embryonic cells into hemogenic endothelium or hematopoietic stem cells. Most of these protocols can successfully reproduce the EHT process that occurs in embryonic sites, but cannot reproducibly generate HSCs. Thus, in vitro differentiation of PS cells is likely reproducing the first embryonic hematopoietic waves that do not produce HSCs. With these results, scientists have turned the attention to the stromal signals and the AGM niche and obtained a successful long-term repopulating HSC activity using different stromal-incubation strategies [37]. Within this scenario, the role of Notch ligands and Notch signals will be further developed in this review.

12.1.2 The Niche for HSC Specification and Generation: AGM

As mentioned, HSC generation is spatially and temporarily restricted during embryonic development. The AGM region, which corresponds to the caudal part of the dorsal aorta, shelters the endothelial-like precursors that will undergo endothelial to hematopoietic transition. Only few of these cells, which constitute the also called hemogenic endothelium, will become HSCs. However, to date there are no specific markers that single out HSC precursors from the rest of the hemogenic endothelium. This fact has greatly postponed defining the signals that affect HSC and HSC precursors directly from those affecting other cells in the AGM niche that can also influence HSC formation. Some of the identified cellular elements that are important in this process are endothelial/arterial cells, macrophages, mesenchyme, and neuronal/adrenal gland cells.

12.1.2.1 Endothelial/Arterial Cells in the AGM

Endothelial cells are important elements in the process of HSC formation for several reasons. First of all, there is a common ancestor of both lineages that, based on recent investigations, could be previous to the commitment of hemogenic endothelium and arterial specification [21, 30]. Secondly, hemogenic endothelium is immersed in the endothelial layer of the dorsal aorta at the time of HSC commitment. Third, the endothelial cell layers deliver signals that can activate Notch and Wnt pathways, which are essential for HSC commitment but also arterial specification [72, 76]. Moreover, arterial and HSC specification in the embryonic dorsal aorta occurs simultaneously or at least in the same time frame (for more details, see Sect. 12.2.1).

12.1.2.2 Subaortic Cells

The aorta is surrounded by mesenchymal cells originated from the splanchnic lateral plate and is later replaced by the sclerotomal-derived mesenchyme [68, 69, 92, 96]. Detection of cells expressing Gata2 and Gata3 mRNA or CD41 within the mesenchymal layer supported the idea that HSC precursors are located in the subaortic patches [8]. However, other structures also stain for these genes being difficult to interpret this result. For example, the adrenal gland precursors also express and depend on Gata3. Alternative attempts to demonstrate the putative mesenchymal origin of HSCs have also failed [68, 104]. It is likely that mesenchymal cells may serve as signal-sending cells required for hematopoietic development as was recently shown for BMP regulatory molecules [55]. In fact, stromal cell lines that have been obtained from AGM and support HSC development display mesenchymal features [16, 62]. However, the composition of this mesenchymal layer is not resolved, and cells with hemogenic characteristics with capability to become HSCs have been described (Rybtsov, Medvinsky). It is then conceivable that pre-HSC cells are intermingled in the mesenchyme in the subluminal layer of the aorta or that cells from the committed pre-HSC cells from the endothelial layer migrate to the subaortic layers.

12.1.2.3 Sympathetic Nervous System

A connection between the AGM niche and the nervous system was found by analyzing the Gata3 mutant embryos, which lack functional HSCs. Neuronal precursors for the adrenal gland are Gata3-expressing cells, reside in the subaortic mesenchyme, and are not found in the absence of Gata3. Thus, defective HSC formation in the GATA3-null mice was due to the absence of a catecholamine, which is normally synthesized by these neuronal precursors and required for the survival of nascent HSC. As a proof of concept, addition of exogenous catecholamines partially rescued the production of transplantable Gata3-deficient HSCs [28]. Interestingly, the production of adrenal gland derivatives and components of the nervous system are also critical in the migration and homing of adult HSCs to the bone marrow niche [40].

12.1.2.4 Macrophages

Macrophages are key cellular elements for the remodeling of developing tissues and during adulthood (rev. [97]). Studies with $CSF^{op/op}$ mice lacking macrophages due to a mutation in the colony-stimulating factor-1 gene (CSF-1 or M-CSF) were crucial to understand the role in osteogenesis, remodeling of bone marrow cavities, and the hematopoietic system [5]. More recently, macrophages were found to play an essential function in HSC emergence in zebrafish [85]. In this study, it was elegantly demonstrated that primitive macrophages are responsible for extracellular matrix degradation that permits the migration of HSPC through the AGM stroma to the posterior cardinal vein. Although one could argue that migration of the newly formed HSPC through the AGM stroma is a unique trait of the zebrafish system, the fact that CD68+ macrophages are also detected among the CD34+ human aortic clusters supports the possibility that this is a more general HSC regulatory mechanism.

12.1.3 The Niche for HSC Expansion: Fetal Liver and Placenta

HSCs are first detected in the AGM, but soon after, the placenta contains much higher HSC activity (about 15-fold compared to the AGM) [31, 63]. This observation revealed that the placenta was an important site for HSC amplification, before or simultaneous to the fetal liver [31]. Since circulation from the placenta to the embryo occurs through the umbilical artery, just upstream of the fetal liver, and HSC number in the placenta decreases concomitant to the increase in the fetal liver HSC potential, it was suggested that placenta-derived HSCs (and not the AGM-produced HSCs) colonize the fetal liver. Moreover, mutant embryos with heartbeat and circulation defects (ncx mutants) can produce lymphoid and myeloid cells, thus suggesting that HSCs may not only be generated in the AGM [71]. Moreover, some pre-HSCs present in the AGM require a maturation step in the fetal liver to become functional HSCs [10], but it is possible that the placenta can serve as a maturation niche similar to the fetal liver. In any case, the fetal liver is unequivocally a HSC expansion organ, as shown by detailed limiting dilution transplantation assays [11]. In these assays, fetal liver HSCs displayed a higher transplantation capacity than adult bone marrow cells that was directly linked to differences in their expression profile [41].

In the human embryo, the site of origin of the HSCs is uniquely associated with the AGM region as early as 32–33 days postfertilization [38], but it is not until week 9 of gestation that HSCs are robustly detected [75].

12.1.4 Bone Marrow Niche: Maintenance of HSC

Close to birth, HSCs migrate to the bone marrow where they reside all through adulthood. A tightly controlled balance between self-renewal and differentiation is required to avoid life-threatening hematopoietic malignancies. For this reason, the detailed characterization of the elements that compose the bone marrow niche and the signals that control hematopoietic homeostasis is still an important topic of investigation.

Inside the long and flat bones, there is soft tissue formed by an endosteal layer that recovers the osteoblast tissue. This endosteal tissue and the endothelium of the small vessels contain the cells that more closely associate with the HSCs and regulate their functions [15, 42, 100]. Discussion on the nature of the bona fide HSC niche is still ongoing although imaging technology is rapidly developing and its application to bone marrow imaging is already happening [52]. For example, it was recently shown that different types of capillary structures affect HSC activity [1]. Current and future studies using this technology should be able to uncover most of these questions.

Other elements of the bone marrow niche include the arterioles, which are surrounded by sympathetic nerves, smooth muscle cells, and matrix components and differ from other venule sinusoids. They express specific markers such as sca1 and NG2+ and localize adjacent to the HSCs. Other stromal cell types that are also important in the maintenance of HSCs are mesenchymal stem cells characterized by nestin expression [58].

The bone marrow contains not only the HSC population but also most of the differentiating hematopoietic cell types that originate from them. Importantly, HSC, progenitors, and differentiated cells were shown to send signals to the HSCs, thus regulating its self-renewal capacity and differentiation [12, 103]. Recently, the identification of dormant HSC (in comparison to the active HSCs) has provided valuable data in relation with stromal specific cells that may regulate particular HSC stages. Dormant HSCs divide about five to six times in the whole life of a mouse in homeostatic conditions; however, they become crucial in stress conditions such as bone marrow transplantation or hematopoietic recovery after insults (infections or chemotherapy). Arterioles have been shown to be essential to maintain HSC quiescence, in the dormant population [47].

12.1.5 *Ex Vivo Production of HSC*

Since the discovery of ES cells (mouse and human), many efforts have concentrated on using them as a source of HSC. Although ES cells can produce many types of hematopoietic cells and progenitors, no reliable protocols are currently available to generate cells with engraftment capacity or HSC activity. In fact, hematopoietic production from ES cells closely resembles the primitive hematopoietic wave that occurs in the yolk sac. This observation strongly suggests that signals required for HSC specification are different from that required for hematopoietic production and highlights the need for their identification. Recently, different reprogramming strategies have been more successful in obtaining cells with hematopoietic transplantation capacity. For example, some HSPC activity has been obtained from fibroblasts reprogrammed with the transcription factors Gata2, Gfi1b, cFos, and Etv1 [67] or Erg, Lmo2, Runx1, Gata2, and SCL [3]. However, only in one study in which murine B cells were reprogrammed using Runt1t1, Hlf, Lmo2, Pbx1, and Zfp37 has reported long-term repopulation capacity [91]. Another recent report has been able to induce ESC differentiation into HSC by using a combination of another seven transcription factors (erg, HoxA5, HoxA9, HoxA10, LCOR, Runx1, and Spi1) [81]. Lastly, a very promising strategy has come from direct conversion of human adult endothelial cells into long-term engrafting HSCs, which was achieved by Rafii's group. By exploring combinations of transcription factors, they found that Fosb, Gfi1, Runx1, and Spi1 (FGRS) can reprogram endothelial cells, generating HSCs with engraftment potential [77] and T-cell immunity potential [49].

Together these studies show that de novo generation of HSCs in vitro is feasible, but the translation into clinical application resides in activating and controlling the expression of endogenous transcription factors without genetic manipulation. In this sense, the control of developmental pathways (Notch, Wnt, HH, or FGF) that respond to extracellular cues should be crucial to achieve this regulation.

12.2 Notch and Notch Ligands in Hematopoietic Stem Cell Niches

From development to adulthood, each hematopoietic wave and process has a different requirement for Notch activity. Since Notch activation is governed by cell-cell interaction and ligand-receptor availability, the specific Notch activity is delivered and controlled by the niche.

12.2.1 Notch Ligands in HSC Specification

Work from different groups unequivocally shows that Notch is required for the proper development of the hematopoietic system. Although this is still a matter of investigation, data in mouse and zebrafish embryos demonstrated that Notch is essential to specify the hemogenic endothelium and/or HSCs [14, 46, 74]. Notch is however dispensable for the generation of primitive and definitive blood cells in the yolk sac [7, 36, 73]. The pioneer study from Hirai's lab in 2003 analyzed Notch1- and Notch2-deficient embryos and observed a profound hematopoietic defect with lack of HSC activity specifically in the Notch1-deficient embryos. Other studies in mouse and zebrafish models confirmed that definitive hematopoiesis was impaired in Notch mutants [14]. The fact that Notch loss-of-function embryos also lacked arterial identity, which disturbs the niche for nascent HSCs, was not appropriately considered by most of these studies. However, in the zebrafish embryo, the ectopic activation of Notch in the vein resulted in hematopoietic production, which suggests that the preexistence of arterial identity was not required [14]. In 2008, we found that Jag1 mutant embryos preserved the arterial identity but lacked definitive hematopoiesis in the AGM [74]. This observation was crucial in the understanding of Notch signaling in HSC determination, allowed uncoupling the role of Notch in arterial and HSC specification, and demonstrated that a productive Notch signal was required for both processes. The latter was confirmed by analyzing Notch target genes that are important for the correct specification of HSC [34, 35]. However, Notch signals are not just on and off but rather defined by levels of activity. Using Notch activity reporters with different sensitivities, we have recently confirmed that HSC precursors in the AGM do not experience high Notch activity as opposed to the arterial cells, but they descend from cells that experienced low Notch activity [30]. The right Notch activity level is achieved by the interplay of Jag1- and Dll4-delivered signals, being Jag1 required to maintain low Notch active levels and prevent arterial specification in the hemogenic precursors. Recently, other mechanisms involved in maintaining lower levels of Notch activity have been described in EHT. For example, inhibition of sox17 is required to downregulate Notch1 transcriptionally [51], while G-protein-coupled receptor (gpr) 183 contributes to Notch degradation [101]. These results can be reconciled in a model in which hemogenic endothelial precursors refrain from turning on the arterial program by partially inhibiting the Notch pathway. Afterward, they will require Notch activation (at a lower level) to activate HSC-specific Notch-dependent target genes such as Gata2 [35]. Finally, hematopoietic development will become Notch independent at the end of HSC maturation [79].

12.2.2 Notch Signaling in the Fetal Liver

As mentioned, the fetal liver is the main site for HSC amplification during embryonic development. The understanding of this process is crucial for improving protocols for HSC expansion. Until recently, the role of Notch in this process has remained unknown. Evidence that Notch is not only involved in HSC determination but also in HSC amplification comes from the analysis of a Notch1 hypomorphic mutant, carrying a deletion of the transcriptional activation domain (TAD) [32]. In this model, the amount of Notch1 signal is enough to allow the generation of the HSC in the AGM, but it is not enough for proper expansion of the HSC pool in the liver. This activity has not been associated with any specific ligand yet although early studies did show the presence of Jag1 and Delta1 expression in the E12–E17 murine fetal liver by in situ hybridization [90], while Delta4 and Jag2 were not determined. Different ligands seem to signal similarly downstream of Notch receptor; however, they exhibit different efficiencies in activating Notch, which results in different Notch signal strengths [86]. Taking into account results from other cell types, the strength of Notch activity delivered by Dll4 is higher than that delivered by Dll1, which is also higher than that induced by Jagged ligands. We speculate that Dll1 ligand is a good candidate for regulating Notch-mediated fetal liver HSC amplification. In fact, most of the in vitro amplification studies have been performed with Dll1 (see Sect. 12.3).

Furthermore, several tissues simultaneously express two or more Notch ligands, and it is the activity of fringe glycosyltransferases that modulate the ability of the Notch receptor to interact with each individual ligand [98]. For example, it was first described in the Drosophila wing margin formation that glycosylated Notch has higher affinity to bind to Delta but lower affinity to bind to Serrate (orthologue for Jagged) [29]. This observation has been reproduced in vertebrates, not only involving trans-activation but also cis-inhibition of Notch signals, which result in several Notch-sending and Notch-receiving cellular states [48]. In mammals, four Notch receptors, five Notch ligands, and three different fringes can produce a whole range of Notch states that can explain several contradictory observations for Notch phenotypes. Further research in this direction should help to elucidate the appropriate Notch state that is compatible with HSC formation and HSC expansion.

12.2.3 Notch Ligands in the Bone Marrow

The bone marrow niche is involved in maintaining the HSC fitness during the lifespan of an organism. As described above, different cellular components residing in the bone marrow are involved in this function through both cell-cell interactions and secreted molecules. As example, the Notch ligand Jag1 that is present in the surface of the endosteal cells has indirectly been associated with the maintenance of the quiescent state of LT-HSC [15]. However, other studies using loss-of-function mouse models did not confirm the requirement for Notch in the adult HSC compartment. These studies include the Notch1- [70] and Jagged1 [54]-deficient mice, the dominant-negative of mastermind transgenic (blocks Notch signaling), and the RBPj-deficient mice [53]. Interestingly, detailed analysis of Notch2 mutant mice revealed a role for Notch2 in the proliferation and myeloid differentiation of short-term HSC that affected regeneration of the bone marrow after 5-FU treatment [88]. In contrast, the best characterized effect of Notch1 activity disruption is the impairment of T-cell development, which is also observed after specific Notch pathway abrogation in the hematopoietic system [70].

Analysis of other Notch pathway mutants uncovers the presence of myeloid proliferative defects, which are both cell autonomous and non-cell autonomous. This is the case of hematopoietic deletion of Nicastrin; compound Notch1, Notch2, and Notch3; RBPj [44]; presenilin [78]; and pofut [99]. Thus, although interpretation of all these data remains controversial, it highlights the importance of Notch in the regulation of hematopoietic homeostasis.

12.2.4 Notch in Hematopoietic Differentiation and Leukemia

Notch1 and Notch3 are required to control T-cell development, and their constitutive activation in hematopoietic progenitors unequivocally results in T-cell leukemia [6, 65]. During normal T-cell differentiation, cells need to activate Notch at the double-negative (DN) 1 stage and turn it off after the DN3 stage. This is a tightly regulated process that involves essential transcriptional Notch targets such as hes1, il7r, and deltex.

Following the initial cloning of Notch1 as a rare translocation present in T-ALL patients [23], its pathological relevance was confirmed by the identification of

Notch1 mutations in more than 60% of all T-ALL patient samples [94]. This finding has been extensively confirmed, and it is now evidenced that most T-cell transformation requires Notch activity to occur. However, which are the mechanisms and the downstream effectors of Notch in this disease is not totally understood. Many Notch target genes have been identified in T-ALL models including Myc [95], CCR7 [13], IL7 receptor alpha [33], Hes1 [93], and Notch3 itself [66], among others. The relevance of these targets in T-ALL has been confirmed in different experimental models, and each one has a specific impact on the leukemic process. For example, CCR7 is responsible for the infiltration of tumor cells in the central nervous system (CNS). Hes1 is involved in repressing important tumor suppressor genes such as PTEN [64] and CYLD [24], which directly impinge on the PI3K/Akt and NF-κB pathways, respectively. Surprisingly, several years after the identification of Notch as a tumor driver in T-ALL, it is now clear that Notch mutations confer good prognosis in response to current chemotherapy treatment protocols [26].

In addition to its role in T-ALL, Notch has also some effect on myeloid differentiation and can affect early erythropoiesis and/or megakaryopoiesis [59, 61], as it has been mentioned. Also, recent data suggests that Notch is essential for hematopoietic regeneration after immunodepletion [43, 88].

12.3 Manipulation of Notch Signal Ex Vivo

12.3.1 Notch Ligands in the Expansion of HSC and Progenitors

Notch activity associates with stem cell self-renewal and inhibition of cell differentiation in many different tissues (reviewed in [9]. More recently, endosomal segregation of Notch components has been found to regulate stem cell fate in the drosophila CNS and the gut but also in the neural precursors of the spinal cord in zebrafish [18, 45]. These observations have led to nominate Notch as a good candidate to promote HSC self-renewal and amplification, although the experimental evidences for this assumption are still weak. Among them, early studies showed that constitutive activation of Notch in the murine hematopoietic precursors (lin-sca1 + kit+ cells) resulted in a self-renewal multipotent cell line capable of lymphoid and myeloid reconstitution [89]. This result was a proof of concept that Notch could be used to amplify HSPC. In this line, the Bernstein group has pioneered studies demonstrating the possibility to expand hematopoietic progenitors, and to improve their engraftment capacity, by culturing them on recombinant ligands such as Delta1 (the most used in these studies) [87]. Of special interest is the expansion of cord blood (CB) progenitors on Delta1 ligand as described below [20].

12.3.2 Notch Ligands in Hematopoietic Transplantation

The number of putative clinical application for recombinant Notch ligands is rapidly increasing, and in fact, there is an ongoing clinical trial for CB expansion and transplantation. Among the advantages of CB as a potential source of hematopoietic progenitor cells for transplantation are the availability and the easy access to HLA-compatible units worldwide. However, the limited number of transplantable cells that are provided from each cord blood unit is still a problem that can lead to engraftment failure. One approach to circumvent this problem has been the transplantation of double CB (dCB) units, which has greatly improved the donor engraftment but not neutrophil recovery. Thus, dCB transplantation is becoming a fantastic model to functionally test expansion protocols. Based on promising preclinical studies, Bernstein and colleagues have now designed a phase 1 clinical trial for patients undergoing CB transplantation. In this trial, one non-manipulated CB unit is transplanted along with a second CB unit (CD34+ cells) that has undergone ex vivo expansion on Delta1. This trial is still ongoing, but some early conclusions have already been reported from the first ten patients such as the short-term engraftment and the faster recovery of absolute neutrophil count [19].

In addition to HSC expansion, Notch signaling could be modified to prevent graft-versus-host disease (GVHD) in transplantation procedures. In this sense, different biochemical and genetic approaches in several models showed that Notch depletion in the T cells efficiently protects from acute GVHD in allo-HCT recipients [102]. Mechanistically, Notch inhibition blocked the production of multiple inflammatory cytokines by alloreactive T cells. In addition, Notch-depleted T cells retained potent cytotoxic effects against allogeneic targets and were able to eliminate host-type leukemic cells, leading to long-term disease-free survival while preventing GVHD. More recently, Maillard and colleagues have identified Dll4 as the ligand responsible for alloreactivity in T cells. This is therapeutically relevant since blockage of Dll4 with antibodies at early time points after transplantation of allo-HCT in murine models decreased GVHD incidence and severity without causing global immunosuppression [84].

12.3.3 Notch Ligands in HSC Generation

Notch is essential for the first steps of HSC development in vivo, although the mechanistic base is not completely understood (see Sect. 12.1.2.1). The lack of knowledge and the complexity of HSC specification have delayed the success of reproducing this process in vitro from ESC or iPS. To gain light into the HSC specification process, Daley and colleagues have compared the transcriptome of different embryo-derived subpopulations of cells with HSC potential and ES-derived cells with HSC phenotype (CD41+, CD45+, CD34+) [56]. One of the conclusions of this study was that ESC-derived HSC lacked the activation of the Notch pathway when compared with their embryo-derived counterparts. This pioneer study was performed before the general implementation of RNA-Seq, and the authors needed more than 2,500 embryos to perform the analysis. Thus, although the reported observation highlighted the importance of Notch signaling in the generation of actual HSCs, improvement of current genomic techniques should provide more accurate information on this process, especially at a single-cell level. In a more

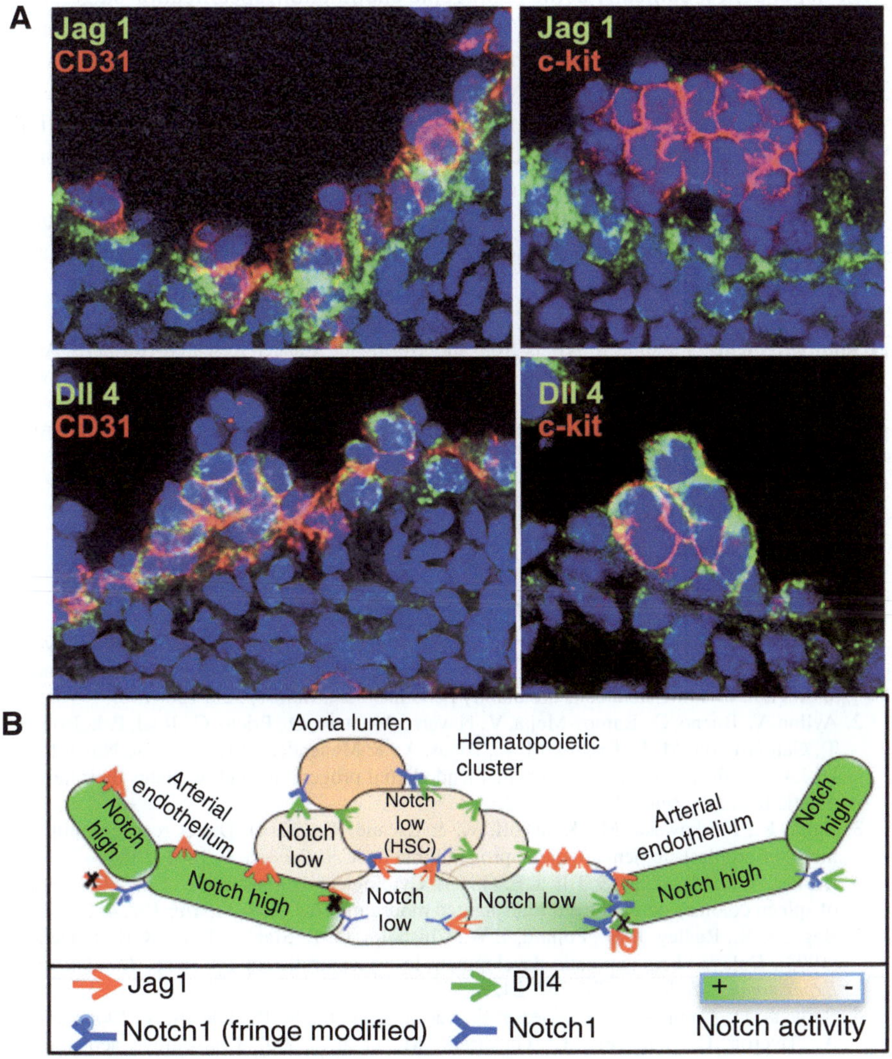

Fig. 12.2 Model for Notch signaling in HSC specification. (**a**) Notch ligands (Jag1 and Dll4) distribution in embryonic aortic endothelium (expressing CD31) and cluster cells (expressing c-kit and CD31). (**b**) Model for HSC and arterial endothelium specification in the embryonic aorta (AGM)

comprehensive characterization of cells arising in the ESC-derived cultures, Menendez and colleagues observed that embryo body-derived cells with endothelial or hematopoietic potential can be separated by the levels of the Dll4 protein [2].

On the other hand, studies from the Keller lab have been essential to improve the current protocols for ESC-HSC development. By using activin/nodal/TGFb and Wnt-b-catenin activation, they distinguished between primitive and definitive hematopoieses [80] and found that definitive hematopoiesis with lymphoid capacity was Wnt-dependent specifically at the hemogenic endothelium specification stage. More recently, this precursor was shown to be different from the one undergoing arterial/venous fate decision. Moreover, the definitive hemogenic precursor was shown to be Notch dependent [21]. These observations are in agreement with our results obtained with the Notch activation reporters N1::CRE [50], which can differentially report Notch activity levels. Our conclusions from the analysis of these embryos were that arteries require high Notch activity levels, whereas in hematopoietic precursors, Notch levels are kept low (only reported with the more sensitive mouse, N1::Cre^{HI}) to induce/preserve the hematopoietic commitment while preventing arterial specification [30] (see model in Fig. 12.2).

Acknowledgments Funding to AB is from the Worldwide Cancer Research (formerly AICR, 13-0064), Fundación AECC (Cancer infantil), Ministerio de Economía y Competitividad (SAF2013-40922-R and SAF2016-75613-R), Red Temática de Investigación Cooperativa en Cáncer (RD12/0036/0054), and Agència de Gestió d'Ajuts Universitaris i de Recerca (AGAUR) (2014SGR-124).

References

1. Acar, M., Kocherlakota, K. S., Murphy, M. M., Peyer, J. G., Oguro, H., Inra, C. N., Jaiyeola, C., Zhao, Z., Luby-Phelps, K., & Morrison, S. J. (2015). Deep imaging of bone marrow shows non-dividing stem cells are mainly perisinusoidal. *Nature, 526*, 126–130.
2. Ayllon, V., Bueno, C., Ramos-Mejia, V., Navarro-Montero, O., Prieto, C., Real, P. J., Romero, T., Garcia-Leon, M. J., Toribio, M. L., Bigas, A., & Menendez, P. (2015). The Notch ligand DLL4 specifically marks human hematoendothelial progenitors and regulates their hematopoietic fate. *Leukemia, 29*, 1741–1753.
3. Batta, K., Florkowska, M., Kouskoff, V., & Lacaud, G. (2014). Direct reprogramming of murine fibroblasts to hematopoietic progenitor cells. *Cell Reports, 9*, 1871–1884.
4. Becker, A. J., Mc, C. E., & Till, J. E. (1963). Cytological demonstration of the clonal nature of spleen colonies derived from transplanted mouse marrow cells. *Nature, 197*, 452–454.
5. Begg, S. K., Radley, J. M., Pollard, J. W., Chisholm, O. T., Stanley, E. R., & Bertoncello, I. (1993). Delayed hematopoietic development in osteopetrotic (op/op) mice. *The Journal of Experimental Medicine, 177*, 237–242.
6. Bellavia, D., Campese, A. F., Alesse, E., Vacca, A., Felli, M. P., Balestri, A., Stoppacciaro, A., Tiveron, C., Tatangelo, L., Giovarelli, M., et al. (2000). Constitutive activation of NF-kappaB and T-cell leukemia/lymphoma in notch3 transgenic mice. *The EMBO Journal, 19*, 3337–3348.
7. Bertrand, J. Y., Cisson, J. L., Stachura, D. L., & Traver, D. (2010). Notch signaling distinguishes 2 waves of definitive hematopoiesis in the zebrafish embryo. *Blood, 115*, 2777–2783.

8. Bertrand, J. Y., Giroux, S., Golub, R., Klaine, M., Jalil, A., Boucontet, L., Godin, I., & Cumano, A. (2005). Characterization of purified intraembryonic hematopoietic stem cells as a tool to define their site of origin. *Proceedings of the National Academy of Sciences of the United States of America, 102*, 134–139.
9. Bigas, A., & Espinosa, L. (2012). Hematopoietic stem cells: To be or Notch to be. *Blood, 119*, 3226–3235.
10. Boisset, J. C., Clapes, T., Klaus, A., Papazian, N., Onderwater, J., Mommaas-Kienhuis, M., Cupedo, T., & Robin, C. (2015). Progressive maturation toward hematopoietic stem cells in the mouse embryo aorta. *Blood, 125*, 465–469.
11. Bowie, M. B., Kent, D. G., Dykstra, B., McKnight, K. D., McCaffrey, L., Hoodless, P. A., & Eaves, C. J. (2007). Identification of a new intrinsically timed developmental checkpoint that reprograms key hematopoietic stem cell properties. *Proceedings of the National Academy of Sciences of the United States of America, 104*, 5878–5882.
12. Bruns, I., Lucas, D., Pinho, S., Ahmed, J., Lambert, M. P., Kunisaki, Y., Scheiermann, C., Schiff, L., Poncz, M., Bergman, A., & Frenette, P. S. (2014). Megakaryocytes regulate hematopoietic stem cell quiescence through CXCL4 secretion. *Nature Medicine, 20*, 1315–1320.
13. Buonamici, S., Trimarchi, T., Ruocco, M. G., Reavie, L., Cathelin, S., Mar, B. G., Klinakis, A., Lukyanov, Y., Tseng, J. C., Sen, F., et al. (2009). CCR7 signalling as an essential regulator of CNS infiltration in T-cell leukaemia. *Nature, 459*, 1000–1004.
14. Burns, C. E., Traver, D., Mayhall, E., Shepard, J. L., & Zon, L. I. (2005). Hematopoietic stem cell fate is established by the Notch-Runx pathway. *Genes & Development, 19*, 2331–2342.
15. Calvi, L. M., Adams, G. B., Weibrecht, K. W., Weber, J. M., Olson, D. P., Knight, M. C., Martin, R. P., Schipani, E., Divieti, P., Bringhurst, F. R., et al. (2003). Osteoblastic cells regulate the haematopoietic stem cell niche. *Nature, 425*, 841–846.
16. Charbord, P., Pouget, C., Binder, H., Dumont, F., Stik, G., Levy, P., Allain, F., Marchal, C., Richter, J., Uzan, B., et al. (2014). A systems biology approach for defining the molecular framework of the hematopoietic stem cell niche. *Cell Stem Cell, 15*, 376–391.
17. Chen, M. J., Li, Y., De Obaldia, M. E., Yang, Q., Yzaguirre, A. D., Yamada-Inagawa, T., Vink, C. S., Bhandoola, A., Dzierzak, E., & Speck, N. A. (2011). Erythroid/myeloid progenitors and hematopoietic stem cells originate from distinct populations of endothelial cells. *Cell Stem Cell, 9*, 541–552.
18. Coumailleau, F., Furthauer, M., Knoblich, J. A., & Gonzalez-Gaitan, M. (2009). Directional Delta and Notch trafficking in Sara endosomes during asymmetric cell division. *Nature, 458*, 1051–1055.
19. Dahlberg, A., Delaney, C., & Bernstein, I. D. (2011). Ex vivo expansion of human hematopoietic stem and progenitor cells. *Blood, 117*, 6083–6090.
20. Delaney, C., Heimfeld, S., Brashem-Stein, C., Voorhies, H., Manger, R. L., & Bernstein, I. D. (2010). Notch-mediated expansion of human cord blood progenitor cells capable of rapid myeloid reconstitution. *Nature Medicine, 16*, 232–236.
21. Ditadi, A., Sturgeon, C. M., Tober, J., Awong, G., Kennedy, M., Yzaguirre, A. D., Azzola, L., Ng, E. S., Stanley, E. G., French, D. L., et al. (2015). Human definitive haemogenic endothelium and arterial vascular endothelium represent distinct lineages. *Nature Cell Biology, 17*, 580–591.
22. Dzierzak, E., & Speck, N. A. (2008). Of lineage and legacy: The development of mammalian hematopoietic stem cells. *Nature Immunology, 9*, 129–136.
23. Ellisen, L. W., Bird, J., West, D. C., Soreng, A. L., Reynolds, T. C., Smith, S. D., & Sklar, J. (1991). TAN-1, the human homolog of the Drosophila Notch gene, is broken by chromosomal translocations in T lymphoblastic neoplasms. *Cell, 66*, 649–661.
24. Espinosa, L., Cathelin, S., D'Altri, T., Trimarchi, T., Statnikov, A., Guiu, J., Rodilla, V., Ingles-Esteve, J., Nomdedeu, J., Bellosillo, B., et al. (2010). The Notch/Hes1 pathway sustains NF-kappaB activation through CYLD repression in T cell leukemia. *Cancer Cell, 18*, 268–281.

25. Evans, M. J., & Kaufman, M. H. (1981). Establishment in culture of pluripotential cells from mouse embryos. *Nature, 292*, 154–156.
26. Ferrando, A. (2010). NOTCH mutations as prognostic markers in T-ALL. *Leukemia, 24*, 2003–2004.
27. Ferrebee, J. W., Lochte, H. L., Jr., Jaretzki, A., 3rd, Sahler, O. D., & Thomas, E. D. (1958). Successful marrow homograft in the dog after radiation. *Surgery, 43*, 516–520.
28. Fitch, S. R., Kimber, G. M., Wilson, N. K., Parker, A., Mirshekar-Syahkal, B., Gottgens, B., Medvinsky, A., Dzierzak, E., & Ottersbach, K. (2012). Signaling from the sympathetic nervous system regulates hematopoietic stem cell emergence during embryogenesis. *Cell Stem Cell, 11*, 554–566.
29. Fleming, R. J., Gu, Y., & Hukriede, N. A. (1997). Serrate-mediated activation of Notch is specifically blocked by the product of the gene fringe in the dorsal compartment of the Drosophila wing imaginal disc. *Development, 124*, 2973–2981.
30. Gama-Norton, L., Ferrando, E., Ruiz-Herguido, C., Liu, Z., Guiu, J., Islam, A. B., Lee, S. U., Yan, M., Guidos, C. J., Lopez-Bigas, N., et al. (2015). Notch signal strength controls cell fate in the haemogenic endothelium. *Nature Communications, 6*, 8510.
31. Gekas, C., Dieterlen-Lievre, F., Orkin, S. H., & Mikkola, H. K. (2005). The placenta is a niche for hematopoietic stem cells. *Developmental Cell, 8*, 365–375.
32. Gerhardt, D. M., Pajcini, K. V., D'Altri, T., Tu, L., Jain, R., Xu, L., Chen, M. J., Rentschler, S., Shestova, O., Wertheim, G. B., et al. (2014). The Notch1 transcriptional activation domain is required for development and reveals a novel role for Notch1 signaling in fetal hematopoietic stem cells. *Genes & Development, 28*, 576–593.
33. Gonzalez-Garcia, S., Garcia-Peydro, M., Martin-Gayo, E., Ballestar, E., Esteller, M., Bornstein, R., de la Pompa, J. L., Ferrando, A. A., & Toribio, M. L. (2009). CSL-MAML-dependent Notch1 signaling controls T lineage-specific IL-7R{alpha} gene expression in early human thymopoiesis and leukemia. *The Journal of Experimental Medicine, 206*, 779–791.
34. Guiu, J., Bergen, D. J., De Pater, E., Islam, A. B., Ayllon, V., Gama-Norton, L., Ruiz-Herguido, C., Gonzalez, J., Lopez-Bigas, N., Menendez, P., et al. (2014). Identification of Cdca7 as a novel Notch transcriptional target involved in hematopoietic stem cell emergence. *The Journal of Experimental Medicine, 211*, 2411–2423.
35. Guiu, J., Shimizu, R., D'Altri, T., Fraser, S. T., Hatakeyama, J., Bresnick, E. H., Kageyama, R., Dzierzak, E., Yamamoto, M., Espinosa, L., & Bigas, A. (2013). Hes repressors are essential regulators of hematopoietic stem cell development downstream of Notch signaling. *The Journal of Experimental Medicine, 210*, 71–84.
36. Hadland, B. K., Huppert, S. S., Kanungo, J., Xue, Y., Jiang, R., Gridley, T., Conlon, R. A., Cheng, A. M., Kopan, R., & Longmore, G. D. (2004). A requirement for Notch1 distinguishes 2 phases of definitive hematopoiesis during development. *Blood, 104*, 3097–3105.
37. Hadland, B. K., Varnum-Finney, B., Poulos, M. G., Moon, R. T., Butler, J. M., Rafii, S., & Bernstein, I. D. (2015). Endothelium and NOTCH specify and amplify aorta-gonad-mesonephros-derived hematopoietic stem cells. *The Journal of Clinical Investigation, 125*, 2032–2045.
38. Ivanovs, A., Rybtsov, S., Anderson, R. A., Turner, M. L., & Medvinsky, A. (2014). Identification of the niche and phenotype of the first human hematopoietic stem cells. *Stem Cell Reports, 2*, 449–456.
39. Ivanovs, A., Rybtsov, S., Welch, L., Anderson, R. A., Turner, M. L., & Medvinsky, A. (2011). Highly potent human hematopoietic stem cells first emerge in the intraembryonic aorta-gonad-mesonephros region. *The Journal of Experimental Medicine, 208*, 2417–2427.
40. Katayama, Y., Battista, M., Kao, W. M., Hidalgo, A., Peired, A. J., Thomas, S. A., & Frenette, P. S. (2006). Signals from the sympathetic nervous system regulate hematopoietic stem cell egress from bone marrow. *Cell, 124*, 407–421.
41. Kent, D. G., Copley, M. R., Benz, C., Wohrer, S., Dykstra, B. J., Ma, E., Cheyne, J., Zhao, Y., Bowie, M. B., Zhao, Y., et al. (2009). Prospective isolation and molecular characterization of hematopoietic stem cells with durable self-renewal potential. *Blood, 113*, 6342–6350.

42. Kiel, M. J., Yilmaz, O. H., Iwashita, T., Yilmaz, O. H., Terhorst, C., & Morrison, S. J. (2005). SLAM family receptors distinguish hematopoietic stem and progenitor cells and reveal endothelial niches for stem cells. *Cell, 121*, 1109–1121.
43. Kim, J. H., Thimmulappa, R. K., Kumar, V., Cui, W., Kumar, S., Kombairaju, P., Zhang, H., Margolick, J., Matsui, W., Macvittie, T., et al. (2014). NRF2-mediated Notch pathway activation enhances hematopoietic reconstitution following myelosuppressive radiation. *The Journal of Clinical Investigation, 124*, 730–741.
44. Klinakis, A., Lobry, C., Abdel-Wahab, O., Oh, P., Haeno, H., Buonamici, S., van De Walle, I., Cathelin, S., Trimarchi, T., Araldi, E., et al. (2011). A novel tumour-suppressor function for the Notch pathway in myeloid leukaemia. *Nature, 473*, 230–233.
45. Kressmann, S., Campos, C., Castanon, I., Furthauer, M., & Gonzalez-Gaitan, M. (2015). Directional Notch trafficking in Sara endosomes during asymmetric cell division in the spinal cord. *Nature Cell Biology, 17*, 333–339.
46. Kumano, K., Chiba, S., Kunisato, A., Sata, M., Saito, T., Nakagami-Yamaguchi, E., Yamaguchi, T., Masuda, S., Shimizu, K., Takahashi, T., et al. (2003). Notch1 but not Notch2 is essential for generating hematopoietic stem cells from endothelial cells. *Immunity, 18*, 699–711.
47. Kunisaki, Y., Bruns, I., Scheiermann, C., Ahmed, J., Pinho, S., Zhang, D., Mizoguchi, T., Wei, Q., Lucas, D., Ito, K., et al. (2013). Arteriolar niches maintain haematopoietic stem cell quiescence. *Nature, 502*, 637–643.
48. LeBon, L., Lee, T. V., Sprinzak, D., Jafar-Nejad, H., & Elowitz, M. B. (2014). Fringe proteins modulate Notch-ligand cis and trans interactions to specify signaling states. *eLife, 3*, e02950.
49. Lis, R., Karrasch, C. C., Poulos, M. G., Kunar, B., Redmond, D., Duran, J. G. B., Badwe, C. R., Schachterle, W., Ginsberg, M., Xiang, J., et al. (2017). Conversion of adult endothelium to immunocompetent haematopoietic stem cells. *Nature, 545*, 439–445.
50. Liu, Z., Brunskill, E., Boyle, S., Chen, S., Turkoz, M., Guo, Y., Grant, R., & Kopan, R. (2015). Second-generation Notch1 activity-trap mouse line (N1IP::CreHI) provides a more comprehensive map of cells experiencing Notch1 activity. *Development, 142*, 1193–1202.
51. Lizama, C. O., Hawkins, J. S., Schmitt, C. E., Bos, F. L., Zape, J. P., Cautivo, K. M., Borges Pinto, H., Rhyner, A. M., Yu, H., Donohoe, M. E., et al. (2015). Repression of arterial genes in hemogenic endothelium is sufficient for haematopoietic fate acquisition. *Nature Communications, 6*, 7739.
52. Lo Celso, C., Fleming, H. E., Wu, J. W., Zhao, C. X., Miake-Lye, S., Fujisaki, J., Cote, D., Rowe, D. W., Lin, C. P., & Scadden, D. T. (2009). Live-animal tracking of individual haematopoietic stem/progenitor cells in their niche. *Nature, 457*, 92–96.
53. Maillard, I., Koch, U., Dumortier, A., Shestova, O., Xu, L., Sai, H., Pross, S. E., Aster, J. C., Bhandoola, A., Radtke, F., & Pear, W. S. (2008). Canonical notch signaling is dispensable for the maintenance of adult hematopoietic stem cells. *Cell Stem Cell, 2*, 356–366.
54. Mancini, S. J., Mantei, N., Dumortier, A., Suter, U., MacDonald, H. R., & Radtke, F. (2005). Jagged1-dependent Notch signaling is dispensable for hematopoietic stem cell self-renewal and differentiation. *Blood, 105*, 2340–2342.
55. McGarvey, A. C., Rybtsov, S., Souilhol, C., Tamagno, S., Rice, R., Hills, D., Godwin, D., Rice, D., Tomlinson, S. R., & Medvinsky, A. (2017). A molecular roadmap of the AGM region reveals BMPER as a novel regulator of HSC maturation. *The Journal of Experimental Medicine, 214*, 3731–3751.
56. McKinney-Freeman, S., Cahan, P., Li, H., Lacadie, S. A., Huang, H. T., Curran, M., Loewer, S., Naveiras, O., Kathrein, K. L., Konantz, M., et al. (2012). The transcriptional landscape of hematopoietic stem cell ontogeny. *Cell Stem Cell, 11*, 701–714.
57. Medvinsky, A., & Dzierzak, E. (1996). Definitive hematopoiesis is autonomously initiated by the AGM region. *Cell, 86*, 897–906.
58. Mendez-Ferrer, S., Michurina, T. V., Ferraro, F., Mazloom, A. R., Macarthur, B. D., Lira, S. A., Scadden, D. T., Ma'ayan, A., Enikolopov, G. N., & Frenette, P. S. (2010). Mesenchymal and haematopoietic stem cells form a unique bone marrow niche. *Nature, 466*, 829–834.

59. Mercher, T., Cornejo, M. G., Sears, C., Kindler, T., Moore, S. A., Maillard, I., Pear, W. S., Aster, J. C., & Gilliland, D. G. (2008). Notch signaling specifies megakaryocyte development from hematopoietic stem cells. *Cell Stem Cell, 3*, 314–326.
60. Nostro, M. C., Cheng, X., Keller, G. M., & Gadue, P. (2008). Wnt, activin, and BMP signaling regulate distinct stages in the developmental pathway from embryonic stem cells to blood. *Cell Stem Cell, 2*, 60–71.
61. Oh, P., Lobry, C., Gao, J., Tikhonova, A., Loizou, E., Manent, J., van Handel, B., Ibrahim, S., Greve, J., Mikkola, H., et al. (2013). In vivo mapping of notch pathway activity in normal and stress hematopoiesis. *Cell Stem Cell, 13*, 190–204.
62. Oostendorp, R. A., Harvey, K., & Dzierzak, E. A. (2005). Generation of murine stromal cell lines: Models for the microenvironment of the embryonic mouse aorta-gonads-mesonephros region. *Methods in Molecular Biology, 290*, 163–172.
63. Ottersbach, K., & Dzierzak, E. (2005). The murine placenta contains hematopoietic stem cells within the vascular labyrinth region. *Developmental Cell, 8*, 377–387.
64. Palomero, T., Sulis, M. L., Cortina, M., Real, P. J., Barnes, K., Ciofani, M., Caparros, E., Buteau, J., Brown, K., Perkins, S. L., et al. (2007). Mutational loss of PTEN induces resistance to NOTCH1 inhibition in T-cell leukemia. *Nature Medicine, 13*, 1203–1210.
65. Pear, W. S., Aster, J. C., Scott, M. L., Hasserjian, R. P., Soffer, B., Sklar, J., & Baltimore, D. (1996). Exclusive development of T cell neoplasms in mice transplanted with bone marrow expressing activated notch alleles. *The Journal of Experimental Medicine, 183*, 2283–2291.
66. Pelullo, M., Quaranta, R., Talora, C., Checquolo, S., Cialfi, S., Felli, M. P., te Kronnie, G., Borga, C., Besharat, Z. M., Palermo, R., et al. (2014). Notch3/Jagged1 circuitry reinforces notch signaling and sustains T-ALL. *Neoplasia, 16*, 1007–1017.
67. Pereira, C. F., Chang, B., Qiu, J., Niu, X., Papatsenko, D., Hendry, C. E., Clark, N. R., Nomura-Kitabayashi, A., Kovacic, J. C., Ma'ayan, A., et al. (2013). Induction of a hemogenic program in mouse fibroblasts. *Cell Stem Cell, 13*, 205–218.
68. Pouget, C., Gautier, R., Teillet, M. A., & Jaffredo, T. (2006). Somite-derived cells replace ventral aortic hemangioblasts and provide aortic smooth muscle cells of the trunk. *Development, 133*, 1013–1022.
69. Pouget, C., Pottin, K., & Jaffredo, T. (2008). Sclerotomal origin of vascular smooth muscle cells and pericytes in the embryo. *Developmental Biology, 315*, 437–447.
70. Radtke, F., Wilson, A., Stark, G., Bauer, M., van Meerwijk, J., MacDonald, H. R., & Aguet, M. (1999). Deficient T cell fate specification in mice with an induced inactivation of Notch1. *Immunity, 10*, 547–558.
71. Rhodes, K. E., Gekas, C., Wang, Y., Lux, C. T., Francis, C. S., Chan, D. N., Conway, S., Orkin, S. H., Yoder, M. C., & Mikkola, H. K. (2008). The emergence of hematopoietic stem cells is initiated in the placental vasculature in the absence of circulation. *Cell Stem Cell, 2*, 252–263.
72. Robert-Moreno, A., Espinosa, L., de la Pompa, J. L., & Bigas, A. (2005). RBPjkappa-dependent Notch function regulates Gata2 and is essential for the formation of intra-embryonic hematopoietic cells. *Development, 132*, 1117–1126.
73. Robert-Moreno, A., Espinosa, L., Sanchez, M. J., de la Pompa, J. L., & Bigas, A. (2007). The notch pathway positively regulates programmed cell death during erythroid differentiation. *Leukemia, 21*, 1496–1503.
74. Robert-Moreno, A., Guiu, J., Ruiz-Herguido, C., Lopez, M. E., Ingles-Esteve, J., Riera, L., Tipping, A., Enver, T., Dzierzak, E., Gridley, T., et al. (2008). Impaired embryonic haematopoiesis yet normal arterial development in the absence of the Notch ligand Jagged1. *The EMBO Journal, 27*, 1886–1895.
75. Robin, C., Bollerot, K., Mendes, S., Haak, E., Crisan, M., Cerisoli, F., Lauw, I., Kaimakis, P., Jorna, R., Vermeulen, M., et al. (2009). Human placenta is a potent hematopoietic niche containing hematopoietic stem and progenitor cells throughout development. *Cell Stem Cell, 5*, 385–395.

76. Ruiz-Herguido, C., Guiu, J., D'Altri, T., Ingles-Esteve, J., Dzierzak, E., Espinosa, L., & Bigas, A. (2012). Hematopoietic stem cell development requires transient Wnt/beta-catenin activity. *The Journal of Experimental Medicine, 209*, 1457–1468.
77. Sandler, V. M., Lis, R., Liu, Y., Kedem, A., James, D., Elemento, O., Butler, J. M., Scandura, J. M., & Rafii, S. (2014). Reprogramming human endothelial cells to haematopoietic cells requires vascular induction. *Nature, 511*, 312–318.
78. Shawber, C. J., & Kitajewski, J. (2004). Notch function in the vasculature: Insights from zebrafish, mouse and man. *BioEssays, 26*, 225–234.
79. Souilhol, C., Lendinez, J. G., Rybtsov, S., Murphy, F., Wilson, H., Hills, D., Batsivari, A., Binagui-Casas, A., McGarvey, A. C., MacDonald, H. R., et al. (2016). Developing HSCs become Notch independent by the end of maturation in the AGM region. *Blood, 128*, 1567–1577.
80. Sturgeon, C. M., Ditadi, A., Awong, G., Kennedy, M., & Keller, G. (2014). Wnt signaling controls the specification of definitive and primitive hematopoiesis from human pluripotent stem cells. *Nature Biotechnology, 32*, 554–561.
81. Sugimura, R., Jha, D. K., Han, A., Soria-Valles, C., da Rocha, E. L., Lu, Y. F., Goettel, J. A., Serrao, E., Rowe, R. G., Malleshaiah, M., et al. (2017). Haematopoietic stem and progenitor cells from human pluripotent stem cells. *Nature, 545*, 432–438.
82. Takahashi, K., & Yamanaka, S. (2006). Induction of pluripotent stem cells from mouse embryonic and adult fibroblast cultures by defined factors. *Cell, 126*, 663–676.
83. Thomson, J. A., Itskovitz-Eldor, J., Shapiro, S. S., Waknitz, M. A., Swiergiel, J. J., Marshall, V. S., & Jones, J. M. (1998). Embryonic stem cell lines derived from human blastocysts. *Science, 282*, 1145–1147.
84. Tran, I. T., Sandy, A. R., Carulli, A. J., Ebens, C., Chung, J., Shan, G. T., Radojcic, V., Friedman, A., Gridley, T., Shelton, A., et al. (2013). Blockade of individual Notch ligands and receptors controls graft-versus-host disease. *The Journal of Clinical Investigation, 123*, 1590–1604.
85. Travnickova, J., Tran Chau, V., Julien, E., Mateos-Langerak, J., Gonzalez, C., Lelievre, E., Lutfalla, G., Tavian, M., & Kissa, K. (2015). Primitive macrophages control HSPC mobilization and definitive haematopoiesis. *Nature Communications, 6*, 6227.
86. Van de Walle, I., Waegemans, E., De Medts, J., De Smet, G., De Smedt, M., Snauwaert, S., Vandekerckhove, B., Kerre, T., Leclercq, G., Plum, J., et al. (2013). Specific Notch receptor-ligand interactions control human TCR-alphabeta/gammadelta development by inducing differential Notch signal strength. *The Journal of Experimental Medicine, 210*, 683–697.
87. Varnum-Finney, B., Brashem-Stein, C., & Bernstein, I. D. (2003). Combined effects of Notch signaling and cytokines induce a multiple log increase in precursors with lymphoid and myeloid reconstituting ability. *Blood, 101*, 1784–1789.
88. Varnum-Finney, B., Halasz, L. M., Sun, M., Gridley, T., Radtke, F., & Bernstein, I. D. (2011). Notch2 governs the rate of generation of mouse long- and short-term repopulating stem cells. *The Journal of Clinical Investigation, 121*, 1207–1216.
89. Varnum-Finney, B., Xu, L., Brashem-Stein, C., Nourigat, C., Flowers, D., Bakkour, S., Pear, W. S., & Bernstein, I. D. (2000). Pluripotent, cytokine-dependent, hematopoietic stem cells are immortalized by constitutive notch1 signaling. *Nature Medicine, 6*, 1278–1281.
90. Walker, L., Carlson, A., Tan-Pertel, H. T., Weinmaster, G., & Gasson, J. (2001). The notch receptor and its ligands are selectively expressed during hematopoietic development in the mouse. *Stem Cells, 19*, 543–552.
91. Warren, L., Manos, P. D., Ahfeldt, T., Loh, Y. H., Li, H., Lau, F., Ebina, W., Mandal, P. K., Smith, Z. D., Meissner, A., et al. (2010). Highly efficient reprogramming to pluripotency and directed differentiation of human cells with synthetic modified mRNA. *Cell Stem Cell, 7*, 618–630.
92. Wasteson, P., Johansson, B. R., Jukkola, T., Breuer, S., Akyurek, L. M., Partanen, J., & Lindahl, P. (2008). Developmental origin of smooth muscle cells in the descending aorta in mice. *Development, 135*, 1823–1832.

93. Wendorff, A. A., Koch, U., Wunderlich, F. T., Wirth, S., Dubey, C., Bruning, J. C., MacDonald, H. R., & Radtke, F. (2010). Hes1 is a critical but context-dependent mediator of canonical Notch signaling in lymphocyte development and transformation. *Immunity, 33*, 671–684.
94. Weng, A. P., Ferrando, A. A., Lee, W., Morris, J. P. T., Silverman, L. B., Sanchez-Irizarry, C., Blacklow, S. C., Look, A. T., & Aster, J. C. (2004). Activating mutations of NOTCH1 in human T cell acute lymphoblastic leukemia. *Science, 306*, 269–271.
95. Weng, A. P., Millholland, J. M., Yashiro-Ohtani, Y., Arcangeli, M. L., Lau, A., Wai, C., Del Bianco, C., Rodriguez, C. G., Sai, H., Tobias, J., et al. (2006). c-Myc is an important direct target of Notch1 in T-cell acute lymphoblastic leukemia/lymphoma. *Genes & Development, 20*, 2096–2109.
96. Wiegreffe, C., Christ, B., Huang, R., & Scaal, M. (2007). Sclerotomal origin of smooth muscle cells in the wall of the avian dorsal aorta. *Developmental Dynamics, 236*, 2578–2585.
97. Wynn, T. A., Chawla, A., & Pollard, J. W. (2013). Macrophage biology in development, homeostasis and disease. *Nature, 496*, 445–455.
98. Yang, L. T., Nichols, J. T., Yao, C., Manilay, J. O., Robey, E. A., & Weinmaster, G. (2005). Fringe glycosyltransferases differentially modulate Notch1 proteolysis induced by Delta1 and Jagged1. *Molecular Biology of the Cell, 16*, 927–942.
99. Yao, D., Huang, Y., Huang, X., Wang, W., Yan, Q., Wei, L., Xin, W., Gerson, S., Stanley, P., Lowe, J. B., & Zhou, L. (2011). Protein O-fucosyltransferase 1 (Pofut1) regulates lymphoid and myeloid homeostasis through modulation of notch receptor ligand interactions. *Blood, 117*, 5652–5662.
100. Zhang, J., Niu, C., Ye, L., Huang, H., He, X., Tong, W. G., Ross, J., Haug, J., Johnson, T., Feng, J. Q., et al. (2003). Identification of the haematopoietic stem cell niche and control of the niche size. *Nature, 425*, 836–841.
101. Zhang, P., He, Q., Chen, D., Liu, W., Wang, L., Zhang, C., Ma, D., Li, W., Liu, B., & Liu, F. (2015). G protein-coupled receptor 183 facilitates endothelial-to-hematopoietic transition via Notch1 inhibition. *Cell Research, 25*, 1093–1107.
102. Zhang, Y., Sandy, A. R., Wang, J., Radojcic, V., Shan, G. T., Tran, I. T., Friedman, A., Kato, K., He, S., Cui, S., et al. (2011). Notch signaling is a critical regulator of allogeneic CD4+ T-cell responses mediating graft-versus-host disease. *Blood, 117*, 299–308.
103. Zhou, B. O., Ding, L., & Morrison, S. J. (2015). Hematopoietic stem and progenitor cells regulate the regeneration of their niche by secreting Angiopoietin-1. *eLife, 4*, e05521.
104. Zovein, A. C., Hofmann, J. J., Lynch, M., French, W. J., Turlo, K. A., Yang, Y., Becker, M. S., Zanetta, L., Dejana, E., Gasson, J. C., et al. (2008). Fate tracing reveals the endothelial origin of hematopoietic stem cells. *Cell Stem Cell, 3*, 625–636.

Chapter 13
Notch Signaling in the Normal Intestine and Intestinal Cancer

Lluís Espinosa, Erika López-Arribillaga, Oriol Bachs, and Anna Bigas

Abstract The intestinal epithelium is a highly proliferative tissue whose integrity depends on the function of *intestinal stem cells* residing at the bottom of the crypts. The Notch pathway is essential for ISC maintenance and normal tissue differentiation, and it is activated by Delta-like ligands present in the Paneth cells. In intestinal cancer Notch activity is also essential, with Notch signal inhibition leading to a reduction on tumor growth and/or tumor formation associated with enforced differentiation toward the postmitotic secretory lineage. However, general Notch inhibitors are highly toxic, which precludes using them for anticancer therapy. Several strategies are now being tested to reduce Notch inhibitor toxicity such as glucocorticoid co-treatment or intermittent dosing. The use of blocking antibodies against particular ligands or receptors that specifically function in CRC, or in particular CRC subtypes, would represent a novel low-toxicity therapeutic strategy for anticancer treatment. This possibility requires a better understanding of the mechanisms regulating Notch/Notch ligand selectivity in CRC. All these issues are analyzed and discussed in the current chapter.

Keywords Stem cells · Intestine · Intestinal cancer · Cancer initiation · Notch-based therapy · Antibodies

---

L. Espinosa (✉) · E. López-Arribillaga · A. Bigas
Program in Cancer Research, Institut Hospital del Mar d'Investigacions Mèdiques (IMIM), CIBERONC, Barcelona, Spain
e-mail: lespinosa@imim.es

O. Bachs
Department of Biomedical Sciences, (CIBERONC), University of Barcelona, Barcelona, Spain

L. Miele, S. Artavanis-Tsakonas (eds.), *Targeting Notch in Cancer*,
https://doi.org/10.1007/978-1-4939-8859-4_13

13.1 The Gastrointestinal Tissue

13.1.1 Overview of the Gastrointestinal System

13.1.1.1 Structure and Function of the Intestine

The digestive system is a broad term that refers to the gastrointestinal (GI) tract and their accessories such as the liver, gallbladder, and pancreas. The main function of the GI tract is to digest and absorb nutrients from the diet, but it also plays a major role in immunity and as a defensive barrier. Anatomically, the GI tract is divided in the upper GI tract including the esophagus and the stomach and the lower tract that consists of the *small* and *large intestines.*

The *small intestine* is subdivided in the duodenum, jejunum, and ileum (from proximal to distal) and plays a principal function in absorbing the products of digestion.

The large intestine is primarily responsible for absorbing water and electrolytes, and it includes the cecum, *colon*, rectum, and anal canal.

Transversally, the GI tract is formed by *a* series of concentric layers that surround the lumen. The *mucosa* is the innermost layer of the gut that is in contact with the food and other elements such as mucosa-associated microorganisms. It is further divided in the *epithelium*, the lamina propria, and a thin layer of smooth muscle. In the stomach and the intestine, the epithelial layer is simple and columnar and vastly protected by a cover of mucus that is secreted by specialized epithelial cells. Other GI tract layers are the submucosa, muscularis externa, a single layer of mesothelial cells, and several strata of connective tissue.

13.1.1.2 The Intestinal Epithelium

The epithelial component of the small and large intestine is highly similar, and the cellular components are essentially the same. However, it exhibits some particularities associated with its function: the most characteristic is the presence of a succession of fingerlike structures (*villus*) and adjacent invaginations (crypts of Lieberkühn) in the small intestine, which are not present in the colon. In contrast, the colonic epithelium is arranged in deeper invaginations that represent a compressed version of this architecture.

In general, the intestinal epithelial cells belong to two principal functional categories:

The *absorptive* epithelial cells (*enterocytes* and *colonocytes*) represent the majority of the epithelial component in the intestinal mucosa and are responsible for the absorption and transport of nutrients. They are polarized cells with membranous protrusions in their apical surface called microvilli, which increase the absorptive area. Microvilli are also covered by a glycocalyx, which is a layer of glycoproteins enriched in digestive enzymes.

The *secretory* cells include a collection of cell lineages that are further classified according to the molecules that they secrete. The *goblet cell*s are localized and scattered among the enterocytes with a frequency that increases along the anterior-posterior axis of the gut [1]. They produce a protective mucus layer that allows for the smooth passage of the intestinal contents and acts as a protective barrier for bacteria [2, 3]. The *enteroendocrine* cells produce peptidic hormones and digestive enzymes and are characterized by the presence of secretory vesicles. They localize along the GI tract, but some subtypes are intestine-specific (reviewed in [4]). The *tuft cells* [5] are characterized by their long and blunt microvilli and a well-developed tubulovesicular system. They produce and secrete opioids such as β-endorphin and display absorptive and chemoreception functions (reviewed in [6]). The *Paneth cells* reside at the bottom of the intestinal crypts and are characterized by the presence of large apical granules with antimicrobial peptides such as lysozyme [7] and α-defensins [8], which are secreted to the intestinal lumen as part of the innate immune response [9]. These cells are now emerging as functional constituents of the stem cell niche in the small intestine (reviewed in [10]). Interestingly, *Paneth cells* are aberrantly found in the colon [11] and the esophagus [12] in conditions of chronic inflammation.

13.1.2 Intestinal Stem Cells

13.1.2.1 Diverse Intestinal Stem Cell Populations

The intestinal epithelium is a highly self-renewing tissue that in the mouse turns over entirely within 3–5 days [13]. *Intestinal stem cells* (ISCs), residing at the bottom of the crypts, are the source of a highly proliferative transit-amplifying (TA) cell compartment responsible to replenish all mature epithelial lineages. Intestinal epithelial cell differentiation and maturation are associated with the upward migration of TA descendants with the exception of *Paneth cells* that migrate downward, thus accumulating at the bottom of the crypt compartment [14].

The *crypt base columnar* (CBC) cells, located at the bottom of the crypts intermingled with the Paneth cells, were identified as the first ISC compartment [14]. These same cells were later rediscovered as long-lived, multipotent, actively proliferating ISCs, which express the Lgr5 marker [15] and are capable of generating self-renewing structures that recapitulate the intestinal architecture (called organoids or miniguts) [16] (see 1.2.4). However, organoid formation is more efficient when Lgr5+ cells are co-cultured with Paneth cells, indicating that the latter represent a putative ISC niche [17]. In the colon, where Paneth cells are very infrequent, cells expressing CD24 [17] and c-Kit [18] may represent their functional equivalents. Later on, a second population of label-retaining ISCs that gave rise to all epithelial lineages was identified located at the +4 position above the crypt base [19]. These cells express the Bmi1 marker [20] and can replenish the Lgr5+ pool in response to damage [21], indicating a role in the maintenance of tissue homeostasis under stress conditions [22]. However, Bmi1 expression is not restricted to the +4 cells, but it spreads throughout the crypt compartment of the small intestine and the colon [23, 24]. Other markers for quiescent ISCs are mTert [25], Lrig1 [26], and Hopx [27], while Olfm4 [28] and Ascl2 [29] are preferentially expressed in actively cycling ISCs, although individual crypt cells can simultaneously express several of these markers [30]. Interestingly enough, most of these stem cell genes are under the transcriptional control of Wnt and Notch pathways (see Sect. 13.2.2).

13.1.2.2 Functional Contribution of Particular ISC Markers

Understanding how particular markers contribute to the ISC function is a relevant issue. The *Lgr5* protein is a leucine-rich repeat-containing G protein-coupled receptor [31] that negatively acts on Wnt signaling. However, inhibition of Wnt by Lgr5 is reverted in the presence of the Lgr5 ligands R-spondins (RSPO) [32–35]. Activation of Wnt by Lgr5 depends on the interaction RSPO with the ZNRF3/RNF43 complex in the ISC compartment [36, 37]. *Ascl2* also modulates Wnt/β-catenin-dependent transcription in the *Lgr5*+ ISC compartment [29, 38]. The murine telomerase reverse transcriptase, *mTert*, is required for telomere integrity maintenance, which directly impacts on the self-renewal capacity of the stem cells. *Lrig1* is a negative-feedback regulator of the ErbB receptor family that controls the size of the intestinal stem cell niche [39]. *Bmi1* is a member of the polycomb group (PcG) of transcriptional repressors that promotes specific gene silencing through histone H2A ubiquitination [40–43]. Bmi1 plays an essential function in different stem cell compartments, and Bmi1-null mice die around 2–3 months of age, displaying progressive hematopoietic and neurological abnormalities [44]. We previously found that Bmi1 is downstream of Notch in the ISCs and its depletion results in reduced proliferation and impaired DNA-damage repair in this compartment [24].

13.1.2.3 Ex Vivo ISC Production

In 2009, two different groups established the in vitro conditions to reproducibly grow ISCs while maintaining their self-renewal and multi-lineage differentiation capacity [16, 45, 46]. As mentioned, ISC-derived structures were called organoids and can be generated from isolated Lgr5+ cells, although this capacity was improved in the Paneth cell co-cultures. Recently, several combinations of factors such as IL22 have been found to enhance Lgr5+-derived organoid formation in the absence of Paneth cells. Similar culture conditions support the growing of mouse and human intestinal adenoma or carcinoma cells, which then generate spherical structures (spheroids) [47], mostly composed of highly proliferative and undifferentiated Bmi1-positive cells [24]. As intestinal organoids and spheroids can be passaged indefinitely, they are powerful tools for testing pharmacologic and genetic interventions against normal or tumor stem cells [48–51].

13.2 Notch Signaling in the Normal Intestine

The Notch pathway is crucial in the delivery of signals from neighboring cells, which directly impact on embryonic development and the maintenance of tissue and stem cell homeostasis. Notch receptors comprise a family of transmembrane proteins that contain an extracellular N-terminal domain (N^{EC}) and a C-terminal portion (N^{TM}, including the transmembrane and intracellular domains) that are cleaved apart during Notch protein maturation in the Golgi. Notch activation is achieved by the interaction of N^{EC} with a Notch ligand of the Jagged or Delta families. The correct folding of the NRR region in the linkage region and the addition of sugar moieties during Notch maturation will determine the activation capacity of the receptor as well as its ligand selectivity. In this regard, the Fringe family of glycosyltransferases exerts a crucial function, with Fringe-mediated glycosylation enhancing Notch association with Delta while reducing responsiveness to Jagged [52, 53].

Once activated, Notch translocates to the nucleus, where it interacts with the DNA-binding protein RBPj to promote specific gene transcription. Most Notch-dependent genes are context specific with the exception of the Hes family of transcriptional repressors that are recurrently induced by Notch in different cell types. The activation of hes genes is also important to limit the extent of Notch activation [24, 54]. In the normal intestine, Notch signaling promotes specification of the absorptive lineage in the intestine through an axis involving Hes1 and Math1 (ATOH1), but it is also essential in the regulation of the stem and progenitor compartments [24, 55–57].

13.2.1 Notch Receptors and Ligands in the Small Intestine and Colon

According to their critical contribution to intestinal homeostasis, two different Notch receptors, Notch1 and Notch2, are expressed all along the villus-crypt axis including the crypt stem cells. By lineage tracing analysis, it was formally proved that Notch activity was restricted to the stem and progenitor cells of both the small intestine and the colon [55, 58, 59]. Unexpectedly, Jagged1, which is ubiquitously detected in most of the intestinal epithelial cells including the stem and progenitor compartments, does not contribute to Notch activation in the normal intestine and in the maintenance of intestinal homeostasis [55]. In contrast, Delta1 and Delta4 that are expressed in the Paneth cell lineage [17] are required and sufficient to support intestinal-specific Notch activation [55], likely related with the Paneth cell function on the ISC compartment. The mechanisms regulating Notch ligand selectivity in the intestinal epithelium are primarily unknown, but they may involve the activity of Fringe glycosyltransferases that are distinctively expressed at particular intestinal compartments [60].

13.2.2 Genetic Models to Study Notch Function in the Murine Intestine

The first evidence that Notch signaling plays a role in the intestinal tissue arose from the *Hes1* knockout mice [61]. Hes1 belongs to the Hes family of transcriptional repressors, which are conserved transcriptional Notch targets and are generally required for the Notch function in different tissues. In the intestine, Hes1 deficiency led to a massive differentiation into the secretory lineages (most predominantly the postmitotic *goblet cells*), a phenotype that was mimicked by pharmacologic Notch signal inhibition [62]. Similar results were obtained by knocking out critical elements of the Notch pathway such as RBPj [63], Notch1 and Notch2 [56], and the O-fucosyltransferase for Notch Pofut1 [64]. Mechanistically, Hes1 is induced by active Notch in the intestinal tissue [65] and imposes the repression of *Math1* (*ATOH1*), which is a master transcription factor of the secretory lineages [66].

It is because of the strong phenotype of its inhibition on lineage determination that the identification of Notch functions in the ISC compartment has been delayed. Nevertheless, genetic data have demonstrated that Notch is required to induce Hes1 in the crypt cells, which transcriptionally represses the CDK inhibitors *p27Kip1* and *p57Kip2*, thus allowing cell proliferation [56]. Notch also controls the expression of the ISC markers Olfm4 [57] and Bmi1, which is essential to maintain several ISC functions (see Sect. 13.1.2.3) (see model in Fig. 13.1). Activation of Notch in stem and progenitor cells is dependent on Dll1 and Dll4 ligands [55] that are present in the Paneth cells. Surprisingly, ISCs from *Math1*-deficient mice are unresponsive to Notch inhibition [67], a subject that remains mechanistically unexplored.

13.3 Notch and Intestinal Cancer

13.3.1 Colorectal Cancer

13.3.1.1 Incidence and Mortality

According to a recent Globocan project report [68], *colorectal cancer* (CRC) is the third most common cancer in men (12.4% of the total) and second in women (12% of the total) in industrialized countries, only outranked by breast cancer in females and prostate and lung cancer in males. Regarding its mortality, CRC is the second leading cause of death due to cancer in men (175.000 deaths per year, 11% of the total) and third in women (158.000 deaths per year, 12.3% of the total).

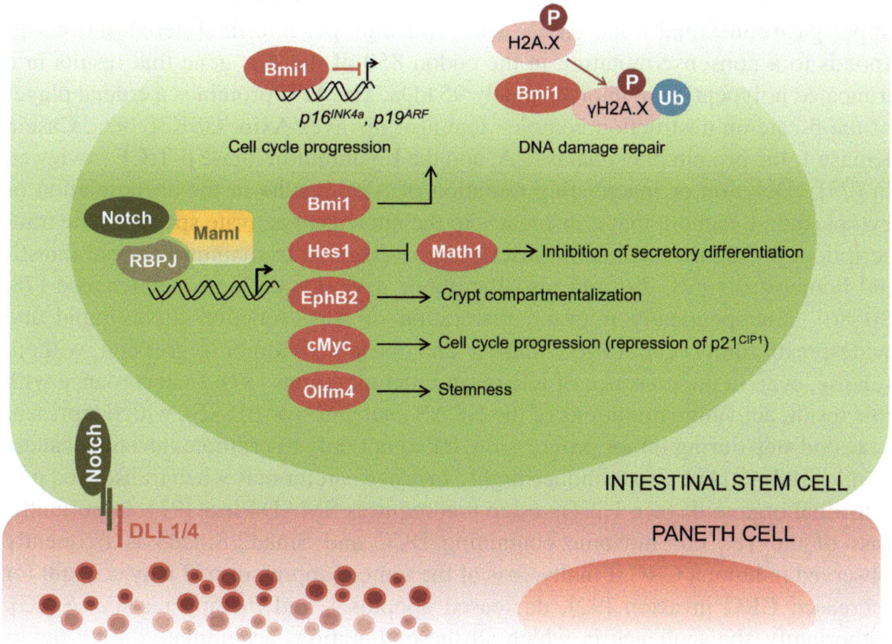

Fig. 13.1 Schematic representation of how Notch gets activated and contributes to specific intestinal stem cell functions

13.3.1.2 The Adenoma-Carcinoma Sequence

Formation of aberrant intestinal crypt foci is the earliest manifestation of an intestinal neoplasia. These foci can then progress to become polyps, benign tumors that protrude into the lumen from the intestinal epithelium, which can be classified into two different subtypes: *hyperplastic* polyps, which preserve their normal architecture and cellular morphology, and *adenomatous* polyps, characterized by the presence of organizational abnormalities. *Invasive carcinomas* evolve from adenomatous polyps through the acquisition of specific mutations [69]. The genetic model for *colorectal cancer progression* was proposed in 1990 by Fearon and Vogelstein [70] and has remained mostly unchanged for the last 25 years.

In brief, CRC (both hereditary and non-hereditary) is initiated by the inactivation of both *adenomatous polyposis coli (APC)* alleles [71]. About 80% of all sporadic intestinal adenomas and CRC cases contain inactive forms of the APC protein [72] that are also responsible for the majority of inherited familial adenomatous polyposis (FAP) syndrome cases [73–75]. APC disruption is also sufficient to promote the formation of adenomatous polyps, as it was originally demonstrated in the Apc^{Min}

mouse, generated by random ethylnitrosourea mutagenesis [76] and characterized by the presence of more than 100 intestinal tumors per animal, mainly located in the upper gastrointestinal tract. APC "Min" (for *m*ultiple *i*ntestinal *n*eoplasia) corresponds to a nonsense mutation in the codon 850 of the *Apc* gene that results in a truncated polypeptide of approximately 95 kDa. The APC protein is a crucial player of the β-catenin destruction complex that also involves Axin, GSK3β beta, Casein Kinase 1, the protein phosphatase 2A, and the E3 ubiquitin ligase β-TrCP (reviewed in [77]). Deletion or inactivating mutation of APC results in the accumulation of cytoplasmic β-catenin that translocates to the nucleus to activate specific gene transcription. β-Catenin-mediated transcription is essential to maintain normal intestinal homeostasis [78, 79] and also for tumor development and maintenance [78, 80–86]. Therapeutically relevant, restoration of APC function drives rapid and widespread tumor cell differentiation and sustained tumor regression without relapse, even in the presence of KRAS and p53 mutations [87]. In accordance with this result, activating mutations of the KRAS oncogene (or BRAF), which represent a second step during tumor progression, failed not only to promote intestinal cancer in mice [88–90] but also to induce highly invasive carcinomas when transduced into intestinal organoids (see 1.2.4), a step that requires SMAD4 loss [91]. Importantly, loss of the 18q chromosome containing DCC and Smad2/Smad4 is frequently observed in human CRC. Finally, loss of the tumor suppressor p53 may account for increased CRC invasion [92], decreased apoptosis, and therapy resistance [93]. Importantly, the sequence in which all these alterations accumulate during tumor progression is nonrandom, further supporting the argument that certain mutations confer selective advantages at a given stage of the tumor's natural history. Relevant for this review, mutations in the Notch target *CMYC* gene but also in the negative regulator of Notch, FBXW7, have been consistently identified in a significant proportion of human CRC cases (reviewed in [94]).

Recently, a novel molecular classification has been established that permits the stratification of most CRCs in four subtypes with distinguishable features [95]: *CMS1* (for *c*onsensus *m*olecular *s*ubtype 1) includes tumors with microsatellite instability and an important immune activation; *CMS2*, the most frequent (37%), is characterized by an epithelial phenotype and a marked activation of the WNT and MYC pathways; *CMS3* is still epithelial but with significant metabolic alterations; and *CMS4* includes the more mesenchymal tumors, with high TGF activity and stromal and vascular invasion. Of note, different subtypes can coexist, indicating the existence of transition phenotypes or tumor heterogeneity. This fact suggests that further stratification is still possible that can improve the prognostic significance.

13.3.1.3 Cancer Stem Cells

It is becoming evident that cancers, either leukemia or solid tumors, are heterogeneous and primarily sustained by specific populations of self-renewing cells (reviewed in [96–98]). There are two principal models that explain intra-tumor heterogeneity: the *stochastic model* predicts that a tumor is biologically homogeneous and the behavior of cancer cells is influenced by intrinsic or extrinsic factors, resulting in differences in cell surface marker expression, entry to cell cycle, or tumor initiation capacity. In contrast, the *hierarchy model* predicts that the tumor mimics the hierarchical organization of the normal tissue with *cancer stem cells* (CSCs) being a distinct population that can be identified and isolated. The clinical implication of the hierarchy model is the possibility to specifically target CSCs as an effective method to revert tumor growth and to eliminate the possibility of relapse. This is not so evident in a stochastic model where every tumor cell has the potential to behave as cancer stem cell (reviewed in [99]).

Validation of particular tumor cell populations for their CSC capacity has classically been done using different approaches. The more in vivo approach involves the purification of specific cell populations (by the presence of cell surface markers) and testing their tumor initiation activity, as determined by their capacity to form serially transplantable xenografts in mice. Alternatively, cells can be tested for their stem cell capacity in vitro by culturing as spheroids in non-adherent serum-free conditions. Recent identification and phenotypic characterization of such populations from CRC samples have reinforced the concept of CSC in this particular tumor type. However, there is no clear consensus on what the intestinal CSC is, as multiple subpopulations follow these same criteria. This is the case of CRC cells expressing CD133 [100, 101], CD44 [102, 103], ALDH1 [104], CD26 [105], EPHB2 [106], Lgr5 [107], Krt119 [108], or PTK7 [109]. Further experimental data have directly demonstrated the capacity of Lgr5+ and CD133+ cells to initiate tumors in vivo [110, 111].

In any case, the fact that CSCs are likely responsible for tumor initiation, metastasis, and therapy resistance identifies them as preferential targets for novel anticancer drugs.

13.3.2 Notch in Intestinal Cancer

13.3.2.1 Notch in Murine Intestinal Cancer Models

Although mutations of Notch or Notch family members have never been included in the intestinal cancer acquisition and progression models, it was initially demonstrated that Notch signaling abrogation in the Wnt/β-catenin-active *Apc*^{Min} mice model imposed differentiation of the adenoma cells into the secretory lineage, thus limiting tumor progression [62]. Notch signaling is also important for regulating adenoma formation and tumor cell proliferation, and in mice carrying active Notch1, adenomas arise at earlier age [59, 112]. Therapeutically relevant, Jagged1 is a transcriptional target of Wnt/β-catenin in the intestinal adenoma cells and plays a crucial role in the pathologic activation of Notch at least in the *Apc*-mutated cancer models. Thus, reducing Jagged1 levels (i.e., in the heterozygous Jagged1-deficient mice) was sufficient to attenuate tumor load in the *Apc*^{Min} background with no apparent effects on the normal intestinal homeostasis [59]. Conversely, genetic deletion of the Aes gene, which is a negative regulator of Notch activation, promotes tumor progression and metastatic invasion in the presence of mutant *Apc* [113]. As part of the mechanism that connects Notch with intestinal cancer progression, it was found that DAB1 is a transcriptional target of Notch in murine intestinal tumors leading to the activation of ABL, which then induces phosphorylation of the RAC/RHOGEF protein TRIO at Tyr 2681. Unphosphorylatable mutation of TRIO at this particular residue (Y2681F) reduces RHOGEF activity and inhibits invasion of colorectal cancer cells [114]. Recently, we demonstrated that Jagged1 expressed in the epithelial cells from *Apc*-mutated mouse tumors is required for Notch activation and adenoma cell survival. The absence of Manic Fringe (MFNG) in the adenoma cells is at the base of Jagged1 addiction that was reverted by ectopic MFNG [115]. Specific activation of Notch by Jagged1 is also essential in other cancer systems such as metastatic breast tumors [116].

13.3.2.2 Notch in Human CRC

In human CRC, Notch1 activation was found to be increased [117], with total Notch1 levels correlating with tumor progression, tumor grade, and metastatic capacity [118]. Active Notch1 and Notch2 were also detected in tumors arising in familial adenomatous polyposis (FAP) patients, which carry frequent mutation in the APC gene associated with increased amounts of membranous Jagged1 [59]. Moreover, endothelial cells can produce soluble forms of Jagged1 that activate Notch and enhance the stem cell phenotype of CRC cells [119]. Further demonstrating the functional relevance of Notch activity in human CRC and in intestinal CSCs, Notch1 depletion was sufficient to promote apoptosis and inhibit the formation of tumorspheres from human CRC cell lines [118]. Moreover, Jagged1 knockdown induced G0/G1 phase cell cycle arrest, reduced the migratory and invasive capacity of CRC cells in vitro, and reduced tumor growth, proliferation, and expression of metastasis markers in a xenograft mouse model in vivo [120]. The impact of Notch activity in tumor-initiating cell activity (TIC) has been also demonstrated in a human CRC xenograft model using specific antibodies against Dll4 expressed in either the tumor cells (human) or in the murine stromal cells. In this work, antibody treatment decreased HES1 levels, the frequency of TICs, and the tumorigenic capacity of the transplanted tissue [121]. Together these data indicate that Notch signaling is relevant for CRC initiation and progression and it can be activated by Delta or Jagged ligands in specific CRC subgroups. Considering the recently published classification of CRC subtypes [95], it is tempting to speculate that *CMS2* tumors that are associated with high WNT activity would be more Jagged1-dependent, being Jagged1 a target of β-catenin, whereas *CMS4* tumors would depend on Delta ligands that are highly expressed in the endothelial infiltrate that is a characteristic of this tumor subtype [122].

13.3.2.3 Notch Effectors in Human CRC

The mechanisms underlying Notch dependence for CRC initiation and/or progression can vary in a context-dependent manner. For example, Notch1 can promote cell proliferation by repressing Kruppel-like factor (KLF4) [123], which is a well-known tumor suppressor in human CRC [124]. Phosphorylation of TRIO at Y2681, which lays downstream of Notch in the Aes-mutated mouse model of intestinal cancer (see Sect. 13.3.2.1), has been detected in CRC patient samples and associated with poorer prognosis after surgery [114]. Notch also increased the levels of the stem cell-like marker CD44 and promotes the transcriptional induction of Snail and Slug, two potent and evolutionarily conserved mediators of EMT in many tissues and tumor types including CRC [125, 126]. Combined detection of the Notch target proteins HEY1, HES1, and SOX9 significantly predicts reduced survival after chemotherapy in a study including 441 CRC patients, when compared with each marker alone with a hazard ratio of 2.09 and a significance of $p = 0.01$ [127]. Moreover, several of these genes are co-regulated by Notch and the inhibitor of kappaB kinase (IKK) [128], which is also involved in human CRC progression and metastasis [129].

13.3.3 Notch-Based Therapy for Treating Human CRC

13.3.3.1 State of the Art

Surgery is the primary choice for the treatment of nonmetastatic CRC patients, in combination with adjuvant therapies, which essentially consist of chemotherapy and radiotherapy. Typically, the first-line drug regimens used in the treatment of CRC are 5-fluorouracil together with leucovorin and irinotecan or oxaliplatin and can also be combined with specific antibodies against VEGF such as bevacizumab [130]. Cetuximab, a monoclonal antibody against the epidermal growth factor receptor (EGFR), is also used in CRC treatment in combination with irinotecan in patients that relapsed after first-line therapy but also in aggressive primary tumors [131, 132]. Even following surgery and chemotherapy treatment, about 30–40% of newly diagnosed stage II and III patients will develop distant metastasis that will finally lead to patient death [133, 134]. Moreover, the presence of KRAS and BRAF mutations in the tumors precludes the use of antibodies against EGFR. Hence, there is a clear need to identify additional targeted therapies to limit progression of the disease and to better treat patients with advanced metastasis.

13.3.3.2 Targeting the γ-Secretase Complex

Due to the essential role of Notch in intestinal tumor initiation and progression, different compounds inhibiting Notch have been (and are being) tested for their competence as anti-CRC agents. The first evidence that Notch inhibition protected from intestinal cancer was obtained using general Notch/γ-secretase activity inhibitors (GSI) [62], as mentioned in Sect. 13.3.2. Subsequent preclinical research has consistently shown that GSI reverts tumorigenesis through a mechanism involving both anti-angiogenic and anti-CSC activities [76, 135–138]. GSI treatment also prevented Notch1 activation by chemotherapy, thus sensitizing colon cancer cells to the treatment with oxaliplatin and 5-FU [139]. Recently, antibody fragments targeting Nicastrin, a component of the γ-secretase complex, were found to specifically prevent Notch activation in mammalian cells [140] similar to quinomycin A, which reduced the levels of γ-secretase complex components [141].

Because Notch is required to maintain the homeostasis of multiple tissues in the adult organisms, GSI-associated toxicity is still a major obstacle that needs further investigation. In mice, the most prominent toxicities associated with GSI treatment arise in the gastrointestinal tract and result in intractable diarrheas, especially when using continuous dosing schedules. Importantly, GSI toxicity is reduced by intermittent dosing and ameliorated by glucocorticoid co-treatment [142–144]. In fact, glucocorticoids have demonstrated their efficacy even when administered after GSI treatment [145].

13.3.3.3 Targeting Notch Receptors

Recently, interventions leading to inhibition of specific Notch receptors or ligands have demonstrated less toxic effects than general Notch signaling blockage. Based on this observation, several monoclonal antibodies selectively targeting particular Notch receptors have been already generated by different groups and tested for clinical applications [146–148]. For example, antibodies targeting the extracellular negative regulator region (NRR) of Notch were found to inhibit the conformational change that allows ADAM protease cleavage. NRR anti-Notch-specific antibodies have been developed for Notch1, Notch2, and Notch3 [149, 150]. Other anti-Notch antibodies have been designed to block the ligand-binding domain (LBD), thereby competitively inhibiting the Notch ligands by binding to their EGF repeats [151]. In general, antibodies that efficiently inhibit Notch signaling are currently being tested in clinical trials on patients with solid tumors and metastatic disease who have previously undergone chemotherapy.

13.3.3.4 Targeting Notch Ligands

In addition, antibodies targeting Notch ligands are also being investigated for their therapeutic potential. Among them, demcizumab (OMP-21M18), a humanized monoclonal antibody targeting DLL4, has demonstrated a significant antitumor activity in patients with previously treated solid tumors [152]. Combination of anti-DLL4 antibodies with irinotecan produced a significant decrease of TIC activity and promoted apoptosis in a xenograft model of early passage patient-derived CRC [153]. Other antibodies against Dll4 (REGN1035 and REGN421) revealed a potent antitumor activity in renal carcinoma patient-derived tumors that was enhanced by

VEGF signaling inhibition [154], likely related with reduced angiogenesis. Neutralizing Dll4 signal with a humanized anti-Dll4-selective antibody (YW152F) caused defective endothelial cell differentiation both in vitro and in vivo and inhibited tumor growth in several tumor models without affecting intestinal differentiation [155]. These particular effects could be therapeutically exploited for treating the *CMS4* subtype of CRC. However, DLL4 blockade can also disrupt normal organ homeostasis and induce vascular tumors [156], thus raising serious concerns about its therapeutic potential. Recently, we found that high Jagged1 levels in the absence of MFNG predict poor survival in a subset of CRC patients. Moreover patient-derived tumors lacking MFNG were particularly sensitive to specific antibodies targeting Jagged1 in an orthoxenograft mouse model [115].

Soluble forms of Jagged-1 and Dll-1 have also been designed that can either reduce [157] or enhance Notch signaling [158]. Importantly, the smaller size of these molecules compared to the monoclonal antibodies would represent a clear advantage for their bio-distribution, thus improving their therapeutic efficiency.

13.3.3.5 Disrupting the Active Notch Complex

Finally, another attractive method for inhibiting Notch signal is by blocking its nuclear transcriptional complex. In this sense, it was initially shown that a 62-amino acid peptide derived from the NOTCH coactivator MAML1 was capable to form a transcriptionally inert nuclear complex with NOTCH1 and CSL and specifically inhibits the growth of murine and human NOTCH1-transformed T-ALL cells [159]. More recently, a synthetic peptide called SAHM1 has been shown to prevent the assembly of a transcriptionally active Notch1 complex in T-ALL cells. Treatment of leukemic cells with SAHM1 resulted in the transcriptional suppression of NOTCH-dependent transcription and showed a specific antiproliferative effect in both cultured cells and in a mouse model of NOTCH1-driven T-ALL [160]. Cell-permeable peptides such as SAHM1, which impede the formation of protein complexes, could be extremely advantageous owing to their small size and their ability to interfere with specific protein surfaces, which should impact on their target selectivity.

Acknowledgments This work has been supported by grants 20131210 from the Fundació la Marató de TV3; PI16/00437, PIE15/00008, and RD12/0036/0054 from the Instituto de Salud Carlos III/FEDER; and 2017 SGR 135 from the Agència de Gestió Ajuts Universitaris de Recerca.

References

1. Paulus, U., et al. (1993). The differentiation and lineage development of goblet cells in the murine small intestinal crypt: Experimental and modelling studies. *Journal of Cell Science, 106*(Pt 2), 473–483.
2. Pelaseyed, T., et al. (2014). The mucus and mucins of the goblet cells and enterocytes provide the first defense line of the gastrointestinal tract and interact with the immune system. *Immunological Reviews, 260*(1), 8–20.

3. Shan, M., et al. (2013). Mucus enhances gut homeostasis and oral tolerance by delivering immunoregulatory signals. *Science, 342*(6157), 447–453.
4. Engelstoft, M. S., et al. (2013). Enteroendocrine cell types revisited. *Current Opinion in Pharmacology, 13*(6), 912–921.
5. Jarvi, O., & Keyrilainen, O. (1956). On the cellular structures of the epithelial invasions in the glandular stomach of mice caused by intramural application of 20-methylcholantren. *Acta Pathologica et Microbiologica Scandinavica. Supplement, 39*(Suppl 111), 72–73.
6. Gerbe, F., Legraverend, C., & Jay, P. (2012). The intestinal epithelium tuft cells: Specification and function. *Cellular and Molecular Life Sciences, 69*(17), 2907–2917.
7. Deckx, R. J., Vantrappen, G. R., & Parein, M. M. (1967). Localization of lysozyme activity in a Paneth cell granule fraction. *Biochimica et Biophysica Acta, 139*(1), 204–207.
8. Ouellette, A. J., et al. (1992). Purification and primary structure of murine cryptdin-1, a Paneth cell defensin. *FEBS Letters, 304*(2–3), 146–148.
9. Bevins, C. L. (2004). The Paneth cell and the innate immune response. *Current Opinion in Gastroenterology, 20*(6), 572–580.
10. Clevers, H. C., & Bevins, C. L. (2013). Paneth cells: Maestros of the small intestinal crypts. *Annual Review of Physiology, 75*, 289–311.
11. Cunliffe, R. N., et al. (2001). Human defensin 5 is stored in precursor form in normal Paneth cells and is expressed by some villous epithelial cells and by metaplastic Paneth cells in the colon in inflammatory bowel disease. *Gut, 48*(2), 176–185.
12. Shen, B., et al. (2005). Human defensin 5 expression in intestinal metaplasia of the upper gastrointestinal tract. *Journal of Clinical Pathology, 58*(7), 687–694.
13. Potten, C. S., & Loeffler, M. (1987). A comprehensive model of the crypts of the small intestine of the mouse provides insight into the mechanisms of cell migration and the proliferation hierarchy. *Journal of Theoretical Biology, 127*(4), 381–391.
14. Cheng, H., & Leblond, C. P. (1974). Origin, differentiation and renewal of the four main epithelial cell types in the mouse small intestine. V. Unitarian theory of the origin of the four epithelial cell types. *The American Journal of Anatomy, 141*(4), 537–561.
15. Barker, N., et al. (2007). Identification of stem cells in small intestine and colon by marker gene Lgr5. *Nature, 449*(7165), 1003–1007.
16. Sato, T., et al. (2009). Single Lgr5 stem cells build crypt-villus structures in vitro without a mesenchymal niche. *Nature, 459*(7244), 262–265.
17. Sato, T., et al. (2011). Paneth cells constitute the niche for Lgr5 stem cells in intestinal crypts. *Nature, 469*(7330), 415–418.
18. Rothenberg, M. E., et al. (2012). Identification of a cKit(+) colonic crypt base secretory cell that supports Lgr5(+) stem cells in mice. *Gastroenterology, 142*(5), 1195–1205 e6.
19. Bjerknes, M., & Cheng, H. (1981). The stem-cell zone of the small intestinal epithelium. III. Evidence from columnar, enteroendocrine, and mucous cells in the adult mouse. *The American Journal of Anatomy, 160*(1), 77–91.
20. Sangiorgi, E., & Capecchi, M. R. (2008). Bmi1 is expressed in vivo in intestinal stem cells. *Nature Genetics, 40*(7), 915–920.
21. Tian, H., et al. (2011). A reserve stem cell population in small intestine renders Lgr5-positive cells dispensable. *Nature, 478*(7368), 255–259.
22. Li, L., & Clevers, H. (2010). Coexistence of quiescent and active adult stem cells in mammals. *Science, 327*(5965), 542–545.
23. Munoz, J., et al. (2012). The Lgr5 intestinal stem cell signature: Robust expression of proposed quiescent '+4' cell markers. *The EMBO Journal, 31*(14), 3079–3091.
24. Lopez-Arribillaga, E., et al. (2015). Bmi1 regulates murine intestinal stem cell proliferation and self-renewal downstream of Notch. *Development, 142*(1), 41–50.
25. Montgomery, R. K., et al. (2011). Mouse telomerase reverse transcriptase (mTert) expression marks slowly cycling intestinal stem cells. *Proceedings of the National Academy of Sciences of the United States of America, 108*(1), 179–184.

26. Powell, A. E., et al. (2012). The pan-ErbB negative regulator Lrig1 is an intestinal stem cell marker that functions as a tumor suppressor. *Cell, 149*(1), 146–158.
27. Takeda, N., et al. (2011). Interconversion between intestinal stem cell populations in distinct niches. *Science, 334*(6061), 1420–1424.
28. van der Flier, L. G., et al. (2009). OLFM4 is a robust marker for stem cells in human intestine and marks a subset of colorectal cancer cells. *Gastroenterology, 137*(1), 15–17.
29. van der Flier, L. G., et al. (2009). Transcription factor achaete scute-like 2 controls intestinal stem cell fate. *Cell, 136*(5), 903–912.
30. Itzkovitz, S., et al. (2012). Single-molecule transcript counting of stem-cell markers in the mouse intestine. *Nature Cell Biology, 14*(1), 106–114.
31. Hsu, S. Y., Liang, S. G., & Hsueh, A. J. (1998). Characterization of two LGR genes homologous to gonadotropin and thyrotropin receptors with extracellular leucine-rich repeats and a G protein-coupled, seven-transmembrane region. *Molecular Endocrinology, 12*(12), 1830–1845.
32. de Lau, W. B., Snel, B., & Clevers, H. C. (2012). The R-spondin protein family. *Genome Biology, 13*(3), 242.
33. Glinka, A., et al. (2011). LGR4 and LGR5 are R-spondin receptors mediating Wnt/beta-catenin and Wnt/PCP signalling. *EMBO Reports, 12*(10), 1055–1061.
34. Carmon, K. S., et al. (2011). R-spondins function as ligands of the orphan receptors LGR4 and LGR5 to regulate Wnt/beta-catenin signaling. *Proceedings of the National Academy of Sciences of the United States of America, 108*(28), 11452–11457.
35. Walker, F., et al. (2011). LGR5 is a negative regulator of tumourigenicity, antagonizes Wnt signalling and regulates cell adhesion in colorectal cancer cell lines. *PLoS One, 6*(7), e22733.
36. Hao, H. X., et al. (2012). ZNRF3 promotes Wnt receptor turnover in an R-spondin-sensitive manner. *Nature, 485*(7397), 195–200.
37. Koo, B. K., et al. (2012). Tumour suppressor RNF43 is a stem-cell E3 ligase that induces endocytosis of Wnt receptors. *Nature, 488*(7413), 665–669.
38. Schuijers, J., et al. (2015). Ascl2 acts as an R-spondin/Wnt-responsive switch to control stemness in intestinal crypts. *Cell Stem Cell, 16*(2), 158–170.
39. Wong, V. W., et al. (2012). Lrig1 controls intestinal stem-cell homeostasis by negative regulation of ErbB signalling. *Nature Cell Biology, 14*(4), 401–408.
40. Wang, H., et al. (2004). Role of histone H2A ubiquitination in Polycomb silencing. *Nature, 431*(7010), 873–878.
41. de Napoles, M., et al. (2004). Polycomb group proteins Ring1A/B link ubiquitylation of histone H2A to heritable gene silencing and X inactivation. *Developmental Cell, 7*(5), 663–676.
42. Cao, R., Tsukada, Y., & Zhang, Y. (2005). Role of Bmi-1 and Ring1A in H2A ubiquitylation and Hox gene silencing. *Molecular Cell, 20*(6), 845–854.
43. Buchwald, G., et al. (2006). Structure and E3-ligase activity of the Ring-Ring complex of polycomb proteins Bmi1 and Ring1b. *The EMBO Journal, 25*(11), 2465–2474.
44. van der Lugt, N. M., et al. (1994). Posterior transformation, neurological abnormalities, and severe hematopoietic defects in mice with a targeted deletion of the bmi-1 proto-oncogene. *Genes & Development, 8*(7), 757–769.
45. Jung, P., et al. (2011). Isolation and in vitro expansion of human colonic stem cells. *Nature Medicine, 17*(10), 1225–1227.
46. Ootani, A., et al. (2009). Sustained in vitro intestinal epithelial culture within a Wnt-dependent stem cell niche. *Nature Medicine, 15*(6), 701–706.
47. Sato, T., et al. (2011). Long-term expansion of epithelial organoids from human colon, adenoma, adenocarcinoma, and Barrett's epithelium. *Gastroenterology, 141*(5), 1762–1772.
48. Dekkers, J. F., et al. (2013). A functional CFTR assay using primary cystic fibrosis intestinal organoids. *Nature Medicine, 19*(7), 939–945.
49. Lindemans, C. A., et al. (2015). Interleukin-22 promotes intestinal-stem-cell-mediated epithelial regeneration. *Nature, 528*(7583), 560–564.

50. Schwank, G., et al. (2013). Functional repair of CFTR by CRISPR/Cas9 in intestinal stem cell organoids of cystic fibrosis patients. *Cell Stem Cell, 13*(6), 653–658.
51. VanDussen, K. L., et al. (2015). Development of an enhanced human gastrointestinal epithelial culture system to facilitate patient-based assays. *Gut, 64*(6), 911–920.
52. Stanley, P. (2007). Regulation of Notch signaling by glycosylation. *Current Opinion in Structural Biology, 17*(5), 530–535.
53. Stanley, P., & Okajima, T. (2010). Roles of glycosylation in Notch signaling. *Current Topics in Developmental Biology, 92*, 131–164.
54. Guiu, J., et al. (2013). Hes repressors are essential regulators of hematopoietic stem cell development downstream of Notch signaling. *The Journal of Experimental Medicine, 210*(1), 71–84.
55. Pellegrinet, L., et al. (2011). Dll1- and dll4-mediated notch signaling are required for homeostasis of intestinal stem cells. *Gastroenterology, 140*(4), 1230–1240.e1–7.
56. Riccio, O., et al. (2008). Loss of intestinal crypt progenitor cells owing to inactivation of both Notch1 and Notch2 is accompanied by derepression of CDK inhibitors p27Kip1 and p57Kip2. *EMBO Reports, 9*(4), 377–383.
57. VanDussen, K. L., et al. (2012). Notch signaling modulates proliferation and differentiation of intestinal crypt base columnar stem cells. *Development, 139*(3), 488–497.
58. Fre, S., et al. (2011). Notch lineages and activity in intestinal stem cells determined by a new set of knock-in mice. *PLoS One, 6*(10), e25785.
59. Rodilla, V., et al. (2009). Jagged1 is the pathological link between Wnt and Notch pathways in colorectal cancer. *Proceedings of the National Academy of Sciences of the United States of America, 106*(15), 6315–6320.
60. Schroder, N., & Gossler, A. (2002). Expression of Notch pathway components in fetal and adult mouse small intestine. *Gene Expression Patterns, 2*(3–4), 247–250.
61. Jensen, J., et al. (2000). Control of endodermal endocrine development by Hes-1. *Nature Genetics, 24*(1), 36–44.
62. van Es, J. H., et al. (2005). Notch/gamma-secretase inhibition turns proliferative cells in intestinal crypts and adenomas into goblet cells. *Nature, 435*(7044), 959–963.
63. Fre, S., et al. (2005). Notch signals control the fate of immature progenitor cells in the intestine. *Nature, 435*(7044), 964–968.
64. Guilmeau, S., et al. (2008). Intestinal deletion of Pofut1 in the mouse inactivates notch signaling and causes enterocolitis. *Gastroenterology, 135*(3), 849–860.e1–6.
65. Jarriault, S., et al. (1995). Signalling downstream of activated mammalian notch. *Nature, 377*(6547), 355–358.
66. Yang, Q., et al. (2001). Requirement of Math1 for secretory cell lineage commitment in the mouse intestine. *Science, 294*(5549), 2155–2158.
67. van Es, J. H., et al. (2010). Intestinal stem cells lacking the Math1 tumour suppressor are refractory to Notch inhibitors. *Nature Communications, 1*, 18.
68. Ferlay, J., et al. (2013). Cancer incidence and mortality patterns in Europe: Estimates for 40 countries in 2012. *European Journal of Cancer, 49*(6), 1374–1403.
69. Fodde, R., & Smits, R. (2001). Disease model: Familial adenomatous polyposis. *Trends in Molecular Medicine, 7*(8), 369–373.
70. Fearon, E. R., & Vogelstein, B. (1990). A genetic model for colorectal tumorigenesis. *Cell, 61*(5), 759–767.
71. Levy, D. B., et al. (1994). Inactivation of both APC alleles in human and mouse tumors. *Cancer Research, 54*(22), 5953–5958.
72. Gregorieff, A., & Clevers, H. (2005). Wnt signaling in the intestinal epithelium: From endoderm to cancer. *Genes & Development, 19*(8), 877–890.
73. Albuquerque, C., et al. (2002). The 'just-right' signaling model: APC somatic mutations are selected based on a specific level of activation of the beta-catenin signaling cascade. *Human Molecular Genetics, 11*(13), 1549–1560.

74. Crabtree, M., et al. (2003). Refining the relation between 'first hits' and 'second hits' at the APC locus: The 'loose fit' model and evidence for differences in somatic mutation spectra among patients. *Oncogene, 22*(27), 4257–4265.
75. Ichii, S., et al. (1993). Detailed analysis of genetic alterations in colorectal tumors from patients with and without familial adenomatous polyposis (FAP). *Oncogene, 8*(9), 2399–2405.
76. Su, L. K., et al. (1992). Multiple intestinal neoplasia caused by a mutation in the murine homolog of the APC gene. *Science, 256*(5057), 668–670.
77. Stamos, J. L., & Weis, W. I. (2013). The beta-catenin destruction complex. *Cold Spring Harbor Perspectives in Biology, 5*(1), a007898.
78. Batlle, E., et al. (2002). Beta-catenin and TCF mediate cell positioning in the intestinal epithelium by controlling the expression of EphB/ephrinB. *Cell, 111*(2), 251–263.
79. van de Wetering, M., et al. (2002). The beta-catenin/TCF-4 complex imposes a crypt progenitor phenotype on colorectal cancer cells. *Cell, 111*(2), 241–250.
80. Sancho, E., Batlle, E., & Clevers, H. (2004). Signaling pathways in intestinal development and cancer. *Annual Review of Cell and Developmental Biology, 20*, 695–723.
81. Korinek, V., et al. (1997). Constitutive transcriptional activation by a beta-catenin-Tcf complex in APC-/- colon carcinoma. *Science, 275*(5307), 1784–1787.
82. Morin, P. J., et al. (1997). Activation of beta-catenin-Tcf signaling in colon cancer by mutations in beta-catenin or APC. *Science, 275*(5307), 1787–1790.
83. Rubinfeld, B., et al. (1993). Association of the APC gene product with beta-catenin. *Science, 262*(5140), 1731–1734.
84. Su, L. K., Vogelstein, B., & Kinzler, K. W. (1993). Association of the APC tumor suppressor protein with catenins. *Science, 262*(5140), 1734–1737.
85. Hinck, L., et al. (1994). Beta-catenin: A common target for the regulation of cell adhesion by Wnt-1 and Src signaling pathways. *Trends in Biochemical Sciences, 19*(12), 538–542.
86. Cortina, C., et al. (2007). EphB-ephrin-B interactions suppress colorectal cancer progression by compartmentalizing tumor cells. *Nature Genetics, 39*(11), 1376–1383.
87. Dow, L. E., et al. (2015). Apc restoration promotes cellular differentiation and reestablishes crypt homeostasis in colorectal cancer. *Cell, 161*(7), 1539–1552.
88. Feng, Y., et al. (2011). Mutant KRAS promotes hyperplasia and alters differentiation in the colon epithelium but does not expand the presumptive stem cell pool. *Gastroenterology, 141*(3), 1003–1013.e1–10.
89. Luo, F., et al. (2007). Conditional expression of mutated K-ras accelerates intestinal tumorigenesis in Msh2-deficient mice. *Oncogene, 26*(30), 4415–4427.
90. Luo, F., et al. (2011). Synergism between K-rasVal12 and mutant Apc accelerates murine large intestinal tumourigenesis. *Oncology Reports, 26*(1), 125–133.
91. Drost, J., et al. (2015). Sequential cancer mutations in cultured human intestinal stem cells. *Nature, 521*(7550), 43–47.
92. Sui, X., et al. (2015). p53 controls colorectal cancer cell invasion by inhibiting the NF-kappaB-mediated activation of Fascin. *Oncotarget, 6*(26), 22869–22879.
93. Benhattar, J., et al. (1996). p53 mutations as a possible predictor of response to chemotherapy in metastatic colorectal carcinomas. *International Journal of Cancer, 69*(3), 190–192.
94. Fearon, E. R. (2011). Molecular genetics of colorectal cancer. *Annual Review of Pathology, 6*, 479–507.
95. Guinney, J., et al. (2015). The consensus molecular subtypes of colorectal cancer. *Nature Medicine, 21*(11), 1350–1356.
96. Clevers, H. (2011). The cancer stem cell: Premises, promises and challenges. *Nature Medicine, 17*(3), 313–319.
97. Dick, J. E. (2008). Stem cell concepts renew cancer research. *Blood, 112*(13), 4793–4807.
98. Visvader, J. E., & Lindeman, G. J. (2008). Cancer stem cells in solid tumours: Accumulating evidence and unresolved questions. *Nature Reviews Cancer, 8*(10), 755–768.
99. Colak, S., & Medema, J. P. (2014). Cancer stem cells – Important players in tumor therapy resistance. *The FEBS Journal, 281*(21), 4779–4791.

100. O'Brien, C. A., et al. (2007). A human colon cancer cell capable of initiating tumour growth in immunodeficient mice. *Nature, 445*(7123), 106–110.
101. Ricci-Vitiani, L., et al. (2007). Identification and expansion of human colon-cancer-initiating cells. *Nature, 445*(7123), 111–115.
102. Dalerba, P., et al. (2007). Phenotypic characterization of human colorectal cancer stem cells. *Proceedings of the National Academy of Sciences of the United States of America, 104*(24), 10158–10163.
103. Todaro, M., et al. (2014). CD44v6 is a marker of constitutive and reprogrammed cancer stem cells driving colon cancer metastasis. *Cell Stem Cell, 14*(3), 342–356.
104. Huang, E. H., et al. (2009). Aldehyde dehydrogenase 1 is a marker for normal and malignant human colonic stem cells (SC) and tracks SC overpopulation during colon tumorigenesis. *Cancer Research, 69*(8), 3382–3389.
105. Pang, R., et al. (2010). A subpopulation of CD26+ cancer stem cells with metastatic capacity in human colorectal cancer. *Cell Stem Cell, 6*(6), 603–615.
106. Merlos-Suarez, A., et al. (2011). The intestinal stem cell signature identifies colorectal cancer stem cells and predicts disease relapse. *Cell Stem Cell, 8*(5), 511–524.
107. Schepers, A. G., et al. (2012). Lineage tracing reveals Lgr5+ stem cell activity in mouse intestinal adenomas. *Science, 337*(6095), 730–735.
108. Asfaha, S., et al. (2015). Krt19(+)/Lgr5(-) cells are radioresistant cancer-initiating stem cells in the colon and intestine. *Cell Stem Cell, 16*(6), 627–638.
109. Jung, P., et al. (2015). Isolation of human colon stem cells using surface expression of PTK7. *Stem Cell Reports, 5*(6), 979–987.
110. Barker, N., et al. (2009). Crypt stem cells as the cells-of-origin of intestinal cancer. *Nature, 457*(7229), 608–611.
111. Zhu, L., et al. (2009). Prominin 1 marks intestinal stem cells that are susceptible to neoplastic transformation. *Nature, 457*(7229), 603–607.
112. Fre, S., et al. (2009). Notch and Wnt signals cooperatively control cell proliferation and tumorigenesis in the intestine. *Proceedings of the National Academy of Sciences of the United States of America, 106*(15), 6309–6314.
113. Sonoshita, M., et al. (2011). Suppression of colon cancer metastasis by Aes through inhibition of Notch signaling. *Cancer Cell, 19*(1), 125–137.
114. Sonoshita, M., et al. (2015). Promotion of colorectal cancer invasion and metastasis through activation of NOTCH-DAB1-ABL-RHOGEF protein TRIO. *Cancer Discovery, 5*(2), 198–211.
115. Lopez-Arribillaga, E. (2018). Manic Fringe deficiency imposes Jagged1 addiction to intestinal tumor cells. *Nature Communications, 9*(1), 2992.
116. Zheng, H., et al. (2017). Therapeutic antibody targeting tumor- and osteoblastic niche-derived Jagged1 sensitizes bone metastasis to chemotherapy. *Cancer Cell, 32*(6), 731–747 e6.
117. Reedijk, M., et al. (2008). Activation of Notch signaling in human colon adenocarcinoma. *International Journal of Oncology, 33*(6), 1223–1229.
118. Zhang, Y., et al. (2010). Notch1 regulates the growth of human colon cancers. *Cancer, 116*(22), 5207–5218.
119. Lu, J., et al. (2013). Endothelial cells promote the colorectal cancer stem cell phenotype through a soluble form of Jagged-1. *Cancer Cell, 23*(2), 171–185.
120. Dai, Y., et al. (2014). Silencing of Jagged1 inhibits cell growth and invasion in colorectal cancer. *Cell Death & Disease, 5*, e1170.
121. Hoey, T., et al. (2009). DLL4 blockade inhibits tumor growth and reduces tumor-initiating cell frequency. *Cell Stem Cell, 5*(2), 168–177.
122. Mailhos, C., et al. (2001). Delta4, an endothelial specific notch ligand expressed at sites of physiological and tumor angiogenesis. *Differentiation, 69*(2–3), 135–144.
123. Ghaleb, A. M., et al. (2008). Notch inhibits expression of the Kruppel-like factor 4 tumor suppressor in the intestinal epithelium. *Molecular Cancer Research, 6*(12), 1920–1927.

124. Zhao, W., et al. (2004). Identification of Kruppel-like factor 4 as a potential tumor suppressor gene in colorectal cancer. *Oncogene, 23*(2), 395–402.
125. Timmerman, L. A., et al. (2004). Notch promotes epithelial-mesenchymal transition during cardiac development and oncogenic transformation. *Genes & Development, 18*(1), 99–115.
126. Fender, A. W., et al. (2015). Notch-1 promotes stemness and epithelial to mesenchymal transition in colorectal cancer. *Journal of Cellular Biochemistry, 116*(11), 2517–2527.
127. Candy, P. A., et al. (2013). Notch-induced transcription factors are predictive of survival and 5-fluorouracil response in colorectal cancer patients. *British Journal of Cancer, 109*(4), 1023–1030.
128. Fernandez-Majada, V., et al. (2007). Nuclear IKK activity leads to dysregulated notch-dependent gene expression in colorectal cancer. *Proceedings of the National Academy of Sciences of the United States of America, 104*(1), 276–281.
129. Margalef, P., et al. (2015). BRAF-induced tumorigenesis is IKKalpha-dependent but NF-kappaB-independent. *Science Signaling, 8*(373), ra38.
130. Van Cutsem, E., et al. (2009). Cetuximab and chemotherapy as initial treatment for metastatic colorectal cancer. *The New England Journal of Medicine, 360*(14), 1408–1417.
131. Cunningham, D., et al. (2004). Cetuximab monotherapy and cetuximab plus irinotecan in irinotecan-refractory metastatic colorectal cancer. *The New England Journal of Medicine, 351*(4), 337–345.
132. Lenz, H. J., et al. (2006). Multicenter phase II and translational study of cetuximab in metastatic colorectal carcinoma refractory to irinotecan, oxaliplatin, and fluoropyrimidines. *Journal of Clinical Oncology, 24*(30), 4914–4921.
133. Boland, P. M., & Fakih, M. (2014). The emerging role of neoadjuvant chemotherapy for rectal cancer. *Journal of Gastrointestinal Oncology, 5*(5), 362–373.
134. Pita-Fernandez, S., et al. (2015). Intensive follow-up strategies improve outcomes in non-metastatic colorectal cancer patients after curative surgery: A systematic review and meta-analysis. *Annals of Oncology, 26*(4), 644–656.
135. Hassan, K. A., et al. (2013). Notch pathway activity identifies cells with cancer stem cell-like properties and correlates with worse survival in lung adenocarcinoma. *Clinical Cancer Research, 19*(8), 1972–1980.
136. Kalen, M., et al. (2011). Gamma-secretase inhibitor treatment promotes VEGF-A-driven blood vessel growth and vascular leakage but disrupts neovascular perfusion. *PLoS One, 6*(4), e18709.
137. Miyamoto, S., Nakanishi, M., & Rosenberg, D. W. (2013). Suppression of colon carcinogenesis by targeting Notch signaling. *Carcinogenesis, 34*(10), 2415–2423.
138. Palagani, V., et al. (2012). Epithelial mesenchymal transition and pancreatic tumor initiating CD44+/EpCAM+ cells are inhibited by gamma-secretase inhibitor IX. *PLoS One, 7*(10), e46514.
139. Meng, R. D., et al. (2009). gamma-Secretase inhibitors abrogate oxaliplatin-induced activation of the Notch-1 signaling pathway in colon cancer cells resulting in enhanced chemosensitivity. *Cancer Research, 69*(2), 573–582.
140. Zhang, X., et al. (2014). A synthetic antibody fragment targeting nicastrin affects assembly and trafficking of gamma-secretase. *The Journal of Biological Chemistry, 289*(50), 34851–34861.
141. Ponnurangam, S., et al. (2016). Quinomycin A targets Notch signaling pathway in pancreatic cancer stem cells. *Oncotarget, 7*(3), 3217–3232.
142. Real, P. J., & Ferrando, A. A. (2009). NOTCH inhibition and glucocorticoid therapy in T-cell acute lymphoblastic leukemia. *Leukemia, 23*(8), 1374–1377.
143. Real, P. J., et al. (2009). Gamma-secretase inhibitors reverse glucocorticoid resistance in T cell acute lymphoblastic leukemia. *Nature Medicine, 15*(1), 50–58.
144. Samon, J. B., et al. (2012). Preclinical analysis of the gamma-secretase inhibitor PF-03084014 in combination with glucocorticoids in T-cell acute lymphoblastic leukemia. *Molecular Cancer Therapeutics, 11*(7), 1565–1575.

145. Wei, P., et al. (2010). Evaluation of selective gamma-secretase inhibitor PF-03084014 for its antitumor efficacy and gastrointestinal safety to guide optimal clinical trial design. *Molecular Cancer Therapeutics, 9*(6), 1618–1628.
146. Wu, Y., et al. (2010). Therapeutic antibody targeting of individual Notch receptors. *Nature, 464*(7291), 1052–1057.
147. Lafkas, D., et al. (2015). Therapeutic antibodies reveal Notch control of transdifferentiation in the adult lung. *Nature, 528*(7580), 127–131.
148. Tran, I. T., et al. (2013). Blockade of individual Notch ligands and receptors controls graft-versus-host disease. *The Journal of Clinical Investigation, 123*(4), 1590–1604.
149. Tiyanont, K., et al. (2013). Insights into Notch3 activation and inhibition mediated by antibodies directed against its negative regulatory region. *Journal of Molecular Biology, 425*(17), 3192–3204.
150. Falk, R., et al. (2012). Generation of anti-Notch antibodies and their application in blocking Notch signalling in neural stem cells. *Methods, 58*(1), 69–78.
151. Aste-Amezaga, M., et al. (2010). Characterization of Notch1 antibodies that inhibit signaling of both normal and mutated Notch1 receptors. *PLoS One, 5*(2), e9094.
152. Smith, D. C., et al. (2014). A phase I dose escalation and expansion study of the anticancer stem cell agent demcizumab (anti-DLL4) in patients with previously treated solid tumors. *Clinical Cancer Research, 20*(24), 6295–6303.
153. Fischer, M., et al. (2011). Anti-DLL4 inhibits growth and reduces tumor-initiating cell frequency in colorectal tumors with oncogenic KRAS mutations. *Cancer Research, 71*(5), 1520–1525.
154. Miles, K. M., et al. (2014). Dll4 blockade potentiates the anti-tumor effects of VEGF inhibition in renal cell carcinoma patient-derived xenografts. *PLoS One, 9*(11), e112371.
155. Ridgway, J., et al. (2006). Inhibition of Dll4 signalling inhibits tumour growth by deregulating angiogenesis. *Nature, 444*(7122), 1083–1087.
156. Yan, M., et al. (2010). Chronic DLL4 blockade induces vascular neoplasms. *Nature, 463*(7282), E6–E7.
157. Klose, R., et al. (2015). Soluble Notch ligand and receptor peptides act antagonistically during angiogenesis. *Cardiovascular Research, 107*(1), 153–163.
158. Yan, X., et al. (2015). Endothelial cells-targeted soluble human Delta-like 4 suppresses both physiological and pathological ocular angiogenesis. *Science China Life Sciences, 58*(5), 425–431.
159. Weng, A. P., et al. (2003). Growth suppression of pre-T acute lymphoblastic leukemia cells by inhibition of notch signaling. *Molecular and Cellular Biology, 23*(2), 655–664.
160. Moellering, R. E., et al. (2009). Direct inhibition of the NOTCH transcription factor complex. *Nature, 462*(7270), 182–188.

Chapter 14
Notch Signaling in Estrogen-Dependent Cancers

Judy S. Crabtree

Abstract Prolonged lifetime estrogen exposure due to early puberty, delayed menopause, environmental estrogen/phytoestrogen exposure, and/or exogenous hormone therapy has been correlated with an increased risk of estrogen-responsive cancers including breast, endometrial, and ovarian carcinomas. Accumulating evidence links aberrant Notch signaling with these estrogen-responsive cancers, and mechanisms of cross talk between the estrogen signaling pathway and Notch are beginning to emerge. Notch signaling is a tightly regulated process that is controlled temporally and spatially by the cellular environment, and Notch can behave as an oncogene or as a tumor suppressor in a cell-, tissue-, and timing-specific manner. The role played by Notch in cancer stem cells as a mediator of hormone therapy resistance is becoming increasingly clear, most notably in breast cancer, wherein combinatorial therapeutic strategies are being designed to target not only the bulk of tumor cells but also endocrine-resistant cancer stem cells. This chapter seeks to outline the recent history and current state of the estrogen-Notch interaction in estrogen-dependent cancers.

Keywords Notch · Estrogen · Breast · Endometriosis · Endometrial cancer · Ovarian · Estrogen receptor · Estrogen-related receptor · Cancer · Angiogenesis · Stem Cell

14.1 Introduction to Estrogen Signaling

Mechanisms of hormone action were first proposed by Jensen over 50 years ago and included a description of direct hormone binding to nuclear receptors [1]. The role of estrogen and its receptors has since expanded beyond the direct ligand-receptor interaction to include mechanisms of DNA binding, non-genomic effects, and receptor-mediated non-ligand hormone activities. In addition to their role in gonadal

J. S. Crabtree (✉)
Louisiana State University Health Sciences Center, Department of Genetics, New Orleans, LA, USA
e-mail: jcrabt@lsuhsc.edu

L. Miele, S. Artavanis-Tsakonas (eds.), *Targeting Notch in Cancer*,
https://doi.org/10.1007/978-1-4939-8859-4_14

function, estrogens are now known to impact many cellular processes in systems as varied as immune, neuroendocrine, vascular, and skeletal, as well as play a key role in disease such as cancers, endometriosis, uterine fibroids, autoimmune disease, and obesity [2]. Understanding the function of estrogens (and all steroid hormones) in both the normal and diseased state is critical for developing relevant therapeutic strategies for hormone-dependent pathologies.

Estrogens freely cross the cellular membrane to interact with estrogen receptors. Upon ligand binding, these receptors dimerize and activate gene transcription in the nucleus by binding to estrogen response elements (EREs) in the DNA, displacing corepressors and/or recruiting coactivators [3]. In mammals, there are two classical estrogen receptors, ERα and ERβ [4, 5], as well as three orphan nuclear receptors called estrogen-related receptors (ERRα/NR3B1, ERRβ/NR3B2, and ERRγ/NR3B3). ERRs have significant amino acid homology with ERα/β, yet do not bind to naturally occurring estrogens. Elevated expression of ERRα correlates with poor prognosis in breast and ovarian cancers [6, 7] and tumor aggressiveness in ovarian and endometrial cancers [8, 9]. Interestingly, ERRγ expression is linked with favorable outcomes and improved progression-free survival in ovarian and breast cancers [7, 10]. The role of ERRs in cancer has been reviewed recently [11], and this chapter will focus on the role of the classical estrogen receptors, ERα and ERβ.

Estrogens are present in both males and females, and ERα/β are differently distributed across tissues. Estrogen receptors are also present on the cellular membrane where they can initiate rapid, non-genomic signaling [12–14]. Mitochondria-localized estrogen receptor transcription factors have also been described [15], and GPR30/GPER, a G protein-coupled receptor, was identified in the endoplasmic reticulum where it binds estrogen leading to mobilization of intracellular calcium and production of phosphatidylinositol 3,4,5-trisphosphate, an upstream regulator of AKT in the nucleus [16, 17]. A recent review of estrogen biology is available [3].

Prolonged exposure to estrogens due to precocious puberty, delayed menopause, or the presence of environmental estrogens/phytoestrogens is associated with an increased risk of estrogen-responsive cancers [18]. Small molecule agonists and/or antagonists of estrogen receptors have been used as therapeutic strategies for estrogen-responsive cancers, but tumor recurrence and resistance limit the success of these approaches. Additionally, molecules with selective action in particular tissues have also been designed (termed selective estrogen receptor modulators, SERMs). These compounds function as agonists in some tissues and antagonists in others toward the goal of minimizing side effects while maximizing efficacy. For example, tamoxifen is a SERM that is used as a first-line therapy for estrogen receptor-positive breast cancer in premenopausal patients [19]. Tamoxifen is an ER antagonist in the breast but an agonist in other tissues such as the bone, endometrium, and vascular endothelium. Raloxifene, a second-generation SERM with a slightly different estrogenic profile, has decreased side effects compared to tamoxifen and is beneficial in the bone with decreased risk of endometrial cancer and cardiovascular events. Conversely, the pure ER antagonist ICI 182,780 (fulvestrant) is antiestrogenic in all tissues and causes degradation of ER proteins [20]. A complete understanding of the molecular pathways modulated by steroid hormones could lead to improved and novel therapeutics for hormone-related pathologies and prevention of therapy-resistant cancers. The signaling mechanisms by which steroid receptors regulate their many processes have been the subject of a number of reviews [16, 21, 22]. This chapter seeks to highlight data accumulated over the last 20 years on the intersection of estrogen and the Notch signaling pathways.

14.2 Introduction to Notch Signaling

Notch signaling is an evolutionarily conserved pathway that is involved in a number of cellular processes including cell self-renewal, proliferation, differentiation, and death. Notch activation occurs via juxtacrine activation of Notch receptors by ligands present on neighboring cells. In mammals, there are four notch receptors (Notch1–Notch4) and five known Notch ligands (Jagged-1 and Jagged-2 and Delta-like 1, 3, and 4). Of these, Delta-like 1 and 4 are activating ligands, while Delta-like 3 functions as a negative regulator [23]. Notch receptors are synthesized as single-chain proteins and are cleaved into extracellular and transmembrane subunits in the Golgi apparatus. Once present at the cellular membrane, binding to ligand induces a second cleavage event by ADAM10, which removes the extracellular subunit. ADAM17/TACE can also cleave Notch during ligand-independent activation [24, 25]. A third cleavage event by the γ secretase complex releases the Notch intracellular domain (NICD) which translocates into the nucleus and regulates transcription of Notch target genes by interacting with the CSL transcription factor complex. This interaction displaces corepressors and recruits coactivators to regulate the expression of Notch targets such as the HES and HEY families of genes [26]. Notch is known to regulate transcription of many genes involved in the cell cycle [26], apoptosis [27], and stem cell maintenance [28], and recent genome-wide studies suggest the number of Notch transcriptional target genes is even higher than initially thought [29].

Notch can also signal in a noncanonical fashion, wherein Notch affects cell survival and metabolism by interacting with the mitochondria in the cytoplasm, instead of in the nucleus [30]. Posttranslational modifications regulate Notch activity, with phosphorylation, glycosylation, and ubiquitination playing key roles in Notch availability and degradation [31]. Notch is known to cross talk with other important cellular signaling pathways such as the TNFα [32], interleukin 1β [33], VEGF [34], and TGFβ [35] signaling pathways and modulate pathways involved in cell survival and proliferation like NF-κB [36] and ErbB2 [37]. As a result of these layers of regulation, the effects of Notch signaling are tightly controlled in a dose-, time-, and cell context-dependent manner. As a result, Notch signaling in hormone-dependent cancers can have oncogenic or tumor-suppressive activity, depending on the cellular environment, tissue type, and strength of signal. Deregulation of the Notch pathway has been described in a variety of tumors including estrogen-responsive solid tumors of the breast [38, 39], endometrium [40], and ovary [41].

14.3 Notch-Estrogen Cross Talk in Cancers

14.3.1 Breast Cancer

Estrogens play a major role in the proliferation of normal mammary epithelia, and lifetime exposure to unopposed estrogens via early puberty, late menopause, and/or exogenous exposure through oral contraceptives or hormone replacement therapy has been linked to increased breast cancer risk [42]. Breast cancer itself is a heterogeneous disease that is split into clinico-pathological subcategories based on immunohistochemical staining, ERα positive, Her2/neu positive, and triple negative (cancers that lack expression of ERα, progesterone receptor, and Her2/neu), with ERα-positive cancers making up more than 80% of breast malignancies in developed countries. More recently, breast cancers have been further subcategorized at the molecular level by gene expression profiles into luminal A, luminal B, basal-like, Her2-enriched, and claudin-low subtypes [43, 44]. Of these, luminal A and luminal B tumors are ERα positive but have different molecular profiles. Luminal B tumors tend to have a worse prognosis, a higher proliferation rate as measured by Ki67, and a higher likelihood of developing endocrine resistance [45]. An even more granular molecular classification identifies ten subgroups on the basis of mutational and gene expression profiles [46]. Attempts have been made to correlate molecular signatures of breast cancers with patient outcomes for personalized breast cancer therapy. Two gene expression-based tests, Oncotype DX and MammaPrint/BluePrint, do predict clinical outcomes in early-stage breast cancer and provide information on the likelihood of benefit from chemotherapy [47, 48]. However, more complete analyses are required before genetic signatures can guide clinical decision-making processes, especially in late-stage cancers [46, 49].

14.3.1.1 Notch Receptors and Ligands

Aberrant activation of the Notch signaling pathway has been implicated in breast cancer pathogenesis [37, 50] due to elevated levels of Notch signaling pathway components, including Notch receptors, ligands, and target genes [51, 52]. For example, high levels of Jagged-1 and Notch1 expression correlate with poor overall survival [53–55], and loss of the Numb-mediated inhibitory control of Notch signaling is found in 50% of human breast cancers [56]. On the other hand, Notch2 appears to reverse the oncogenic impact of Notch1 and Notch4 in some breast cancer cells [57], and its expression tracks with more differentiated tumors [58].

The first evidence of cross talk between the Notch signaling pathway and estrogens was generated by Rizzo et al. studying breast cancer cell lines [59]. Despite the high expression of Jagged-1 and Notch1 mRNA in breast cancer specimens, Notch transcriptional activity did not correlate with receptor overexpression in breast cancer cell lines. In ERα-positive cells, estrogen inhibited Notch transcriptional activity through decreased Notch1 ICD levels that led to an accumulation of Notch at the cellular membrane. This effect was reversed by treatment with tamoxifen or raloxifene, demonstrating the involvement of ERα [59]. Further, this effect was independent of ligand, since estrogen had no effect on Jagged-1 protein levels, and this effect was also observed upon coculture of MCF7 cells with Jagged-1 overexpressing feeder cells. These data suggested that Notch signaling may be reactivated by the use of common first-line endocrine therapies for breast cancer [59]. Other investigators have generated conflicting results using cDNA arrays followed by semiquantitative RT-PCR, demonstrating an increase in Jagged-1 and Notch1 expression in MCF7 cells [60]. Differences in therapeutic approaches may account for this discrepancy in results. The data by Rizzo et al. were further confirmed through knockdown studies wherein Notch1 and Notch4 were ablated and with studies using γ secretase inhibitors. All of these approaches resulted in significant decreases in endpoints of tumorigenesis and increases in cellular apoptosis [37, 59]. GPER has also been shown to facilitate estrogen-Notch cross talk in breast cancer, independent of ERα. In ERα-negative cells, Pupo et al. report an increase in γ secretase-dependent activation of Notch1 and increased levels of the Notch target gene Hes1 upon stimulation with the GPER ligand G1 or estrogen [61].

Reactivation of Notch in the context of resistance to antiestrogen therapy or estrogen withdrawal results in the activation of ERα target genes, and overexpression of Notch1 has been measured in tamoxifen-resistant breast cancer samples [62]. Notch1 can activate transcription of ERα target genes via recruitment of Notch-CSL-MAML1 transcriptional complexes to promoter regions of ERα target genes [63]. CSL binding elements are frequently in close proximity to EREs, and the presence of ERα recruits p300. Data generated by Hao et al. suggests cross talk between p300 and the Notch transcriptional complex to activate ERα-responsive genes in the absence of estrogen [63]. PKCα overexpression in clinical specimens predicts endocrine therapy resistance [64]. Yun et al. demonstrate that overexpression of PKCα correlates with Notch4 expression. PKCα was shown to selectively increase Notch4, but not Notch1, in endocrine-resistant breast cancer cell lines through an AP-1-dependent mechanism [65]. DMXL2, a modulator of Notch signaling, is overexpressed in ERα-positive metastatic breast cancers that progress after endocrine therapy [66]. Another study reports that elevated levels of nicastrin, a subunit of the γ secretase complex, correlate with elevated Notch4 in estrogen therapy-resistant cells [67]. Treatment of cells with anti-nicastrin monoclonal antibody or a γ secretase inhibitor (GSI) attenuates the invasiveness of endocrine therapy-resistant cells by blocking endothelial to mesenchymal transition. On the other hand, overexpression of nicastrin induces Notch4, resulting in increased tamoxifen resistance and invasiveness [67].

The therapeutic implications of these studies are paramount and suggest that in response to antiestrogen therapy, ERα-positive breast cancers develop additional mechanisms through the Notch pathway to activate estrogen signaling. Therefore, the efficacy of endocrine therapy can be improved by the addition of Notch inhibition, and several studies have been reported which support this hypothesis. Preclinically, MCF7 xenografts treated intratumorally with tamoxifen combined with γ secretase inhibitor decrease tumor growth better than either agent individually [59]. Haughian et al. demonstrate that in luminal breast cancers, there is often an expansion of "luminobasal" cells upon antiestrogen therapy. Notch inhibitors block the expansion of luminobasal cells and increase the efficacy of antiestrogen therapy [68]. Yun et al. demonstrate increased tamoxifen sensitivity in ERα-positive, PKCα overexpressing cells in culture and in vivo that have been treated with Notch inhibitors [65]. Genome-wide chromatin remodeling studies demonstrate that there is a global change in the chromatin landscape in resistant breast cancers. Classical ERα signaling is "epigenetically disengaged," while Notch signaling is hyperactive. Blocking Notch signaling with γ secretase inhibitors attenuated growth of endocrine-resistant breast cancer cells [69]. Activation of the Notch pathway in serial xenografts in mice results in acquired resistance to tamoxifen, which can then be reversed by treatment with γ secretase inhibitors [62].

14.3.1.2 Stem Cells in Breast Cancer

Cancer stem cells (CSC) have been identified in breast cancer and are generally accepted to be responsible for tumor recurrence [70]. Despite being ERα negative, the growth of breast CSCs is affected by estrogen, and both tamoxifen and siRNA silencing of ERα inhibit the proliferation of breast cancer cell lines enriched with cancer stem cells. This signaling is thought to occur between non-CSC and CSC, similar to the paracrine communication between stromal and stem cells in the tumor microenvironment. Notch signaling was investigated by Harrison et al., and treatment with a γ secretase inhibitor blocked the response of CSCs to estrogen both in vitro and in vivo [71]. In contrast, Simoes et al. report a decrease in the number of CSCs in response to estrogen. In this study, the embryonic stem cell genes NANOG, OCT4, and SOX2 decreased upon estrogen treatment, implying differentiation and hence a decrease of the available CSC pool [72]. Other studies report that antagonism of ERα increases the number and self-renewing capability of CSCs and suggest that this activity may be responsible for endocrine therapy resistance. For example, tamoxifen treatment increased the number of MCF7 mammospheres [72], and in a different study, mammospheres were resistant to high doses of tamoxifen [73]. In preclinical in vitro and clinical studies after endocrine or chemotherapy, resistant cells and tumor biopsies are enriched for tumor-initiating cells as measured by markers of breast CSCs [74, 75].

Notch signaling is also required for proliferation of breast CSCs and is strongly linked to endocrine therapy resistance [76, 77]. Short-term treatment with endocrine therapies enriches for Jagged-1/Notch4 activated CSCs in patient tumor samples as well as PDX models. Two independent ERα-positive patient cohorts demonstrate that a Notch4/Hes/Hey gene signature predicts poor response to hormone therapy [77]. Further, hormone therapy has been reported to promote resistant, self-renewing CSCs through a mechanism involving Notch and ERα switching. In this study, initial responses to hormone therapy abrogated oxidative phosphorylation, increased paracrine levels of IL6, and resulted in a population of cells that were deficient in self-renewal, $CD133^{hi}/ER^{lo}/OXPHOS^{lo}$. These cells become metabolically active and utilize oxidative phosphorylation in the absence of ERα. Inhibition of IL6-Notch switches the $CD133^{hi}$ CSC dependence on IL6/Notch to dependence on ER by activating expression of ERα. Thus, through an oxidative phosphorylation mechanism presumably regulated by Notch, hormone therapy drives self-renewal of dormant CSCs and mediates metastatic progression [78].

Clinically, there are a number of trials investigating the combination of Notch inhibitors with tamoxifen and other standard of care chemotherapeutics to increase sensitivity of bulk tumor cells while simultaneously targeting CSCs. Studies have been performed to investigate the safety and target engagement profiles of γ secretase inhibitors MK-0752 (Merck), RO4929097 (Roche), and PF03084014 (Pfizer) in combination therapy with tamoxifen or letrozole for breast cancer. Additional phase II/III studies are in the planning stages. Second generation GSIs such as LY3039478 are currently being investigated in breast cancer in combination with endocrine therapy. For a comprehensive list of current breast cancer clinical trials, see clinicaltrials.gov.

14.3.2 Endometriosis/Endometrial Cancer

Endometrial cancer is the most common gynecological malignancy in the United States with an estimated 60,000 new cases diagnosed and more than 10,000 deaths in 2016 alone [79]. Endometrial cancers are classified by histological staging and appearance. Approximately 70–80% of endometrial cancers are estrogen-dependent and are classified as endometrioid adenocarcinoma, type I [80]. The remaining 20–30% are type II non-endometrioid cancers (typically serous papillary and clear cell carcinoma along with mixed Müllerian tumors) and are estrogen independent. The 5-year survival rate in patients with low-grade, localized disease is approximately 80%, with 15–20% of patients developing metastasis and tumor recurrence. Treatments have limited efficacy for advanced-stage disease due to chemoresistance [81]. Approximately 90% of endometrial cancers are sporadic, and 10% are inherited. Genetic mutations in PTEN, PI3CA and K-ras have been identified in endometrioid endometrial cancer along with alterations in DNA repair pathways involving MLH1, MSH6, and microsatellite instability [82, 83]. Mutation in p53 is associated with type II endometrial cancer, along with inactivating mutations in p16 and overexpression of Her2/neu [82].

During the reproductive years, normal uterine endometrium undergoes regular cycles of differentiation and remodeling throughout the menstrual cycle. This process is mediated by a variety of factors including hormones (specifically estrogen, progesterone, and chorionic gonadotropin), changes in cell cycle activities, differentiation of endometrial cells, and vascular remodeling to produce a receptive environment for implantation. Notch pathway components are present in the endometrium throughout the menstrual cycle [84–86], and the dysregulation of Notch signaling has been implicated in this tumor type.

14.3.2.1 Notch Receptors and Ligands in the Endometrium

In endometrial carcinoma, the presence/absence of individual Notch receptors and ligands remains an area of active debate. Reported results appear to be extremely dependent on the Notch receptor analyzed, menopausal state of the patient, phase of menstrual cycle at time of analysis, and tumor stage. Using immunohistochemistry, Mitsuhashi et al. reported elevated levels of Notch1, Notch3, Jagged-1, and Delta-like-4 in endometrial cancer ($n = 76$) versus normal endometrium from unmatched, non-cancer patients ($n = 37$) [85]. Further, the elevation of Notch1 increased in later-stage cancers and correlated with cancer aggressiveness measures such as ovarian metastasis and invasion into the myometrial layer of the uterus. Elevated Notch3 remained constant across all cancer stages and did not correlate with metastasis or invasion; however, elevation of Notch1 and Notch3 correlated with poorer patient outcomes [85]. The Mitsuhashi study did not analyze Notch4.

Another study by Cobellis et al. examined the levels of Notch1, Notch4, and Jagged-1 by immunohistochemistry in normal endometrial samples ($n = 60$) of pre- and postmenopausal women, along with unmatched pathologic endometrial samples ($n = 60$) from patients with polyps, endometrial hyperplasia, and carcinoma. In this study, Notch1 and Notch4 had equivalent expression in the normal proliferative phase, while Notch1 increased and Notch4 decreased in the normal secretory phase. The authors propose that this result indicates a key role for Notch4 in cellular proliferation as characterized by the proliferative phase of the menstrual cycle, while Notch1 plays a more significant role in cellular differentiation as is characteristic of the secretory phase. These results are consistent with the notion of unopposed estrogen inhibiting Notch1 activation, as Rizzo et al. observed in breast cancer cells [84]. Further, Notch1, Notch4, and Jagged-1 all decreased significantly in normal menopausal endometrium indicating a decreased role for Notch signaling in the normal postmenopausal endometrium. In pathologies, Notch1 demonstrated elevated expression in hyperplasia and carcinoma compared to polyps, whereas Notch4 and Jagged-1 displayed striking decreases with increasing histological grade. Notch often functions as an oncogene in tissues where its normal role is a regulator of progenitor or stem cell fate and as a tumor suppressor in cases when normal function is the induction of terminal differentiation. In the Cobellis study, the decrease in Notch4 and Jagged-1 protein from polyps to carcinoma suggests a role for Notch4 signaling as a tumor suppressor and perhaps Notch1 as an oncogene in endometrial carcinoma [84]. This study did not analyze Notch3, and there is no data on the menopausal status of the patients from whom pathological endometrial samples were obtained.

The Didžiapetrienė laboratory reports that Notch receptors (Notch1-4), ligands (Jagged-1, Jagged-2, and Delta-like 1), and target gene Hes1 are all significantly decreased at the RNA level (via q-PCR) in endometrial carcinoma ($n = 20$) when compared to matched, adjacent non-tumor endometrium ($n = 20$). This suggests that Notch signaling plays a tumor-suppressive role in endometrial cancers [87]. Further, at the RNA level, Notch1, Notch4, and Delta-like 1 were decreased significantly more in stage IB than stage 1A cancers. At the protein level as measured by Western blot, only Notch4 and Jagged-1 were decreased in endometrial cancer, leading the authors to propose that a change in the stability of Notch receptors and ligands may happen in the cancerous state [88]. A comprehensive, complete evaluation of known Notch receptors, ligands, and target genes is still necessary in a larger, well-controlled study of matched tumor/normal sample pairs of known estrogen status to understand the role of the different Notch receptors in endometrial pathology.

Endometrioid endometrial cancers are typically estrogen receptor positive and proliferate in response to estrogen. As mentioned above, aberrant Notch signaling has been proposed as a key mechanism in endometrial cancer. Wei et al. performed studies in Ishikawa (ER-positive) endometrial carcinoma cells and demonstrated that estrogen stimulated cell proliferation due to induction of Notch1 and that this effect could be abolished by using the γ secretase inhibitor, N-[N-(3,5-difluorophenacetyl)-L-alanyl]-S-phenylglycine t-butyl ester (DAPT). Blocking with the ER antagonist ICI 182,780 also blocked Notch signaling and induced growth arrest.

MicroRNAs are a class of small, non-coding RNAs that inhibit gene expression. Jurcevic et al. identified 138 miRNAs that were differentially expressed in endometrial carcinoma in comparison to normal endometrium [89]. One of these miRNAs, miR-34a, regulates the Notch signaling pathway by targeting both Notch1 and Delta-like 1. Using miR-34a mimetics and inhibitors, the effect of miR-34a on Notch1 and Delta-like 1 was confirmed in Ishikawa cells in vitro, suggesting that miR-34a mimetics may be another future avenue of therapeutic potential.

14.3.2.2 Stem Cells in Endometrial Carcinoma

Endometrial carcinoma stem-like cells are identified by the cell surface marker CD133. $CD133^+$ cells have active Notch signaling resulting in increased proliferation and low rates of apoptosis and play a critical role in retaining the self-renewing properties of cancer stem cells. Epidermal growth factor receptor (EGFR) is overexpressed, mutated, or otherwise functionally altered in many epithelial malignancies, including endometrial carcinoma. EGFR is an important histological marker for invasive potential and is predictive of recurrence and overall outcomes of endometrial cancers [90]. EGFR is also a therapeutic target for endometrial carcinoma through antibody or small molecule-based therapies. Treatment of Ishikawa cells with DAPT or AG1478 was more efficacious than treating with either compound alone suggesting that combination therapy targeting Notch and EGFR may have improved outcomes in endometrial cancer [91].

Another stem cell marker in endometrial carcinoma is Musashi-1 [92]. Endometrial carcinomas have significantly more Musashi-1 positive cells than normal endometrium. SiRNA knockdown of Musashi-1 resulted in increased expression of Notch1 mRNA. However, since Musashi-1 is a transcriptional repressor of Numb, which induces Notch internalization and degradation by ubiquitination, the loss of Musashi-1 resulted in significantly decreased levels of Notch1 and Hes1 protein. Further, the loss of Musashi-1 resulted in an accumulation of cells in the G1 phase indicating a block in cell cycle progression [92]. Musashi-1 may emerge as a putative therapeutic target for endometrial carcinoma stem cell therapy.

The expression of microRNAs may also play a role in regulating endometrial cancer stem cells. miRNA-134 is significantly downregulated in endometrial cancer stem cells. miRNA-134 is a member of the genetically imprinted DLK1-DIO3 region present on 14q23 which contains genes for large and small RNAs, for paternally expressed genes such as Delta-like homolog 1 (*DLK1*) and iodothyronine deiodinase 3 (*DIO3*) and also the maternally expressed genes *MEG3, MEG8,* and the antisense retrotransposon-like 1 (*RTL1*) [93]. Overexpression of miR-134 decreased proliferation, decreased the cell's ability to develop chemoresistance, and suppressed the migratory ability of human endometrial cancer stem cells. Further, overexpression of miR-134 decreased Notch pathway signaling in human endometrial cancer stem cells [94]. Whereas this miRNA has only been tested in stem cells from type II endometrial carcinoma, this pathway may also have utility in type I endometrial cancers. Additional studies are required to further elucidate the direct target(s) of miR-134 and their role in endometrial carcinoma.

14.3.2.3 Endometriosis and Infertility

Endometriosis is the aberrant overgrowth of hormonally responsive endometrial cells outside the uterine cavity that results in severe pelvic pain, dysmenorrhea, and infertility. Endometriosis affects one in ten women of childbearing age [95]. During the mid- to late secretory phase of the menstrual cycle, estrogen and progesterone induce the stromal cells of the endometrium to differentiate such that pregnancy will ensue if implantation occurs [96]. Notch is regulated by chorionic gonadotropin and progesterone to mediate uterine stromal differentiation and decidualization via several mechanisms [97, 98]. In mice, the lack of Notch1 decreases cellular proliferation by altering the activity of cell cycle proteins and by increasing apoptosis, suggesting that Notch signaling is crucial to promoting successful implantation. Given the role of Notch1 in decidualization, Su et al. studied the role of Notch1 in women with endometriosis, as well as in a baboon model of spontaneous endometriosis. They demonstrated that receptors Notch1 and Notch4, ligands Jagged-2 and Delta-like 4, and Notch target genes HES5 and HEY1 were decreased in endometriosis compared to normal endometrial tissue, suggesting that suppressed Notch signaling is responsible for decreased fertility in patients with endometriosis [99]. Additionally, one of the early genes activated in decidualization is FOXO1 [100], which acts as a Notch1 coactivator by interacting with CSL. In the endometrium, FOXO1 expression is also regulated by Notch1 such that in the case of endometriosis, suppression of the Notch signaling pathway also suppresses FOXO1 and inhibits decidualization [99]. Interestingly in normal endometrium, the mechanism through which Notch1 activates FOXO1 expression is by cross talk with the liganded progesterone receptor at the promoter of FOXO1 [97]. However, in endometriosis, progesterone resistance inhibits Notch1 activity, results in decreased FOXO1 expression and decidualization failure [99].

14.3.3 Ovarian Cancer

Ovarian cancer is by far the most lethal gynecologic cancer in the United States. It is estimated that over 22,000 new cases will be diagnosed in 2017, and ovarian cancer will be responsible for over 14,000 deaths [101]. This mortality rate is due in part to the lack of molecular markers to identify early ovarian cancers and the observation that more than 75% of patients present at diagnosis with stage III or IV disease. First-line therapy often involves debulking surgery followed by aggressive chemotherapy, but recurrence rates are high, and tumors are often resistant to further chemotherapy, resulting in a 5-year survival rate of 46.5% [101]. Treatment options for recurrent, resistant ovarian cancer are few, highlighting the necessity for new, targeted molecular therapies for this devastating disease.

The majority of ovarian cancers are classified as ovarian adenocarcinomas that derive from the ovarian surface epithelium. There are numerous histological subtypes, of which the most common is serous adenocarcinoma, followed by endometrioid and mucinous carcinomas as well as other, less common subtypes [102]. Although the etiology of ovarian cancer is unknown, there are several loss-of-function mutations in well-described tumor suppressor genes that have been correlated with ovarian cancer, for example, *TP53* [103], *PTEN* [104], and *BRCA1/2* in familial cancer [105, 106]. Similarly, overexpression or gene duplication of oncogenes has also been described for *PI3K* [107], *AKT2* [108], *EFGR* [109], *c-Myc* [110], *K-ras* [111], and *Her2/neu* [112]. Disruptions in the Notch signaling pathway have also been correlated with ovarian cancer formation.

14.3.3.1 Notch1

Initial studies of Notch1 signaling in ovarian cancer were performed by Hopfer et al. [113] on a collection of 32 ovarian cancers (17 ovarian adenocarcinoma, 12 ovarian adenoma, 3 borderline tumors), 3 ovarian cancer-derived cell lines (A2780, OVCAR-3, 2008), and 1 ovarian surface epithelial cell line (IOSE-144). At both the mRNA and protein levels, the group demonstrated a consistent increase in Jagged-2, DLL-1, and Manic Fringe in adenocarcinoma compared to adenoma. Overexpression of the Notch1 ICD in ovarian cancer cells led to an increase in proliferation and anchorage-independent growth, suggesting a role for Notch1 in ovarian tumorigenesis [113]. Analysis of Notch1 by Rose et al. demonstrates that NICD is overexpressed in 76% of human ovarian adenocarcinomas when measured by Western blotting and is consistent with the expression of NICD measured in ovarian cancer cell lines [114]. Knockdown of NICD using siRNAs to Notch1 ICD resulted in decreased proliferation in three ovarian cancer cell lines [114]. Further, Notch1 expression was shown to correlate with the stage and differentiation status of ovarian cancers. Using immunohistochemistry, Wang et al. demonstrated elevated expression of Notch1 in 95% of ovarian cancers compared to patient-matched opposite side normal ovarian tissue. These results were confirmed using RT-PCR and Western blotting, and additional stratification of these data indicates Notch1 expression increased in samples with poor differentiation and elevated FIGO staging scores [115]. Additionally, Notch1, Notch3, and Notch ligand DLL4 were elevated in 18 ovarian cancers compared to healthy ovarian tissues [116], and in a smaller study ($n = 10$), Notch1, Jagged-1, and DLL1 were elevated and correlated with metastatic ovarian cancers [117]. However, conflicting data has also been reported. Using a novel immunohistochemical method to detect Notch1 ICD in 147 ovarian cancer samples, none demonstrated increased Notch1, even though NICD was detected in other cancers with known Notch activation [118]. More recently, the prognostic utility of Notch receptors and ligands was assessed and correlated with patient outcomes using the Kaplan-Meier plotter [119] (http://kmplot.com) to analyze publically available ovarian cancer gene expression datasets from the Cancer Biomedical Informatics Grid (caBIG, https://biospecimens.cancer.gov/relatedinitiatives/overview/caBIG.asp), the Gene Expression Omnibus (GEO; http://www.ncbi.nlm.nih.gov/geo), and The Cancer Genome Atlas (TCGA; https://cancergenome.nih.gov) [120]. Elevated Notch2 and Notch3 expression was correlated with poor progression-free survival, whereas high Notch4 expression was associated with overall survival. These results suggest that the different Notch receptors may have different prognostic value in ovarian cancers.

Next-generation sequencing has also been performed to identify a molecular signature specific for a subtype of ovarian cancer that is associated with endometriosis termed endometriosis-associated ovarian cancer or EAOC. Recent studies have suggested that endometriosis may be a precursor lesion to this form of ovarian cancer and a molecular profile would aid diagnosis in preneoplastic lesions. Notch1, Notch2, and Notch4 showed recurrent missense mutations in EAOC specimens [121].

14.3.3.2 Notch3

Notch3 was also initially identified through studies designed to identify early biomarkers of ovarian cancer. In one study, Affymetrix microarrays were used to analyze transcriptional profiles of 42 ovarian cancers versus normal ovarian epithelium; Notch3 was upregulated more than threefold in this sample set [122]. Another study in ovarian cancer cell lines identified Jagged-2 when compared to immortalized ovarian surface epithelial cell lines [123]. Gene amplification was studied by Park et al. to identify chromosomal regions with copy number variations in 31 late-stage ovarian cancers [124]. Single nucleotide polymorphism (SNP) array and digital karyotyping both identified an amplified region on chromosome 19 – the region containing Notch3. Amplification of Notch3 was identified in 20% of the samples and was confirmed by increased protein expression as measured by fluorescent in situ hybridization and immunohistochemistry [124]. Notch3 knockdown by siRNA or inhibition of γ secretase decreased DNA synthesis as a measure of proliferation and increased apoptosis in ovarian cancer cell lines [124] suggesting that Notch3 activation may play an important role in ovarian cancer development. A similar study confirmed these results in a different sample set [125], while a genome-wide study of ovarian carcinoma conducted by The Cancer Genome Atlas (TCGA) revealed similar results with *Notch3* genetic changes identified in 50% of ovarian cancer cases [41]. Further studies implicated Notch3 as a prognostic indicator, demonstrating that elevated mRNA for *Notch3*, *Jagged-1*, and *Jagged-2* as well as elevated Notch3 protein correlated with chemoresistance and poor overall survival [126, 127].

The identification of Notch3 as a prognostic marker and driver of ovarian carcinoma led to mechanistic studies aimed at identifying the primary Notch ligand responsible for Notch3 activation. Choi et al. analyzed the expression levels of all known Notch ligands in ovarian cancer and found Jagged-1 to have the highest expression. Knockout of Jagged-1 in feeder cell cocultures negatively impacted the proliferative and adhesive properties of ovarian cancer cells, whereas constitutive expression of Notch3 ICD had the reverse effect [128]. Further studies confirm the presence of Notch3 and Jagged-1 expression in ovarian cancer samples and propose that dynamin-dependent endocytosis is a key step in the Jagged-1 activation of Notch3 [129].

Notch3 was found to exert its effect through the actions of target genes such as Pbx1. Pbx1 is a known proto-oncogene that has been studied in leukemias and was recently identified as a Notch3 target gene in ovarian cancer [130]. Chen et al. used a systems biology approach to identify Notch3 target genes by combining transcriptome analysis with ChIP-on-chip analysis. From this, they were able to demonstrate that the target genes identified by ChIP were often the same transcriptional regions regulated by Notch3 in ovarian cancer cells and were able to identify DLGAP5 as a new Notch3 target gene in ovarian cancer [131].

Studies of the epigenetic regulation and gene methylation modifications present in ovarian cancer were performed by Ivan et al. [132]. These studies used TCGA data to highlight the clinical relevance of epigenetic modification of genes in the Notch signaling pathway by examining the overlap between epigenetic regulation by methylation and miRNAs and overall patient survival. Using this approach, the authors found an inverse relationship between DNA methylation and the gene expression of *CCND1*, *PPARG*, and *RUNX1*, all genes involved in the Notch pathway. Further, the expression level of these genes along with the DNA methylation status was predictive of patient outcomes with low DNA methylation/high expression being indicative of poorer overall survival. miRNA correlations demonstrated a similar trend with an inverse relationship between miRNA levels and gene expression of *CCND1*, *PPARG*, and *RUNX1*. As with DNA methylation, patients with low miRNA expression/high gene expression demonstrated poorer overall survival [132].

In an effort to identify proteins involved in modulating the Notch3 signaling pathway in ovarian cancer, Jung et al. used a human proteome microarray to screen for Notch3-ICD interacting proteins [133]. The E3 ubiquitin-protein ligase WWP2 was identified as an interacting partner of Notch3 that specifically binds Notch3 over the other Notch receptors. Further, WWP2 attenuates Notch3 pathway activity and leads to cell cycle arrest. Analysis of TCGA data revealed that the majority of ovarian carcinomas carry inactivating mutations in WWP2, suggesting that in the normal ovarian epithelium, WWP2 acts as a tumor suppressor by inhibiting Notch3 activity [133].

14.3.3.3 Angiogenesis in Ovarian Cancer

In general, Notch is actively involved in angiogenesis and vessel patterning [134, 135], with Notch1, Notch4, DLL1, DLL4, and Jagged-1 being the most highly expressed Notch pathway components involved in the differentiation between the tip and tube cellular phenotype in a developing vessel [136–140]. In ovarian cancer, Lu et al. specifically examined the gene expression profiles of endothelial cells from normal ovarian tissue or aggressive ovarian cancer and detected 2.5X elevated expression of Jagged-1 among other genes [141]. Jagged-1 has been shown to be a critical regulator of tip formation and sprouting through competitive, antagonistic regulation of DLL4-activated Notch signaling [142], confirming hypotheses that the equilibrium between available Notch ligands can have significant effects on the outcome of pathway activation. DLL4 has been extensively studied as a regulator of angiogenic activities in ovarian tumor endothelium [135, 143, 144] and other tumors [145]. In one study, DLL4 was overexpressed in 72% of tumors analyzed and correlated with poor clinical outcomes. The investigators noted that DLL4 was lowest in tumors responding to anti-VEGF therapies and that the combination of anti-VEGF therapies plus knockdown of DLL4 in mouse models decreased tumor proliferation better than either therapy alone [146]. Subsequently, Kuhnert et al. reported efficacy using a humanized DLL4 monoclonal antibody (REGN421) in mouse xenograft models of ovarian cancer. Antagonism of DLL4 in this system led not only to a reduction in tumor volume but also the formation of nonfunctional blood vessels. As with the Hu study, combination of DLL4 monoclonal antibody with anti-VEGF therapy showed decreased tumor proliferation and decreased angiogenesis than either therapy alone [143]. Additionally, use of a γ secretase inhibitor in a mouse model of ovarian cancer resulted in decreased microvessel density, suggesting that Notch pathway inhibition by these compounds may also be a mechanism to block angiogenesis in tumors resistant to anti-VEGF therapies [147]. Estrogen also enhances angiogenic branching via signaling of the VEGF-DLL4/Notch pathway in human umbilical vein endothelial cells [148]. This effect is attenuated by inhibition of Notch signaling further supporting the combination of anti-DLL4/Notch and anti-VEGF as a putative therapy for estrogen-dependent cancers.

14.3.3.4 Stem Cells in Ovarian Carcinoma

Aberrant activation of the Notch signaling pathway plays a key role in chemoresistance and recurrence in ovarian cancer. This is generally attributed to the presence of a population of cancer stem cells (CSCs) that have the capacity to initiate tumor formation and self-renew through asymmetric division [149]. Cancer stem-like cells in ovarian cancer are identified by a variety of cell surface markers including CD44, CD24, CD117, CD133, and ALDH1. Depending on the published series, combinations of these various markers exhibit different CSC characteristics. For example, in a recent publication, $CD133^+$ and $ALDH1^+$ cells were implicated as CSCs, with the presence of $CD133^+$ cells in a primary ovarian cancer strongly correlating with poor survival and the coexpression of both $CD133^+$ and $ALDH1^+$ indicative of a decreased progression-free interval and poor overall survival [150]. Interestingly, of patients with CD133/ALDH1 positivity in primary tumors, 85% lost these surface markers in recurrent tumors where cancer stem-like cells would be expected to be more prominent. This may represent cellular differentiation or other changes that would lead to the loss of CSC surface markers [150]. Further studies are warranted to clarify this issue. In earlier studies, Bapat et al. reported a subpopulation of $CD44^+$ stem-like cells with tumor-initiating activity [151], and Zhang et al. isolated $CD44^+$ and $CD117^+$ cells from ovarian tumors with self-renewing and tumor-initiating properties [152]. This diversity in surface and functional markers may reflect the heterogeneity of ovarian cancer and ovarian CSC, and further studies are necessary to clarify this issue. Comprehensive reviews of the many stem cell marker studies have been recently published [153, 154].

Notch signaling is one of the signal transduction pathways that has been implicated in CSC stemness, along with Wnt/β-catenin, IL6/JAK/STAT, Hedgehog, NF-kB, and PI3K/AKT [28, 155, 156]. In a study of 45 matched primary and recurrent tumor samples, genes involved in these pathways, including Notch, were significantly increased in recurrent disease [157]. More recently, Kang et al. demonstrated that galectin-3 supports CSC stemness by activating Notch signaling via Notch1 ICD. Galectin-3 was overexpressed in advanced-stage ovarian cancers, and in vitro modulation of galectin-3 reduced the levels of cleaved Notch1 ICD and expression of Notch target genes Hes1 and Hey1 [158].

14.3.3.5 Epithelial-to-Mesenchymal Transition

Another characteristic of CSCs is their ability to acquire mesenchymal traits and the ability of cells to develop increased migratory and invasiveness characteristics. Notch signaling is an inducer of the epithelial-to-mesenchymal transition (EMT) along with TGFβ, Hedgehog, and Wnt signaling pathways and promotes tumor invasion, metastasis, and chemoresistance through the activation of EMT-associated transcription factors such as Snail, Slug, Twist, and ZEB [159, 160]. Notch3 was demonstrated to induce EMT, block carboplatin-induced apoptosis, and attenuate ERK phosphorylation in ovarian cancer cell lines [161]. Subsequent studies implicated Ras-associated protein Rap1A as the upstream activator of ERK and Notch in EMT [162]. Further accumulated evidence suggests that EMT can be blocked by Notch inhibition as a therapeutic strategy [163, 164]. Indeed, the γ secretase inhibitor DAPT blocked TGFβ-induced EMT in ovarian cancer cell lines [165, 166].

14.3.3.6 Targeting Notch in Ovarian Cancer

Preclinical studies demonstrate that inhibition of Notch pathway components is a viable strategy in ovarian cancer. Inhibition of Jagged-1 by siRNA delivered intravenously by chitosan nanoparticle delivery in an orthotopic mouse model of ovarian cancer demonstrated significant reductions in tumor volume and microvessel density. Further, knockdown of Jagged-1 sensitized cells to subsequent docetaxel treatment [167]. Several studies have demonstrated that Notch inhibition sensitizes ovarian cancer cells (particularly CSCs) to chemotherapy [168–173]. McAuliffe et al. show that overexpression of Notch3 results in the expansion of CSCs and increased resistance to platinum-based chemotherapy [170]. Treatment with a γ secretase inhibitor had the reverse effect, leading to depleted CSCs and increased sensitivity to platinum therapy. Importantly, the combination of γ secretase inhibitor and cisplatin was a synergistic effect that eliminated CSC and bulk tumor cells through enhanced DNA damage response, cell cycle arrest, and apoptosis [170]. Inhibition with the MRK-003 γ secretase inhibitor in combination with standard chemotherapy agent paclitaxel demonstrated decreases in Notch signaling and paclitaxel resistance in ovarian cancer model systems [169]. Pretreatment of chemotherapy-resistant ovarian cancer cell lines with the γ secretase inhibitors DAPT or MK-0752 also downregulates Notch and decreases proliferation [168, 171]. Yen et al. presented a novel strategy by inhibiting Notch2/3 with an antagonist antibody alone or in combination with paclitaxel [174]. Again, inhibition of Notch signaling in addition to standard chemotherapy demonstrated a decrease in CSCs and a delay in tumor recurrence in preclinical models. Similarly, inhibition of DLL4 with anti-DLL4 antibodies in combination with anti-VEGF therapy aflibercept was efficacious in reducing tumor volume in preclinical models of ovarian cancer [143, 175]. Finally, combination of Notch inhibition by DAPT in combination with Bay11-7085 decreased proliferation of ovarian cancer cell lines suggesting that this combination therapy may have efficacy in ovarian cancer [176].

The preclinical successes with Notch inhibition have led to clinical trials of Notch γ secretase inhibitors alone and in combination with other therapies. Several phase I trials have been reported, including the use of enoticumab, a humanized DLL4 monoclonal antibody [177], and three γ secretase inhibitors (MK-0752, RO4929097, and LY900009) [178–180]. The RO4929097 γ secretase inhibitor has completed a phase II clinical trial in patients with platinum therapy-resistant ovarian cancer but demonstrated insufficient activity to warrant further study as a monotherapy [181]. For a complete, up-to-date listing of clinical trials in progress, visit www.clinicaltrials.gov.

14.4 Conclusions

The regulation of estrogen signaling in cancers encompasses a much broader range of pathways than initially appreciated, and there is still much to be learned. The newly discovered mechanisms of cross talk between Notch and estrogen signaling pathways that have been identified in breast cancers may also be applicable and relevant to other estrogen-dependent cancers such as endometrial and ovarian cancers. The intersection of estrogen and Notch signaling pathways has opened up a new direction for future investigation into the etiology of hormone-dependent cancers. More importantly, these new studies are offering translational approaches that may have clinical utility in the form of combination therapies utilizing Notch inhibitors along with traditional chemotherapy regimens.

References

1. Jensen, E. V. (1962). On the mechanism of estrogen action. *Perspectives in Biology and Medicine, 6*, 47–59.
2. Burns, K. A., & Korach, K. S. (2012). Estrogen receptors and human disease: An update. *Archives of Toxicology, 86*, 1491–1504.
3. Hamilton, K. J., Hewitt, S. C., Arao, Y., & Korach, K. S. (2017). Estrogen hormone biology. *Current Topics in Developmental Biology, 125*, 109–146.
4. Kuiper, G. G., Enmark, E., Pelto-Huikko, M., Nilsson, S., & Gustafsson, J. A. (1996). Cloning of a novel receptor expressed in rat prostate and ovary. *Proceedings of the National Academy of Sciences of the United States of America, 93*, 5925–5930.
5. Mangelsdorf, D. J., Thummel, C., Beato, M., Herrlich, P., Schutz, G., Umesono, K., Blumberg, B., Kastner, P., Mark, M., Chambon, P., & Evans, R. M. (1995). The nuclear receptor superfamily: The second decade. *Cell, 83*, 835–839.
6. Ariazi, E. A., & Jordan, V. C. (2006). Estrogen-related receptors as emerging targets in cancer and metabolic disorders. *Current Topics in Medicinal Chemistry, 6*, 203–215.
7. Sun, P., Sehouli, J., Denkert, C., Mustea, A., Konsgen, D., Koch, I., Wei, L., & Lichtenegger, W. (2005). Expression of estrogen receptor-related receptors, a subfamily of orphan nuclear receptors, as new tumor biomarkers in ovarian cancer cells. *Journal of Molecular Medicine (Berlin), 83*, 457–467.
8. Fujimoto, J., Alam, S. M., Jahan, I., Sato, E., Sakaguchi, H., & Tamaya, T. (2007). Clinical implication of estrogen-related receptor (ERR) expression in ovarian cancers. *The Journal of Steroid Biochemistry and Molecular Biology, 104*, 301–304.
9. Fujimoto, J., & Sato, E. (2009). Clinical implication of estrogen-related receptor (ERR) expression in uterine endometrial cancers. *The Journal of Steroid Biochemistry and Molecular Biology, 116*, 71–75.
10. Ariazi, E. A., Clark, G. M., & Mertz, J. E. (2002). Estrogen-related receptor alpha and estrogen-related receptor gamma associate with unfavorable and favorable biomarkers, respectively, in human breast cancer. *Cancer Research, 62*, 6510–6518.
11. Tam, I. S., & Giguere, V. (2016). There and back again: The journey of the estrogen-related receptors in the cancer realm. *The Journal of Steroid Biochemistry and Molecular Biology, 157*, 13–19.
12. Gu, S., Papadopoulou, N., Gehring, E. M., Nasir, O., Dimas, K., Bhavsar, S. K., Foller, M., Alevizopoulos, K., Lang, F., & Stournaras, C. (2009). Functional membrane androgen recep-

tors in colon tumors trigger pro-apoptotic responses in vitro and reduce drastically tumor incidence in vivo. *Molecular Cancer, 8*, 114.
13. Gustafsson, K. L., Farman, H., Henning, P., Lionikaite, V., Moverare-Skrtic, S., Wu, J., Ryberg, H., Koskela, A., Gustafsson, J. A., Tuukkanen, J., Levin, E. R., Ohlsson, C., & Lagerquist, M. K. (2016). The role of membrane ERalpha signaling in bone and other major estrogen responsive tissues. *Scientific Reports, 6*, 29473.
14. Valadez-Cosmes, P., Vazquez-Martinez, E. R., Cerbon, M., & Camacho-Arroyo, I. (2016). Membrane progesterone receptors in reproduction and cancer. *Molecular and Cellular Endocrinology, 434*, 166–175.
15. Sepuri, N. B., Tammineni, P., Mohammed, F., & Paripati, A. (2017). Nuclear transcription factors in the Mitochondria: A new paradigm in fine-tuning Mitochondrial metabolism. *Handbook of Experimental Pharmacology, 240*, 3–20.
16. Shi, H., Kumar, S. P., & Liu, X. (2013). G protein-coupled estrogen receptor in energy homeostasis and obesity pathogenesis. *Progress in Molecular Biology and Translational Science, 114*, 193–250.
17. Revankar, C. M., Cimino, D. F., Sklar, L. A., Arterburn, J. B., & Prossnitz, E. R. (2005). A transmembrane intracellular estrogen receptor mediates rapid cell signaling. *Science, 307*, 1625–1630.
18. Key, T. J., Appleby, P. N., Reeves, G. K., Travis, R. C., Alberg, A. J., Barricarte, A., Berrino, F., Krogh, V., Sieri, S., Brinton, L. A., Dorgan, J. F., Dossus, L., Dowsett, M., Eliassen, A. H., Fortner, R. T., Hankinson, S. E., Helzlsouer, K. J., Hoff man-Bolton, J., Comstock, G. W., Kaaks, R., Kahle, L. L., Muti, P., Overvad, K., Peeters, P. H., Riboli, E., Rinaldi, S., Rollison, D. E., Stanczyk, F. Z., Trichopoulos, D., Tworoger, S. S., & Vineis, P. (2013). Sex hormones and risk of breast cancer in premenopausal women: A collaborative reanalysis of individual participant data from seven prospective studies. *The Lancet Oncology, 14*, 1009–1019.
19. Maximov, P. Y., Lee, T. M., & Jordan, V. C. (2013). The discovery and development of selective estrogen receptor modulators (SERMs) for clinical practice. *Current Clinical Pharmacology, 8*, 135–155.
20. Jia, M., Dahlman-Wright, K., & Gustafsson, J. A. (2015). Estrogen receptor alpha and beta in health and disease. *Best Practice & Research. Clinical Endocrinology & Metabolism, 29*, 557–568.
21. Gustafsson, J. A. (2016). Historical overview of nuclear receptors. *The Journal of Steroid Biochemistry and Molecular Biology, 157*, 3–6.
22. Schwartz, N., Verma, A., Bivens, C. B., Schwartz, Z., & Boyan, B. D. (2016). Rapid steroid hormone actions via membrane receptors. *Biochimica et Biophysica Acta, 1863*, 2289–2298.
23. Zhang, J., Gao, H., & Zhang, Y. (2017). Differential expression of the Notch1 receptor, and its ligands Dll1, Dll3 and Dll4 in distinct human pituitary adenoma subtypes. *Oncology Letters, 13*, 4533–4539.
24. Hirata, N., Yamada, S., Shoda, T., Kurihara, M., Sekino, Y., & Kanda, Y. (2014). Sphingosine-1-phosphate promotes expansion of cancer stem cells via S1PR3 by a ligand-independent Notch activation. *Nature Communications, 5*, 4806.
25. Palmer, W. H., & Deng, W. M. (2015). Ligand-independent mechanisms of Notch activity. *Trends in Cell Biology, 25*, 697–707.
26. Crabtree, J. S., Singleton, C. S., & Miele, L. (2016). Notch signaling in neuroendocrine tumors. *Frontiers in Oncology, 6*, 94.
27. Afshar, Y., Stanculescu, A., Miele, L., & Fazleabas, A. T. (2007). The role of chorionic gonadotropin and Notch1 in implantation. *Journal of Assisted Reproduction and Genetics, 24*, 296–302.
28. Takebe, N., Miele, L., Harris, P. J., Jeong, W., Bando, H., Kahn, M., Yang, S. X., & Ivy, S. P. (2015). Targeting Notch, Hedgehog, and Wnt pathways in cancer stem cells: Clinical update. *Nature Reviews. Clinical Oncology, 12*, 445–464.

29. Guruharsha, K. G., Kankel, M. W., & Artavanis-Tsakonas, S. (2012). The Notch signalling system: Recent insights into the complexity of a conserved pathway. *Nature Reviews. Genetics, 13*, 654–666.
30. Ayaz, F., & Osborne, B. A. (2014). Non-canonical notch signaling in cancer and immunity. *Frontiers in Oncology, 4*, 345.
31. Borggrefe, T., & Liefke, R. (2012). Fine-tuning of the intracellular canonical Notch signaling pathway. *Cell Cycle, 11*, 264–276.
32. Quillard, T., Devalliere, J., Chatelais, M., Coulon, F., Seveno, C., Romagnoli, M., Barille Nion, S., & Charreau, B. (2009). Notch2 signaling sensitizes endothelial cells to apoptosis by negatively regulating the key protective molecule survivin. *PLoS One, 4*, e8244.
33. Verginelli, F., Adesso, L., Limon, I., Alisi, A., Gueguen, M., Panera, N., Giorda, E., Raimondi, L., Ciarapica, R., Campese, A. F., Screpanti, I., Stifani, S., Kitajewski, J., Miele, L., Rota, R., & Locatelli, F. (2015). Activation of an endothelial Notch1-Jagged1 circuit induces VCAM1 expression, an effect amplified by interleukin-1beta. *Oncotarget, 6*, 43216–43229.
34. Gu, J. W., Rizzo, P., Pannuti, A., Golde, T., Osborne, B., & Miele, L. (2012). Notch signals in the endothelium and cancer "stem-like" cells: Opportunities for cancer therapy. *Vascular Cell, 4*, 7.
35. Kurpinski, K., Lam, H., Chu, J., Wang, A., Kim, A., Tsay, E., Agrawal, S., Schaffer, D. V., & Li, S. (2010). Transforming growth factor-beta and notch signaling mediate stem cell differentiation into smooth muscle cells. *Stem Cells, 28*, 734–742.
36. Osipo, C., Golde, T. E., Osborne, B. A., & Miele, L. A. (2008). Off the beaten pathway: The complex cross talk between Notch and NF-kappaB. *Laboratory Investigation; A Journal of Technical Methods and Pathology, 88*, 11–17.
37. Rizzo, P., Osipo, C., Pannuti, A., Golde, T., Osborne, B., & Miele, L. (2009). Targeting Notch signaling cross-talk with estrogen receptor and ErbB-2 in breast cancer. *Advances in Enzyme Regulation, 49*, 134–141.
38. Miele, L., Golde, T., & Osborne, B. (2006). Notch signaling in cancer. *Current Molecular Medicine, 6*, 905–918.
39. Stylianou, S., Clarke, R. B., & Brennan, K. (2006). Aberrant activation of notch signaling in human breast cancer. *Cancer Research, 66*, 1517–1525.
40. Daley-Brown, D., Oprea-Ilies, G. M., Lee, R., Pattillo, R., & Gonzalez-Perez, R. R. (2015). Molecular cues on obesity signals, tumor markers and endometrial cancer. *Hormone Molecular Biology and Clinical Investigation, 21*, 89–106.
41. N. Cancer Genome Atlas Research. (2011). Integrated genomic analyses of ovarian carcinoma. *Nature, 474*, 609–615.
42. Rice, M. S., Eliassen, A. H., Hankinson, S. E., Lenart, E. B., Willett, W. C., & Tamimi, R. M. (2016). Breast cancer research in the nurses' health studies: Exposures across the life course. *American Journal of Public Health, 106*, 1592–1598.
43. Herschkowitz, J. I., Simin, K., Weigman, V. J., Mikaelian, I., Usary, J., Hu, Z., Rasmussen, K. E., Jones, L. P., Assefnia, S., Chandrasekharan, S., Backlund, M. G., Yin, Y., Khramtsov, A. I., Bastein, R., Quackenbush, J., Glazer, R. I., Brown, P. H., Green, J. E., Kopelovich, L., Furth, P. A., Palazzo, J. P., Olopade, O. I., Bernard, P. S., Churchill, G. A., Van Dyke, T., & Perou, C. M. (2007). Identification of conserved gene expression features between murine mammary carcinoma models and human breast tumors. *Genome Biology, 8*, R76.
44. Perou, C. M., Sorlie, T., Eisen, M. B., van de Rijn, M., Jeffrey, S. S., Rees, C. A., Pollack, J. R., Ross, D. T., Johnsen, H., Akslen, L. A., Fluge, O., Pergamenschikov, A., Williams, C., Zhu, S. X., Lonning, P. E., Borresen-Dale, A. L., Brown, P. O., & Botstein, D. (2000). Molecular portraits of human breast tumours. *Nature, 406*, 747–752.
45. Sorlie, T., Perou, C. M., Tibshirani, R., Aas, T., Geisler, S., Johnsen, H., Hastie, T., Eisen, M. B., van de Rijn, M., Jeffrey, S. S., Thorsen, T., Quist, H., Matese, J. C., Brown, P. O., Botstein, D., Lonning, P. E., & Borresen-Dale, A. L. (2001). Gene expression patterns of breast carcinomas distinguish tumor subclasses with clinical implications. *Proceedings of the National Academy of Sciences of the United States of America, 98*, 10869–10874.

46. Curtis, C., Shah, S. P., Chin, S. F., Turashvili, G., Rueda, O. M., Dunning, M. J., Speed, D., Lynch, A. G., Samarajiwa, S., Yuan, Y., Graf, S., Ha, G., Haffari, G., Bashashati, A., Russell, R., McKinney, S., M. Group, Langerod, A., Green, A., Provenzano, E., Wishart, G., Pinder, S., Watson, P., Markowetz, F., Murphy, L., Ellis, I., Purushotham, A., Borresen-Dale, A. L., Brenton, J. D., Tavare, S., Caldas, C., & Aparicio, S. (2012). The genomic and transcriptomic architecture of 2,000 breast tumours reveals novel subgroups. *Nature, 486*, 346–352.
47. Paik, S., Shak, S., Tang, G., Kim, C., Baker, J., Cronin, M., Baehner, F. L., Walker, M. G., Watson, D., Park, T., Hiller, W., Fisher, E. R., Wickerham, D. L., Bryant, J., & Wolmark, N. (2004). A multigene assay to predict recurrence of tamoxifen-treated, node-negative breast cancer. *The New England Journal of Medicine, 351*, 2817–2826.
48. Cardoso, F., van't Veer, L. J., Bogaerts, J., Slaets, L., Viale, G., Delaloge, S., Pierga, J. Y., Brain, E., Causeret, S., DeLorenzi, M., Glas, A. M., Golfinopoulos, V., Goulioti, T., Knox, S., Matos, E., Meulemans, B., Neijenhuis, P. A., Nitz, U., Passalacqua, R., Ravdin, P., Rubio, I. T., Saghatchian, M., Smilde, T. J., Sotiriou, C., Stork, L., Straehle, C., Thomas, G., Thompson, A. M., van der Hoeven, J. M., Vuylsteke, P., Bernards, R., Tryfonidis, K., Rutgers, E., Piccart, M., & Investigators, M. (2016). 70-gene signature as an aid to treatment decisions in early-stage breast cancer. *The New England Journal of Medicine, 375*, 717–729.
49. Rivenbark, A. G., O'Connor, S. M., & Coleman, W. B. (2013). Molecular and cellular heterogeneity in breast cancer: Challenges for personalized medicine. *The American Journal of Pathology, 183*, 1113–1124.
50. Miele, L. (2006). Notch signaling. *Clinical Cancer Research, 12*, 1074–1079.
51. Yao, K., Rizzo, P., Rajan, P., Albain, K., Rychlik, K., Shah, S., & Miele, L. (2011). Notch-1 and notch-4 receptors as prognostic markers in breast cancer. *International Journal of Surgical Pathology, 19*, 607–613.
52. Bednarz-Knoll, N., Efstathiou, A., Gotzhein, F., Wikman, H., Mueller, V., Kang, Y., & Pantel, K. (2016). Potential involvement of Jagged1 in metastatic progression of human breast carcinomas. *Clinical Chemistry, 62*, 378–386.
53. Reedijk, M., Odorcic, S., Chang, L., Zhang, H., Miller, N., McCready, D. R., Lockwood, G., & Egan, S. E. (2005). High-level coexpression of JAG1 and NOTCH1 is observed in human breast cancer and is associated with poor overall survival. *Cancer Research, 65*, 8530–8537.
54. Dickson, B. C., Mulligan, A. M., Zhang, H., Lockwood, G., O'Malley, F. P., Egan, S. E., & Reedijk, M. (2007). High-level JAG1 mRNA and protein predict poor outcome in breast cancer. *Modern Pathology, 20*, 685–693.
55. Reedijk, M., Pinnaduwage, D., Dickson, B. C., Mulligan, A. M., Zhang, H., Bull, S. B., O'Malley, F. P., Egan, S. E., & Andrulis, I. L. (2008). JAG1 expression is associated with a basal phenotype and recurrence in lymph node-negative breast cancer. *Breast Cancer Research and Treatment, 111*, 439–448.
56. Pece, S., Serresi, M., Santolini, E., Capra, M., Hulleman, E., Galimberti, V., Zurrida, S., Maisonneuve, P., Viale, G., & Di Fiore, P. P. (2004). Loss of negative regulation by Numb over Notch is relevant to human breast carcinogenesis. *The Journal of Cell Biology, 167*, 215–221.
57. O'Neill, C. F., Urs, S., Cinelli, C., Lincoln, A., Nadeau, R. J., Leon, R., Toher, J., Mouta-Bellum, C., Friesel, R. E., & Liaw, L. (2007). Notch2 signaling induces apoptosis and inhibits human MDA-MB-231 xenograft growth. *The American Journal of Pathology, 171*, 1023–1036.
58. Parr, C., Watkins, G., & Jiang, W. G. (2004). The possible correlation of Notch-1 and Notch-2 with clinical outcome and tumour clinicopathological parameters in human breast cancer. *International Journal of Molecular Medicine, 14*, 779–786.
59. Rizzo, P., Miao, H., D'Souza, G., Osipo, C., Song, L. L., Yun, J., Zhao, H., Mascarenhas, J., Wyatt, D., Antico, G., Hao, L., Yao, K., Rajan, P., Hicks, C., Siziopikou, K., Selvaggi, S., Bashir, A., Bhandari, D., Marchese, A., Lendahl, U., Qin, J. Z., Tonetti, D. A., Albain, K., Nickoloff, B. J., & Miele, L. (2008). Cross-talk between notch and the estrogen receptor in breast cancer suggests novel therapeutic approaches. *Cancer Research, 68*, 5226–5235.

60. Soares, R., Balogh, G., Guo, S., Gartner, F., Russo, J., & Schmitt, F. (2004). Evidence for the notch signaling pathway on the role of estrogen in angiogenesis. *Molecular Endocrinology, 18*, 2333–2343.
61. Pupo, M., Pisano, A., Abonante, S., Maggiolini, M., & Musti, A. M. (2014). GPER activates Notch signaling in breast cancer cells and cancer-associated fibroblasts (CAFs). *The International Journal of Biochemistry & Cell Biology, 46*, 56–67.
62. Martz, C. A., Ottina, K. A., Singleton, K. R., Jasper, J. S., Wardell, S. E., Peraza-Penton, A., Anderson, G. R., Winter, P. S., Wang, T., Alley, H. M., Kwong, L. N., Cooper, Z. A., Tetzlaff, M., Chen, P. L., Rathmell, J. C., Flaherty, K. T., Wargo, J. A., McDonnell, D. P., Sabatini, D. M., & Wood, K. C. (2014). Systematic identification of signaling pathways with potential to confer anticancer drug resistance. *Science Signaling, 7*, ra121.
63. Hao, L., Rizzo, P., Osipo, C., Pannuti, A., Wyatt, D., Cheung, L. W., Sonenshein, G., Osborne, B. A., & Miele, L. (2010). Notch-1 activates estrogen receptor-alpha-dependent transcription via IKKalpha in breast cancer cells. *Oncogene, 29*, 201–213.
64. Assender, J. W., Gee, J. M., Lewis, I., Ellis, I. O., Robertson, J. F., & Nicholson, R. I. (2007). Protein kinase C isoform expression as a predictor of disease outcome on endocrine therapy in breast cancer. *Journal of Clinical Pathology, 60*, 1216–1221.
65. Yun, J., Pannuti, A., Espinoza, I., Zhu, H., Hicks, C., Zhu, X., Caskey, M., Rizzo, P., D'Souza, G., Backus, K., Denning, M. F., Coon, J., Sun, M., Bresnick, E. H., Osipo, C., Wu, J., Strack, P. R., Tonetti, D. A., & Miele, L. (2013). Crosstalk between PKCalpha and Notch-4 in endocrine-resistant breast cancer cells. *Oncogene, 2*, e60.
66. Faronato, M., Nguyen, V. T., Patten, D. K., Lombardo, Y., Steel, J. H., Patel, N., Woodley, L., Shousha, S., Pruneri, G., Coombes, R. C., & Magnani, L. (2015). DMXL2 drives epithelial to mesenchymal transition in hormonal therapy resistant breast cancer through Notch hyper-activation. *Oncotarget, 6*, 22467–22479.
67. Lombardo, Y., Faronato, M., Filipovic, A., Vircillo, V., Magnani, L., & Coombes, R. C. (2014). Nicastrin and Notch4 drive endocrine therapy resistance and epithelial to mesenchymal transition in MCF7 breast cancer cells. *Breast Cancer Research, 16*, R62.
68. Haughian, J. M., Pinto, M. P., Harrell, J. C., Bliesner, B. S., Joensuu, K. M., Dye, W. W., Sartorius, C. A., Tan, A. C., Heikkila, P., Perou, C. M., & Horwitz, K. B. (2012). Maintenance of hormone responsiveness in luminal breast cancers by suppression of Notch. *Proceedings of the National Academy of Sciences of the United States of America, 109*, 2742–2747.
69. Magnani, L., Stoeck, A., Zhang, X., Lanczky, A., Mirabella, A. C., Wang, T. L., Gyorffy, B., & Lupien, M. (2013). Genome-wide reprogramming of the chromatin landscape underlies endocrine therapy resistance in breast cancer. *Proceedings of the National Academy of Sciences of the United States of America, 110*, E1490–E1499.
70. Reya, T., Morrison, S. J., Clarke, M. F., & Weissman, I. L. (2001). Stem cells, cancer, and cancer stem cells. *Nature, 414*, 105–111.
71. Harrison, H., Simoes, B. M., Rogerson, L., Howell, S. J., Landberg, G., & Clarke, R. B. (2013). Oestrogen increases the activity of oestrogen receptor negative breast cancer stem cells through paracrine EGFR and Notch signalling. *Breast Cancer Research, 15*, R21.
72. Simoes, B. M., Piva, M., Iriondo, O., Comaills, V., Lopez-Ruiz, J. A., Zabalza, I., Mieza, J. A., Acinas, O., & Vivanco, M. D. (2011). Effects of estrogen on the proportion of stem cells in the breast. *Breast Cancer Research and Treatment, 129*, 23–35.
73. Cariati, M., Naderi, A., Brown, J. P., Smalley, M. J., Pinder, S. E., Caldas, C., & Purushotham, A. D. (2008). Alpha-6 integrin is necessary for the tumourigenicity of a stem cell-like subpopulation within the MCF7 breast cancer cell line. *International Journal of Cancer, 122*, 298–304.
74. Creighton, C. J., Li, X., Landis, M., Dixon, J. M., Neumeister, V. M., Sjolund, A., Rimm, D. L., Wong, H., Rodriguez, A., Herschkowitz, J. I., Fan, C., Zhang, X., He, X., Pavlick, A., Gutierrez, M. C., Renshaw, L., Larionov, A. A., Faratian, D., Hilsenbeck, S. G., Perou, C. M., Lewis, M. T., Rosen, J. M., & Chang, J. C. (2009). Residual breast cancers after conven-

tional therapy display mesenchymal as well as tumor-initiating features. *Proceedings of the National Academy of Sciences of the United States of America, 106*, 13820–13825.
75. Kabos, P., Haughian, J. M., Wang, X., Dye, W. W., Finlayson, C., Elias, A., Horwitz, K. B., & Sartorius, C. A. (2011). Cytokeratin 5 positive cells represent a steroid receptor negative and therapy resistant subpopulation in luminal breast cancers. *Breast Cancer Research and Treatment, 128*, 45–55.
76. Harrison, H., Farnie, G., Howell, S. J., Rock, R. E., Stylianou, S., Brennan, K. R., Bundred, N. J., & Clarke, R. B. (2010). Regulation of breast cancer stem cell activity by signaling through the Notch4 receptor. *Cancer Research, 70*, 709–718.
77. Simoes, B. M., O'Brien, C. S., Eyre, R., Silva, A., Yu, L., Sarmiento-Castro, A., Alferez, D. G., Spence, K., Santiago-Gomez, A., Chemi, F., Acar, A., Gandhi, A., Howell, A., Brennan, K., Ryden, L., Catalano, S., Ando, S., Gee, J., Ucar, A., Sims, A. H., Marangoni, E., Farnie, G., Landberg, G., Howell, S. J., & Clarke, R. B. (2015). Anti-estrogen resistance in human breast tumors is driven by JAG1-NOTCH4-dependent cancer stem cell activity. *Cell Reports, 12*, 1968–1977.
78. Sansone, P., Ceccarelli, C., Berishaj, M., Chang, Q., Rajasekhar, V. K., Perna, F., Bowman, R. L., Vidone, M., Daly, L., Nnoli, J., Santini, D., Taffurelli, M., Shih, N. N., Feldman, M., Mao, J. J., Colameco, C., Chen, J., DeMichele, A., Fabbri, N., Healey, J. H., Cricca, M., Gasparre, G., Lyden, D., Bonafe, M., & Bromberg, J. (2016). Self-renewal of CD133(hi) cells by IL6/Notch3 signalling regulates endocrine resistance in metastatic breast cancer. *Nature Communications, 7*, 10442.
79. Siegel, R. L., Miller, K. D., & Jemal, A. (2016). Cancer statistics, 2016. *CA: a Cancer Journal for Clinicians, 66*, 7–30.
80. Evans, T., Sany, O., Pearmain, P., Ganesan, R., Blann, A., & Sundar, S. (2011). Differential trends in the rising incidence of endometrial cancer by type: Data from a UK population-based registry from 1994 to 2006. *British Journal of Cancer, 104*, 1505–1510.
81. Amant, F., Moerman, P., Neven, P., Timmerman, D., Van Limbergen, E., & Vergote, I. (2005). Endometrial cancer. *Lancet, 366*, 491–505.
82. Bansal, N., Yendluri, V., & Wenham, R. M. (2009). The molecular biology of endometrial cancers and the implications for pathogenesis, classification, and targeted therapies. *Cancer Control, 16*, 8–13.
83. Hecht, J. L., & Mutter, G. L. (2006). Molecular and pathologic aspects of endometrial carcinogenesis. *Journal of Clinical Oncology, 24*, 4783–4791.
84. Cobellis, L., Caprio, F., Trabucco, E., Mastrogiacomo, A., Coppola, G., Manente, L., Colacurci, N., De Falco, M., & De Luca, A. (2008). The pattern of expression of Notch protein members in normal and pathological endometrium. *Journal of Anatomy, 213*, 464–472.
85. Mitsuhashi, Y., Horiuchi, A., Miyamoto, T., Kashima, H., Suzuki, A., & Shiozawa, T. (2012). Prognostic significance of Notch signalling molecules and their involvement in the invasiveness of endometrial carcinoma cells. *Histopathology, 60*, 826–837.
86. Van Sinderen, M., Cuman, C., Gamage, T., Rainczuk, K., Osianlis, T., Rombauts, L., & Dimitriadis, E. (2014). Localisation of the Notch family in the human endometrium of fertile and infertile women. *Journal of Molecular Histology, 45*, 697–706.
87. Jonusiene, V., Sasnauskiene, A., Lachej, N., Kanopiene, D., Dabkeviciene, D., Sasnauskiene, S., Kazbariene, B., & Didziapetriene, J. (2013). Down-regulated expression of Notch signaling molecules in human endometrial cancer. *Medical Oncology, 30*, 438.
88. Sasnauskiene, A., Jonusiene, V., Krikstaponiene, A., Butkyte, S., Dabkeviciene, D., Kanopiene, D., Kazbariene, B., & Didziapetriene, J. (2014). NOTCH1, NOTCH3, NOTCH4, and JAG2 protein levels in human endometrial cancer. *Medicina (Kaunas, Lithuania), 50*, 14–18.
89. Jurcevic, S., Olsson, B., & Klinga-Levan, K. (2014). MicroRNA expression in human endometrial adenocarcinoma. *Cancer Cell International, 14*, 88.

90. Cai, S., Zhang, Y. X., Han, K., & Ding, Y. Q. (2017). Expressions and clinical significance of COX-2, VEGF-C, and EFGR in endometrial carcinoma. *Archives of Gynecology and Obstetrics, 296*, 93–98.
91. Shang, C., Lang, B., & Meng, L. R. (2016). Blocking NOTCH pathway can enhance the effect of EGFR inhibitor through targeting CD133+ endometrial cancer cells. *Cancer Biology & Therapy, 19*(2), 113–119.
92. Gotte, M., Greve, B., Kelsch, R., Muller-Uthoff, H., Weiss, K., Kharabi Masouleh, B., Sibrowski, W., Kiesel, L., & Buchweitz, O. (2011). The adult stem cell marker Musashi-1 modulates endometrial carcinoma cell cycle progression and apoptosis via Notch-1 and p21WAF1/CIP1. *International Journal of Cancer, 129*, 2042–2049.
93. Benetatos, L., Hatzimichael, E., Londin, E., Vartholomatos, G., Loher, P., Rigoutsos, I., & Briasoulis, E. (2013). The microRNAs within the DLK1-DIO3 genomic region: Involvement in disease pathogenesis. *Cellular and Molecular Life Sciences, 70*, 795–814.
94. Gao, Y., Liu, T., & Huang, Y. (2015). MicroRNA-134 suppresses endometrial cancer stem cells by targeting POGLUT1 and Notch pathway proteins. *FEBS Letters, 589*, 207–214.
95. Eskenazi, B., & Warner, M. L. (1997). Epidemiology of endometriosis. *Obstetrics and Gynecology Clinics of North America, 24*, 235–258.
96. Ramathal, C. Y., Bagchi, I. C., Taylor, R. N., & Bagchi, M. K. (2010). Endometrial decidualization: Of mice and men. *Seminars in Reproductive Medicine, 28*, 17–26.
97. Afshar, Y., Miele, L., & Fazleabas, A. T. (2012). Notch1 is regulated by chorionic gonadotropin and progesterone in endometrial stromal cells and modulates decidualization in primates. *Endocrinology, 153*, 2884–2896.
98. Afshar, Y., Jeong, J. W., Roqueiro, D., DeMayo, F., Lydon, J., Radtke, F., Radnor, R., Miele, L., & Fazleabas, A. (2012). Notch1 mediates uterine stromal differentiation and is critical for complete decidualization in the mouse. *The FASEB Journal, 26*, 282–294.
99. Su, R. W., Strug, M. R., Joshi, N. R., Jeong, J. W., Miele, L., Lessey, B. A., Young, S. L., & Fazleabas, A. T. (2015). Decreased Notch pathway signaling in the endometrium of women with endometriosis impairs decidualization. *The Journal of Clinical Endocrinology and Metabolism, 100*, E433–E442.
100. Brar, A. K., Handwerger, S., Kessler, C. A., & Aronow, B. J. (2001). Gene induction and categorical reprogramming during in vitro human endometrial fibroblast decidualization. *Physiological Genomics, 7*, 135–148.
101. National Cancer Institute SEER Program website at https://seer.cancer.gov/statfacts/html/ovary.html, accessed on 21 June 2017.
102. Koshiyama, M., Matsumura, N., & Konishi, I. (2017). Subtypes of ovarian cancer and ovarian cancer screening. *Diagnostics (Basel)*, Mar 2;7(1). pii: E12. doi: https://doi.org/10.3390/diagnostics7010012. Review.PMID:28257098
103. Kupryjanczyk, J., Thor, A. D., Beauchamp, R., Merritt, V., Edgerton, S. M., Bell, D. A., & Yandell, D. W. (1993). p53 gene mutations and protein accumulation in human ovarian cancer. *Proceedings of the National Academy of Sciences of the United States of America, 90*, 4961–4965.
104. Obata, K., Morland, S. J., Watson, R. H., Hitchcock, A., Chenevix-Trench, G., Thomas, E. J., & Campbell, I. G. (1998). Frequent PTEN/MMAC mutations in endometrioid but not serous or mucinous epithelial ovarian tumors. *Cancer Research, 58*, 2095–2097.
105. Ford, D., Easton, D. F., Stratton, M., Narod, S., Goldgar, D., Devilee, P., Bishop, D. T., Weber, B., Lenoir, G., Chang-Claude, J., Sobol, H., Teare, M. D., Struewing, J., Arason, A., Scherneck, S., Peto, J., Rebbeck, T. R., Tonin, P., Neuhausen, S., Barkardottir, R., Eyfjord, J., Lynch, H., Ponder, B. A., Gayther, S. A., Zelada-Hedman, M., et al. (1998). Genetic heterogeneity and penetrance analysis of the BRCA1 and BRCA2 genes in breast cancer families. The Breast Cancer Linkage Consortium. *American Journal of Human Genetics, 62*, 676–689.
106. Kote-Jarai, Z., & Eeles, R. A. (1999). BRCA1, BRCA2 and their possible function in DNA damage response. *British Journal of Cancer, 81*, 1099–1102.

107. Philp, A. J., Campbell, I. G., Leet, C., Vincan, E., Rockman, S. P., Whitehead, R. H., Thomas, R. J., & Phillips, W. A. (2001). The phosphatidylinositol 3′-kinase p85alpha gene is an oncogene in human ovarian and colon tumors. *Cancer Research, 61*, 7426–7429.
108. Cheng, J. Q., Godwin, A. K., Bellacosa, A., Taguchi, T., Franke, T. F., Hamilton, T. C., Tsichlis, P. N., & Testa, J. R. (1992). AKT2, a putative oncogene encoding a member of a subfamily of protein-serine/threonine kinases, is amplified in human ovarian carcinomas. *Proceedings of the National Academy of Sciences of the United States of America, 89*, 9267–9271.
109. Kohler, M., Janz, I., Wintzer, H. O., Wagner, E., & Bauknecht, T. (1989). The expression of EGF receptors, EGF-like factors and c-myc in ovarian and cervical carcinomas and their potential clinical significance. *Anticancer Research, 9*, 1537–1547.
110. Tashiro, H., Miyazaki, K., Okamura, H., Iwai, A., & Fukumoto, M. (1992). c-myc overexpression in human primary ovarian tumours: Its relevance to tumour progression. *International Journal of Cancer, 50*, 828–833.
111. Enomoto, T., Weghorst, C. M., Inoue, M., Tanizawa, O., & Rice, J. M. (1991). K-ras activation occurs frequently in mucinous adenocarcinomas and rarely in other common epithelial tumors of the human ovary. *The American Journal of Pathology, 139*, 777–785.
112. Slamon, D. J., Godolphin, W., Jones, L. A., Holt, J. A., Wong, S. G., Keith, D. E., Levin, W. J., Stuart, S. G., Udove, J., Ullrich, A., et al. (1989). Studies of the HER-2/neu proto-oncogene in human breast and ovarian cancer. *Science, 244*, 707–712.
113. Hopfer, O., Zwahlen, D., Fey, M. F., & Aebi, S. (2005). The Notch pathway in ovarian carcinomas and adenomas. *British Journal of Cancer, 93*, 709–718.
114. Rose, S. L., Kunnimalaiyaan, M., Drenzek, J., & Seiler, N. (2010). Notch 1 signaling is active in ovarian cancer. *Gynecologic Oncology, 117*, 130–133.
115. Wang, M., Wang, J., Wang, L., Wu, L., & Xin, X. (2010). Notch1 expression correlates with tumor differentiation status in ovarian carcinoma. *Medical Oncology, 27*, 1329–1335.
116. Wang, H., Huang, X., Zhang, J., Shao, N., Chen, L. O., Ma, D., & Ji, C. (2014). The expression of VEGF and Dll4/Notch pathway molecules in ovarian cancer. *Clinica Chimica Acta, 436*, 243–248.
117. Oktem, G., Sanci, M., Bilir, A., Yildirim, Y., Kececi, S. D., Ayla, S., & Inan, S. (2012). Cancer stem cell and embryonic development-associated molecules contribute to prognostic significance in ovarian cancer. *International Journal of Gynecological Cancer, 22*, 23–29.
118. Kluk, M. J., Ashworth, T., Wang, H., Knoechel, B., Mason, E. F., Morgan, E. A., Dorfman, D., Pinkus, G., Weigert, O., Hornick, J. L., Chirieac, L. R., Hirsch, M., Oh, D. J., South, A. P., Leigh, I. M., Pourreyron, C., Cassidy, A. J., Deangelo, D. J., Weinstock, D. M., Krop, I. E., Dillon, D., Brock, J. E., Lazar, A. J., Peto, M., Cho, R. J., Stoeck, A., Haines, B. B., Sathayanrayanan, S., Rodig, S., & Aster, J. C. (2013). Gauging NOTCH1 activation in cancer using immunohistochemistry. *PLoS One, 8*, e67306.
119. Szasz, A. M., Lanczky, A., Nagy, A., Forster, S., Hark, K., Green, J. E., Boussioutas, A., Busuttil, R., Szabo, A., & Gyorffy, B. (2016). Cross-validation of survival associated biomarkers in gastric cancer using transcriptomic data of 1,065 patients. *Oncotarget, 7*, 49322–49333.
120. Chen, C., Wang, X., Huang, S., Wang, L., Han, L., & Yu, S. (2017). Prognostic roles of Notch receptor mRNA expression in human ovarian cancer. *Oncotarget, 8*, 32731–32740.
121. Er, T. K., Su, Y. F., Wu, C. C., Chen, C. C., Wang, J., Hsieh, T. H., Herreros-Villanueva, M., Chen, W. T., Chen, Y. T., Liu, T. C., Chen, H. S., & Tsai, E. M. (2016). Targeted next-generation sequencing for molecular diagnosis of endometriosis-associated ovarian cancer. *Journal of Molecular Medicine (Berlin), 94*, 835–847.
122. Lu, K. H., Patterson, A. P., Wang, L., Marquez, R. T., Atkinson, E. N., Baggerly, K. A., Ramoth, L. R., Rosen, D. G., Liu, J., Hellstrom, I., Smith, D., Hartmann, L., Fishman, D., Berchuck, A., Schmandt, R., Whitaker, R., Gershenson, D. M., Mills, G. B., & Bast, R. C., Jr. (2004). Selection of potential markers for epithelial ovarian cancer with gene expression arrays and recursive descent partition analysis. *Clinical Cancer Research, 10*, 3291–3300.

123. Euer, N. I., Kaul, S., Deissler, H., Mobus, V. J., Zeillinger, R., & Weidle, U. H. (2005). Identification of L1CAM, Jagged2 and Neuromedin U as ovarian cancer-associated antigens. *Oncology Reports, 13*, 375–387.
124. Park, J. T., Li, M., Nakayama, K., Mao, T. L., Davidson, B., Zhang, Z., Kurman, R. J., Eberhart, C. G., Shih Ie, M., & Wang, T. L. (2006). Notch3 gene amplification in ovarian cancer. *Cancer Research, 66*, 6312–6318.
125. Nakayama, K., Nakayama, N., Jinawath, N., Salani, R., Kurman, R. J., Shih Ie, M., & Wang, T. L. (2007). Amplicon profiles in ovarian serous carcinomas. *International Journal of Cancer, 120*, 2613–2617.
126. Jung, S. G., Kwon, Y. D., Song, J. A., Back, M. J., Lee, S. Y., Lee, C., Hwang, Y. Y., & An, H. J. (2010). Prognostic significance of Notch 3 gene expression in ovarian serous carcinoma. *Cancer Science, 101*, 1977–1983.
127. Rahman, M. T., Nakayama, K., Rahman, M., Katagiri, H., Katagiri, A., Ishibashi, T., Ishikawa, M., Iida, K., Nakayama, S., Otsuki, Y., & Miyazaki, K. (2012). Notch3 overexpression as potential therapeutic target in advanced stage chemoresistant ovarian cancer. *American Journal of Clinical Pathology, 138*, 535–544.
128. Choi, J. H., Park, J. T., Davidson, B., Morin, P. J., Shih Ie, M., & Wang, T. L. (2008). Jagged-1 and Notch3 juxtacrine loop regulates ovarian tumor growth and adhesion. *Cancer Research, 68*, 5716–5723.
129. Hu, W., Liu, T., Ivan, C., Sun, Y., Huang, J., Mangala, L. S., Miyake, T., Dalton, H. J., Pradeep, S., Rupaimoole, R., Previs, R. A., Han, H. D., Bottsford-Miller, J., Zand, B., Kang, Y., Pecot, C. V., Nick, A. M., Wu, S. Y., Lee, J. S., Sehgal, V., Ram, P., Liu, J., Tucker, S. L., Lopez-Berestein, G., Baggerly, K. A., Coleman, R. L., & Sood, A. K. (2014). Notch3 pathway alterations in ovarian cancer. *Cancer Research, 74*, 3282–3293.
130. Park, J. T., Shih Ie, M., & Wang, T. L. (2008). Identification of Pbx1, a potential oncogene, as a Notch3 target gene in ovarian cancer. *Cancer Research, 68*, 8852–8860.
131. Chen, X., Thiaville, M. M., Chen, L., Stoeck, A., Xuan, J., Gao, M., Shih Ie, M., & Wang, T. L. (2012). Defining NOTCH3 target genes in ovarian cancer. *Cancer Research, 72*, 2294–2303.
132. Ivan, C., Hu, W., Bottsford-Miller, J., Zand, B., Dalton, H. J., Liu, T., Huang, J., Nick, A. M., Lopez-Berestein, G., Coleman, R. L., Baggerly, K. A., & Sood, A. K. (2013). Epigenetic analysis of the Notch superfamily in high-grade serous ovarian cancer. *Gynecologic Oncology, 128*, 506–511.
133. Jung, J. G., Stoeck, A., Guan, B., Wu, R. C., Zhu, H., Blackshaw, S., Shih Ie, M., & Wang, T. L. (2014). Notch3 interactome analysis identified WWP2 as a negative regulator of Notch3 signaling in ovarian cancer. *PLoS Genetics, 10*, e1004751.
134. Phng, L. K., Potente, M., Leslie, J. D., Babbage, J., Nyqvist, D., Lobov, I., Ondr, J. K., Rao, S., Lang, R. A., Thurston, G., & Gerhardt, H. (2009). Nrarp coordinates endothelial Notch and Wnt signaling to control vessel density in angiogenesis. *Developmental Cell, 16*, 70–82.
135. Li, J. L., Sainson, R. C., Shi, W., Leek, R., Harrington, L. S., Preusser, M., Biswas, S., Turley, H., Heikamp, E., Hainfellner, J. A., & Harris, A. L. (2007). Delta-like 4 Notch ligand regulates tumor angiogenesis, improves tumor vascular function, and promotes tumor growth in vivo. *Cancer Research, 67*, 11244–11253.
136. Favre, C. J., Mancuso, M., Maas, K., McLean, J. W., Baluk, P., & McDonald, D. M. (2003). Expression of genes involved in vascular development and angiogenesis in endothelial cells of adult lung. *American Journal of Physiology. Heart and Circulatory Physiology, 285*, H1917–H1938.
137. Hofmann, J. J., & Iruela-Arispe, M. L. (2007). Notch signaling in blood vessels: Who is talking to whom about what? *Circulation Research, 100*, 1556–1568.
138. Villa, N., Walker, L., Lindsell, C. E., Gasson, J., Iruela-Arispe, M. L., & Weinmaster, G. (2001). Vascular expression of Notch pathway receptors and ligands is restricted to arterial vessels. *Mechanisms of Development, 108*, 161–164.

139. Xie, Q., Cheng, Z., Chen, X., Lobe, C. G., & Liu, J. (2017). The role of Notch signalling in ovarian angiogenesis. *Journal of Ovarian Research, 10*, 13.
140. Vorontchikhina, M. A., Zimmermann, R. C., Shawber, C. J., Tang, H., & Kitajewski, J. (2005). Unique patterns of Notch1, Notch4 and Jagged1 expression in ovarian vessels during folliculogenesis and corpus luteum formation. *Gene Expression Patterns, 5*, 701–709.
141. Lu, C., Bonome, T., Li, Y., Kamat, A. A., Han, L. Y., Schmandt, R., Coleman, R. L., Gershenson, D. M., Jaffe, R. B., Birrer, M. J., & Sood, A. K. (2007). Gene alterations identified by expression profiling in tumor-associated endothelial cells from invasive ovarian carcinoma. *Cancer Research, 67*, 1757–1768.
142. Benedito, R., Roca, C., Sorensen, I., Adams, S., Gossler, A., Fruttiger, M., & Adams, R. H. (2009). The notch ligands Dll4 and Jagged1 have opposing effects on angiogenesis. *Cell, 137*, 1124–1135.
143. Kuhnert, F., Chen, G., Coetzee, S., Thambi, N., Hickey, C., Shan, J., Kovalenko, P., Noguera-Troise, I., Smith, E., Fairhurst, J., Andreev, J., Kirshner, J. R., Papadopoulos, N., & Thurston, G. (2015). Dll4 blockade in stromal cells mediates antitumor effects in preclinical models of ovarian cancer. *Cancer Research, 75*, 4086–4096.
144. Patel, N. S., Li, J. L., Generali, D., Poulsom, R., Cranston, D. W., & Harris, A. L. (2005). Up-regulation of delta-like 4 ligand in human tumor vasculature and the role of basal expression in endothelial cell function. *Cancer Research, 65*, 8690–8697.
145. Trindade, A., Djokovic, D., Gigante, J., Mendonca, L., & Duarte, A. (2017). Endothelial Dll4 overexpression reduces vascular response and inhibits tumor growth and metastasization in vivo. *BMC Cancer, 17*, 189.
146. Hu, W., Lu, C., Dong, H. H., Huang, J., Shen, D. Y., Stone, R. L., Nick, A. M., Shahzad, M. M., Mora, E., Jennings, N. B., Lee, S. J., Roh, J. W., Matsuo, K., Nishimura, M., Goodman, B. W., Jaffe, R. B., Langley, R. R., Deavers, M. T., Lopez-Berestein, G., Coleman, R. L., & Sood, A. K. (2011). Biological roles of the Delta family Notch ligand Dll4 in tumor and endothelial cells in ovarian cancer. *Cancer Research, 71*, 6030–6039.
147. Shah, M. M., Zerlin, M., Li, B. Y., Herzog, T. J., Kitajewski, J. K., & Wright, J. D. (2013). The role of Notch and gamma-secretase inhibition in an ovarian cancer model. *Anticancer Research, 33*, 801–808.
148. Caliceti, C., Aquila, G., Pannella, M., Morelli, M. B., Fortini, C., Pinton, P., Bonora, M., Hrelia, S., Pannuti, A., Miele, L., Rizzo, P., & Ferrari, R. (2013). 17beta-estradiol enhances signalling mediated by VEGF-A-delta-like ligand 4-notch1 axis in human endothelial cells. *PLoS One, 8*, e71440.
149. Lupia, M., & Cavallaro, U. (2017). Ovarian cancer stem cells: Still an elusive entity? *Molecular Cancer, 16*, 64.
150. Ruscito, I., Cacsire Castillo-Tong, D., Vergote, I., Ignat, I., Stanske, M., Vanderstichele, A., Ganapathi, R. N., Glajzer, J., Kulbe, H., Trillsch, F., Mustea, A., Kreuzinger, C., Benedetti Panici, P., Gourley, C., Gabra, H., Kessler, M., Sehouli, J., Darb-Esfahani, S., & Braicu, E. I. (2017). Exploring the clonal evolution of CD133/aldehyde-dehydrogenase-1 (ALDH1)-positive cancer stem-like cells from primary to recurrent high-grade serous ovarian cancer (HGSOC). A study of the Ovarian Cancer Therapy-Innovative Models Prolong Survival (OCTIPS) Consortium. *European Journal of Cancer, 79*, 214–225.
151. Bapat, S. A., Mali, A. M., Koppikar, C. B., & Kurrey, N. K. (2005). Stem and progenitor-like cells contribute to the aggressive behavior of human epithelial ovarian cancer. *Cancer Research, 65*, 3025–3029.
152. Zhang, S., Balch, C., Chan, M. W., Lai, H. C., Matei, D., Schilder, J. M., Yan, P. S., Huang, T. H., & Nephew, K. P. (2008). Identification and characterization of ovarian cancer-initiating cells from primary human tumors. *Cancer Research, 68*, 4311–4320.
153. Foster, R., Buckanovich, R. J., & Rueda, B. R. (2013). Ovarian cancer stem cells: Working towards the root of stemness. *Cancer Letters, 338*, 147–157.
154. Ottevanger, P. B. (2017). Ovarian cancer stem cells more questions than answers. *Seminars in Cancer Biology, 44*, 67–71.

155. Iqbal, W., Alkarim, S., AlHejin, A., Mukhtar, H., & Saini, K. S. (2016). Targeting signal transduction pathways of cancer stem cells for therapeutic opportunities of metastasis. *Oncotarget, 7*, 76337–76353.
156. Matsui, W. H. (2016). Cancer stem cell signaling pathways. *Medicine (Baltimore), 95*, S8–S19.
157. Steg, A. D., Bevis, K. S., Katre, A. A., Ziebarth, A., Dobbin, Z. C., Alvarez, R. D., Zhang, K., Conner, M., & Landen, C. N. (2012). Stem cell pathways contribute to clinical chemoresistance in ovarian cancer. *Clinical Cancer Research, 18*, 869–881.
158. Kang, H. G., Kim, D. H., Kim, S. J., Cho, Y., Jung, J., Jang, W., & Chun, K. H. (2016). Galectin-3 supports stemness in ovarian cancer stem cells by activation of the Notch1 intracellular domain. *Oncotarget, 7*, 68229–68241.
159. Singh, A., & Settleman, J. (2010). EMT, cancer stem cells and drug resistance: An emerging axis of evil in the war on cancer. *Oncogene, 29*, 4741–4751.
160. Marchini, S., Fruscio, R., Clivio, L., Beltrame, L., Porcu, L., Fuso Nerini, I., Cavalieri, D., Chiorino, G., Cattoretti, G., Mangioni, C., Milani, R., Torri, V., Romualdi, C., Zambelli, A., Romano, M., Signorelli, M., di Giandomenico, S., & D'Incalci, M. (2013). Resistance to platinum-based chemotherapy is associated with epithelial to mesenchymal transition in epithelial ovarian cancer. *European Journal of Cancer, 49*, 520–530.
161. Gupta, N., Xu, Z., El-Sehemy, A., Steed, H., & Fu, Y. (2013). Notch3 induces epithelial-mesenchymal transition and attenuates carboplatin-induced apoptosis in ovarian cancer cells. *Gynecologic Oncology, 130*, 200–206.
162. Lu, L., Wang, J., Wu, Y., Wan, P., & Yang, G. (2016). Rap1A promotes ovarian cancer metastasis via activation of ERK/p38 and notch signaling. *Cancer Medicine, 5*, 3544–3554.
163. Espinoza, I., & Miele, L. (2013). Deadly crosstalk: Notch signaling at the intersection of EMT and cancer stem cells. *Cancer Letters, 341*, 41–45.
164. Espinoza, I., Pochampally, R., Xing, F., Watabe, K., & Miele, L. (2013). Notch signaling: Targeting cancer stem cells and epithelial-to-mesenchymal transition. *OncoTargets and Therapy, 6*, 1249–1259.
165. Pazos, M. C., Abramovich, D., Bechis, A., Accialini, P., Parborell, F., Tesone, M., & Irusta, G. (2017). Gamma secretase inhibitor impairs epithelial-to-mesenchymal transition induced by TGF-beta in ovarian tumor cell lines. *Molecular and Cellular Endocrinology, 440*, 125–137.
166. Zhou, J., Jain, S., Azad, A. K., Xu, X., Yu, H. C., Xu, Z., Godbout, R., & Fu, Y. (2016). Notch and TGFbeta form a positive regulatory loop and regulate EMT in epithelial ovarian cancer cells. *Cellular Signalling, 28*, 838–849.
167. Steg, A. D., Katre, A. A., Goodman, B., Han, H. D., Nick, A. M., Stone, R. L., Coleman, R. L., Alvarez, R. D., Lopez-Berestein, G., Sood, A. K., & Landen, C. N. (2011). Targeting the notch ligand JAGGED1 in both tumor cells and stroma in ovarian cancer. *Clinical Cancer Research, 17*, 5674–5685.
168. Chen, X., Gong, L., Ou, R., Zheng, Z., Chen, J., Xie, F., Huang, X., Qiu, J., Zhang, W., Jiang, Q., Yang, Y., Zhu, H., Shi, Z., & Yan, X. (2016). Sequential combination therapy of ovarian cancer with cisplatin and gamma-secretase inhibitor MK-0752. *Gynecologic Oncology, 140*, 537–544.
169. Groeneweg, J. W., DiGloria, C. M., Yuan, J., Richardson, W. S., Growdon, W. B., Sathyanarayanan, S., Foster, R., & Rueda, B. R. (2014). Inhibition of notch signaling in combination with Paclitaxel reduces platinum-resistant ovarian tumor growth. *Frontiers in Oncology, 4*, 171.
170. McAuliffe, S. M., Morgan, S. L., Wyant, G. A., Tran, L. T., Muto, K. W., Chen, Y. S., Chin, K. T., Partridge, J. C., Poole, B. B., Cheng, K. H., Daggett, J., Jr., Cullen, K., Kantoff, E., Hasselbatt, K., Berkowitz, J., Muto, M. G., Berkowitz, R. S., Aster, J. C., Matulonis, U. A., & Dinulescu, D. M. (2012). Targeting Notch, a key pathway for ovarian cancer stem cells, sensitizes tumors to platinum therapy. *Proceedings of the National Academy of Sciences of the United States of America, 109*, E2939–E2948.

171. Wang, M., Ma, X., Wang, J., Wang, L., & Wang, Y. (2014). Pretreatment with the gamma-secretase inhibitor DAPT sensitizes drug-resistant ovarian cancer cells to cisplatin by down-regulation of Notch signaling. *International Journal of Oncology, 44*, 1401–1409.
172. Feng, Z., Xu, W., Zhang, C., Liu, M., & Wen, H. (2017). Inhibition of gamma-secretase in Notch1 signaling pathway as a novel treatment for ovarian cancer. *Oncotarget, 8*, 8215–8225.
173. Kang, H., Jeong, J. Y., Song, J. Y., Kim, T. H., Kim, G., Huh, J. H., Kwon, A. Y., Jung, S. G., & An, H. J. (2016). Notch3-specific inhibition using siRNA knockdown or GSI sensitizes paclitaxel-resistant ovarian cancer cells. *Molecular Carcinogenesis, 55*, 1196–1209.
174. Yen, W. C., Fischer, M. M., Axelrod, F., Bond, C., Cain, J., Cancilla, B., Henner, W. R., Meisner, R., Sato, A., Shah, J., Tang, T., Wallace, B., Wang, M., Zhang, C., Kapoun, A. M., Lewicki, J., Gurney, A., & Hoey, T. (2015). Targeting Notch signaling with a Notch2/Notch3 antagonist (tarextumab) inhibits tumor growth and decreases tumor-initiating cell frequency. *Clinical Cancer Research: An Official Journal of the American Association for Cancer Research, 21*, 2084–2095.
175. Huang, J., Hu, W., Hu, L., Previs, R. A., Dalton, H. J., Yang, X. Y., Sun, Y., McGuire, M., Rupaimoole, R., Nagaraja, A. S., Kang, Y., Liu, T., Nick, A. M., Jennings, N. B., Coleman, R. L., Jaffe, R. B., & Sood, A. K. (2016). Dll4 inhibition plus aflibercept markedly reduces ovarian tumor growth. *Molecular Cancer Therapeutics, 15*, 1344–1352.
176. Majidinia, M., Alizadeh, E., Yousefi, B., Akbarzadeh, M., Mihanfar, A., Rahmati-Yamchi, M., & Zarghami, N. (2017). Co-inhibition of Notch and NF-kappaB signaling pathway decreases proliferation through downregulating IkappaB-alpha and Hes-1 expression in human ovarian cancer OVCAR-3 cells. *Drug Research (Stuttg), 67*, 13–19.
177. Chiorean, E. G., LoRusso, P., Strother, R. M., Diamond, J. R., Younger, A., Messersmith, W. A., Adriaens, L., Liu, L., Kao, R. J., DiCioccio, A. T., Kostic, A., Leek, R., Harris, A., & Jimeno, A. (2015). A phase I first-in-human study of enoticumab (REGN421), a fully human Delta-like ligand 4 (Dll4) monoclonal antibody in patients with advanced solid tumors. *Clinical Cancer Research, 21*, 2695–2703.
178. Brana, I., Berger, R., Golan, T., Haluska, P., Edenfield, J., Fiorica, J., Stephenson, J., Martin, L. P., Westin, S., Hanjani, P., Jones, M. B., Almhanna, K., Wenham, R. M., Sullivan, D. M., Dalton, W. S., Gunchenko, A., Cheng, J. D., Siu, L. L., & Gray, J. E. (2014). A parallel-arm phase I trial of the humanised anti-IGF-1R antibody dalotuzumab in combination with the AKT inhibitor MK-2206, the mTOR inhibitor ridaforolimus, or the NOTCH inhibitor MK-0752, in patients with advanced solid tumours. *British Journal of Cancer, 111*, 1932–1944.
179. Pant, S., Jones, S. F., Kurkjian, C. D., Infante, J. R., Moore, K. N., Burris, H. A., McMeekin, D. S., Benhadji, K. A., Patel, B. K., Frenzel, M. J., Kursar, J. D., Zamek-Gliszczynski, M. J., Yuen, E. S., Chan, E. M., & Bendell, J. C. (2016). A first-in-human phase I study of the oral Notch inhibitor, LY900009, in patients with advanced cancer. *European Journal of Cancer, 56*, 1–9.
180. Richter, S., Bedard, P. L., Chen, E. X., Clarke, B. A., Tran, B., Hotte, S. J., Stathis, A., Hirte, H. W., Razak, A. R., Reedijk, M., Chen, Z., Cohen, B., Zhang, W. J., Wang, L., Ivy, S. P., Moore, M. J., Oza, A. M., Siu, L. L., & McWhirter, E. (2014). A phase I study of the oral gamma secretase inhibitor R04929097 in combination with gemcitabine in patients with advanced solid tumors (PHL-078/CTEP 8575). *Investigational New Drugs, 32*, 243–249.
181. Diaz-Padilla, I., Wilson, M. K., Clarke, B. A., Hirte, H. W., Welch, S. A., Mackay, H. J., Biagi, J. J., Reedijk, M., Weberpals, J. I., Fleming, G. F., Wang, L., Liu, G., Zhou, C., Blattler, C., Ivy, S. P., & Oza, A. M. (2015). A phase II study of single-agent RO4929097, a gamma-secretase inhibitor of Notch signaling, in patients with recurrent platinum-resistant epithelial ovarian cancer: A study of the Princess Margaret, Chicago and California phase II consortia. *Gynecologic Oncology, 137*, 216–222.

Index

L. Miele, S. Artavanis-Tsakonas (eds.), *Targeting Notch in Cancer*,
https://doi.org/10.1007/978-1-4939-8859-4

MIX
Papier aus verantwortungsvollen Quellen
Paper from responsible sources
FSC® C105338

If you have any concerns about our products,
you can contact us on
ProductSafety@springernature.com

In case Publisher is established outside the EU,
the EU authorized representative is:
Springer Nature Customer Service Center GmbH
Europaplatz 3, 69115 Heidelberg, Germany

Printed by Libri Plureos GmbH
in Hamburg, Germany